DIAGNOSTIC IMAGING

DIAGNOSTIC IMAGING

PETER ARMSTRONG

MB, BS, FRCR

Professor of Radiology
Medical College of St Bartholomew's
and the Royal London Hospitals, London
Formerly Professor and Vice-Chairman
Department of Radiology, University of Virginia
Charlottesville, Virginia, USA

MARTIN L. WASTIE

MB, BChir, FRCP, FRCR

Consultant Radiologist
University Hospital, Nottingham

FOURTH EDITION

b

**Blackwell
Science**

© 1981, 1987, 1992, 1998 by
Blackwell Science Ltd
Editorial Offices:
Osney Mead, Oxford OX2 0EL
25 John Street, London WC1N 2BL
23 Ainslie Place, Edinburgh EH3 6AJ
350 Main Street, Malden
  MA 02148 5018, USA
54 University Street, Carlton
  Victoria 3053, Australia
10, rue Casimir Delavigne
  75006 Paris, France

Other Editorial Offices:
Blackwell Wissenschafts-Verlag GmbH
Kurfürstendamm 57
10707 Berlin, Germany

Blackwell Science KK
MG Kodenmacho Building
7–10 Kodenmacho Nihombashi
Chuo-ku, Tokyo 104, Japan

First published as *X-ray Diagnosis* 1981
Reprinted 1982, 1983 (twice), 1985
Second edition published as
Diagnostic Imaging 1987
Reprinted 1989
International Student Edition 1989
Indonesian translation 1990
Third edition 1992
Four Dragons edition 1992
Reprinted 1993, 1994
Chinese translation 1994
Fourth edition 1998
International edition 1998

Set by Excel Typesetters Co., Hong Kong
Origination by Tenon and Polert, Hong Kong
Printed and bound in Great Britain
at the Alden Press, Oxford and
Northampton

A catalogue record for this title
is available from the British Library

ISBN 0 86542 696 1 (BSL).
      0 632 04846 8 (International Edition)

Library of Congress
Cataloging-in-publication Data

Armstrong, Peter, 1940–
    Diagnostic imaging / Peter Armstrong,
Martin Wastie. – 4th ed.
        p.   cm.
    Includes bibliographical references
and index.
    ISBN 0-86542-696-1 (BSL). –
ISBN 0-632-04846-8 (international ed.)
    1. Diagnostic imaging.
I. Wastie, Martin L.   II. Title.
    [DNLM: 1. Diagnostic Imaging.
WN 180 A737d 1997]
RC78.7.D53A76   1997
616.07′54 – dc21
DNLM/DLC
for Library of Congress   97-23281
                                   CIP

DISTRIBUTORS

Marston Book Services Ltd
PO Box 269
Abingdon, Oxon OX14 4YN
(*Orders*: Tel: 01235 465500
          Fax: 01235 465555)

USA
Blackwell Science, Inc.
Commerce Place
350 Main Street
Malden, MA 02148 5018
(*Orders*: Tel: 800 759 6102
               781 388 8250
          Fax: 781 388 8255)

Canada
  Login Brothers Book Company
  324 Saulteaux Grescent
  Winnipeg, Manitoba R3J 3T2
  (*Orders*: Tel: 204 224-4068)

Australia
  Blackwell Science Pty Ltd
  54 University Street
  Carlton, Victoria 3053
  (*Orders*: Tel: 3 9347 0300
            Fax: 3 9347 5001)

For further information on
Blackwell Science, visit our website:
www. blackwell-science. com

Contents

Preface

The role of imaging is becoming ever more important in patient management and medical students can be forgiven their bewilderment when faced with the daunting array of information which goes under the heading 'Diagnostic Imaging'. As conventional radiology remains the mainstay of most imaging departments we have once again given it due emphasis in this edition of *Diagnostic Imaging*. Since the previous edition was published six years ago there has been a steady increase in the use of ultrasound and computed tomography (CT) but the growth of magnetic resonance imaging (MRI) has been dramatic. MRI now impinges upon many fields of medicine and surgery and for some conditions has become the imaging modality of choice. Interventional radiology is also gaining more and more importance with radiologists carrying out therapeutic procedures that were formerly in the province of the surgeon.

With the now widespread use of the various different imaging techniques it has become apparent that there are different ways of investigating the same condition. We have avoided being too prescriptive as practice in each hospital differs and so much depends on the personal preference of clinicians and radiologists as well as on the available equipment and expertise.

We have once again tried to meet the needs of the medical student and young doctor in training by explaining the techniques used in diagnostic imaging and the indications for their use. As before, much of the book is devoted to helping the reader understand the principles of interpretation, both of plain films and the images obtained with other imaging modalities.

It is, unfortunately, beyond the scope of a small book such as this one, to describe fully the pathology responsible for the various appearances. Similarly, to have dealt adequately with the role of imaging in clinical management would have necessitated large sections on surgery, medicine and pathology. Consequently, this book cannot be read in isolation; it must be accompanied by the study of these other subjects.

Peter Armstrong
Martin L. Wastie

Acknowledgements

It would not have been possible to prepare this edition without the help of the many radiologists who have given ideas, valuable comments and inspiration. We would like to thank particularly the staff of the Radiology Departments at the University Hospital, Nottingham and St Bartholomew's Hospital, London. We would also like to thank Jackie Chambers, Rachel Vincent, Professors Rodney Reznek, Geraint Roberts and Alan Wilson, Drs Gnana Kumar, Roger Gregson, Bryan Preston, Robert Kerslake, Stewart Dawson, Simon Whitaker, Ian Holland, Sat Amar, John Somers, Tim Jaspan, Judith Webb, and Nick Perry for their help in providing pictures.

We would like to thank many other people who in the past have provided illustrations: Drs Theodore Keats, Robin Wilson, Philip McMillan, Janet Dacie, Wayne Cail, Keith Dewberry, Paul Dee, Spencer Gay, Denny Watson, Brent Harrison, Scott McPherson, Professors Paramsothy, Joginder Singh, Donald Longmore, Andreas Adam and Janet Husband, Drs Norman Brenbridge, Tony Buschi, Andrew McLeod, Mark Monaghan, Olle Nylén and Björn Lindén.

We must also thank sincerely the photographers in the Departments of Medical Illustration at the University Hospital, Nottingham and at St Bartholomew's Hospital, London.

This work would have been totally impossible without the superb secretarial help undertaken by Linda Hopkinson of Nottingham and Julie Jessop of St Bartholomew's Hospital. Secretarial assistance was also provided by Veronica Nettleship and Tiina Wastie and we thank them all most heartily for all their help.

Finally, we would like to express our gratitude to Alice Emmott and the staff of Blackwell Science Ltd.

1

Introduction

The use of the imaging department

Imaging departments need to be well run and efficiently utilized in order to minimize radiation hazard and be cost-effective. Organizing a department is in the hands of radiologists and radiographers, but the use to which it is put is largely decided by referring clinicians. Good communication between clinician and radiologist is vital. The radiology staff need to understand the clinical problem in order to carry out appropriate tests and to interpret the results in a meaningful way. Clinicians need to understand the strengths and limitations of the answers provided.

Sensible selection of imaging investigations is of great importance. There are two opposing philosophies. One approach is to request a battery of investigations, aimed vaguely in the direction of the patient's symptoms, in the hope that something will turn up. The other approach is 'trial and error': decide one or two likely diagnoses and carry out the appropriate test to support or refute these possibilities. Each course has its proponents; we favour the selective approach since there is little doubt that the answers are obtained usually less expensively and with less distress to the patient. This approach depends on critical clinical evaluation; the more experienced the doctor, the more accurate he or she becomes in choosing appropriate tests.

Laying down precise guidelines for requesting imaging examinations is difficult because patients are managed differently in different centres and the information required varies significantly.

• An examination should only be requested when there is a reasonable chance that it will affect the management of the patient. There should be a question attached to every request, e.g. for a chest radiograph – what is the cause of this patient's haemoptysis?

• The time interval between follow-up examinations should be sensible, e.g. once pneumonia has been diagnosed, chest films to assess progress can safely be left 7–10 days, unless clinical features suggest a complication.

• Be specific about the localization of problems. X-raying the clavicle, shoulder, humerus, elbow and forearm is clearly inappropriate for a patient whose symptoms are clinically those of an abnormality in or immediately adjacent to the shoulder. It may be reasonable to construct a programme of investigations but the radiologist should always be asked to cancel any remaining tests once the desired positive result is obtained.

• Consider carefully which diagnostic imaging procedure will give the relevant information most easily, e.g. radionuclide bone scans should be the initial screening method in a search for asymptomatic bone metastases rather than skeletal survey.

• Choose an examination, whenever possible, which minimizes or avoids ionising radiation.

X-rays

Production of x-rays (Fig. 1.1)

X-rays are used for all conventional radiography and for computed tomography (CT). They are produced by passing a very high voltage across two tungsten terminals within an evacuated tube. One terminal, the cathode, is heated to incandescence so that it liberates free electrons. When a high voltage, usually in the range of 50–150 kV, is applied across the two terminals, the electrons are attracted towards the

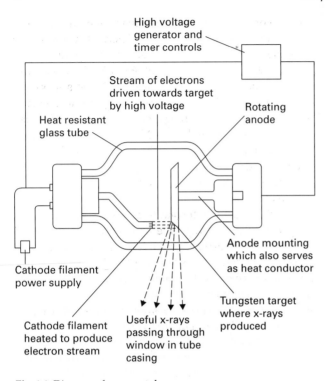

High voltage
generator and
timer controls

Stream of electrons
driven towards target
by high voltage

Rotating
anode

Heat resistant
glass tube

Anode mounting
which also serves
as heat conductor

Cathode filament
power supply

Tungsten target
where x-rays
produced

Cathode filament
heated to produce
electron stream

Useful x-rays
passing through
window in tube
casing

Fig. 1.1 Diagram of an x-ray tube.

anode at high speed. When the electrons hit the anode
target, x-rays are produced.

Absorption of x-rays

Radiographic and CT images depend on the fact that x-rays
are absorbed to a variable extent as they pass through the
body. The visibility of normal structures and of disease
depends on this differential absorption.

Conventional radiography

With conventional radiography there are four basic densities – gas, fat, all other soft tissues and calcified structures.
X-rays that pass through air are least absorbed and therefore
cause the most blackening of the radiograph, whereas
calcium absorbs the most and so the bones and other calcified structures appear virtually white. The soft tissues, with

the exception of fat, e.g. the solid viscera, muscle, blood,
fluids, bowel wall, etc., all have similar absorptive capacity
and appear the same shade of grey on the conventional
radiograph. Fat absorbs slightly fewer x-rays and therefore
appears a little blacker than the other soft tissues.

Projections in conventional radiography

Projections are usually described by the path of the x-ray
beam. Thus the term PA (posteroanterior) view designates
that the beam passes from the back to the front, the standard
projection for a routine chest film. An AP (anteroposterior)
view is one taken from the front. The term 'frontal' refers to
either PA or AP projection.

The image on an x-ray film is two-dimensional. All the
structures along the path of the beam are projected on to the
same portion of the film. Therefore it is often necessary to
take at least two views to gain information about the third
dimension. These two views are usually at right-angles to
one another, e.g. the PA and lateral chest film. Sometimes
two views at right-angles are not appropriate and oblique
views are substituted.

Horizontal ray films

Air–fluid levels are an important radiological sign. Their
detection requires a projection using a horizontal x-ray
beam, e.g. an erect or a lateral decubitus film. The reason
that air–fluid levels can only be seen on a film taken with a
horizontal beam can best be understood by analogy with
the fluid level in a glass of water. The only way to see the
air–fluid level is to look at it from the side, i.e. in a horizontal
direction.

Portable films

Portable x-ray machines can be used to take films of patients
in bed or in the operating theatres. Such machines have
limitations on the exposures they can achieve. This usually
means longer exposure times and poorer quality films. The
positioning and radiation protection of patients in bed is
often inferior to that which can be achieved within the x-ray
department. Consequently, portable films should only be
requested when the patient cannot be moved safely or comfortably to the x-ray department.

Magnification in radiography

All conventional x-ray images show some magnification, because the x-ray tube sends out a diverging beam of x-rays. The closer the object is to the film, the less the magnification.

Conventional tomography

Tomograms blur out overlying structures, but keep a selected plane of interest in sharp focus when the x-ray tube and film are moved about an axis which can be located at the level of interest.

Computed tomography has now replaced most conventional tomographic examinations.

Computed tomography

Computed tomography, like conventional radiography, relies on x-rays transmitted through the body. Computed tomography differs from conventional radiography in that it uses a more sensitive x-ray detection system than photographic film, namely gas or crystal detectors, and manipulates the data using a computer. The x-ray tube and detectors rotate around the patient (Fig. 1.2). The outstanding feature of CT is that very small differences in x-ray absorption values can be visualized. Compared to conventional radiography, the range of densities recorded is increased approximately 10-fold. Not only can fat be distinguished from other soft tissues, but gradations of density within soft tissues can also be recognized, e.g. brain substance from cerebrospinal fluid, or tumour from surrounding normal tissues.

The patient lies with the part to be examined within the gantry housing the x-ray tube and detectors. Although other planes are sometimes practicable, axial sections are by far the most frequent. The section level and thickness to be imaged are selected by the operator: the usual thickness is between 1.0 and 10 mm. By moving the patient through the gantry, multiple adjacent sections can be imaged allowing a picture of the body to be built up. Thinner sections provide

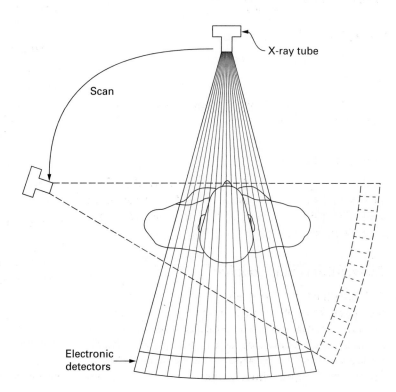

Fig. 1.2 Principle of CT. The x-ray tube and detectors move around the patient enabling a picture of x-ray absorption in different parts of the body to be built up. The time taken for the exposure is in the order of a second or so.

more accurate information, but more sections are then required for a given volume of tissue.

There are two methods of CT scanning: slice-by-slice (usually known as 'conventional' CT) and volume acquisition (usually known as 'spiral' or 'helical' CT) (Fig. 1.3). In the conventional slice-by-slice method, the table top supporting the patient comes to a stop for each section. In spiral (helical) CT, the patient is transported continuously through the scanner, so in effect the x-ray beam traces a

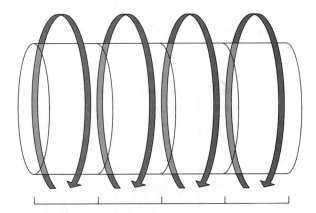

(a)   Slice-by-slice conventional CT scanning, slices at
        specific positions

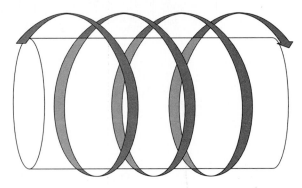

(b)   Spiral CT scanning

Fig. 1.3 Two methods of CT data collection are in common use: (a) conventional slice-by-slice scanning and (b) spiral (helical) CT, whereby the tube rotates continuously and the patient moves gradually through the scanner, so that the effective path of the x-ray beam is a spiral.

spiral path, while the data are collected continuously, to create a 'volume of data' within the computer memory. The advantages of spiral CT are:
• a significant reduction in scan times, so much so that whole organs can be scanned during a single breath-hold;
• the imaged sections are truly contiguous without gaps or overlaps due to inconsistent breathing;
• better reconstruction to other planes and the possibility for three-dimensional reconstruction.

The data obtained from each set of exposures are reconstructed into an image by computer manipulation. The computer calculates the attenuation (absorption) value of each picture element (known in computer jargon as a pixel). Each pixel is 0.25–0.6 mm in diameter, depending on the resolution of the machine, with a height corresponding to the chosen section thickness. Since each pixel has a definite volume, the attenuation value represents the mean value in that volume of tissue (voxel). The resulting images are displayed on a television monitor and photographs of the images are used for the permanent record. Additionally, the basic data can be stored on an optical disc or on magnetic tape.

The attenuation values are expressed on an arbitrary scale (Hounsfield units) with water density being zero, air density being minus 1000 units and bone density being plus 1000 units (Fig. 1.4). The range and level of densities to be displayed can be selected by controls on the computer. The range of densities visualized on a particular image is known as the *window width* and the mean level as the *window level* or *window centre*.

The human eye can only appreciate a limited number of shades of grey. With a wide window all the structures are visible, but fine details of density difference cannot be appreciated. With a narrow window width, variations of just a few Hounsfield units can be seen, but much of the image is either totally black or totally white and in these areas no useful information is provided. The effects of varying window width and level are illustrated in Figs 1.5 and 2.6 (p. 23).

Reconstruction to other planes

Computed tomography is usually performed in the axial plane. It is possible, however, to reconstruct images in other planes. The computer has in its memory attenuation values

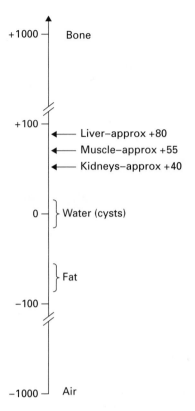

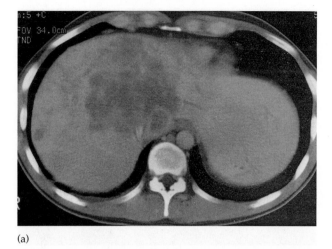

(a)

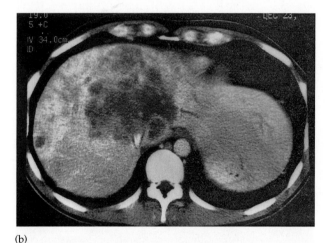

(b)

Fig. 1.4 Scale depicting the CT density (Hounsfield units) of various normal tissues in the body.

Fig. 1.5 Effect of varying window widths. In (a) and (b) the level has been kept constant at 65 Hounsfield units (HU). The window width in (a) is 500 whereas in (b) it is only 150 HU. Note that in the narrow window image (b), the metastases are better seen, but that structures other than the liver are better seen in (a).

for every voxel and can present the data in any desired plane, e.g. coronal or sagittal. With the usual 8–10 mm sections the voxel is composed of long narrow blocks and consequently has poor spatial resolution. If, however, the section thickness is very small, e.g. 1.0 mm, then reconstructions of reasonable spatial resolution can be obtained.

Spiral (helical) CT allows substantially improved reconstruction to other planes and even three-dimensional image reconstruction (Fig. 1.6), because the image data are collected in a continuous spiral as opposed to discrete section blocks.

Partial volume effect

Since each voxel has a definite height, often 10 mm, a structure or lesion may be partly in and partly out of the section.

The image displayed uses the mean attenuation for the entire voxel, so the density of a structure 'partially in the volume' may not be truly representative and its size may be incorrectly represented (Fig. 1.7).

Artefacts

There are numerous CT artefacts. Two that are frequently

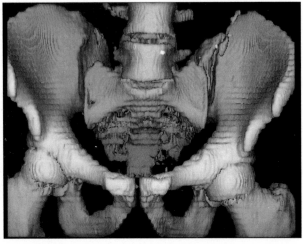

(a)

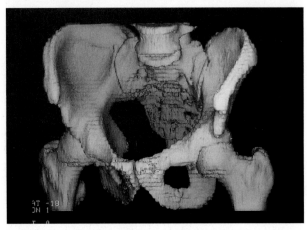

(b)

Fig. 1.6 Three-dimensional reconstructions from spiral CT data (a, b). The pelvic bones, lower spine and femora are shown in three-dimensional reconstruction. The data can be viewed from any desired direction by appropriately instructing the computer.

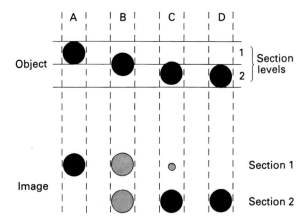

Fig. 1.7 Partial volume effect. Objects A and D occupy the full height of the section and, therefore, their diameter and density are accurately represented on the images of Sections 1 and 2. Object B lies half in Section 1 and half in Section 2. Its image will indicate the correct diameter, but the density will be half the true density of the object on *both* images. Object C lies largely in Section 2 but projects into Section 1. The upper image will underestimate the diameter *and* the density, whereas the lower image will be accurate apart from a minor underestimate of density. By using narrower sections, 'partial volume' inaccuracies are reduced, but more sections are then necessary to cover the same volum of tissue.

Contrast agents in conventional radiography and CT

Radiographic contrast agents are used to visualize structures or disease processes that would otherwise be invisible or difficult to see. Barium is widely used to outline the gastrointestinal tract; all the other radio-opaque media rely on iodine in solution to absorb x-rays and so act as contrast agents. Iodine-containing solutions are used for urography, angiography and intravenous contrast enhancement at computed tomography. Usually they are given in large doses, often with rapid rates of injection. Since their only purpose is to produce opacification, ideally they should be pharmacologically inert. This has not yet been totally achieved, though the introduction of low-osmolality agents, such as the non-ionic media, is a big step in the right direction. Many of the adverse effects are intimately related to the osmolality of the agent and with the new low-osmolality media these effects are much less frequent and often much less severe. The following discussion applies

seen are those produced by movement (each exposure usually takes 1–2 s) and those from objects of very high density such as barium in the bowel, metal implants, dental fillings or surgical clips. Both types give rise to radiating linear streaks. The major problem is the resulting degradation of the image.

particularly to the older ionic agents. The disadvantage of the newer agents is that they are considerably more expensive than their predecessors and the high cost has led some institutions to introduce limitations on their use.

Most patients experience a feeling of warmth spreading over the body as the contrast medium is injected; a few find this feeling objectionable. Sometimes, particularly with slow injections of the more concentrated ionic solutions, pain occurs in the upper arm and shoulder due to stasis in the veins; this can be alleviated by raising the patient's arm at the end of the injection. Contrast inadvertently injected outside the vein is very painful indeed and should be carefully guarded against.

Nausea, vomiting or light-headedness are experienced by a few patients and some will develop an urticarial rash. All these phenomena usually subside spontaneously.

Bronchospasm, laryngeal oedema or hypotension occasionally develop and may be so severe as to be life threatening. It is therefore essential to be prepared for these dangerous reactions and to have available appropriate resuscitation equipment and drugs. Approximately one in 160 000 patients dies as a consequence of ionic contrast agents, a risk which, although small, should not be ignored.

Patients with known allergic manifestations, particularly asthma, are more likely to have an adverse reaction. Similarly, patients who have had a previous reaction to contrast agents have a higher than average risk of problems during the examination. Such patients are usually given non-ionic agents and premedicated with steroids, preferably for at least 18 hours prior to the examination. Antihistamine drugs may also be given shortly before the contrast injection.

Patients with a higher than average risk of complications from intravenous contrast injections include:
• infants, who are at risk from a rapid rise in plasma osmolality because of the high osmolality of the injected contrast agent; even with low-osmolality agents the injection rate in infants should, when possible, be slow;
• elderly patients, who often tolerate the injected contrast medium poorly;
• those with known heart disease; arrhythmias are a risk in patients with heart disease;
• those with renal failure, myeloma or severe diabetes; such patients are more likely to show a deterioration of renal function owing to the contrast medium if they are deprived of fluids prior to the examination.

These high-risk groups are given low-osmolality agents to help minimize complications.

Ultrasound

In diagnostic ultrasound examinations, very high frequency sound is directed into the body from a transducer placed in contact with the skin. In order to make good acoustic contact, the skin is smeared with a jelly-like substance. As the sound travels through the body, it is reflected by the tissue interfaces to produce echoes which are picked up by the same transducer and converted into an electrical signal.

Since air, bone and other heavily calcified materials absorb nearly all the ultrasound beam, ultrasound plays little part in the diagnosis of lung or bone disease. The information from abdominal examinations may be significantly impaired by gas in the bowel which interferes with the transmission of sound.

Fluid is a good conductor of sound, and ultrasound is therefore a particularly good imaging modality for diagnosing cysts, examining fluid-filled structures such as the bladder and biliary system, and demonstrating the fetus in

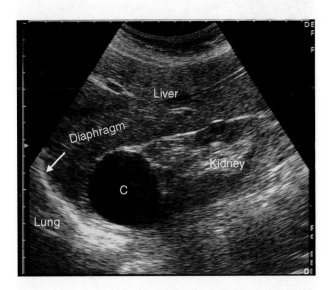

Fig. 1.8 Ultrasound scan of longitudinal section through the liver and right kidney. A cyst (C) is present in the upper pole of the kidney.

its amniotic sac. Ultrasound can also be used to demonstrate solid structures that have a different acoustic impedance from adjacent normal tissues, e.g. metastases.

Ultrasound is often used to determine whether a structure is solid or cystic (Fig. 1.8). Cysts or other fluid-filled structures produce large echoes from their walls but no echoes from the fluid contained within them. Also, more echoes than usual are received from the tissues behind the cyst, an effect known as *acoustic enhancement*. Conversely, with a calcified structure, e.g. a gall stone (Fig. 1.9), there is a great reduction in the sound that will pass through, so a band of reduced echoes, referred to as an *acoustic shadow*, is seen behind the stone.

Ultrasound is produced by causing a special crystal to oscillate at a predetermined frequency. Very short pulses of sound lasting about a millionth of a second are transmitted approximately 500 times each second. The crystal not only transmits the pulses of sound but also 'listens' to the returning echoes, which are electronically amplified to be

recorded as signals on a television monitor. Photographic reproductions of the image can provide a permanent record.

The time taken for each echo to return to the transducer is proportional to the distance travelled. Knowledge of the depth of the interface responsible for the echoes allows an image to be produced. Also by knowing the velocity of sound in tissues it is possible to measure the distance between interfaces. This is of great practical importance in obstetrics, for example, where the measurement of the fetal head has become the standard method of estimating fetal age.

During the scan, the ultrasound beam is electronically swept through the patient's body and a section of the internal anatomy is instantaneously displayed. The resulting image is a slice, so in order to obtain a three-dimensional assessment a number of slices must be created by moving or angling the transducer.

Unlike other imaging modalities there are no fixed projections and the production of the images and their subsequent interpretation depend very much on the observations of the operator during the examination. Ultrasound images are capable of providing highly detailed information: for example, very small lesions can be demonstrated (Fig. 1.10).

A recent advance is the development of small ultrasound probes which may be placed very close to the region of interest thus producing highly detailed images but with a limited range of a few centimetres. Examples are rectal probes for examining the prostate and transvaginal probes for the examination of the pelvic structures. Tiny ultrasound probes may be incorporated in the end of an endoscope. Lesions of the oesophagus, heart and aorta may be demonstrated with an endoscope placed in the oesophagus and lesions of the pancreas may be detected with an endoscope passed into the stomach and duodenum.

At the energies and doses currently used in diagnostic ultrasound, no harmful effects on any tissues have been demonstrated.

Ultrasound contrast agents are currently being developed. These agents contain microscopic air bubbles which enhance the echoes received by the probe. The air bubbles are held in a stabilized form, so they persist for the duration of the examination.

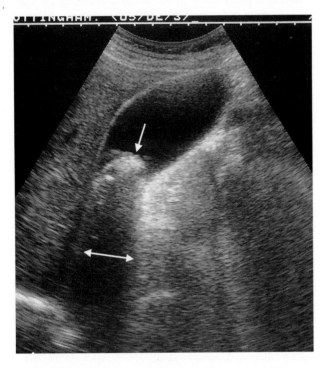

Fig. 1.9 Ultrasound scan of gall bladder showing a large stone in the neck of the gall bladder (white arrow). Note the acoustic shadow behind the stone (horizontal arrows).

Doppler effect

Sound reflected from a mobile structure shows a variation

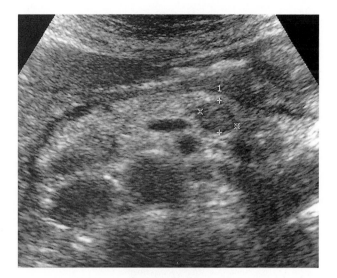

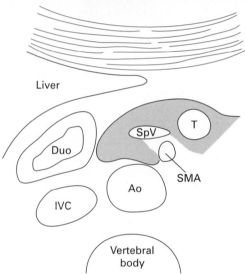

Fig. 1.10 Ultrasound scan of pancreas showing 1 cm tumour (T) (an insulinoma) at the junction of the head and body of the pancreas. The pancreas is shaded in the diagram, Ao, aorta; Duo, duodenum; IVC, inferior vena cava; SMA, superior mesenteric artery; SpV, splenic vein.

in frequency which corresponds to the speed of movement of the structure. This shift in frequency, which can be converted to an audible signal, is the principle underlying the Doppler probe used in obstetrics to listen to the fetal heart.

The Doppler effect can also be exploited to image blood flowing through the heart or blood vessels. Here the sound is reflected from the blood cells flowing in the vessels (Plate 1, opposite p. 14). If blood is flowing towards the transducer the received signal is of higher frequency than the transmitted frequency, whilst the opposite pertains if blood is flowing away from the transducer. The difference in frequency between the sound transmitted and received is known as the Doppler frequency shift.* The direction of blood flow can readily be determined and flow towards the transducer is by convention coloured red, whereas blue indicates flow away from the transducer.

When a patient is being scanned, the Doppler information in colour is superimposed onto a standard ultrasound image (Plate 2 opposite p. 14).

During the examination the flow velocity waveform can be displayed and recorded. As the waveforms from specific arteries and veins have characteristic shapes, flow abnormalities can be detected. If the Doppler angle (Plate 1) is known then the velocity of the flowing blood can be calculated and blood flow can be calculated provided the diameter of the vessel is also known.

Doppler studies are used to detect venous thrombosis, arterial stenosis and occlusion, particularly in the carotid arteries. In the abdomen, Doppler techniques can determine whether a structure is a blood vessel and can help in assessing tumour blood flow. In obstetrics, Doppler ultrasound is used particularly to determine fetal blood flow through the umbilical artery. With Doppler echocardiography it is possible to demonstrate regurgitation through incompetent valves and pressure gradients across valves can be calculated.

Radionuclide imaging

The radioactive isotopes used in diagnostic imaging emit gamma rays as they decay. Gamma rays are electromagnetic radiation, similar to x-rays, produced by radioactive decay

---

* The formula is:

$$\text{frequency shift} = \frac{2Fi \times V \times \cos\Theta}{c}$$

(As c, the speed of sound in tissues, and Fi, the incident frequency of sound, are constant and if Θ, the Doppler angle is kept constant, the frequency shift depends directly on the blood flow velocity V.)

of the nucleus. Many naturally occurring radioactive isotopes, e.g. potassium-40, uranium-235, have half lives of hundreds of years and are, therefore, unsuitable for diagnostic imaging. The radioisotopes used in medical diagnosis are artificially produced and most have short half lives, usually a few hours or days. To keep the radiation dose to the patient to a minimum, the smallest possible dose of an isotope with a short half life should be used. Clearly, the radiopharmaceuticals should have no undesirable biological effects and should be rapidly excreted from the body following completion of the investigation.

Radionuclide imaging depends on the fact that certain substances concentrate selectively in different parts of the body. Radionuclides can be chemically tagged to these substances. Occasionally, the radionuclide in its ionic form will selectively concentrate in an organ, so there is no need to attach it to another compound. The radionuclide most commonly used is technetium-99m (^{99m}Tc). It is readily prepared, has a convenient half life of 6 hours and emits gamma radiation of a suitable energy for easy detection. Other radionuclides that are used include indium-111, gallium-67, iodine-123 and thallium-201.

Technetium-99m can be used in ionic form (as the pertechnetate) for thyroid and vascular imaging, or ^{99m}Tc can be tagged to other substances. For example a complex organic phosphate labelled with ^{99m}Tc will be taken up by the bones and can be used to visualize the skeleton (Fig. 1.11). Particles are used in lung perfusion images; macroaggregates of albumin with a particle size of 10–75 μm when injected intravenously are trapped in the pulmonary capillaries. If the macroaggregates are labelled with ^{99m}Tc, then the blood flow to the lungs can be visualized. It is also possible to label the patient's own red blood cells with ^{99m}Tc to assess cardiac function, or the white cells with indium-111 or ^{99m}Tc for abscess detection. Small quantities of radioactive gases, such as xenon-133, xenon-127 or krypton-81m can be inhaled to assess ventilation of the lungs. All these radiopharmaceuticals are free of side-effects.

The gamma rays emitted by the isotope are detected by a gamma camera enabling an image to be produced. A gamma camera consists of a large sodium iodide crystal, usually 40 cm in diameter coupled to a number of photomultiplier tubes. Light is produced when the gamma rays strike and activate the sodium iodide crystal, and the light is then electronically amplified and converted to an electrical

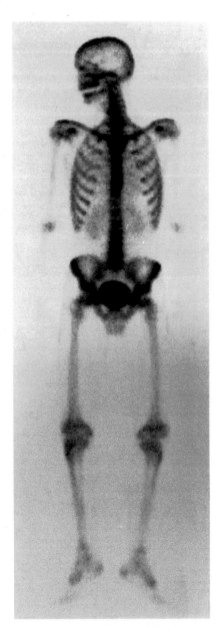

Fig. 1.11 Normal radionuclide bone scan. The patient has received an intravenous injection of a ^{99m}Tc-labelled bone scanning agent (a complex organic phosphate). This agent is taken up by the bone in proportion to bone turnover and blood flow.

pulse. The electrical pulse is further amplified and analysed by a processing unit so that a recording can be made. Invariably, some form of computer is linked to the gamma camera to enable rapid serial images to be taken and to perform computer enhancement of the images when relevant.

In selected cases emission tomography is performed. In this technique the gamma camera moves around the patient. A computer can analyse the information and produce sectional images similar to CT. Emission tomography can detect lesions not visible on the standard views. Because only one usable photon for each disintegration is emitted, this technique is also known as single photon emission computed tomography (SPECT).

Nuclear medicine techniques are used to measure function and to produce anatomical images. Even the anatomical images are dependent on function; for example, a bone scan depends on bone turnover. The anatomical information they provide, however, is limited by the relatively poor spatial resolution of the gamma camera compared to conventional radiography, ultrasound or CT.

Positron emission tomography

Positron emission tomography (PET) uses short-lived positron-emitting isotopes. Two gamma rays are produced from the annihilation of each positron which can be detected by a specialized gamma camera. The resulting images reflect the distribution of the isotope. By using isotopes of biologically important elements such as carbon or oxygen, PET can be used to study physiological processes such as blood perfusion of tissues, metabolism of substances such as glucose, as well as complex biochemical pathways such as neurotransmitter storage and binding. Changes in metabolism of diseased tissue can also be studied.

A cyclotron is needed to produce the necessary isotopes, and, therefore, PET is currently restricted to large research centres.

Magnetic resonance imaging

The basic principles of MRI depend on the fact that the nuclei of certain elements align with the magnetic force when placed in a strong magnetic field. At the field strengths currently used in medical imaging, hydrogen nuclei (protons) in water molecules and lipids are responsible for producing anatomical images. If a radiofrequency pulse at an appropriate frequency (resonant frequency) is applied, a proportion of the protons changes alignment, flipping through a preset angle, and rotate in phase with one another. Following this radiofrequency pulse, the protons return to their original positions. As the protons realign (relax) they induce a radio signal which, although very weak, can be detected and localized by coils placed around the patient. An image representing the distribution of the hydrogen protons can be built up (Fig. 1.12). The strength of the signal depends not only on proton density but also on two relaxation times, T1 and T2; T1 depends on the time the protons take to return to the axis of the magnetic field, and T2 depends on the time the protons take to dephase. A T1-weighted image is one in which the contrast between tissues is due mainly to their T1 relaxation properties, while in a T2-weighted image the contrast is due to the T2 relaxation properties. Some sequences produce mixed (often called 'balanced') images which approximate to proton density. Most pathological processes show increased T1 and T2 relaxation times and these processes therefore appear lower in signal (blacker) on a T1-weighted scan and higher in signal (whiter) on a T2-weighted scan than the normal surrounding tissues. The T1 and T2 weighting of an image can be selected by appropriately altering the timing and sequence of radiofrequency pulses.

A typical MRI scanner (Fig. 1.13) consists of a large circular magnet. Inside the magnet are the radiofrequency transmitter and receiver coils, as well as gradient coils to allow spatial localization of the MRI signal. Ancillary equipment converts the radio signal into a digital form which is then processed by a computer to form a final image. One advantage of MRI over CT is that the information can be directly imaged in any plane. In most instances, MRI requires a longer scan time (often several minutes) compared to CT, with the disadvantage that the patient has to keep still during the scanning procedure. Unavoidable movements from breathing, cardiac pulsation and peristalsis often degrade the image. Techniques to speed up scan times and for limiting the effect of motion by the use of various electronic gating devices are being introduced. Cardiac gating is already widely available.

Magnetic resonance imaging gives very different information to CT. The earliest successful application

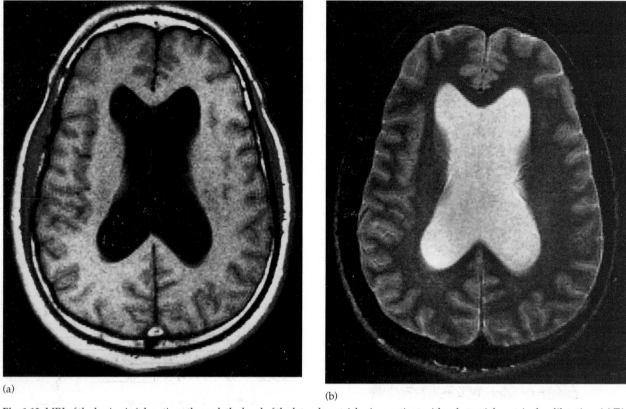

(a)   (b)

Fig. 1.12 MRI of the brain. Axial sections through the level of the lateral ventricles in a patient with substantial ventricular dilatation. (a) T1-weighted image. (b) T2-weighted image. The CSF is dark on the T1-weighted image and white on the T2-weighted image. Note also that the intensity of the white and grey matter of the brain differs on the two images.

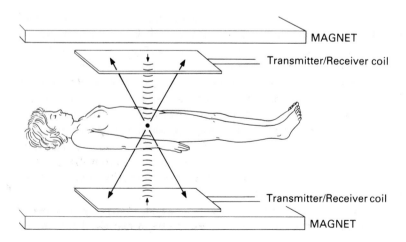

Fig. 1.13 Diagram of an MRI machine. The patient lies within a strong magnet (usually a cylindrical magnet). The radiofrequency transmitter coils send radiowaves into the patient and the same coils receive signals from within the patient. The intensity and source of these signals can be calculated and displayed as an image.

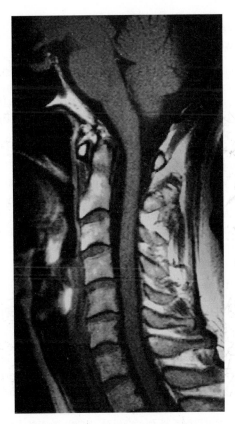

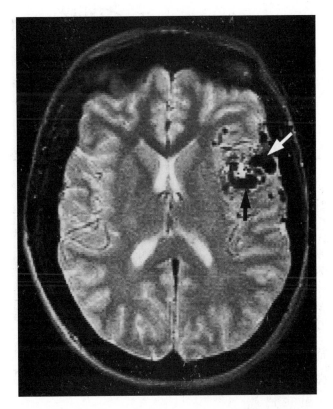

Fig. 1.15 MRI of head showing an arteriovenous malformation (arrows) in the left cerebral hemisphere. The fast-flowing blood in the malformation is responsible for absence of signal (signal void). The image is a T2-weighted image, and is normal apart from the arteriovenous malformation.

Fig. 1.14 Magnetic resonance image: sagittal section of cervical spine and base of brain. On this T1 sequence the brain and spinal cord are grey, CSF is black, fat is white but bone produces no signal. It is the fat in the bone marrow that produces the signal that enables the vertebrae to be visualized.

was for scanning the brain and spinal cord, where MRI has significant advantages over CT and few disadvantages. MRI is now also an established technique for imaging the spine, bones, joints, pelvic organs and heart. At first sight it may seem rather surprising that MRI provides valuable information in skeletal disease since calcified tissues do not generate any signal at MRI. This seeming paradox is explained by the fact that MRI provides images of the bone marrow and the soft tissues inside and surrounding joints (Fig. 1.14).

The physical basis of vascular MRI is complicated and beyond the scope of this book. Suffice it to say that, with some sequences, fast flowing blood produces no signal, whereas with others it produces a bright signal. This 'motion effect' can be exploited to image blood vessels; for example, large arteriovenous malformations can be readily demonstrated without contrast media (Fig. 1.15), hilar vessels can be distinguished from masses, and even stenoses of blood vessels can be demonstrated. Special flow sequences have been developed which give images of vessels, known as magnetic resonance angiography (Fig. 1.16), resembling a conventional angiogram without the need for contrast media. Magnetic resonance angiography may eventually replace conventional angiography.

Magnetic resonance imaging of the heart uses electronic gating to obtain images during a specific portion of the

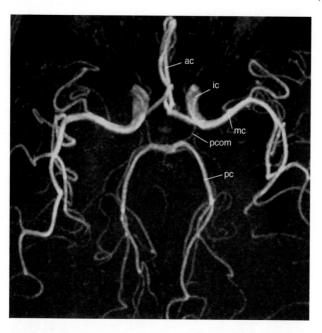

Fig. 1.16 MR angiogram of the intracranial arteries. No contrast, medium was used to obtain this image. ac, anterior cerebral; ic, internal cerebral; mc, middle cerebral; pc, posterior cerebral; pcom, posterior communicating artery.

cardiac cycle. With this technique it is possible to limit the degradation of the image by cardiac motion and therefore demonstrate the cardiac chambers, valves and myocardium. Alternatively, the beating heart can be directly visualized as a cine image.

One of the advantages of MRI is that it involves no ionizing radiation, and no adverse biological effects from diagnostic MRI have been demonstrated. The strong magnetic fields, however, mean that it is at present contraindicated in patients with cardiac pacemakers, intraocular metallic foreign bodies, and certain types of aneurysm clip.

Contrast agents for MRI

Just as contrast media have been of great value in CT, magnetic contrast materials are providing useful diagnostic information with MRI. The most widely used agents are gadolinium compounds which show very high signal intensity (i.e. they appear white) on T1-weighted images.

Picture archiving and communication systems (PACS)

Digital recording has developed dramatically over the past two decades. CT, ultrasound, MRI, nuclear medicine and angiography are nowadays all digital techniques. Even conventional radiographs can be based on digital information.

Digital data can be processed by a computer which allows electronic transmission of images between buildings, towns and even countries, and most importantly allows computer storage. A fully digital department would obviate the need for x-ray films; it would enable images with their reports to be viewed throughout the hospital on television monitors.

Radiation hazards

X-rays used in conventional radiography and CT, as well as gamma rays and other radionuclide emissions, are harmful. Natural radiation from the sun, radioactivity in the environment, together with atmospheric radioactivity from nuclear bombs and other man-made ionizing radiations contribute a genetic risk over which an individual doctor has no control. However, ionizing radiation for medical purposes is of several times greater magnitude than all other sources of man-made radiation and is under the control of doctors. It is their responsibility to limit the use of x-rays and other ionizing radiations to those situations where the benefit clearly outbalances the risks. Unnecessary radiation is to be deplored. The principle to be used is the so-called ALARA principle: 'as low as reasonably achievable'. This is achieved by the use of appropriate equipment and good technique – limiting the size of the x-ray beam to the required areas, limiting the number of films to those that are necessary, keeping repeat examinations to a minimum and ensuring that the examination has not already been performed. Just as important as these factors, all of which are really the province of those who work in the x-ray department, is the avoidance of unnecessary requests for x-ray examinations, particularly those that involve high radiation exposure such as barium enema, lumbar spine x-rays and CT examinations. If possible, alternative techniques such as ultrasound or MRI should be considered.

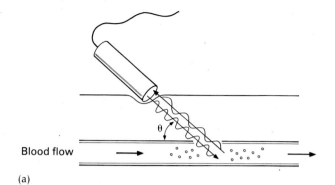

Blood flow

(a)

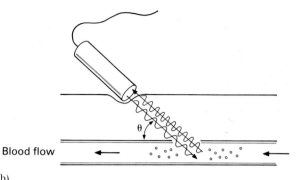

Blood flow

(b)

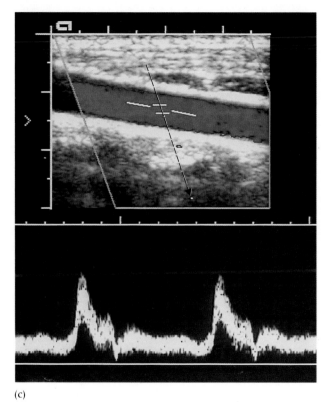

(c)

Plate 1 Principle of Doppler ultrasound. (a) With blood flowing away from the transducer, the frequency of the received sound is reduced. (b) With blood flowing towards the transducer, the frequency of the received sound is increased. (θ is the angle between the vessel and the transmitted sound wave: an angle known as the Doppler angle.) (c) Flow velocity waveform of normal internal carotid artery. The peaks represent systolic blood flow. The waveform has been taken from the gate within the artery shown in the colour Doppler image. The angle of the beam is indicated by the fine zig-zag line.

[*facing page 14*]

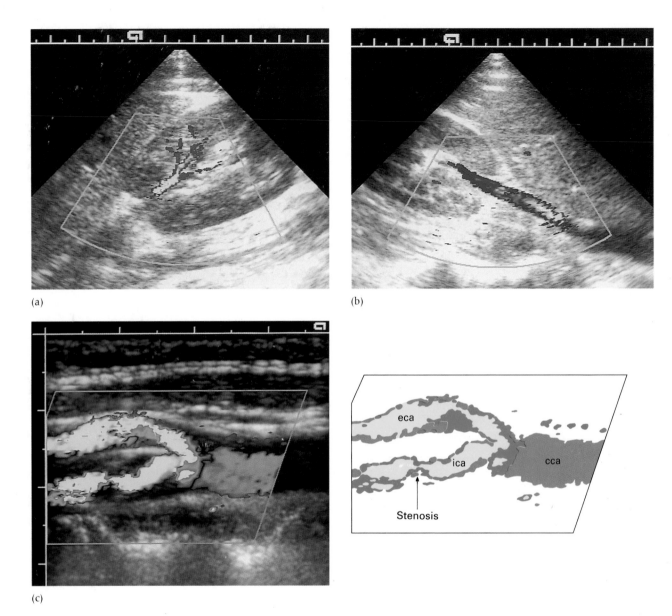

(a)

(b)

(c)

Plate 2 Colour Doppler. (a) Normal renal artery. (b) Normal renal vein. (c) Bifurcation of common carotid artery showing stenosis of internal carotid artery. The flowing blood is revealed by colour. The precise colour depends on the speed and direction of the blood flow. cca, common carotid artery; eca, external carotid artery; ica, internal carotid artery.

Radiation is particularly harmful to dividing cells. Genetically adverse mutations may occur following radiation of the gonads, resulting in congenital malformations and a genetic risk to the population. There is no threshold for the mutation rate, hence there is no such thing as a safe radiation dose.

Radiation to the developing fetus can have catastrophic effects. As well as the increased incidence of malformations induced in the developing fetus, it has been shown that the frequency with which leukaemia and other malignant neoplasms develop within the first 10 years of life is increased in children exposed to diagnostic x-rays while *in utero*, probably by about 40 % compared to the normal population. X-raying a fetus should, therefore, be kept to the absolute minimum and preferably avoided.

Radiation-induced cancer is of general concern. If all radiation reducing methods were followed, including the elimination of unnecessary examinations, then in the UK it might be possible to reduce the number of cancer fatalities by over 100 cases per year.

2

Chest

Imaging techniques

The plain chest radiograph

Routine chest radiography consists of a posteroanterior (PA) and lateral view (Fig. 2.1). Both should be exposed on full inspiration with the patient in the upright position. Films taken on expiration are difficult to interpret, because in expiration the lung bases appear hazy and the heart shadow increases in size (Fig. 2.2).

Even though chest films are the commonest x-ray examinations performed, they are amongst the most difficult to interpret. Trained radiologists often scan films in an apparently random fashion, but when an abnormality is found their thoughts are then structured, thinking of the possibilities for that particular shadow. For example, if a nodule representing a possible lung carcinoma is discovered, the shape of the nodule is analysed and evidence of spread of disease to the hilum, pleura or rib cage, etc., is sought. This problem-orientated approach – the observer constantly asking questions, not only about the shadows but also about the patient's clinical findings – is the quickest and most accurate way of achieving a diagnosis. However, this approach takes time to learn and in the early stages a routine is necessary in order to avoid missing valuable radiological signs. The order in which one looks at the structures is unimportant; what matters is to follow a routine, otherwise important abnormalities will be overlooked. One way of examining the frontal and lateral chest films is presented below.

Trace the diaphragm

The upper surfaces of the diaphragm should be clearly visible from one costophrenic angle to the other, except where the heart and mediastinum are in contact with the diaphragm. On a good inspiratory film, the dome of the right hemidiaphragm is at the level of the anterior end of the sixth rib, the right hemidiaphragm being up to 2.5 cm higher than the left.

Check the size and shape of the heart

See p. 112 for the details.

Check the position of the heart and mediastinum

Normally, the trachea lies midway, or slightly to the right of the midpoint, between the medial ends of the clavicles. The position of the heart is very variable; on average one-third lies to the right of the midline, but anything from one-half to one-fifth of the heart lying to the right of the midline is within the normal range.

Look at the mediastinum

The right superior mediastinal border is usually straight or slightly curved as it passes downwards to merge with the right heart border. The left superior mediastinal border is ill defined above the aortic arch.

The outline of the mediastinum and heart should be clearly seen except where the heart lies in contact with the diaphragm.

In young children, the normal thymus is often clearly

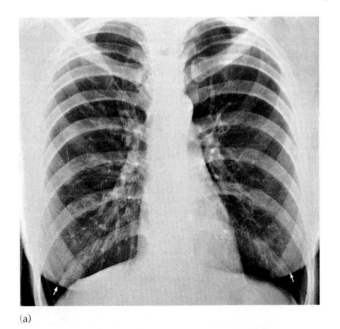

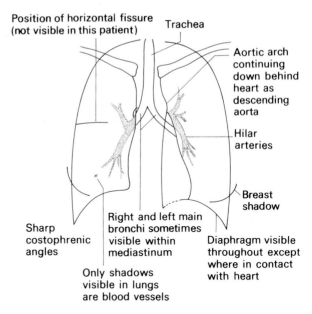

Position of horizontal fissure
(not visible in this patient)   Trachea

Aortic arch
continuing
down behind
heart as
descending
aorta

Hilar
arteries

Breast
shadow

Sharp
costophrenic
angles

Right and left main
bronchi sometimes
visible within
mediastinum

Only shadows
visible in lungs
are blood vessels

Diaphragm visible
throughout except
where in contact
with heart

(a)

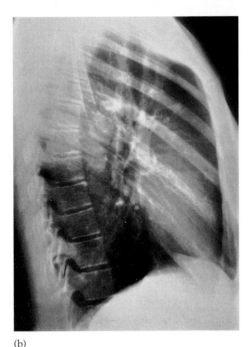

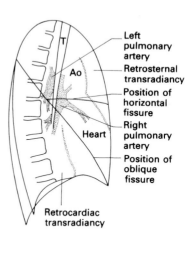

Left
pulmonary
artery

Retrosternal
transradiancy

Position of
horizontal
fissure

Right
pulmonary
artery

Position of
oblique
fissure

Retrocardiac
transradiancy

(b)

Fig. 2.1 Normal chest. (a) PA view. The arrows point to the breast shadows of this female patient. (b) Lateral view. Note that the upper retrosternal area is of the same density as the retrocardiac areas, and the same as over the upper thoracic vertebrae. The vertebrae are more transradiant (i.e. blacker) as the eye travels down the spine, until the diaphragm is reached. Ao, aorta; T, trachea.

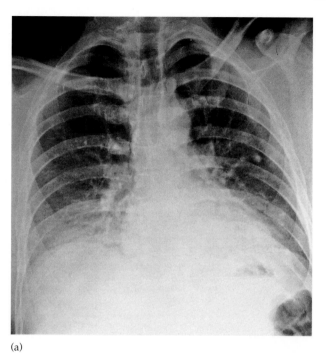 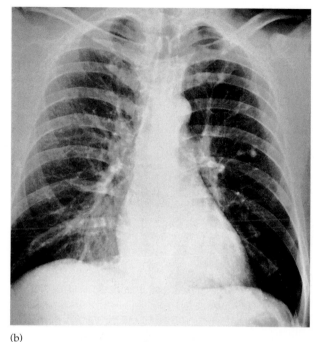

(a)   (b)

Fig. 2.2 Effect of expiration on chest film. Two films of the same patient taken one after the other. (a) Expiration. (b) Inspiration. On expiration the heart appears larger and the lung bases are hazy.

visualized. It may be very large and should not be mistaken for disease (Fig. 2.3).

Examine the hilar shadows

The hilar shadows represent the pulmonary arteries and veins. Air within the major bronchi can be recognised but the walls of the bronchi are not usually visible. The hilar lymph nodes in the normal patient are too small to recognize as discrete shadows.

The left hilum is usually slightly higher in position than the right.

Examine the lungs

The only structures that can be identified within normal lungs are the blood vessels, the interlobar fissures, and the walls of certain larger bronchi seen end-on. The fissures can only be seen if they lie along the line of the x-ray beam; they are after all composed of just two layers of pleura. Usually, only the horizontal fissure (minor fissure) is visible in the

frontal projection, running from the right hilum to the sixth rib in the axilla. There is no equivalent to the horizontal fissure on the left. The oblique fissures (major fissures) are only visible on the lateral view. The fissures form the boundaries of the lobes so a knowledge of their position is essential for an appreciation of lobar anatomy (see Fig. 2.15, p. 30). In about 1% of people there is an extra fissure visible in the frontal view – the so-called azygos lobe fissure (Fig. 2.4).

Look for abnormal pulmonary opacities or translucencies. Do not mistake the pectoral muscles, breasts (Fig. 2.1) or plaits of hair for pulmonary shadows. Skin lumps or the nipples may mimic pulmonary nodules. The nipples are usually in the fifth anterior rib space, but they are, in practice, rarely misdiagnosed because, in general, if one nipple is visible the other will also be seen.

A good method of finding subtle shadows on the frontal film is to compare one lung with the other, zone by zone. Detecting ill-defined shadows on the lateral view can be difficult. A helpful and reliable feature is that as the eye travels down the thoracic vertebral bodies, each vertebral body

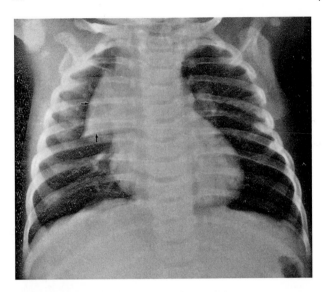

Fig. 2.3 Normal but prominent thymus in a child aged 3 months. The thymus shows the characteristic 'sail shape' projecting to the right of the mediastinum (arrows). This appearance should not be confused with right upper lobe consolidation or collapse.

should appear more lucent than the one above until the diaphragm is reached.

Check the integrity of the ribs, clavicles and spine and examine the soft tissues

In females, check that both breasts are present. Following mastectomy the breast shadow cannot be defined. The reduction in the soft tissue bulk leads to an increased trans-radiancy of that side of the chest, which should not be confused with pulmonary disease.

Assess the technical quality of the film

Technical factors are important since incorrect exposure may hide disease, and faulty centring or projection may mimic pathology. The correctly exposed routine PA chest film is one in which the ribs and spine behind the heart can be identified but the lungs are not overexposed. Unless one can see through the heart, lower lobe lesions may be completely missed. A straight film is one where the medial ends of the clavicles are equidistant from the pedicles of the thoracic vertebrae.

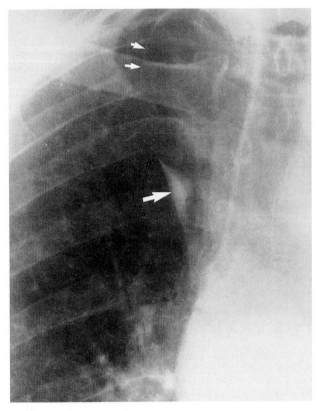

Fig. 2.4 The azygos lobe fissure. During normal intrauterine development the azygos vein migrates through the lung from the chest wall to lie within the mediastinum. In patients with an azygos 'lobe', the vein (large arrow) fails to reach the tracheobronchial angle and, therefore, lies in the lower end of the azygos fissure (small arrows). This variant is of no clinical significance.

Extra views

Oblique views. Films taken with the patient turned deliberately to one or other side are useful for demonstrating the chest wall and, occasionally, for showing intrathoracic shadows to better advantage.

Lateral decubitus views. These are not, as the name would suggest, lateral views; they are frontal projections taken with a horizontal x-ray beam, the patient lying on one or other side. Their purpose is to demonstrate free pleural fluid which will collect along the dependent chest wall (see Fig. 2.44, p. 48).

Expiration films. A frontal film may be deliberately exposed on expiration in order to demonstrate diaphragmatic movement or the ability of the lung to deflate. A pneumothorax may be more obvious on an expiration than an inspiration film.

Fluoroscopy

The image at *fluoroscopy* is poor compared to that which can be achieved with x-ray film. It is rarely used and is limited to observing the movement of the diaphragm and demonstrating air trapping in cases of suspected inhalation of a foreign body.

Computed tomography

There are many advantages to CT in chest disease:
• Showing the presence and extent of mediastinal masses and other mediastinal abnormalities. Computed tomography is widely used to demonstrate enlarged lymph nodes when patients with neoplastic disease are being staged, particularly lung cancer and lymphoma. Sometimes CT can determine the nature of a mediastinal abnormality. Knowing the shape and the precise location of a mediastinal mass may make a particular diagnosis highly likely. One of the advantages of CT is that it can distinguish vascular from non-vascular structures (Fig. 2.5), e.g. an aneurysm from a solid mass. Also, CT allows fat to be recognized, which is useful when fatty tumours are diagnosed. Also, significant abnormalities can be excluded when mediastinal widening is due merely to excess fat deposition.
• Showing the shape of an intrapulmonary or pleural mass and to detect any calcification that may be present in the mass, when this is not evident or doubtful on plain chest radiographs.
• Localizing a mass prior to biopsy.
• Demonstrating the presence of disease when the plain chest radiograph is normal in cases where the possibility of intrathoracic abnormality is suspected on other grounds, e.g. detecting pulmonary metastases; finding a primary carcinoma in patients whose sputum cytology shows neoplastic cells; and demonstrating thymic tumours in patients with myasthenia gravis.

• Documenting the presence, extent and severity of bronchiectasis and certain pulmonary parenchymal processes, such as fibrosing alveolitis.

Technique

A routine examination consists of adjacent sections 8–10 mm thick taken through the area of interest. To examine the entire chest from the posterior costophrenic recesses to the lung apices involves approximately 30 sections. Intravenous contrast medium is given in many cases, particularly when the purpose of the examination is to visualize the mediastinum or hila. The images are usually viewed at two distinct window settings (Fig. 2.6) (see p. 4 for explanation of CT windows and levels). If the CT scan has been performed to see bone lesions then bone settings are used.

Thinner sections can be used to produce images with higher spatial resolution in so-called high resolution CT (HRCT). High resolution CT is a specialized application being used with increasing frequency to show details of pulmonary parenchymal disease and bronchiectasis.

Normal images

Just as on the plain chest radiograph and conventional tomograms, the only structures seen within the normal lungs are the blood vessels, the pleural fissures and the walls of the larger bronchi. Vessels within the lung are recognized by their shape rather than by contrast opacification (Fig. 2.6a). When seen in cross-section they appear round and may be indistinguishable from small lung nodules. Fortunately most metastases and granulomas are located peripherally where the vessels are smallest.

The fissures are seen either as a line or their position may be recognizable only as a relatively avascular zone within the lung. The CT appearances of the normal mediastinum and hila are discussed on p. 57.

Conventional tomography

Conventional tomography has now been almost entirely replaced by CT. It can be used to investigate masses in the lungs and hilum in much the same way as CT, but has few other indications.

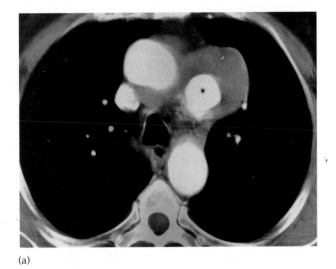

(a)

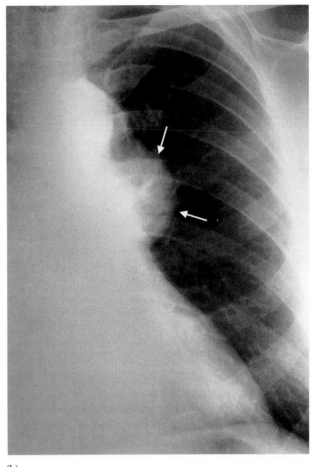

(b)

Fig. 2.5 Aortic aneurysm: example of the use of (a) contrast-enhanced CT to diagnose an aortic aneurysm. The lumen of the aneurysm (*)
enhances brightly. Much of the aneurysm is lined by clot. (b) The plain chest radiograph shows a mass (arrows), but the precise diagnosis of
aortic aneurysm cannot be made.

Magnetic resonance imaging

Magnetic resonance imaging (MRI) has only a very small
role in the management of pulmonary, pleural or mediastinal disease although it is playing an increasingly large part
in the diagnosis of cardiac and aortic diseases. Magnetic
resonance imaging can be useful in selected patients with
lung cancers, notably where the relevant questions cannot
be answered by CT and in showing the intraspinal extent of
neural tumours.

Ultrasound of the thorax

The use of thoracic ultrasound, as opposed to cardiac ultrasound (see Chapter 3), is confined to the demonstration of
processes in contact with the chest wall, notably pleural
effusion and pleural masses. It can be very useful for
guiding a needle to sample or drain loculated pleural fluid
collections and when needle biopsy/aspiration cytology of
masses in contact with the chest wall is being performed.
Since ultrasound is absorbed by air in the lung, conventional ultrasound cannot be used to evaluate processes

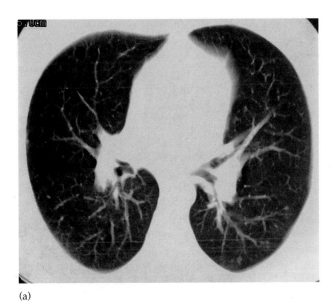
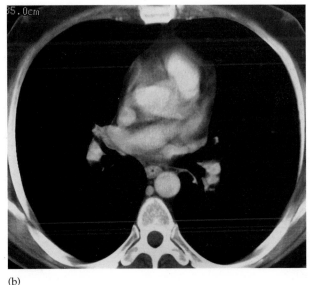

(a)   (b)

Fig. 2.6 Chest CT illustrating the different window centres (levels) used for the lungs and mediastinum. (a) Lung settings.
A negative centre (–700 HU) shows the lungs to advantage, but detail of mediastinal structures is minimal, the mediastinum being virtually white. In this example, the lung vessels are the only identifiable shadows originating from within the lung. (b) Mediastinal settings.
A centre close to average soft-tissue density (35 HU) and a narrow window width (500 HU) shows the structures within the mediastinum clearly, but the lungs are blacked out.

that lie more centrally within the thorax. It is possible to pass a small ultrasound probe through an endoscope to visualize structures immediately adjacent to the oesophagus, e.g. para-oesophageal nodes and the descending aorta.

Radionuclide lung scanning

There are two major types of lung scan: perfusion and ventilation scans.

The perfusion scan uses macroaggregates of albumin with an average particle size of 30 μm, labelled with ^{99m}Tc, injected intravenously. These particles, become trapped in the pulmonary capillaries; the distribution of radioactivity, when imaged by a gamma camera, accurately reflects blood flow (Fig. 2.7).

For ventilation scans, the patient inhales a radioactive gas such as xenon-133, xenon-127 or krypton-81m and the distribution of radioactive gas is imaged using a gamma camera (Fig. 2.8).

The major indication for lung scanning is to diagnose or exclude pulmonary embolism (see p. 88).

Bronchography

Bronchography involves introducing an iodinated contrast material into the bronchial tree, usually as part of a bronchoscopic examination. The only remaining indication is for the assessment of highly selected cases of bronchiectasis.

Pulmonary angiography

The pulmonary arteries and veins can be demonstrated by taking serial films following the rapid injection of angiographic contrast medium into the pulmonary arterial circulation through a catheter. The catheterization is carried out under fluoroscopic control with continuous electrocardiographic and pressure monitoring, by an operator skilled in cardiac catheterization. It carries a small but definite risk to the patient.

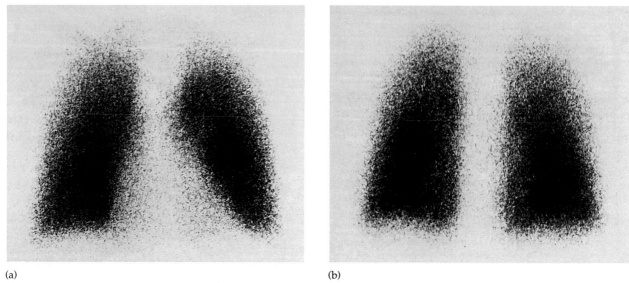

(a)   (b)

Fig. 2.7 Normal radionuclide perfusion scan using ^{99m}Tc-labelled macroaggregates of albumin. (a) Anterior view. (b) Posterior view.

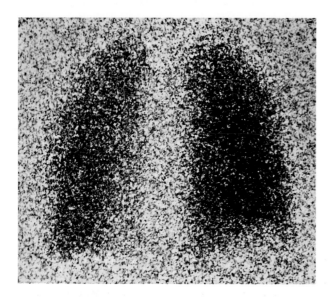

Fig. 2.8 Normal radionuclide ventilation scan using ^{133}Xe; posterior scan.

Its major uses are to diagnose pulmonary emboli or to demonstrate congenital vascular anomalies.

Diseases of the chest with a normal chest radiograph

Serious respiratory disease may exist in patients with a normal chest radiograph. Sometimes it is only possible to detect abnormality by comparison with previous or later examinations, e.g. subtle pulmonary shadows from infection or pulmonary fibrosis.

Respiratory disease with a normal chest radiograph occurs in:

Obstructive airways disease

Asthma and acute bronchiolitis may produce overinflation of the lungs, but in many cases the chest film is normal. Emphysema, when severe, gives rise to the signs described on p. 83 but when the disease is moderate, the chest radiograph may be normal or very nearly so. Uncomplicated acute or chronic bronchitis does not produce any radiological signs, so if a patient with chronic bronchitis has an abnormal film, some other disease or a complication has developed, e.g. pneumonia or cor pulmonale. A proportion of patients with productive cough due to bronchiectasis show no plain film abnormality.

Small lesions

It is usually impossible to see solitary lung masses or consolidations of less than 1 cm in diameter. Even 2–3 cm lung cancers may be very difficult to identify on routine films if they are hidden behind overlapping rib and clavicle shadows or behind the heart or diaphragm.

Endobronchial lesions, such as carcinoma, cannot be diagnosed on routine films unless they cause collapse/consolidation or considerable obstructive emphysema.

Pulmonary emboli without infarction

The chest radiograph is often normal even when life-threatening emboli are present.

Infections

Most patients with acute bacterial pneumonia present with recognizable consolidation, but in other infections, notably *Pneumocystis carinii* pneumonia, obvious pulmonary consolidation may only develop after the onset of symptoms. Patients with miliary tuberculosis may initially have a normal chest film.

Diffuse pulmonary disease

Pulmonary fibrosis in particular, may be responsible for breathlessness with substantial alteration in lung function tests before any clear-cut radiological abnormalities are evident.

Pleural abnormality

Dry pleurisy will not produce any radiological findings; even 300 ml of pleural fluid may be impossible to recognize on standard PA and lateral chest films.

The abnormal chest radiograph

With any abnormal examination of the chest, be it a plain film, CT or MRI scan, the first questions to ask are 'Where is the abnormality?' and 'How extensive is it?' Only then can the question 'What is it?' be asked. Clearly, the differential diagnosis for pulmonary lesions is quite different from that for mediastinal, pleural or chest wall disease. The first step is to examine all available films. Usually, the location of a lesion will then be obvious. If the shadow is surrounded on all sides by aerated lung it must arise within the lung. Similarly, many masses will clearly be within the mediastinum. However, when a lesion is in contact with the pleura or mediastinum it may be difficult to decide its origin.

If the shadow has a broad base with smooth convex borders projecting into the lung and a well-defined outline it is likely to be pleural, extrapleural or mediastinal in origin (Fig. 2.9).

The silhouette sign

The silhouette sign (Fig. 2.10) is an invaluable sign for localizing disease from plain chest radiographs. The information on a chest film is largely dependent on the contrast between the radiolucent air in the lungs compared with the opacity of the heart, blood vessels, mediastinum and diaphragm. An intrathoracic lesion touching a border of the heart, aorta or diaphragm will obliterate that border on the chest radiograph. This sign is known as *the silhouette sign* and has two important applications:

• It is often possible to localize a shadow by observing which borders are lost, e.g. loss of the heart border means that the shadow lies in the anterior half of the chest. Alternatively, loss of part of the diaphragm outline indicates disease of the pleura or of the lung in direct contact with the diaphragm, usually the lower lobes.

• The silhouette sign makes it possible, on occasion, to diagnose disorders such as pulmonary consolidation or collapse even when the presence of an opacity is uncertain. It is a surprising fact that a wedge or lens-shaped opacity may be very difficult to see because of the way the shadow fades out at its margins, but if such a lesion is in contact with the mediastinum or diaphragm it causes loss of their normally sharp outlines.

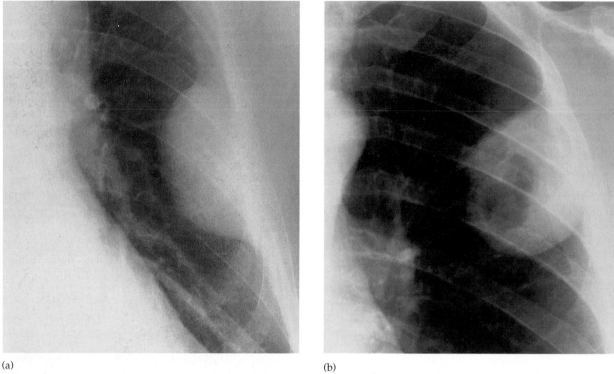

(a)   (b)

Fig. 2.9 (a) Extrapleural mass. The mass has a smooth convex border with a wide base on the chest wall (a myeloma lesion arising in a rib). This shape is quite different from a peripherally located pulmonary mass such as (b) a primary carcinoma of the lung.

Radiological signs of lung disease

Before the appearance of specific disorders is considered, it is worth describing various signs and their differential diagnoses.

With a chest radiograph or a CT scan it is of practical help to try and place any abnormal intrapulmonary shadows into one or more of the following broad categories:
- air-space filling
  (a) pulmonary oedema
  (b) pulmonary consolidation;
- pulmonary collapse (atelectasis);
- spherical shadows;
- line shadows;
- widespread small shadows.

The presence of cavitation or calification should be noted.

Air-space filling

Air-space filling means the replacement of air in the alveoli by fluid or, rarely, by other materials. 'Infiltrate' is a commonly used but less satisfactory term. The fluid can be either a *transudate* (pulmonary oedema) or an *exudate*. The causes of an alveolar exudate include infection, infarction, pulmonary contusion, haemorrhage and immunological disorders, e.g. collagen vascular diseases and extrinsic allergic alveolitis.

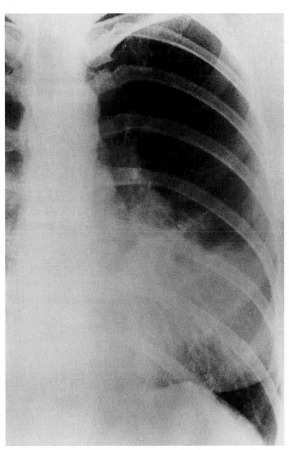

(a)

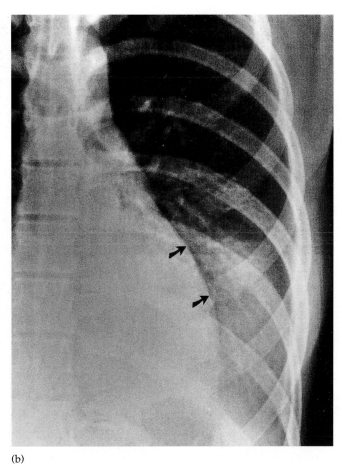

(b)

Fig. 2.10 The silhouette sign. (a) The left heart border is invisible because it is in contact with consolidation in the adjacent lingula. (b) The left heart border can be seen because the consolidation is in the left lower lobe and air in the lingula preserves the visibility of the cardiac silhouette (arrows). Note that now it is the diaphragm outline that is invisible. (c) The relationships of the lingula and lower lobes to the heart and diaphragm are explained by a diagram of the lung viewed from the side.

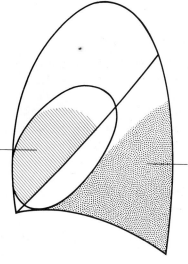

Consolidation in the lingula obliterates the left heart border but leaves the diaphragm visible

Consolidation in the left lower lobe obliterates the diaphragm but leaves the heart border visible

(c)

The signs of air-space filling are:

• A shadow with ill-defined borders (Fig. 2.11) except where the disease process is in contact with a fissure, in which case the shadow has a well-defined edge.

• An air bronchogram (Fig. 2.12). Normally, it is not possible to identify air in the bronchi within normally aerated lung substance because the walls of the bronchi are too thin and air-filled bronchi are surrounded by air in the alveoli, but if the alveoli are filled with fluid, the air in the bronchi contrasts with the fluid in the lung. This sign is seen to great advantage on CT scans (Fig. 2.13).

• The silhouette sign, namely loss of visualization of the adjacent mediastinal or diaphragm outline (see p. 25 for explanation of this sign).

Pulmonary oedema

There are two radiographic patterns of pulmonary oedema: alveolar and interstitial. Since oedema initially collects in the interstitial tissues of the lungs, all patients with alveolar oedema also have interstitial oedema.

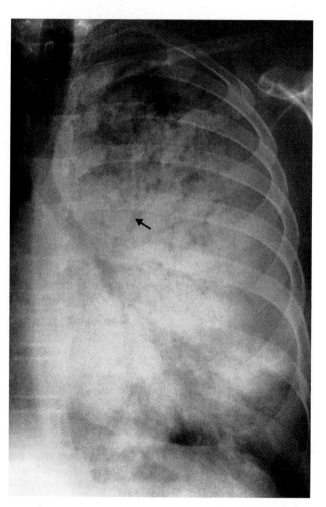

Fig. 2.12 The air bronchogram sign. An extensive air bronchogram is seen in this patient with pneumonia. The arrow points to some bronchi that are particularly well seen.

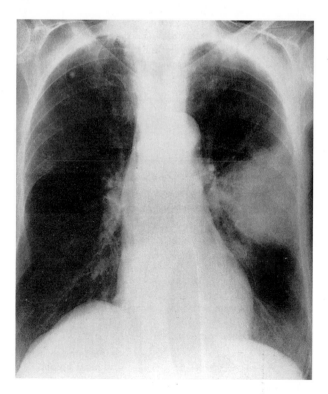

Fig. 2.11 Air-space filling. In this case the consolidation in the left lung is due to a pulmonary infarct.

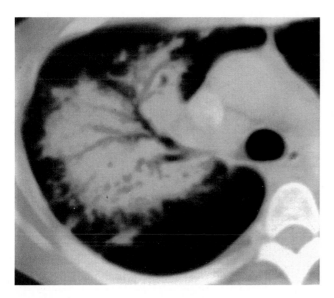

Fig. 2.13 CT scan showing an air bronchogram in an area of pulmonary consolidation from pneumonia.

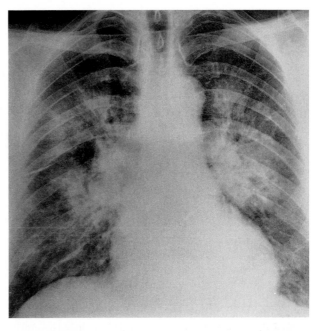

Fig. 2.14 Alveolar pulmonary oedema. Typical 'bat's wing' pattern. The shadows are bilateral and maximal in the perihilar region, fading towards the periphery of the lobes.

Alveolar oedema is always acute. It is almost always bilateral (Fig. 2.14), and involves all the lobes. In the early stages, the shadowing is maximal close to the hila and fades out peripherally, leaving a relatively clear zone around the edges of the lobes. This pattern of oedema is sometimes called the 'butterfly' or the 'bat's wing' pattern.

Interstitial oedema causes thickening of the interstitial tissues of the lungs. The hallmarks of interstitial oedema are septal lines (see p. 42) and thickening of the pleural fissures.

The causes of pulmonary oedema are broadly divided into:
• 'Cardiogenic pulmonary oedema', namely oedema due to circulatory disorders, e.g. acute left ventricular failure, mitral stenosis, renal failure and over-transfusion;
• so-called 'non-cardiogenic pulmonary oedema' in which increased capillary permeability is the important mechanism. This mechanism of oedema is seen in adult respiratory distress syndrome (ARDS), aspiration of gastric contents, and inhalation of noxious gases. The appearance may initially be identical to that seen with cardiogenic pulmonary oedema, but in ARDS (see p. 87) the pulmonary shadowing becomes uniform over a period of days,

until eventually all parts of the lungs are fairly equally affected.

One helpful feature for distinguishing cardiogenic pulmonary oedema from the non-cardiogenic varieties and from widespread exudates, such as pneumonia, is the speed with which cardiogenic oedema appears and disappears. Substantial improvement in a 24-hour period is virtually diagnostic of cardiogenic pulmonary oedema.

Pulmonary consolidation (alveolar infiltrates)

Consolidation of a whole lobe or the majority of a lobe is virtually diagnostic of bacterial pneumonia. The diagnosis of lobar consolidation requires an appreciation of the radiological anatomy of the lobes (Fig. 2.15). Lobar consolidation produces an opaque lobe, except for air in the bronchi (air bronchograms). Because of the silhouette sign, the boundary between the affected lung and the adjacent heart, medi-

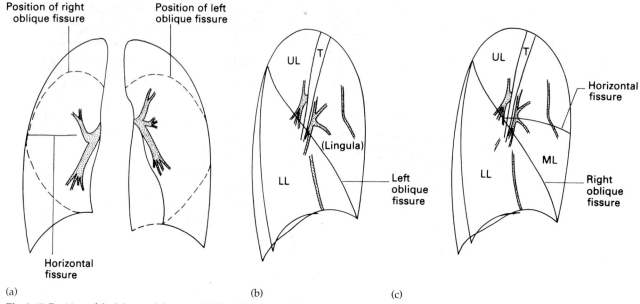

Fig. 2.15 Position of the lobes and fissures. (a) The oblique (major) fissure is similar on the two sides. The oblique fissures are not visible on the frontal view; their position is indicated by the dotted line. (b) In the left lung the oblique fissure separates the upper lobe (UL) and lower lobe (LL). (c) In the right lung, there is an extra fissure – the horizontal (minor) fissure, which separates the upper lobe (UL) and middle lobe (ML). (The lingular segments of the upper lobe are analogous to the segments of the middle lobe.) T, trachea.

astinum and diaphragm will be invisible. An example of lobar consolidation is seen in Fig. 2.16.

Patchy consolidation i.e. one or more patches of ill-defined shadowing (Fig. 2.17), is usually due to:
• pneumonia
• infarction
• contusion
• immunological disorders.

There is no reliable way of telling from the films which of these possibilities is the cause. In most instances the clinical and laboratory findings point to one or other.

Spherical consolidation may be difficult to distinguish from a lung tumour, but usually serial films show a change over a short interval if the shadow is due to consolidation, whereas no change will be apparent if it is due to a tumour. An air bronchogram is a very helpful sign here, since it is common with pneumonia and very rare with tumours.

Cavitation (abscess formation) within consolidated areas in the lung may occur with many bacterial infections (Fig. 2.18), but the organisms that are particularly liable

to produce cavitation are staphylococci, klebsiella, *Mycobacterium tuberculosis*, anaerobic bacteria and various fungi. Abscess formation is only recognizable once there is communication with the bronchial tree, allowing the liquid centre of the abscess to be coughed up and replaced by air. The air is then seen as a transradiancy within the consolidation and an air–fluid level may be present (Fig. 2.19). Computed tomography is better and more sensitive than plain films for demonstrating cavitation (Fig. 2.20).

Cavitation is occasionally seen in other forms of pulmonary consolidation, e.g. infarction and Wegener's granulomatosis.

Pulmonary collapse (atelectasis)

The common causes of collapse (loss of volume of a lobe or lung) are:
• bronchial obstruction;
• pneumothorax or pleural effusion.

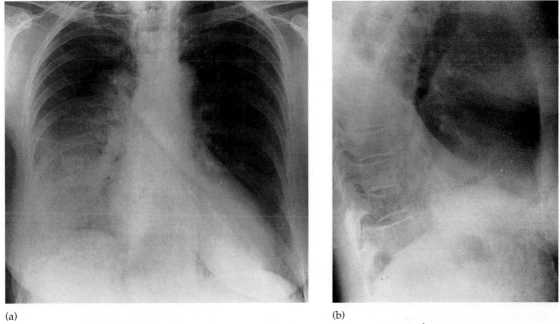

(a) (b)

Fig. 2.16 Consolidation of the right lower lobe. Note the application of the silhouette sign here. (a) PÁ view. The heart border and the medial half of the right hemidiaphragm are visible, whereas the lateral half is invisible. On the lateral view (b), the oblique fissure forms a well-defined anterior boundary and the right hemidiaphragm is ill defined. Only the left hemidiaphragm is seen clearly.

Collapse caused by bronchial obstruction

Collapse caused by bronchial obstruction occurs because air cannot get into the lung in sufficient quantities to replace the air absorbed from the alveoli. The end result is lobar (or lung) collapse.

The signs of lobar collapse are:

• displacement of structures;
• the shadow of the collapsed lobe – consolidation almost invariably accompanies lobar collapse, so the resulting shadow is usually obvious;
• the silhouette sign. The silhouette sign not only helps diagnose lobar collapse when the resulting shadow is difficult to appreciate, it also helps when deciding which lobe is collapsed. Collapse of the anteriorly located lobes (upper

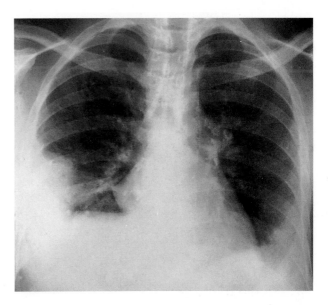

Fig. 2.17 Patchy consolidation in both lower lobes in a patient with bronchopneumonia.

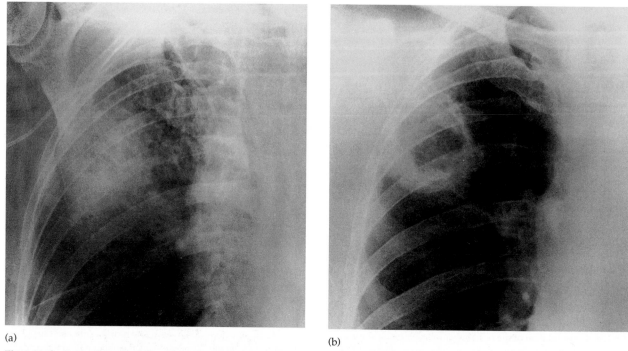

(a)　　　　　　　　　　　　　　　　　　　　　　　　　　(b)

Fig. 2.18 Cavitation in staphylococcal pneumonia. (a) A round area of consolidation which, seven days later (b) shows central translucency due to the development of cavitation.

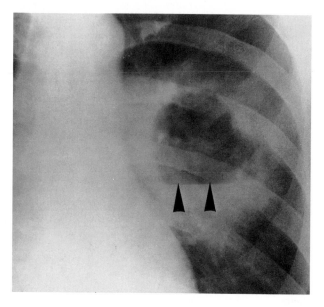

Fig. 2.19 Fluid level (arrows) in a lung abscess. Fluid levels are only visible if the chest radiograph is taken with a horizontal x-ray beam.

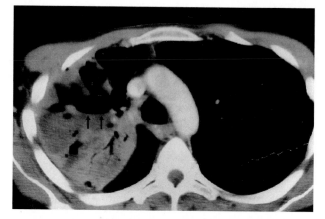

Fig. 2.20 Cavitation with consolidation owing to pneumonia shown by CT. The complex-shaped air–fluid collection is readily seen. The arrows point to an air–fluid level.

and middle) obliterates portions of the mediastinal and heart outlines, whereas collapse of the lower lobes obscures the outline of the adjacent diaphragm and descending aorta.

The commoner causes of lobar collapse are:

1 bronchial wall lesions
   • usually primary carcinoma;
   • rarely, other bronchial tumours such as carcinoid;
   • rarely, endobronchial tuberculosis.

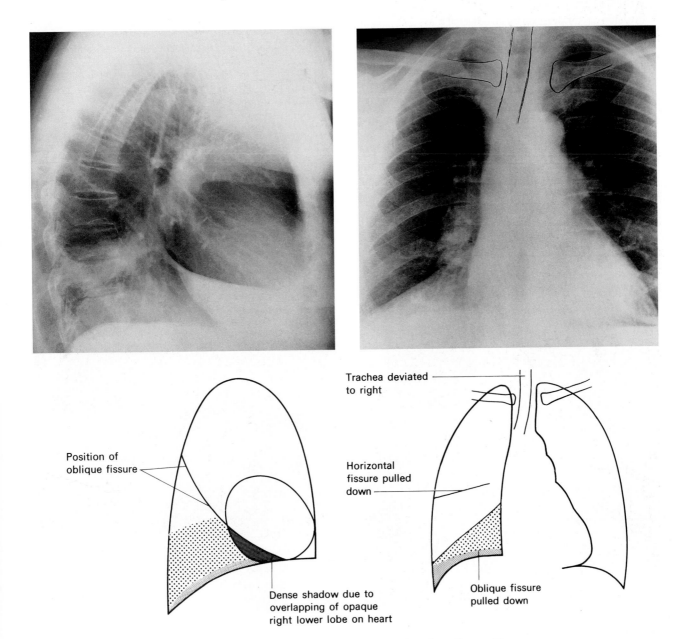

Fig. 2.21 Collapse of the right lower lobe. (In this example the apical segment is relatively well aerated.)

2 Intraluminal occlusion
  - mucus plugging, particularly in postoperative, asthmatic or unconscious patients, or in patients on artificial ventilation;
  - inhaled foreign body.
3 Invasion or compression by an adjacent mass
  - malignant tumour;
  - enlarged lymph nodes.

When a lobe collapses, the unobstructed lobe(s) on the side of the collapse undergo compensatory expansion. The displaced fissure is seen as a well-defined boundary to an airless lobe in one or other view. The mediastinum and diaphragm may move towards the collapsed lobe.

Since lobar collapse is such an important and often difficult diagnosis, it is worth devoting time to study the appearance of collapse of each of the lobes (Figs 2.21–2.25). Computed tomography shows lobar collapse very well

(Figs 2.25, 2.26), but is rarely necessary simply to diagnose a collapsed lobe.

With collapse of the whole of one lung, the entire hemithorax is opaque and there is substantial mediastinal and tracheal shift (Fig. 2.27).

Collapse in association with pneumothorax or pleural effusion

The presence of air or fluid in the pleural cavity will allow the lung to collapse. In pneumothorax, the diagnosis is obvious but if there is a large pleural effusion with underlying pulmonary collapse it may be difficult to diagnose the presence of the collapse on a chest radiograph. This problem does not arise with CT where it is usually easy to recognise pulmonary collapse despite the presence of a pleural effusion (Fig. 2.28). If lobar collapse is identified, it can be difficult to tell whether the collapse is due to pleural

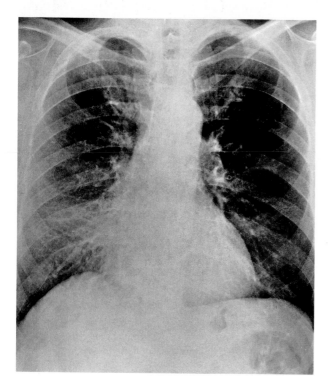
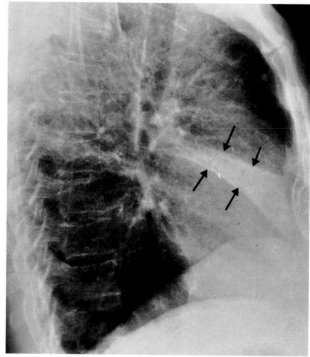

Fig. 2.22 Collapse of the middle lobe. The collapsed lobe is most obvious on the lateral view (arrows). Note the silhouette sign obliterating the lower right heart border.

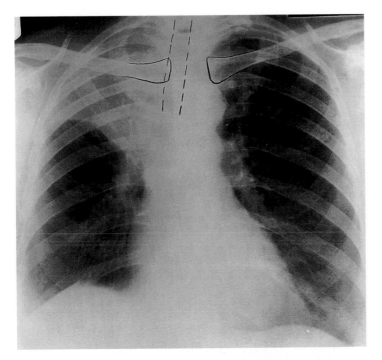
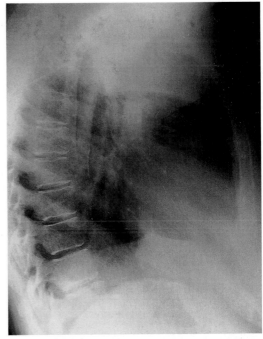

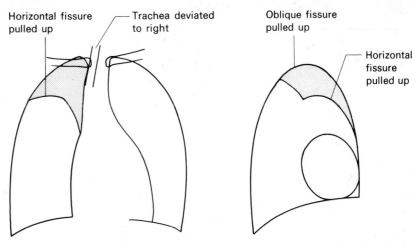

Fig. 2.23 Collapse of the right upper lobe. Note the elevated horizontal fissure.

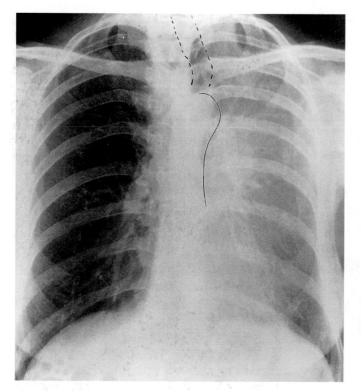

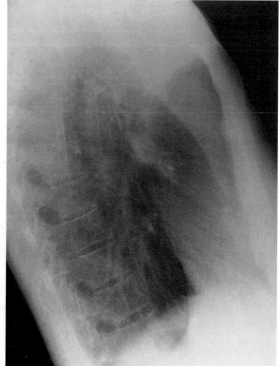

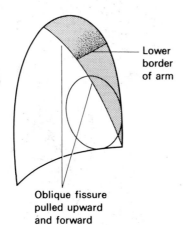

Lower
border
of arm

Oblique fissure
pulled upward
and forward

Fig. 2.24 Collapse of the left upper lobe. Note that the lower
border of the collapsed lobe is ill-defined on the PA view and that
the upper two-thirds of the left mediastinal and heart borders are
invisible, but that the aortic knuckle and descending aorta are
identifiable. (The visible portions of the aorta have been drawn in
for greater clarity.)

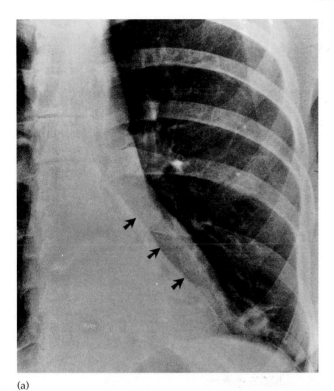

(a)

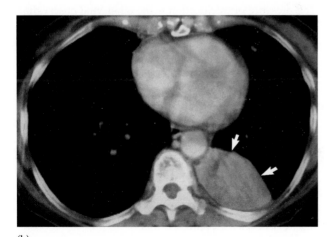

(b)

Fig. 2.25 Collapse of the left lower lobe. (a) Chest radiograph. The triangular shadow of the collapsed lobe is seen through the heart. Its lateral border is formed by the displaced oblique fissure (arrows). (b) CT scan. The collapsed lobe is seen lying posteriorly in the left thorax. The well-defined anterior margin is due to the displaced oblique fissure (arrows).

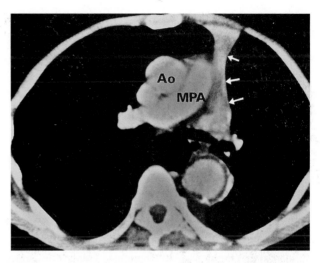

Fig. 2.26 Computed tomography scan of a severely collapsed left upper lobe. Note the smooth lateral border of the collapsed lobe formed by the displaced oblique (major) fissure (arrows). The scan shows compensatory overexpansion of the right upper lobe which has crossed the midline anterior to the ascending aorta (Ao) and main pulmonary artery (MPA).

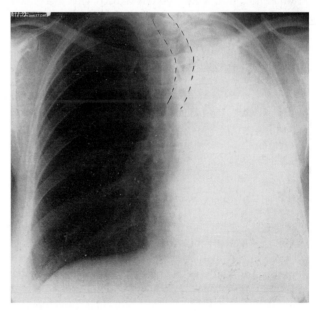

Fig. 2.27 Collapse of left lung showing tracheal and mediastinal displacement.

fluid or whether both the collapse and the effusion are due to the same process, e.g. carcinoma of the bronchus.

Linear (discoid) atelectasis

This topic is discussed on p. 43.

Spherical shadows (lung mass, lung nodule)

The diagnosis of a solitary spherical shadow in the lung (Fig. 2.29) is a common problem.

The usual causes of a solitary pulmonary nodule are:
• bronchial carcinoma/bronchial carcinoid;
• benign tumour of the lung, hamartoma being the most common;
• infective granuloma, tuberculoma being the most common in the UK, fungal granuloma being the most frequent in the USA;
• metastasis;
• lung abscess.

With the exception of lung abscess, the lesions in this list rarely cause symptoms, the mass first being noted on a routine chest film. When a nodule is discovered in a patient who is over 40 and a smoker, bronchial carcinoma becomes the major consideration. In a patient less than 30 years old, primary carcinoma is highly unlikely.

The diagnoses listed for a solitary pulmonary nodule include lesions that require very different forms of management. Hamartomas and granulomas are best left alone, whereas bronchial carcinoma, active tuberculosis and lung abscess require specific treatment. Careful observation of the following features may help in making the diagnosis.

Comparison with previous films

Assessing the rate of growth of a spherical lesion in the lung is one of the most important factors in determining the correct management of the patient. Lack of change over a period of 18 months or more is a strong pointer to either a benign tumour or an inactive granuloma. An enlarging mass is highly likely to be a bronchial carcinoma or a metastasis.

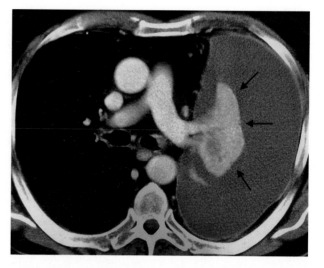

Fig. 2.28 Computed tomography showing pleural effusion and pulmonary collapse. The collapsed lobe (arrows) can be clearly seen beneath the large left pleural effusion.

Calcification

The presence of calcification is the other vital observation, because substantial calcification virtually rules out the diagnosis of a malignant lesion. Calcification is a common finding in hamartomas, tuberculomas and fungal granulomas. In hamartomas it is often of the 'popcorn' type (Fig. 2.30). Computed tomography is of great value in detecting calcification and confirming that the calcification is within the lesion, not just projected over it. Uniform calcification can be difficult to recognize on plain chest radiography. With CT, however, uniform calcification can be diagnosed and in such cases carcinoma of the lung can be excluded from the differential diagnosis (Fig. 2.31).

Involvement of the adjacent chest wall

Destruction of the adjacent ribs is virtually diagnostic of invasion by carcinoma. Tumours of the lung apex are particularly liable to invade the chest wall and adjacent bones (Pancoast's tumour). CT or bone scan may be indicated to demonstrate this invasion (Fig. 2.32).

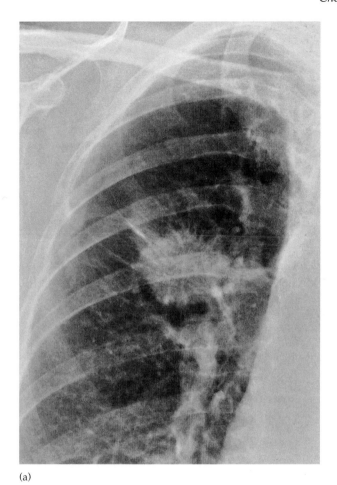

(a)

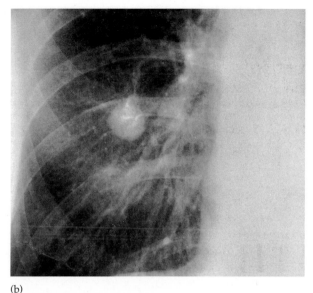

(b)

Fig. 2.29 Solitary spherical shadow. (a) The large size and the irregular infiltrating edge are important diagnostic features suggesting primary carcinoma of the lung. (b) The small size and relatively smooth border leads to a wider differential diagnosis. In this case the diagnosis was bronchial carcinoid.

The shape of the shadow

Primary carcinomas are nearly always rounded with a lobulated, notched or infiltrating outline (Fig. 2.33). Even if only one small portion of the lesion has an irregular or lobular edge the diagnosis of primary carcinoma should be seriously considered.

The shape may be obvious from plain films but CT (or conventional tomography) can be used to confirm the rounded shape. Sometimes a lesion that is rounded and mass-like on chest radiographs is shown to be linear or band-like on CT, in which case the diagnosis is likely to be a focal pulmonary scar of no significance.

Cavitation

If the centre of the mass undergoes necrosis and is coughed up, air is seen within the mass. An air–fluid level may be visible on erect films. These features, which may be difficult to appreciate on plain films, are particularly well seen at CT.

Cavitation almost always indicates a significant lesion. It is very common in lung abscesses (Fig. 2.34), relatively common in primary carcinomas (Fig. 2.35) and occasionally seen with metastases. It does not occur in benign tumours or inactive tuberculomas.

The distinction between cavitating neoplasms and lung

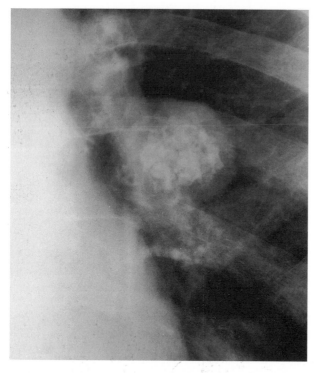

Fig. 2.30 Calcification in a pulmonary hamartoma. The central flocculant ('popcorn') calcification is typical of that seen in hamartomas.

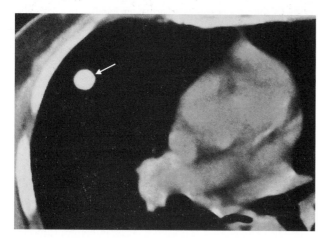

Fig. 2.31 CT of a calcified nodule (arrow). The calcific density of this fungal granuloma is clearly shown by CT. No calcification was evident on plain chest radiographs.

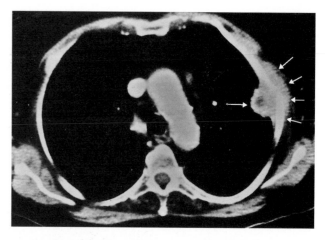

Fig. 2.32 CT showing invasion of chest wall by bronchial carcinoma (single arrow). The soft tissue mass within the chest wall (multiple arrows) is best appreciated by comparison with the normal opposite side.

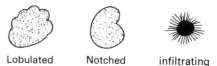

Lobulated   Notched   infiltrating

Fig. 2.33 Outline of primary carcinoma of the lung.

abscesses can be very difficult and sometimes impossible, particularly if the walls are smooth. If, however, either the inner or outer walls are irregular the diagnosis of carcinoma is highly likely.

Size

A solitary mass over 4cm in diameter which does not contain calcium is nearly always either a primary carcinoma or a lung abscess. Lung abscesses of this size, however, virtually always show cavitation.

Other lesions

The rest of the film should be checked carefully after a lung

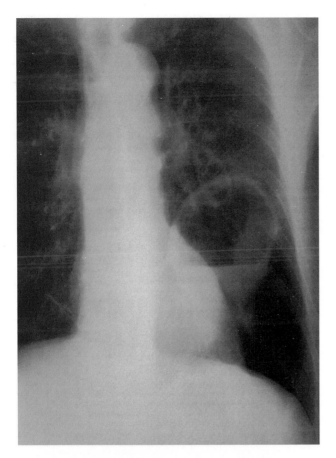

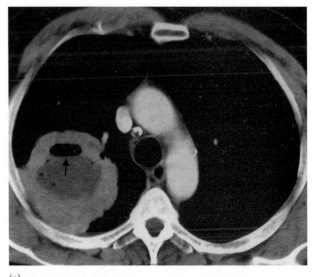

(a)

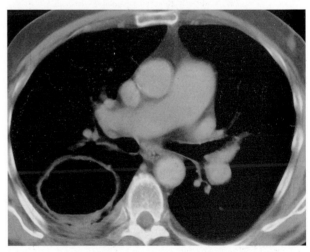

(b)

Fig. 2.34 Cavitation in a lung abscess showing a relatively thin, smooth wall and an air–fluid level.

mass has been found. Metastases are the common cause of multiple nodules and finding a metastasis or a pleural effusion in a patient with primary lung cancer may completely alter the management of the patient.

The role of CT

The role of CT in patients with a solitary pulmonary nodule is to:
• Diagnose the nature of the nodule. The role here is limited since the signs on plain films and knowledge of the rate of growth provide adequate information in most cases. CT is better able to detect calcification in a nodule than con-

Fig. 2.35 CT of cavitating primary carcinoma of the lung. (a) The variable thickness of the cavity wall is a striking feature. The air–fluid level is also well seen (arrow). (b) A case of cavitating primary squamous cell carcinoma showing a very thin wall – a rare but well recognized feature.

ventional films. As mentioned above, extensive calcification of a nodule effectively excludes primary carcinoma of the lung (Fig. 2.31).

• Stage the extent of disease in those cases where the nodule is likely to be a primary carcinoma.

• Localize accurately the nodule prior to bronchoscopic or percutaneous needle biopsy in cases where localization is difficult on conventional films.

• Establish whether or not the nodule is solitary or multiple, when the lesion in question is likely to be a metastasis or when surgical resection of the mass is being considered.

Multiple pulmonary nodules

Multiple well-defined spherical shadows in the lungs are virtually diagnostic of metastases (see Fig. 2.117, p. 97). Occasionally, this pattern is seen with abscesses or with granulomas caused by collagen vascular disorders.

Line or band-like shadows

All line shadows within the lungs, except fissures and the walls of the large central bronchi, are abnormal. Septal lines are by far the most important.

Septal lines

The pulmonary septa are connective tissue planes containing lymph vessels. They are normally invisible. Only thickened pulmonary septa can be seen on a chest film. There are two types of septal lines:

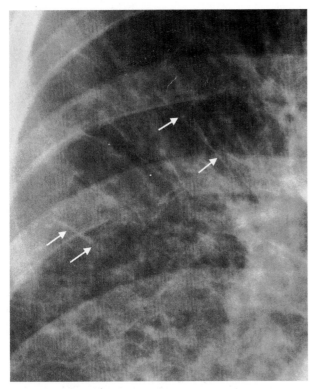

(a)

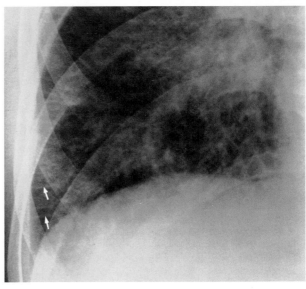

(b)

Fig. 2.36 Septal lines. (a) Kerley A lines (arrows) in a patient with lymphangitis carcinomatosa. (b) Kerley B lines in a patient with pulmonary oedema. The septal lines (arrows) are thinner than the adjacent blood vessels. The B lines are seen in the outer centimetre of lung where blood vessels are invisible or very difficult to identify.

1 Kerley A lines, which radiate towards the hila in the mid and upper zones. These lines are much thinner than the adjacent blood vessels and do not reach the lung edge (Fig. 2.36a).

2 Kerley B lines, which are horizontal, never more than 2 cm in length and best seen at the periphery of the lung. Unlike the blood vessels they often reach the edge of the lung (Fig. 2.36b).

There are two important causes of septal lines:
• pulmonary oedema;
• lymphangitis carcinomatosa.

Pleuropulmonary scars

Scars from previous infection or infarction are a common cause of line or band-like shadows. They usually reach the pleura and are often associated with visible pleural thickening. Such scars are of no clinical significance to the patient.

Linear (discoid) atelectasis

Linear (discoid) atelectasis is a form of collapse that is not secondary to bronchial obstruction. It is due to hypoventilation, the commonest cause of which is postoperative or post-traumatic pain. The result is a horizontally orientated band or disc of collapse (Fig. 2.37).

Emphysematous bullae

Bullae (blebs) are often bounded and traversed by thin line shadows. Bullae have few if any normal vessels within them and this makes the interpretation easy (Fig. 2.38).

The pleural edge in a pneumothorax

The pleural edge in a pneumothorax is seen as a line approximately parallel with the chest wall. No lung vessels can be seen beyond the pleural line. Once the line is spotted the diagnosis is rarely in doubt (see Fig. 2.53, p. 55).

Widespread small shadows

Nodular and reticular shadows

Chest films with widespread small (2–5 mm) pulmonary

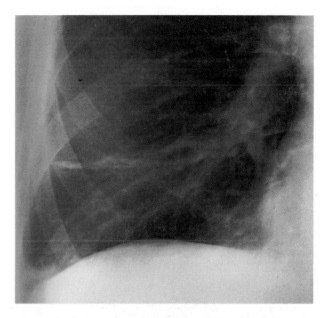

Fig. 2.37 Band-like shadow in right lower lobe caused by discoid atelectasis.

shadows often present a diagnostic problem. With few exceptions it is only possible to give a differential diagnosis when faced with such a film. A final diagnosis can rarely be made without an intimate knowledge of the patient's symptoms, signs and laboratory results.

Many descriptive terms have been applied to these shadows, the commonest being 'mottling', 'honeycomb', 'fine nodular', 'reticular' and 'reticulonodular' shadows. In this book we will use three basic terms: 'nodular', to signify discrete small round shadows (Fig. 2.39) and 'reticular' to discribe a net-like pattern of small lines, and 'reticulonodular', when both patterns are present (Fig. 2.40).

All three patterns are due to very small lesions in the lung, no more than 1 or 2 mm in size. Individual lesions of this size are invisible on a chest film. That these very small lesions are seen at all is explained by the phenomenon of superimposition; when myriads of tiny lesions are present in the lungs it is inevitable that many will lie in line with one another. It follows that when very small non-calcified shadows are visible the lung must be diffusely involved by disease. It is worth noting that the size of the multiple small shadows seen on the x-ray film gives no clue

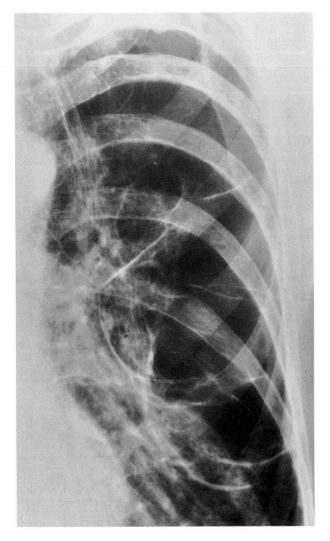

Fig. 2.38 Line shadows caused by walls of bullae (blebs). The bullae are air spaces devoid of blood vessels.

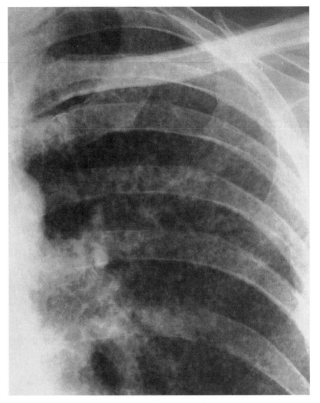

Fig. 2.39 Nodular shadowing in the lung of a patient with miliary tuberculosis.

to the size of the responsible lesions, except to predict that they are small; nor can the shape of the lung shadows be reliably used to predict the shape of the lesions seen at pathology.

How to decide whether or not multiple small pulmonary shadows are present

Often, the greatest problem is to decide whether widespread abnormal shadowing is present at all, since normal blood vessels can appear as nodules and interconnecting lines. To be confident involves looking carefully at many hundreds of normal films to establish a normal pattern in one's mind. Look particularly at the areas between the ribs where the lungs are free of overlying shadows. The normal vessel pattern is a branching system which connects up in an orderly way. The vessels are larger centrally and they become smaller as they travel to the periphery. Vessels seen end-on appear as small nodules, but these nodules are no bigger than vessels seen in the immediate vicinity and their number corresponds to the expected number of vessels in

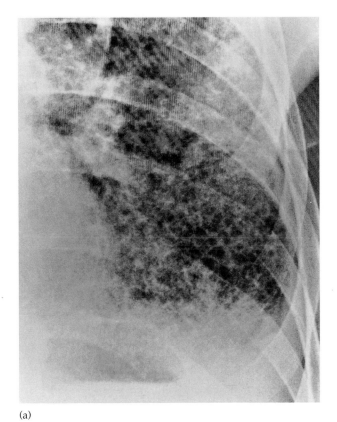

(a)

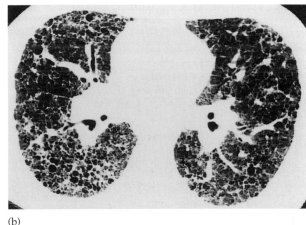

(b)

Fig. 2.40 (a) Reticulonodular shadowing in the lung in a patient with fibrosing alveolitis. (b) Thin-section, high-resolution CT scan of a different patient with cryptogenic (idiopathic) fibrosing alveolitis showing the honeycomb pattern to advantage.

that area. There are no visible vessels in the outer 1–2 cm of the lung.

An important sign in questionable cases is that the abnormal shadows obscure the adjacent vessels and, therefore, the borders of the mediastinum and diaphragm may be less sharp than normal.

When abnormal shadowing is present and its pattern has been determined, the next step is to decide the distribution: is the disease process uniformly distributed, is it more severe in one or other zone, does it extend outward from the hila or is it peripherally predominant? Other abnormalities on the film should then be sought. Once these observations have been made it is possible to produce the differential diagnosis as shown in Table 2.1.

Inevitably, there will be cases when there is doubt, both clinically and radiographically, whether diffuse lung disease is present. In these circumstances, thin-section high-resolution CT (HRCT) can be of considerable help, because the evidence of lung disease may be convincing with CT, even though the chest radiograph is normal or borderline.

High resolution CT can also be of help in defining the character and distribution of the abnormal shadowing (Fig. 2.40b). A few conditions have quite specific appearances, e.g. lymphangitis carcinomatosa (see p. 96) and fibrosing alveolitis, although the precise cause of diffuse pulmonary fibrosis cannot be ascertained by CT scanning.

Multiple ring shadows of 1 cm or larger

Multiple ring shadows larger than 1 cm are diagnostic of bronchiectasis (Fig. 2.41). The shadows represent dilated thick-walled bronchi.

Table 2.1 Commoner causes of nodular and reticular shadowing.

Diagnosis	Radiographic pattern	Distribution of shadows	Other features which may be seen	Thin-section high-resolution CT (HRCT)
Miliary tuberculosis	Small nodules of uniform size	Uniform	± Mediastinal/hilar lymph nodes One or more patches of consolidation	Not necessary
Sarcoidosis	(a) Fine nodular	Uniform	Hilar and paratracheal lymph nodes	Shows disease well but adds little of diagnostic value
	(b) Reticulonodular	Often radiates out from hilar and is predominant in mid and upper zones	Hilar and paratracheal lymph nodes	
Coal miners, pneumoconiosis	Nodular	Predominant in upper zones	Progressive massive fibrosis in the complicated form of the disease Emphysema	Adds little of diagnostic value
Asbestosis	Fine reticulonodular	Predominant in lower zones	Pleural thickening and/or calcification	Useful for documenting the severity of fibrosis, and for showing pleural plaques where the diagnosis is in doubt
Fibrosing alveolitis	Reticulonodular	Often predominant in lower zones, but may show a variety of patterns	Diaphragm often high and indistinct	Characteristically shows basal and peripherally predominant reticulonodular shadowing
Lymphangitis carcinomatosa	Reticulonodular	No predominant distribution	Septal lines Bronchial wall thickening Hilar adenopathy Other sings of carcinoma	The combination of septal lines and small nodules produces a characteristic pattern
Pulmonary oedema	Ill-defined nodules	May show central predominance with clear zone at periphery of lobes	Cardiac enlargement Left atrial enlargement Septal lines	Not indicated

Widespread small pulmonary calcifications

Widespread small pulmonary calcifications may occur following pulmonary infection with tuberculosis, histoplasmosis or chickenpox.

Increased transradiancy of the lungs

Generalized increase in transradiancy

Generalized increased transradiancy of the lungs is one of the signs of emphysema. The other signs are discussed on p. 83.

Localized increase in transradiancy

When only one hemithorax appears more transradiant than normal the following should be considered:

• *Compensatory emphysema.* This occurs when a lobe or lung is collapsed or has been excised and the remaining lung expands to fill the space.

• *Pneumothorax.* The diagnosis of a pneumothorax depends on visualization of the lung edge with air peripheral to it, and checking that the space in question does not contain any vessels (see Fig. 2.54, p. 56).

• *Reduction in the chest wall soft tissues,* e.g. mastectomy.

• *Air-trapping due to central obstruction* (Fig. 2.42). Most obstructing lesions in a major bronchus lead to lobar collapse. Occasionally, particularly with an inhaled foreign body, a check valve mechanism may lead to air-trapping. Inhaled foreign bodies are commonest in children; they usually lodge in a major bronchus. Often, the chest radiograph is normal but sometimes the affected lung becomes abnormally transradiant and the heart is displaced to the opposite side on expiration. Air-trapping is best appreciated at fluoroscopy when the fixed position of the hemidiaphragm is noted and the mediastinum can be seen to swing away from the obstructed side on expiration.

The pleura

Pleural effusion

The chest radiographic appearances of fluid in the pleural cavity are the same regardless of whether the fluid is a transudate, an exudate, pus or blood. On a plain chest radiograph, a large effusion may hide an abnormality in the underlying lung.

Ultrasound is a simple method of determining whether pleural fluid is present. No imaging technique can provide reliable information about the nature of pleural fluid except on rare occasions, e.g. CT, which may show when the fluid is a recent haemorrhage. Imaging does not, in general, obviate the need for diagnostic pleural fluid aspiration.

Free pleural fluid

Plain radiographic findings (Fig. 2.43). Free fluid collects in

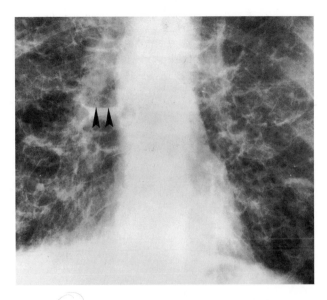

Fig. 2.41 Ring shadows in bronchiectasis. Each ring shadow represents a dilated bronchus. A fluid level in one of the dilated bronchi is arrowed.

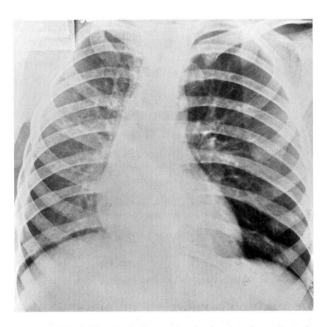

Fig. 2.42 Inhaled foreign body causing check valve obstruction of the left main bronchus. Note the increased transradiancy of the left lung, and the slight displacement of the heart to the right. (The film was exposed in expiration.)

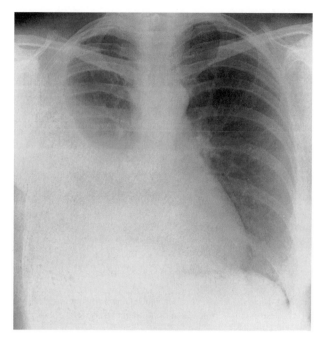

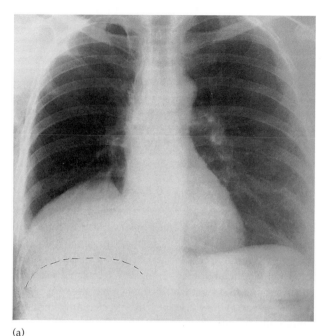

(a)

Fig. 2.43 Large right pleural effusion. The shadow of the pleural fluid is entirely homogeneous and lies outside the lung edge. The fluid appears higher laterally than medially, a point that can be useful in differentiating pleural fluid from pulmonary shadows. In this instance the trachea and heart are in normal position but no pulmonary disease was present.

the most dependent portion of the pleural cavity and always fills in the costophrenic angles. Free pleural effusions assume two basic shapes, usually seen in combination with one another:

1 Usually the fluid surrounds the lung, higher laterally than medially. It also runs into the fissures, particularly into the lower end of the oblique fissures. Very large effusions run over the top of the lung.

The smooth edge between the lung and the fluid can be recognized on an adequately penetrated film, providing that the underlying lung is aerated. This smooth edge should always be looked for: it is diagnostic of pleural pathology.

2 Sometimes, even with a large effusion, little or no fluid is seen running up the chest wall. The fluid is then known as a 'subpulmonary effusion' (Fig. 2.44). The upper border of the

(b)

Fig. 2.44 Large right subpulmonary effusion (the patient has had right mastectomy). Almost all the fluid is between the lung and the diaphragm. The right hemidiaphragm cannot be seen. (a) Its estimated position has been pencilled in. (b) In the lateral decubitus view, the fluid moves to lie between the lateral chest wall and the lung edge (arrows).

fluid is much the same shape as the normal diaphragm, and since the true diaphragm shadow is obscured by the fluid it may be very difficult, or even impossible, to tell from the standard erect film if any fluid is present at all.

It is not always possible to distinguish on chest radiographs whether basal shadowing is due to pleural effusion or to pulmonary collapse/consolidation. If there is doubt, a frontal film taken with the patient lying on one side (a lateral decubitus view) can be of help. The fluid, if free to move, will than lie along the dependent lateral chest wall. This technique is particularly valuable when the effusion is largely subpulmonary.

Since a pleural effusion occupies space in the thorax, compression collapse of the underlying lung is inevitable, the compressed lung being otherwise normal. Alternatively, both the pleural effusion and the pulmonary collapse may be due to the same primary process, e.g. carcinoma of the bronchus.

Computed tomography. Pleural effusions are seen as a homogeneous fluid density between the chest wall and lung (Figs. 2.45 and 2.46). Just as with the plain chest radiograph, it is not possible to distinguish transudate from exudate, nor can one usually tell whether the shadow is due to fluid, blood or pus. Free pleural fluid will move to the dependent portion of the chest and scans are sometimes taken in the lateral decubitus position to demonstrate this movement.

Surprisingly, it is sometimes difficult to determine from CT whether fluid is pleural effusion or ascites. The distinction is made by noting the relationship of the fluid to the diaphragm. Pleural fluid collects outside the diaphragmatic dome and can be seen posterior to the portion of diaphragm that covers the bare area of the liver (Fig. 2.46a).

Distinguishing between pleural effusion and pulmonary consolidation or collapse at CT is relatively easy because the pleural fluid is usually lower in density than the collapsed or consolidated lung, the pleural effusion is of homogeneous density and has a smooth interface with the pleura covering the underlying lung. Air bronchograms are particularly well seen at CT and their presence is unequivocal evidence of collapsed or consolidated lung (see Fig. 2.13, p. 29).

Ultrasound. Pleural fluid can be recognized as a transonic

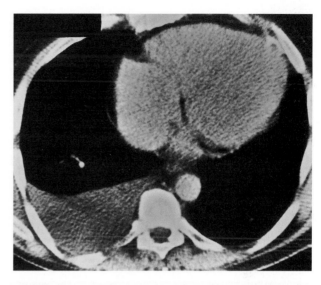

Fig. 2.45 CT of pleural fluid. The right pleural effusion is of homogeneous density, with a CT number between zero and soft tissue. Its well-defined meniscus-shaped border with the lung is typical.

area between the lung and diaphragm (Fig. 2.46b). Since the diaphragm is so well seen there is no confusion with ascites. Ultrasound is a convenient method of imaging control for pleural fluid aspiration or drainage.

Loculated pleural fluid (Fig. 2.47)

Pleural effusions may become loculated by pleural adhesions. Although loculation occurs in all types of effusion, it is a particular feature of empyema. Such loculations may either be at the periphery of the lung or within the fissures between the lobes. A loculated effusion may simulate a lung tumour on chest radiographs.

Ultrasound can be particularly useful in defining the presence, size and shape of any pleural collection loculated against the chest wall or diaphragm. Pleural aspiration and drainage of such collections may be performed under ultrasound guidance.

Computed tomography scanning (Figs 2.48 and 2.49) can be used to distinguish loculation of pleural fluid from adja-

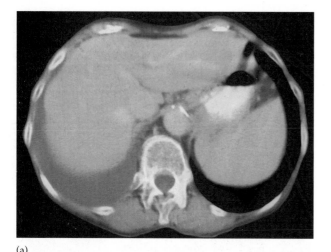

(a)

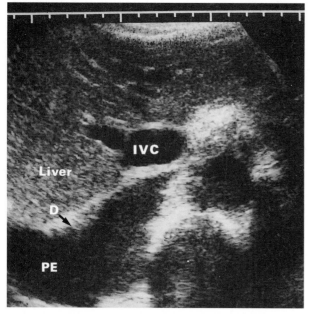

(b)

Fig. 2.46 CT and ultrasound of pleural effusion. (a) CT scan. The section is taken through the lowermost portion of the pleural cavity and at this level the distinction from ascites is a potential problem because the diaphragm itself is not visible. Pleural fluid, as here, is not affected by the peritoneal reflections of the bare area (see Fig. 10.1, p. 285). (b) Ultrasound scan – transverse image. The pleural effusion (PE) is seen as a transonic area behind the diaphragm (D). IVC, inferior vena cava.

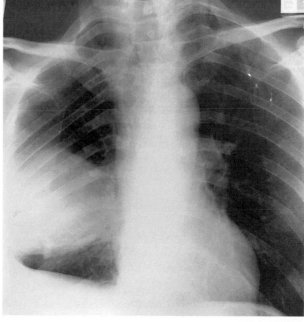

(a)

Fig. 2.47 Loculated pleural fluid. (a) PA and (b) lateral views show an empyema loculated against the posterior chest wall. (c) Fluid loculated in the horizontal (minor) fissure in another patient. Both these fluid collections could be confused with an intrapulmonary mass.

cent pulmonary disease, a distinction that is particularly valuable when empyema formation is suspected. Like ultrasound, CT can be used to direct the placement of drainage tubes.

Causes of pleural effusion

There are many causes for pleural effusion. In some cases the cause is visible on the chest film or CT scan.

Infection. Pleural effusions which are due to pneumonia are on the whole small, and the pneumonia is usually the dominant feature on the chest film. Large loculated effusions in association with pneumonia often indicate empyema formation (Figs 2.48 and 2.49). In some cases of tuberculosis the

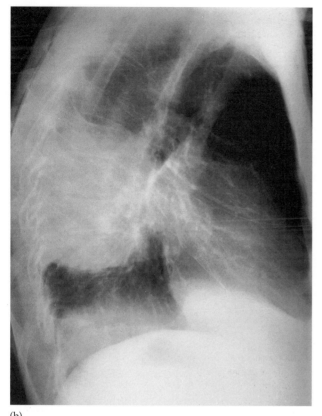

(b)

Fig. 2.47 *Continued*

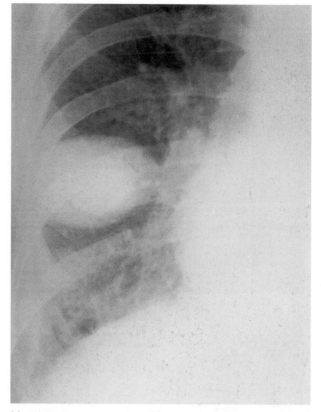

(c)

effusion is the only visible abnormality and the effusion may be large.

Subphrenic abscess nearly always produces a pleural effusion.

Malignant neoplasm. Effusions occur with pleural metastases, but it is unusual to see the pleural deposits themselves on plain chest radiographs. Pleural metastases are occasionally seen on CT, MRI or ultrasound scans as nodular or mass-like pleural thickening. Malignant effusions are frequently large. If the effusion is due to bronchogenic carcinoma or malignant mesothelioma, other signs of the primary tumour are usually, but not always, evident.

Cardiac failure. Small bilateral pleural effusions are fre-

quently seen in acute left ventricular failure. Larger pleural effusions may be present in longstanding congestive cardiac failure. The effusions are usually bilateral, often larger on the right than the left. Other evidence of cardiac failure, such as alteration in the size or shape of the heart, pulmonary oedema or the signs of pulmonary venous hypertension, are usually present.

Pulmonary infarction. This may cause pleural effusion. Such effusions are usually small and accompanied by a lung shadow caused by the pulmonary infarct.

Collagen vascular diseases. Pleural effusions, either unilateral or bilateral, are relatively common in these conditions. They may be the only abnormal features on a chest film.

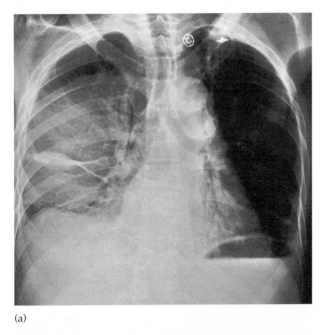

(a)

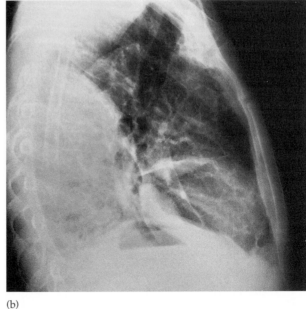

(b)

(c)

Fig. 2.48 Loculated pleural fluid (empyema), showing the value of CT in distinguishing pleural fluid from pulmonary consolidation. The fluid is loculated behind the right lower lobe and in the horizontal (minor) fissure. On the plain chest films (a) and (b) the large posterior collection resembles right lower lobe consolidation. The CT scan (c) clearly shows the characteristic shape and location of loculated pleural fluid.

Nephrotic syndrome, renal failure, ascites and Meig's syndrome. These are all associated with pleural effusion, the cause of which cannot be determined from the chest film.

Pleural thickening (pleural fibrosis) (Fig. 2.50)

Fibrotic pleural thickening, especially in the costophrenic angles, may follow resolution of a pleural effusion, particularly following pleural infection or haemorrhage. The appearances of pleural thickening are similar to pleural fluid but pleural scarring is nearly always much smaller than the original pleural effusion. It is sometimes impossible to distinguish pleural fluid from pleural thickening on conventional projections, especially if comparison with pre-

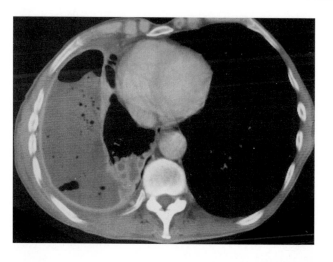 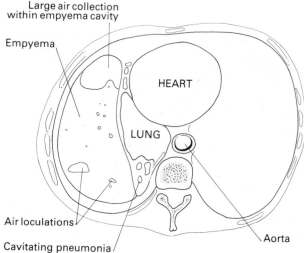

Fig. 2.49 Empyema. CT scan showing loculated air–fluid collection in right pleural cavity. Small loculations of air are seen within the pus.

vious films is not possible. The problem can be resolved by a lateral decubitus view, where free fluid will move to lie along the lateral chest wall, whereas fibrotic thickening is unaltered in appearance.

Localized plaques of pleural thickening along the lateral chest wall commonly indicate asbestos exposure. Such plaques may show irregular calcification.

Pleural tumours (Fig. 2.51)

Pleural tumours produce lobulated masses based on the pleura. Malignant pleural tumours, both primary (malignant mesothelioma) and secondary, frequently cause pleural effusions which may obscure the tumour itself.

Sometimes the predominant feature is pleural effusion with no visible masses on any imaging examinations. The commonest pleural tumours are metastatic carcinoma, breast carcinoma being the most frequent primary tumour to spread to the pleura. Primary pleural tumours are relatively uncommon. Since many malignant mesotheliomas are secondary to asbestos exposure the other features of asbestosis-related disease (pulmonary fibrosis, pleural plaques and pleural calcification) may be seen.

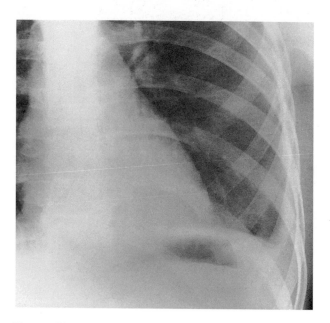

Fig. 2.50 Pleural thickening at the left base. This patient had been treated for a tuberculous pleural effusion, which had resolved leaving pleural thickening, which obliterated the left costophrenic angle.

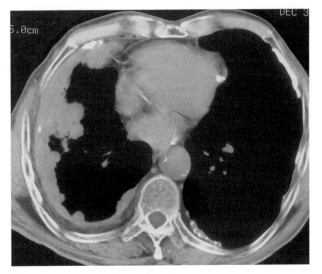

(b)

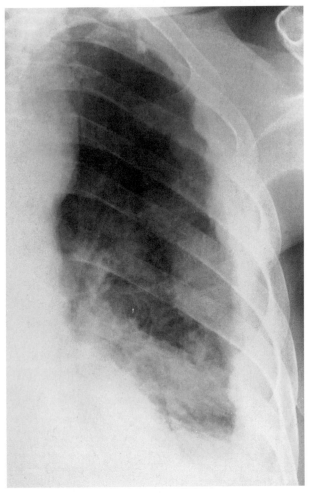

(a)

Fig. 2.51 (a) Lobulated pleural thickening caused by malignant neoplasm. The tumour in this instance was a malignant mesothelioma of the pleura. (b) CT scan of mesothelioma of the pleura. Note also the calcified pleural plaques following asbestos exposure.

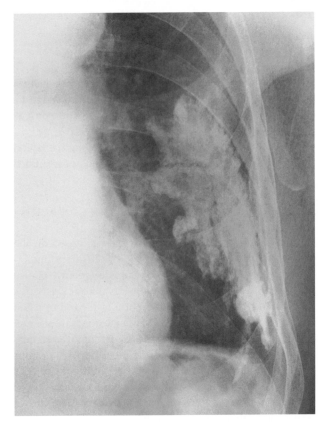

Fig. 2.52 Unilateral pleural calcifications from old tuberculous empyema.

Pleural calcification

Irregular plaques of calcium may be seen with or without accompanying pleural thickening. When unilateral they are likely to be due to either an old empyema, usually tuberculous (Fig. 2.52), or an old haemothorax. Bilateral pleural calcification is often related to asbestos exposure (see Fig. 2.90, p. 80). Sometimes no cause for pleural calcification can be found.

Pneumothorax (Fig. 2.53)

The diagnosis of pneumothorax depends on recognising:
• the line of pleura forming the lung edge separated from the chest wall, mediastinum or diaphragm by air;
• the absence of vessel shadows outside this line.

Lack of vessel shadows alone is insufficient evidence on which to make the diagnosis, since there may be few, or no, visible vessels in emphysematous bullae. Unless the pneumothorax is very large, there may be no appreciable increase in the density of the underlying lung.

The detection of a small pneumothorax can be very difficult. The cortex of the normal ribs takes a similar course to the line of the pleural edge, so the abnormality may not strike the casual observer. Sometimes a pneumothorax is more obvious on a film taken in expiration.

Once the presence of a pneumothorax has been noted, the next step is to decide whether or not it is under tension. This depends on detecting mediastinal shift and flattening or inversion of the hemidiaphragm (Fig. 2.54).

It is worth noting that tension pneumothoraces are usually large because the underlying lung collapses due to increased pressure in the pleural space.

Causes of pneumothorax

The majority of pneumothoraces occur in young people with no recognizable lung disease. These patients have small blebs or bullae at the periphery of their lungs which burst.

Occasionally pneumothorax is due to:
• emphysema
• trauma
• certain forms of pulmonary fibrosis
• *pneumocystis carinii* pneumonia
• metastases, rarely.

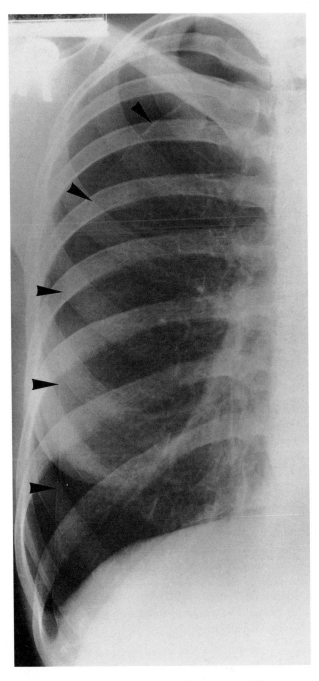

Fig. 2.53 Pneumothorax. The pleural edge is arrowed. The diagnosis of pneumothorax requires the identification of this edge and a clear space beyond it.

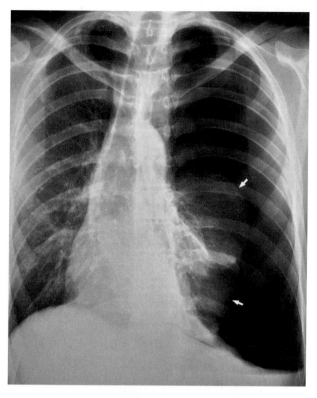

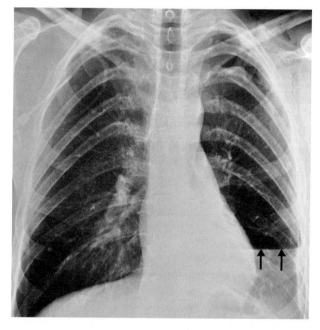

Fig. 2.55 Hydropneumothorax. The arrows point to the air–fluid level in the pleural space. In this case the edge of the lung is difficult to see on the PA view; most of the fluid and air were loculated posteriorly.

Fig. 2.54 Tension pneumothorax. The left hemidiaphragm is depressed and the mediastinum is shifted to the right. The left lung (arrows) is substantially collapsed.

Hydropneumothorax, haemopneumothorax and pyopneumothorax

Fluid in the pleural cavity, whether it be a pleural effusion, blood or pus, assumes a different shape in the presence of a pneumothorax. The diagnostic feature is the air–fluid level (Fig. 2.55).

Some fluid is present in the pleural cavity in most patients with pneumothorax. In spontaneous pneumothorax the amount is usually small.

The mediastinum

The mediastinum is divided into anterior, middle and posterior divisions for descriptive purposes (Fig. 2.56). However, masses often cross from one compartment to the other. Mediastinal widening can be due to many different pathological processes. These are usually classified according to their position in the mediastinum (Fig. 2.57); so if a mediastinal mass is identified on the frontal chest radiograph, the next step must be to attempt to localize it in the lateral view. This may be quite easy, but anterior mediastinal masses are sometimes difficult to visualize on the lateral view (Fig. 2.58). Therefore, if no obvious abnormality is seen on the lateral film, the anterior mediastinum should be carefully reviewed. In most people a transradiant area, known as the retrosternal space, can be identified behind the sternum in front of the ascending aorta. If this space is uniformly opaque there may be anterior mediastinal pathology. However, it is worth noting that this space is sometimes opaque in obese but otherwise normal subjects.

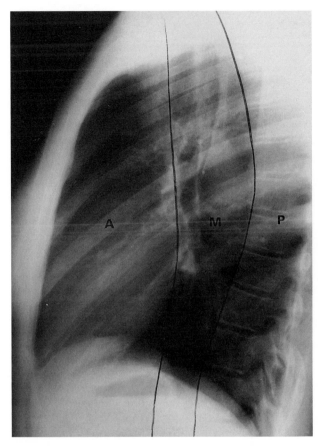

Fig. 2.56 The anterior (A), middle (M) and posterior (P) compartments of the mediastinum. The divisions are arbitrary and do not correspond to those used by anatomists. The anterior mediastinum refers to the structures anterior to the trachea and the major bronchi. The posterior mediastinum refers to structures posterior to a line joining the anterior boundary of the vertebral bodies.

CT and MRI of the normal mediastinum

The greatest impact of CT and MRI in chest radiology has been in imaging the mediastinum, where two major advantages are most apparent: the cross-sectional display of anatomy and the ability to distinguish clearly fat, various soft tissues and blood vessels.

The CT and MRI appearances are illustrated in Figs 2.59 and 2.60. The features to note while viewing these images are:

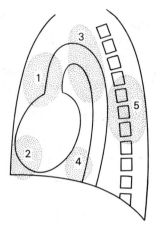

ANTERIOR
1. Thyroid tumour
   Thymic tumour or cyst
   Teratoma/Dermoid cyst
   Lymphadenopathy
   Aortic aneurysm

2. Pericardial cyst
   Fat pad
   Morgagni hernia

MIDDLE
3. Thyroid tumour
   Lymphadenopathy
   Bronchogenic cyst
   Aortic aneurysm

4. Hiatus hernia

POSTERIOR
5. Neurogenic tumours
   Soft tissue mass of vertebral infection or neoplasm
   Lymphadenopathy
   Aortic aneurysm

Fig. 2.57 The causes of mediastinal masses divided according to location. Note that both lymphadenopathy and aortic aneurysms occur in all three major compartments.

1 The bulk of the mediastinum is due to blood vessels. Blood vessels are easy to recognize as tubular structures, retaining a near constant diameter on several adjacent sections. For CT they can be opacified by intravenous contrast medium. (In some centres such opacification is used almost routinely.) At MRI, the larger vessels are readily seen without the need for a contrast agent.
2 The only other normal structures of appreciable size are the thymus, oesophagus, trachea and bronchi. The thymus is the most difficult to assess because it is so variable in size.
3 Normal lymph nodes are small, usually less than 6 mm in diameter (maximum 10 mm) and most are not visible.

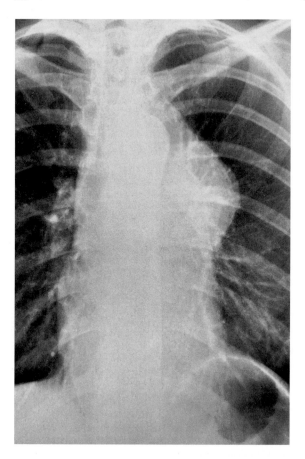
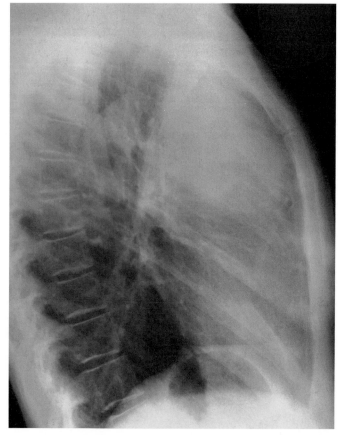

Fig. 2.58 Anterior mediastinal mass. There is a large mass situated anteriorly in the mediastinum projecting to the left side which was due to a mass of lymph nodes involved by malignant lymphoma. Diagnosing the anterior location of the mass depends on noting the density of the retrosternal areas. This area should normally have the same density as the retrocardiac area.

4 The mediastinal structures are surrounded by fat. The sites listed below normally contain nothing but fat or small lymph nodes. They are, therefore, areas in which small masses, particularly enlarged lymph nodes, can be readily recognized:

  • between the right tracheal wall and the adjacent lung (the one exception being the azygos vein which lies in the right tracheobronchial angle);

  • between the right wall of the oesophagus and the adjacent lung all the way down the chest, an anatomical region known as the azygo-oesophageal recess;

  • anterior and to the left of the aorta and main pulmonary artery (other than the thymus and the left brachiocephalic vein).

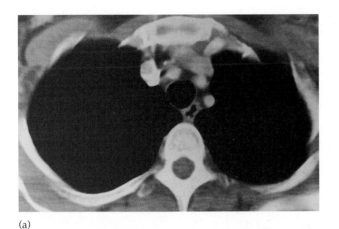

(a)

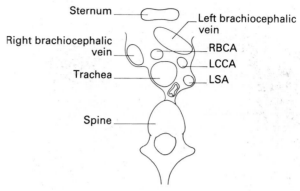

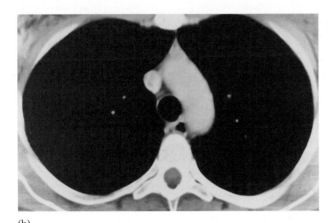

(b)

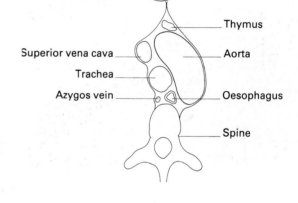

Fig. 2.59 CT of normal mediastinum. The levels at which the four selected levels were taken is shown right. Intravenous contrast has been given; it is particularly concentrated in the right brachiocephalic vein and superior vena cava. Air is present in the oesophagus; this can be a normal finding. LCCA, left common carotid artery; LMB, left main bronchus; LSA, left subclavian artery; RBCA, right brachiocephalic (innominate) artery; RMB, right main bronchus.

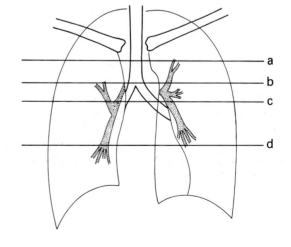

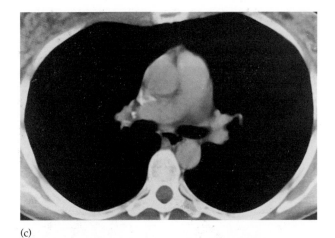

(c)

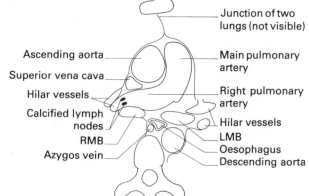

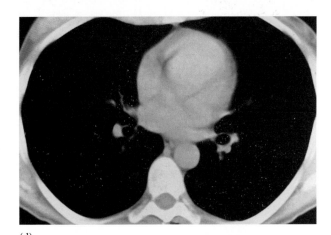

(d)

Fig. 2.59 Continued.

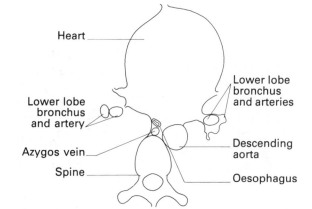

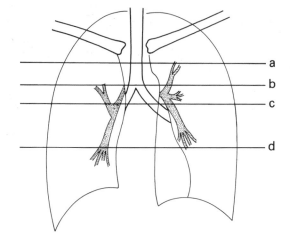

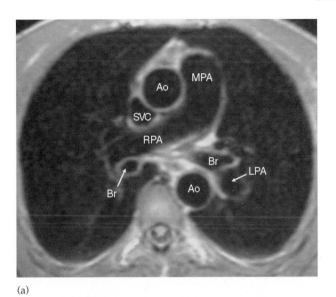

(a)

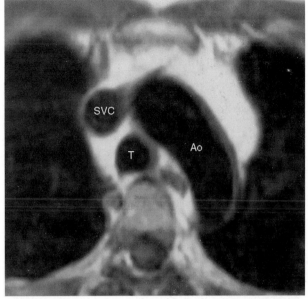

(b)

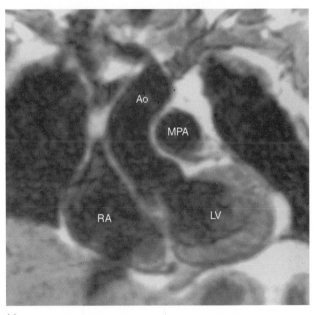

(c)

Fig. 2.60 MRI of normal mediastinum (T1-weighted, cardiac gated). (a) Axial scan through the level of the pulmonary hila. (b) Higher axial section through the level of the aortic arch. (c) Coronal scan. Ao, aorta; Br, bronchi; LPA, left pulmonary artery; LV, left ventricle; MPA, main pulmonary artery; RA, right atrium; RPA, right pulmonary artery; RV, right ventricle; SVC, superior vena cava; T, trachea.

Mediastinal masses

Computed tomography scanning provides a much clearer idea of the position, shape and size of any mass than is possible from the plain chest radiograph; occasionally the CT density even enables a specific diagnosis to be made. Magnetic resonance imaging provides more information than CT only in highly selected cases.

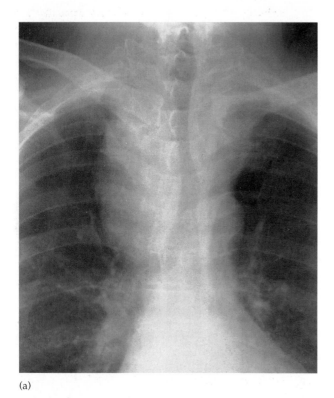

(a)

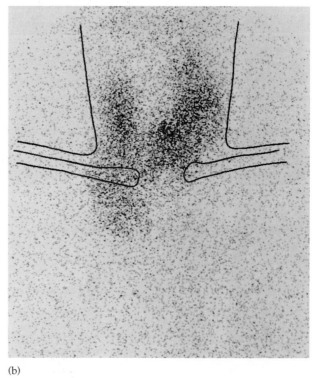

(b)

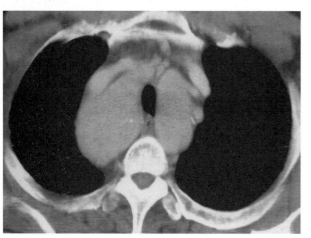

(c)

Fig. 2.61 Retrosternal goitre. (a) The plain chest film shows a large superior mediastinal mass narrowing the trachea. (b) A radionuclide scan in the same patient shows uptake of the ^{123}I below the level of the clavicles on the right, confirming that the mass is due to thyroid tissue. (c) CT scan, in another patient, showing a bilateral superior mediastinal mass that was shown on adjacent sections to be contiguous with the thyroid gland in the neck and to have the same density as thyroid tissue. Note the compression of the trachea.

Plain chest films in mediastinal masses

• Intrathoracic thyroid masses (goitres) are the most frequent cause of a superior mediastinal mass (Fig. 2.61). The characteristic feature is that the mass extends from the superior mediastinum into the neck and almost invariably compresses or displaces the trachea.

• Lymphadenopathy is the next most frequent cause of a mediastinal swelling. Lymphadenopathy may occur in any of the three compartments and it is often possible to diagnose enlarged lymph nodes from their lobulated outlines and the multiple locations involved (Fig. 2.62).

• Neurogenic tumours are by far the commonest causes of a posterior mediastinal mass. Pressure deformity of the adjacent ribs and thoracic spine is often visible.

• Certain tumours, such as dermoid cysts and thymomas, are, for practical purposes, confined to the anterior mediastinum.

• Calcification occurs in many conditions but almost never in malignant lymphadenopathy. Occasionally, the calcification is characteristic in appearance, e.g. in aneurysms of the aorta (Fig. 2.63).

• A mediastinal mass due to a hiatus hernia is usually easy to diagnose on plain films because it often contains air and may have a fluid level, best seen on the lateral view (Fig. 2.64). A film taken after a mouthful of barium has been swallowed will easily confirm or exclude the diagnosis of hiatus hernia.

• Masses in the right cardiophrenic angle anteriorly are virtually never of clinical significance. They are nearly all either large fat pads, benign pericardial cysts or hernias through the foramen of Morgagni (Fig. 2.65).

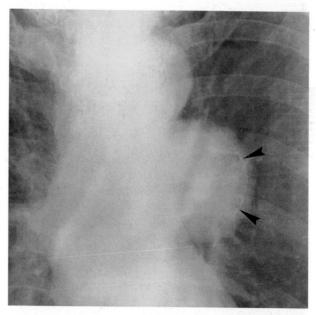

Fig. 2.63 Calcification in an aneurysm arising from the descending aorta. The arrows point to the distinctive curvilinear calcification within the mass, which is in intimate contact with the aorta.

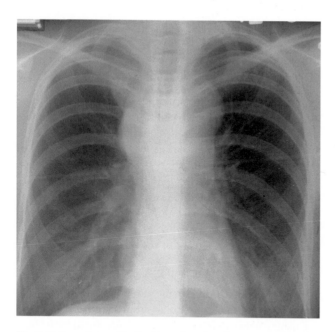

Fig. 2.62 Superior mediastinal lymph node enlargement. Note the bilateral lobular masses.

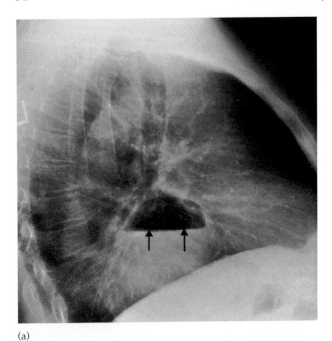

(a)

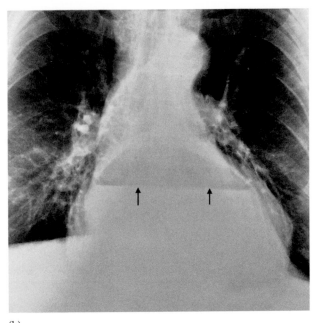

(b)

Fig. 2.64 Hiatus hernia. (a) Lateral and (b) PA chest films show the characteristic retrocardiac density containing an air–fluid level (arrows).

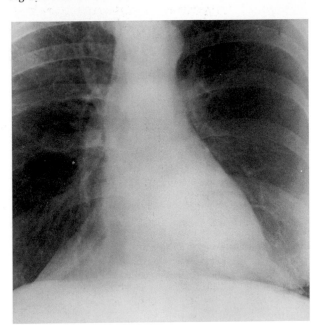

Fig. 2.65 Fat pads in both cardiophrenic angles. Note the loss of clarity of the adjacent cardiac outline – an example of the silhouette sign. The anterior location was confirmed on the lateral view.

Computed tomography of mediastinal masses

Computed tomography scanning is the best method of assessing mediastinal abnormalities when problems remain unanswered from the plain chest radiographs, because:

1 Abnormalities can be accurately localized. Knowledge of the precise shape, position and size of a mediastinal mass frequently narrows the differential diagnosis. For instance, contiguity of the mass with the thyroid in the neck suggests a goitre (Fig. 2.61), and multiple oval-shaped masses suggest lymphadenopathy (Fig. 2.66).

2 Occasionally, the density of the abnormality reveals its nature:

• Fat can be recognized as such. This is useful in distinguishing large cardiophrenic angle fat pads or unusual mediastinal fat collections from tumours, e.g. in Cushing's disease. Cystic teratomas (dermoid cysts) may contain recognizable fat (Fig. 2.67).

• Thyroid tissue has a characteristic density. Beause of its high iodine content, it is of higher attenuation than muscle prior to contrast medium administration. After contrast, it enhances brightly (Fig. 2.61c). (A radio-iodine scan is an alternative to CT for confirming that an intrathoracic mass is a goitre – see Fig. 2. 61.)

• Intravenous contrast enhancement permits ready differentiation of aneurysms (Fig. 2.68) and anomalous blood vessels from other masses.

• Calcification is more readily seen at CT than on plain radiographs. The presence of calcification in a mass excludes untreated malignant neoplastic adenopathy.

• Cysts containing clear fluid, e.g. pericardial cysts and some bronchogenic cysts can be recognized as such by a CT number close to water (0 Hounsfield units).

Magnetic resonance imaging of mediastinal masses

Magnetic resonance imaging gives similar information to CT regarding most mediastinal masses (Fig. 2.69). It is, therefore, rarely indicated. MRI does have certain specific advantages. For example, images can be obtained in any plane and aneurysms and vascular anomalies are readily

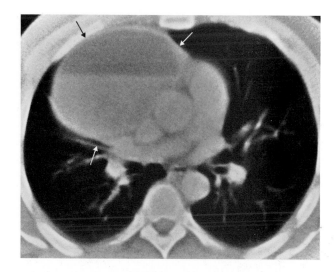

Fig. 2.67 Dermoid cyst (cystic teratoma) (arrows) shown by CT to contain fat. In this cyst the fat can be seen floating in the upper third of the cyst. Note that the density of part of the cyst is the same as subcutaneous fat.

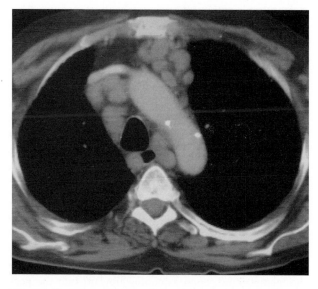

Fig. 2.66 Extensive mediastinal lymphadenopathy (caused by lymphoma) shown by CT scanning.

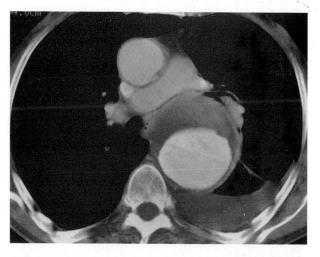

Fig. 2.68 Aneurysm of the descending aorta. The lumen has been opacified by intravenous contrast enhancement. The unopacified component is a blood clot lining the aneurysm.

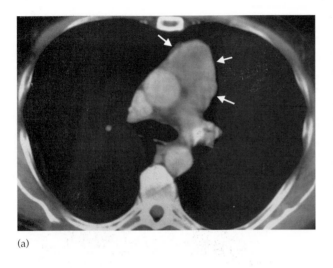

(a)

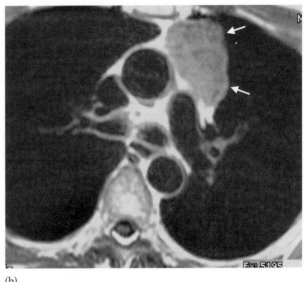

(b)

Fig. 2.69 Thymoma. (a) CT and (b) MRI (T1-weighted) show a lobular mass (arrows) in the left side of the thymus.

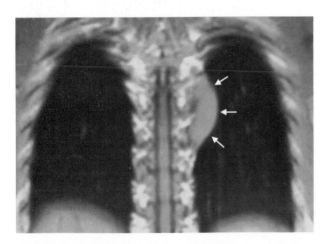

Fig. 2.70 Neurofibroma in posterior mediastinum. The MRI shows the neurofibroma (arrows) lying against the spine, but not growing into the spinal canal.

demonstrable without the need for contrast medium. Also, the relationship of a posterior mass to the spinal canal can be well seen (Fig. 2.70).

Pneumomediastinum

Provided that the air has not tracked into the mediastinum from the root of the neck, adjacent chest wall or retroperitoneum, air in the mediastinum indicates a tear in the oesophagus or an air leak from the bronchi. These tears may be spontaneous or follow trauma, including trauma from endoscopy or swallowed foreign bodies.

Spontaneous leakage from the bronchial tree is most commonly seen in patients with asthma, where the air tracks through the interstitial tissues of the lung into the mediastinum following rupture of a small airway.

The air is seen as fine streaks of transradiancy within the mediastinum, often extending upward into the neck (Fig. 2.71).

Hilar enlargement

The normal hilar shadows are composed of the pulmonary arteries and veins. The hilar lymph nodes cannot be identi-

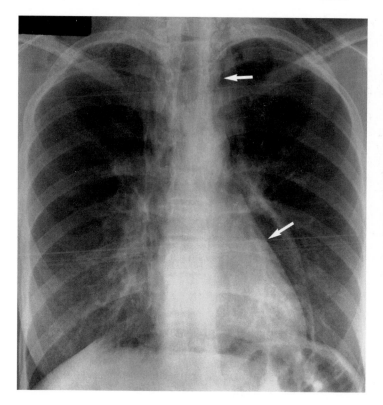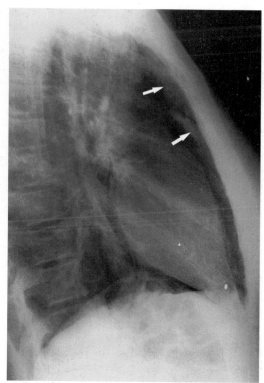

Fig. 2.71 Pneumomediastinum showing air in the mediastinum extending up into the neck.

fied as separate shadows. The walls of the central bronchi are too thin to contribute to any extent to the bulk of the hilar shadows. The main lower lobe arteries are the thickness of an adult's little finger (9–16 mm).

Hilar enlargement (Fig. 2.72) presents two main diagnostic problems. Firstly, is the enlarged hilum due entirely to large blood vessels or to a mass? Secondly, if a hilar mass is present, what is its nature?

It is usually possible to decide from plain films when hilar enlargement is due to enlargement of the pulmonary arteries because (i) both hila show a branching pattern and (ii) vascular enlargement is usually bilateral and accompanied by enlargement of the main pulmonary artery and heart (Fig. 2.73). (The causes of enlargement of the pulmonary artery are discussed on p. 117) On occasion, it is necessary to employ more sophisticated investigations to distinguish between enlarged blood vessels and a mass. The precise tech-

nique employed depends on the availability of specialized equipment. Computed tomography, particularly with the use of intravenous contrast medium, usually answers the question. Computed tomography also demonstrates the mediastinal structures; finding abnormalities within the mediastinum, such as lymphadenopathy, may clarify the nature of the hilar abnormality and may also give important information regarding the extent of disease.

Magnetic resonance imaging is the single best technique for elucidating hilar enlargement. It is rarely required because plain films and CT usually give the necessary information. Its advantage lies in the fact that there is very little signal from the hilar structures in normal individuals using the usual spin-echo sequences; there is no signal from fast-flowing blood in the major hilar vessels and none from the air within the bronchi. Thus, any hilar

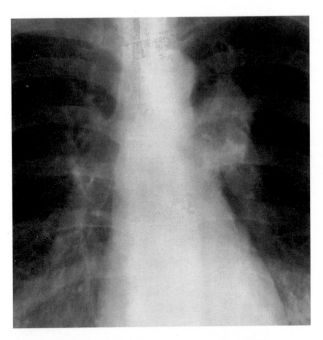

Fig. 2.72 Lobulated mass at left hilum from enlarged lymph nodes. The right hilum is normal. The lymphadenopathy in this case was due to metastases from a bronchial carcinoma in the left lower lobe.

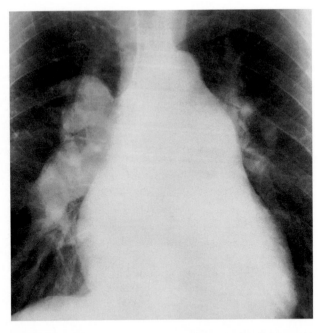

Fig. 2.73 Enlargement of the hilar arteries in a patient with severe pulmonary hypertension. Note that the heart and the main pulmonary artery are also enlarged and that the hilar shadows branch in the manner expected of arteries.

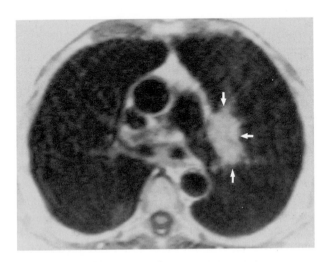

Fig. 2.74 MRI of pulmonary hila. There is a mass (metastatic carcinoma in lymph nodes) at the left hilum (arrows) which stands out clearly, because there is very little signal from normal hilar vessels. The right hilum is normal.

mass stands out clearly against the low signal background (Fig. 2.74).

Hilar masses are nearly always due to either lymph node enlargement or carcinoma of the bronchus.

Lymph node enlargement

Usually more than one lymph node is enlarged, so in patients with lymphadenopathy the hilum appears lobulated in outline (Fig. 2.75). The adjacent bronchi are normal or very slightly narrowed.

Unilateral enlargement of hilar lymph nodes may be due to the following.

• Metastases from carcinoma of the bronchus (Fig. 2.72), in which case the primary tumour is often visible; metastases from other primary sites are rare.

• Malignant lymphoma.

• Infections, particularly tuberculosis and histoplasmosis in endemic areas. Hilar adenopathy is occasionally seen

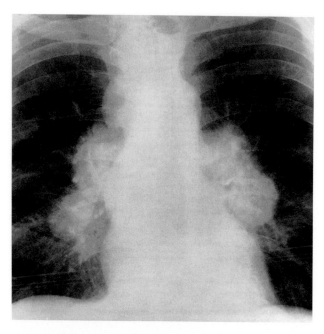

Fig. 2.75 Bilateral hilar adenopathy. The enlarged hila are clearly lobular in outline and there is also enlargement of the right paratracheal nodes (arrow). The diagnosis in this patient was malignant lymphoma.

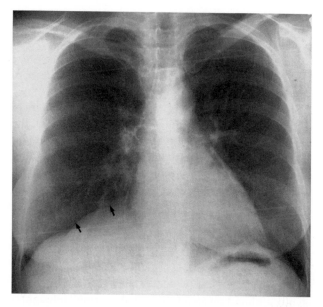

Fig. 2.76 Localized eventration of the diaphragm. There is a smooth localized elevation of the medial half of the right hemidiaphragm (arrows). On the lateral view the eventration involved the anterior half of the right hemidiaphragm.

accompanying acute bacterial infections. Tuberculosis is the commonest cause of unilateral hilar adenopathy in children.

Bilateral enlargement of hilar nodes occurs in:

• Sarcoidosis, which is far and away the commonest cause. The diagnosis is almost certain if the hilar enlargement is symmetrical and if the patient is asymptomatic, or has either erythema nodosum or iridocyclitis (see Fig. 2.87, p. 78). Simultaneous enlargement of the right paratracheal nodes is common. Lung changes are sometimes visible (see p. 77).

• Malignant lymphoma (Fig. 2.75).

• Tuberculosis. African and Asian races show this form of the disease in which substantial nodal enlargement can be a feature. It is rare to see bilateral hilar enlargement due to tuberculosis in Caucasians.

• Fungal diseases, which are rare causes of bilateral hilar enlargement.

Neoplasm

Primary carcinoma of the bronchus frequently presents as a hilar mass. If lobar collapse/consolidation or narrowing of the adjacent bronchus is visible, the diagnosis of carcinoma is virtually certain.

Diaphragm

The position of the diaphragm may reflect disease. Both domes may be pushed up by abdominal distension or they may be high as a result of lung disease. Unilateral elevation of a hemidiaphragm occurs with loss of volume of the ipsilateral lung or it may be due to abdominal pathology, such as an abdominal mass or a subphrenic abscess. In each of these situations, the cause of the elevated hemidiaphragm should be known or suspected from the clinical features or from chest or abdominal films. It should always be borne in mind that subpulmonary effusion may mimic elevation of one or both hemidiaphragms (see Fig. 2.44, p. 48). It is also important to realize that minor elevation of a hemi-diaphragm is a relatively common incidental finding of no significance.

Marked elevation of one hemidiaphragm with no other visible abnormality suggests either paralysis or eventration.

Paralysis of a hemidiaphragm. This results from disorders of the phrenic nerves, e.g. invasion by carcinoma of the bronchus. The signs are elevation of one hemidiaphragm (see Fig. 2.107, p. 92) which on fluoroscopy or ultrasound shows paradoxical movement, i.e. it moves upward on inspiration.

Eventration of the diaphragm. This is a congenital condition in which the diaphragm lacks muscle and becomes a thin membranous sheet. Except in the neonatal period it is almost always an incidental finding and does not cause symptoms. When the whole of one hemidiaphragm is involved, almost invariably the left, that hemidiaphragm is markedly elevated. On fluoroscopy or ultrasound, the hemidiaphragm may remain fixed during inspiration and expiration, but when more severely involved it moves para-doxically and cannot be distinguished from paralysis. The eventration may only involve part of one hemidiaphragm, resulting in a smooth 'hump' (Fig. 2.76).

Rupture of the diaphragm. This is discussed on p. 91.

The chest wall

The chest wall should be examined for evidence of soft tissue swelling or rib abnormality. Because ribs are curved structures, some portions will always be foreshortened on plain chest radiographs. Therefore, if a rib abnormality is suspected, oblique views should be obtained.

Soft tissue swelling occurs with a number of rib lesions: fractures, infections and neoplasms (Fig. 2.77). The soft tissue swelling may be more obvious than the rib lesion on a chest radiograph. If an opacity suggesting soft tissue swelling is seen arising from the chest wall, it is vital to obtain a good view of the underlying ribs using oblique views or CT where necessary.

Clearly, many diseases of bone such as Paget's disease, myeloma and metastases involve the ribs or sternum in much the same way as elsewhere in the skeleton.

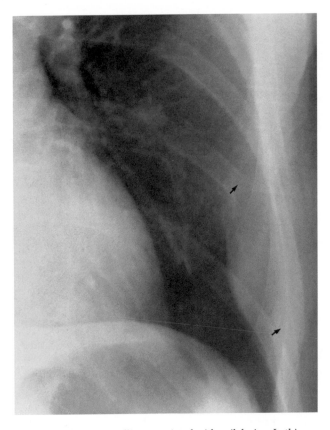

Fig. 2.77 Soft tissue swelling associated with a rib lesion. In this patient with myeloma in a rib, the soft tissue swelling is more obvious than the rib destruction. The bone between the two arrows has been destroyed. This important sign could be easily overlooked unless special attention is paid to identifying rib destruction in the region of soft tissue swelling.

Computed tomography, MRI and ultrasound can be very useful in elucidating chest wall disease, particularly chest wall invasion from an underlying carcinoma of the lung (see p. 94).

Congenital abnormalities of the ribs are common but rarely of clinical significance. It is important not to mistake bifid ribs or fused ribs for lung shadows on plain films.

Specific diseases

The remainder of this chapter is devoted to specific thoracic disorders.

Bacterial pneumonia (see also Pulmonary Tuberculosis, p. 72)

The common feature of all pneumonias is a cellular exudate within the alveoli. The damage to the pulmonary parenchyma varies. With pneumococcal pneumonia, for example, complete resolution usually occurs, whereas with certain other infections, notably staphylococci, klebsiella, anaerobic bacteria and tuberculosis, lung destruction with cavitation is common.

The major purpose of chest radiographs in patients with suspected chest infection is to establish whether or not pneumonia is present. Diagnosing the infective agent on radiological grounds is rarely possible, since there is considerable overlap in the appearance of various bacterial pneumonias and there is even overlap in the appearance of bacterial, fungal and viral pneumonias.

The basic radiological features of pneumonia are one or more areas of consolidation. Cavitation may occur within the consolidated area. Consolidation may be accompanied by loss of volume of the affected lobe, a feature that is particularly common in children.

Pneumonia may be secondary to obstruction of a major bronchus, carcinoma being a common cause of obstruction. Bronchial obstruction should always be considered in any patient presenting with consolidation of one lobe or of two lobes supplied by a common bronchus (e.g. the right middle and lower lobes), particularly if there is associated loss of volume.

The appearance of consolidation varies from a small ill-defined shadow to a large shadow involving the whole of one or more lobes (lobar pneumonia) (see Fig. 2.16, p. 31), the pattern depends on the infecting organism and the integrity of host defences. The common infecting organism in community acquired lobar pneumonia is *Streptococcus pneumoniae*. In pneumococcal pneumonia there is dense consolidation of one lobe, usually without loss of volume. There may be an associated pleural effusion.

When the consolidation is patchy, involving one or more lobes, it is commonly referred to as bronchopneumonia (Fig. 2.78). The most frequent causes of community-acquired bronchopneumonia are *Staphylococcus aureus*, various Gram-negative and anaerobic bacteria, and *Mycoplasma pneumoniae*.

The differentiation between pneumonia and pulmonary

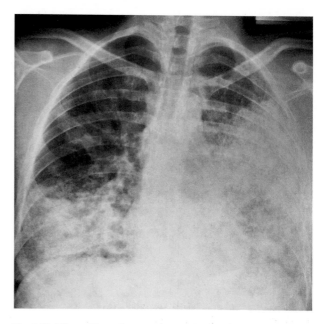

Fig. 2.78 Bilateral bronchopneumonia. There is widespread bilateral patchy consolidation.

oedema or pulmonary infarction may, at times, be difficult or impossible radiographically. The clinical features usually decide the issue.

Viral and mycoplasma pneumonia

Viral pneumonia and pneumonia due to *Mycoplasma pneumoniae* may produce widespread ill-defined consolidation (Fig. 2.79) and loss of clarity of the vascular markings, which on occasion may resemble pulmonary oedema. Alternatively, only a localized area of consolidation may be seen. Pleural effusions are rare. The radiological abnormality may persist for many weeks after clinical recovery.

Lung abscess

A lung abscess is a localized suppurative lesion of the lung parenchyma.

The most frequent causes are:
• aspiration of food or secretions; such abscesses are

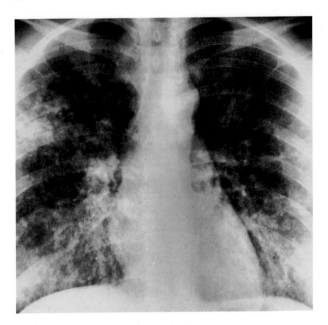

Fig. 2.79 Mycoplasma pneumonia, showing widespread ill-defined consolidation in both lungs.

usually in the apical (superior) segments of the lower lobes or in the posterior segments of the upper lobes;
• infection beyond an obstructing lesion in the bronchus;
• infected emboli, particularly in drug addicts.

A lung abscess is usually seen as a spherical shadow containing a central lucency due to air within the cavity. An air–fluid level may be present. It can be difficult or impossible to distinguish an infective lung abscess from a cavitating lung neoplasm or cavitation in Wegener's granulomatosis.

Pulmonary tuberculosis

Pulmonary tuberculosis is usually divided into primary and postprimary forms even though these divisions are not clear cut. Primary tuberculosis is the result of the first infection with *Mycobacterium tuberculosis* and usually occurs in childhood. Postprimary tuberculosis, the usual form in adults, is believed to be re-infection, the patient having developed relative immunity following the primary infection. Tuberculosis (and atypical mycobacterial infections)

are being seen with considerable frequency in patients with AIDS.

Primary tuberculosis

In primary tuberculosis an area of consolidation, known as the Ghon focus, develops in the periphery of the lung – usually in the mid or upper zones. Usually, the pulmonary shadow is small, but it may occasionally in-volve most of the lobe. Sometimes the pulmonary consolidation is so small that it is nearly invisible. The consolidation is often accompanied by visibly enlarged hilar or mediastinal lymph nodes (Fig. 2.80a). This combination of pulmonary consolidation and lymphadenopathy is known as the *primary complex*. The clinical features of the primary complex vary. The majority of patients have few symptoms and the disease is usually not recognized. The remainder have fever, cough and malaise.

In most cases, whether treated or not, the primary complex heals and often calcifies. A calcified primary complex often remains visible throughout life.

Spread of infection. Spread of infection may occur:
• via the bronchial tree, leading to tuberculous broncho-pneumonia, which appears radiologically as patchy or lobar consolidation; it often involves more than one lobe, may be bilateral and frequently cavitates;
• via the blood stream, resulting in *miliary tuberculosis* (Fig. 2.80b) in which there are innumerable small nodules in the lungs, all much the same size and fairly evenly distributed; usually, the nodules are well defined but in severe cases they become relatively confluent so that the individual nodules are difficult to appreciate; the primary tuberculous focus may be visible and a pleural effusion may be present; it is important to note that early in the course of the illness the chest film may be normal.

Primary tuberculosis may present with a pleural effusion. Occasionally the primary complex is also visible, but more often the effusion is the only visible abnormality.

Postprimary tuberculosis

Postprimary tuberculosis usually presents with cough, haemoptysis, weight loss, night sweats or malaise. Occasionally, the disease is discovered on a routine chest

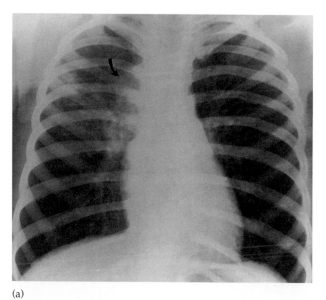

(a)

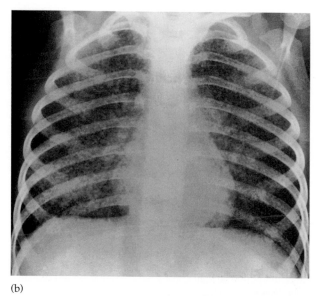

(b)

Fig. 2.80 Tuberculosis. (a) The primary complex. This 7-year-old child shows ill-defined consolidation in the right lung together with enlargement of the draining lymph nodes (arrow). (b) Miliary tuberculosis. The innumerable small nodular shadows uniformly distributed throughout the lungs in this young child are typical of miliary tuberculosis. In this instance, no primary focus of infection is visible.

film. Postprimary tuberculosis is usually confined to the upper posterior portions of the chest, namely the apical and posterior segments of the upper lobes and the apical segments of the lower lobes. The initial lesions are multiple small areas of consolidation (Fig. 2.81a) and are often bilateral. Occasionally, the disease takes the form of lower or middle lobe bronchopneumonia. If the infection progresses the consolidations enlarge and frequently cavitate. Cavities are seen as rounded air spaces (translucencies) completely surrounded by pulmonary shadowing (Fig. 2.81b). The diagnosis of cavitation can be difficult and may require tomography.

The infection may undergo partial or complete healing at any stage. Healing occurs by fibrosis, often with calcification (Fig. 2.82), but both fibrosis and calcification may be seen in the presence of continuing activity.

The predominant or sole feature, particularly in non-Caucasians, may be mediastinal and/or hilar lymphadenopathy. It is not clear whether these cases are primary or postprimary tuberculosis (Fig. 2.83).

As with the primary form, postprimary tuberculosis may spread to give widespread bronchopneumonia or miliary tuberculosis.

Pleural effusions are frequent. They often leave permanent pleural thickening which may calcify.

Tuberculoma. The term tuberculoma refers to a tuberculous granuloma in the form of a spherical mass, usually less than 3 cm in diameter. The edge is usually sharply defined and these lesions are often partly calcified. Conventional or computed tomography may be needed to demonstrate the calcification. Most tuberculomas are inactive but viable tubercle bacilli may be present even in the calcified lesions.

Mycetoma (Fig. 2.84). The fungus *Aspergillus fumigatus* may colonize old tuberculous cavities to produce a ball of fungus (mycetoma) lying free within the cavity. Air is seen between the mycetoma and the wall of the cavity. Cavities containing mycetomas are usually surrounded by other evidence of old tuberculous infection, particularly fibrosis and calcification

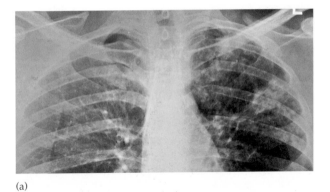

(a)

Fig. 2.81 Postprimary tuberculosis. (a) There are ill-defined consolidations scattered in both upper lobes; their size and distribution should suggest the diagnosis of postprimary tuberculosis. (b) The right upper lobe is consolidated and contains a large central cavity. Patchy consolidation from tuberculous bronchopneumonia is seen in the right mid and lower zones and in the left upper zone.

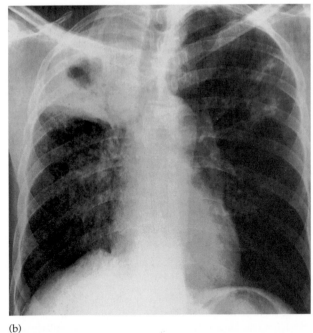

(b)

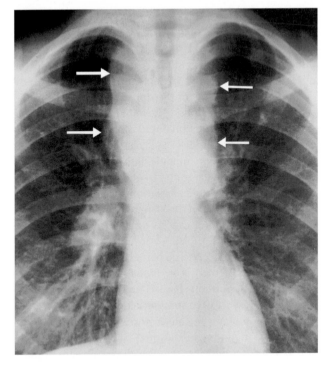

Fig. 2.82 Old calcified tuberculous disease. There are numerous foci of calcification in both lungs. The right upper lobe shows extensive fibrosis and bullae. There was no evidence in this patient that active infection was present. However, given this film in isolation, active disease could not be excluded.

Fig. 2.83 Mediastinal lymphadenopathy (arrows) caused by tuberculosis.

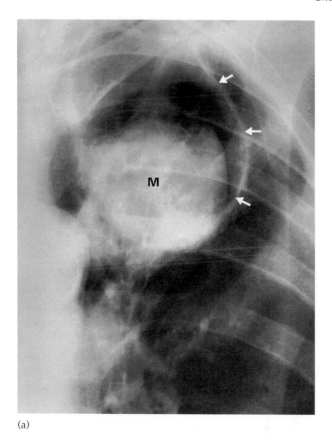

(a)

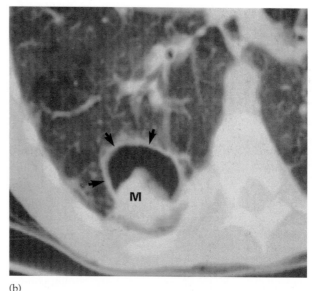

(b)

Fig. 2.84 Mycetoma (M) in pre-existing, old tuberculous cavity, the wall of which is arrowed. (a) Plain film. The fungus ball moved around the cavity when the patient was placed on his side. (b) CT scan of a different patient showing a mycetoma in a pre-existing old tuberculous cavity.

of the adjacent lung. CT often allows a specific diagnosis of mycetoma to be made.

Is the disease active? An important role for radiology in patients with pulmonary tuberculosis is to try and determine whether the disease is active or inactive. This can be very difficult and is sometimes impossible. It is important to realize that there is no way of excluding activity unless serial films over a prolonged period are available. Valuable diagnostic signs of activity are:

• development of new lesions on serial films;
• demonstration of cavities.

Lack of change over a period of years is useful evidence against activity, but the change in serial chest films may be subtle, even with active disease. Remember also that the presence of calcification does not exclude activity.

Many routine chest films in asymptomatic patients show evidence of tuberculosis. In a few, the diagnosis of active disease will be readily apparent by the presence of cavities or by comparison with previous films. In the remainder it can be a considerable problem to decide which patients to investigate further and which to accept as having old inactive infection. The better defined the shadows and the greater the calcification, the less the likelihood of activity. The presence of ill-defined shadows, even if partially calcified, is suggestive of active disease. However, the decision is often largely based on the clinical findings and the results of sputum examination for tubercle bacilli.

Fungal and parasitic diseases

When fungi are inhaled they may produce lung infection. The radiological appearances vary with the particular fungus, but two broad divisions can be made:

• Infection of the otherwise normal patient with histoplasmosis, coccidioidomycosis and blastomycosis (Fig. 2.85). These organisms, which are found chiefly on the continent of North America, produce lesions in the lung that are very similar and often identical to tuberculosis. Cavitation is a particular feature. Healing by fibrosis and calcification is frequent.

• Infection in the immunocompromised host. With impaired immunity, fungi such as *Candida albicans* and *Aspergillus fumigatus* as well as several of the fungi native to North America, may cause widespread pneumonia. It is not possible to predict the infecting organism from the chest film. Indeed, it is usually not possible to distinguish fungal infection from infection with bacteria, viruses and parasites.

Aspergillus fumigatus. This fungus affects the lung in three ways: it may colonize a pre-existing cavity forming a fungus ball or mycetoma (Fig. 2.84); it may infect the lung in an immunocompromised patient causing a severe pneumonia (see below), or it may be responsible for allergic bronchopulmonary aspergillosis, a condition discussed on p. 83.

Hydatid disease

Pulmonary infection with *Echinococcus granulosus* may result in cysts in the lung or pleural cavity. These cysts may be solitary or multiple and are seen as spherical shadows with very well-defined borders. Hydatid cysts occasionally rupture to produce complex cavities.

Pneumonia in the immunocompromised host

Patients who are immunocompromised are not only more susceptible to pulmonary infection, often with unusual organisms, but the pattern of the resulting pneumonia frequently shows an atypical radiographic appearance. Pneumonia in these patients may be due to the usual pathogens, but often it is due to opportunistic fungi, tuberculosis or *Pneumocystis carinii*. *Pneumocystis carinii* pneumonia is a particular scourge in patients with AIDS.

Pneumonia in immunocompresed patients usually causes widespread non-specific pulmonary shadowing. It may not

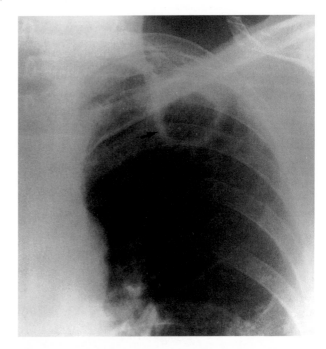

Fig. 2.85 Fungus infection. The cavity (arrow) in this patient from southeast USA was due to North American blastomycosis. Note the similarity to tuberculosis. Other fungi, e.g. histoplasmosis, can give an identical appearance.

even be possible to say whether the shadowing is due to infection or to such conditions as pulmonary oedema or pulmonary haemorrhage, or neoplastic disease.

The predilection of people with AIDS to develop *Pneumocystis carinii* pneumonia means that widespread, uniformly distributed pulmonary shadowing in a patient with AIDS is usually due to this organism (Fig. 2.86), though AIDS patients are also prone to tuberculous infection and the development of extensive Kaposi's sarcoma, both of which can appear similar to *Pneumocystis carinii* pneumonia on plain chest radiography.

Sarcoidosis

Sarcoidosis is characterized pathologically by non-caseating granulomas in many organs including lung, liver, spleen, lymph nodes, skin and bone. The aetiology is unknown and the diagnosis depends on a correlation of the clinical, pathological and radiological manifestations.

The radiological manifestations are largely confined to the chest. The features on plain chest radiograph and CT are:

• Hilar and paratracheal lymphadenopathy. When hilar lymphadenopathy is present it is almost invariably bilateral and usually symmetrical (Fig. 2.87). Mediastinal adenopathy is common and the nodes are large enough to be visible on a plain chest radiograph in about half the patients. The mediastinal lymphadenopathy is most readily recognized in the right paratracheal region. On chest CT, the widespread distribution of the lymphadenopathy is apparent. Unlike lymphoma, the lymph node enlargement is never predominant in the anterior mediastinum.

• Reticulonodular shadowing in the lungs. The pattern varies from uniform small nodular shadows, which may clear on steroid therapy, to coarse reticular shadows maximal in the mid and upper zones, which represent gross pulmonary fibrosis (Fig. 2.88). At this stage the pulmonary disease is often irreversible.

The majority of patients with sarcoidosis of the chest have lymphadenopathy only, which clears without treatment and does not progress to pulmonary involvement. Such patients usually do not have chest symptoms, though they may show non-caseating granulomas on transbronchial biopsy. Some present with iridocyclitis, some with erythema nodosum and fever. A few have, in addition, polyarthritis. Many are discovered on routine chest x-ray and have no symptoms or signs.

Approximately 10% of patients develop lung involvement; some have visibly enlarged lymph nodes at this stage. Often the lymph nodes get smaller and may return to normal, even though the lung changes persist.

Computed tomography, which can demonstrate the hilar/mediastinal adenopathy and the lung shadowing to advantage, does not provide useful extra information and is rarely indicated in sarcoidosis.

Diffuse pulmonary fibrosis

The known causes of diffuse pulmonary fibrosis include: extrinsic allergic alveolitis, collagen vascular diseases (including rheumatoid arthritis), drug-induced fibrosis, pneumoconiosis and sarcoidosis, but a substantial pro-

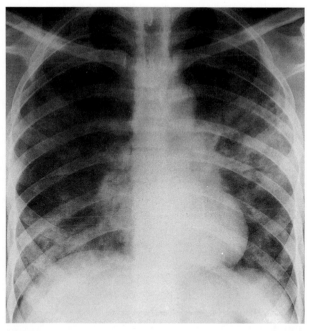

(a)

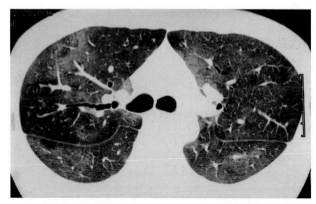

(b)

Fig. 2.86 *Pneumocystis carinii* pneumonia in a patient with AIDS showing (a) typical widespread low-density air space shadowing on chest x-ray; (b) High resolution CT in another patient with similar but less advanced changes.

portion of cases are idiopathic in origin. A variety of names is given to the idiopathic form: idiopathic pulmonary fibrosis, cryptogenic fibrosing alveolitis and usual interstitial pneumonia (UIP).

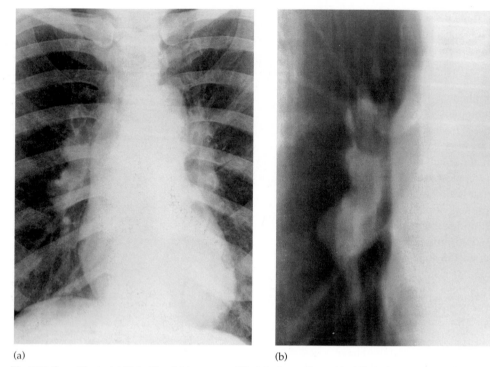

(a)   (b)

Fig. 2.87 Sarcoidosis. (a) Plain film; (b) tomogram. The lobular outline to the hila is characteristic of lymph node enlargement. In this case the paratracheal nodes are not visibly enlarged. This patient had no symptoms or signs, the abnormality being discovered on a routine chest film.

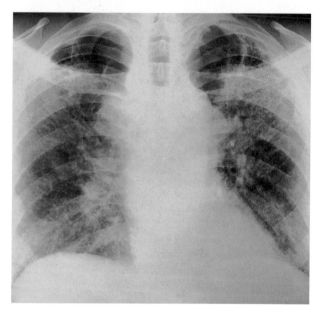

Idiopathic pulmonary fibrosis (cryptogenic fibrosing alveolitis)

In cryptogenic fibrosing alveolitis there is thickening of the alveolar walls with fibrosis and desquamation. The early stage is sometimes known as desquamative interstitial pneumonitis (DIP). As the disease progresses, the alveolar walls break down and rounded air spaces develop. At this stage the appearances are known by the descriptive term 'honeycomb lung'. Fibrosing alveolitis causes a restrictive ventilation defect with severe reduction in gas transfer across the alveolar walls.

The radiological features are:

Fig. 2.88 Late fibrotic stage of sarcoidosis. The dense reticulonodular shadowing radiates outwards from the hila, maximally in the mid and upper zones. Enlarged lymph nodes are still visible at the hila and in the right paratracheal region. Many patients with this degree of pulmonary fibrosis from sarcoidosis will not have visibly enlarged lymph nodes.

• Hazy shadowing at the lung bases leading to a lack of clarity of the vessel outlines known as 'ground-glass shadowing'. Later, ill-defined nodules with connecting lines become discernible.

• Decreased lung volume, often marked, and circular translucencies are seen producing the pattern known as 'honeycomb lung' (Fig. 2.89). Eventually, the heart and pulmonary arteries enlarge from increasingly severe pulmonary hypertension.

These signs are seen on both plain chest radiographs and high resolution CT. HRCT is more sensitive for detecting the changes and demonstrates the distribution and severity of disease to advantage (Fig. 2.89b). Ground-glass shadowing is particularly well seen with HRCT.

Determining the cause of diffuse pulmonary fibrosis

The distribution of the pulmonary shadowing may give a clue to its aetiology. In idiopathic pulmonary fibrosis, the lung shadowing is often maximal at the bases and at the lung periphery, although it may be fairly uniformly distributed in advanced cases (Fig. 2.89). Scleroderma and rheumatoid arthritis give an identical picture.

The combination of pulmonary fibrosis with certain other signs may lead to a specific diagnosis:

• substantial past or present hilar/mediastinal adenopathy suggests sarcoidosis (Fig. 2.88);

• coexistent conglomerate masses in the mid and upper zones are virtually diagnostic of silicosis or coal miners' pneumoconiosis (Fig. 2.93, p. 82);

• coexistent bilateral pleural thickening and calcification are diagnostic of asbestosis (Fig. 2.90);

• past or present pleural effusions are highly suggestive of rheumatoid arthritis.

Radiation pneumonitis (Fig. 2.91)

Radiation pneumonitis may occur following x-ray therapy for intrathoracic neoplasms and breast carcinoma. The response of the lung to radiation varies from patient to patient. Initially, there is no radiological change, but within a few weeks ill-defined small shadows, indistinguishable from infective consolidation, are seen in the radiation field. If the inflammatory change goes on to fibrosis, there is dense coarse shadowing that may be sharply demarcated

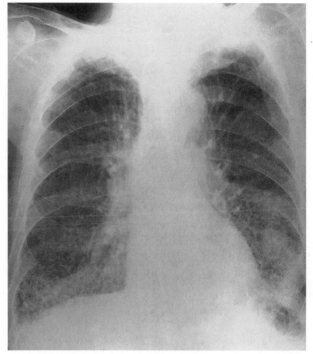

(a)

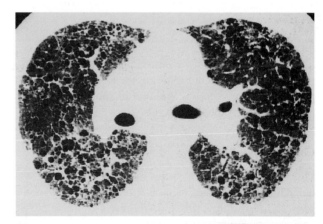

(b)

Fig. 2.89 Idiopathic (cryptogenic) fibrosing alveolitis. (a) In this example there is reticulonodular shadowing (honeycomb lung) with basal predominance. Scleroderma gives a similar picture. Notice that the diaphragm is indistinct because of the changes in the adjacent lungs. (b) High resolution CT scan of a different patient showing the honeycomb pattern in the lungs.

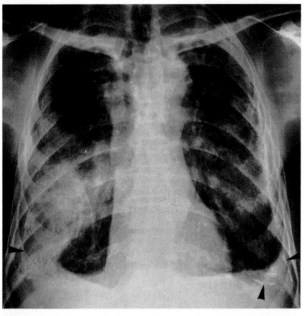

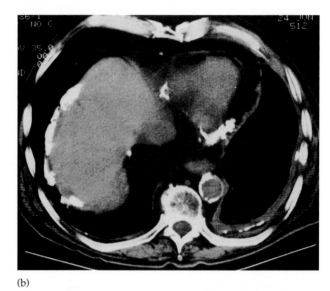

(b)

(a)

Fig. 2.90 Asbestos-related pleural disease. (a) There is extensive bilateral pleural thickening and pleural calcification (arrows) best appreciated along the lateral chest wall. (b) CT scan showing numerous calcified pleural plaques, predominantly over the right hemidiaphragm, but also along the left posterolateral chest wall.

from the normal lung in a geometric fashion, conforming to the field of radiation but ignoring the lobar boundaries of the lung. There is loss of volume of the fibrosed areas. Extensive pleural thickening is also sometimes seen.

Collagen vascular diseases

This group of diseases includes rheumatoid arthritis, systemic lupus erythematosus, polyarteritis nodosa, systemic sclerosis, dermatomyositis and Wegener's granulomatosis. Various radiological signs occur.

Rheumatoid lung

The most common finding in the chest is pleural effusion. Pulmonary fibrosis, often indistinguishable from that seen in cryptogenic fibrosing alveolitis, is another important finding.

An interesting feature of pulmonary involvement in rheumatoid arthritis is the development of rounded granulomas in the periphery of the lung, histologically similar to the subcutaneous nodules seen in this disease. These spherical nodules, which may be single or multiple, rarely exceed 3 cm in size. Eventually, many cavitate and resolve.

Systemic lupus erythematosus

The chest radiograph is usually normal. The commonest abnormalities are pleural effusion and cardiac enlargement due to pericardial effusion. Patchy consolidation in the lungs is occasionally seen.

Scleroderma and dermatomyositis

The cardinal feature is basal reticulonodular shadows from

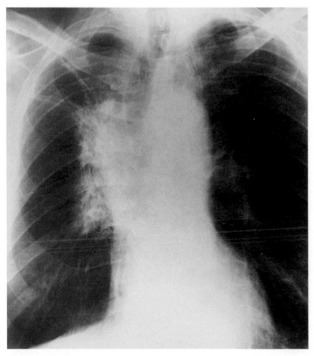

(a)

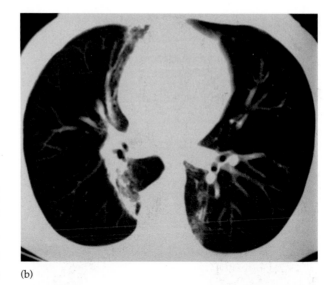

(b)

Fig. 2.91 Postradiation fibrosis. (a) The patient had a carcinoma in the right upper lobe centrally, for which he had received radiation therapy. Notice the geometric outline to the shadowing corresponding to the radiation field. There has been contraction of the irradiated lung resulting in mediastinal deviation and distortion of the pulmonary vessels. (b) Computed tomography scan in a patient treated for lymphoma. Note the linear fibrosis (arrows) in the lungs on either side of the mediastinum.

pulmonary fibrosis, similar to that seen in cryptogenic fibrosing alveolitis. Pleural effusion is rare.

Polyarteritis nodosa

Patchy consolidations, which may be fleeting and repetitive, and pleural effusions are occasionally seen in patients with polyarteritis nodosa.

Wegener's granulomatosis

The lungs may show one or more well-defined consolidations or masses, usually in the mid zones, which may cavitate. These lesions are often difficult to distinguish from bronchogenic carcinoma, when single, or metastases, when multiple, on radiographic grounds alone.

Pneumoconiosis

The pneumoconioses include a group of conditions caused by the inhalation of a variety of dusts.

Coal workers' pneumoconiosis

Simple pneumoconiosis is due to dust retention in the lungs with minor fibrosis. It is recognized radiologically by many small nodules, initially in the mid and upper zones, eventually involving the whole of the lung fields (Fig. 2.92).

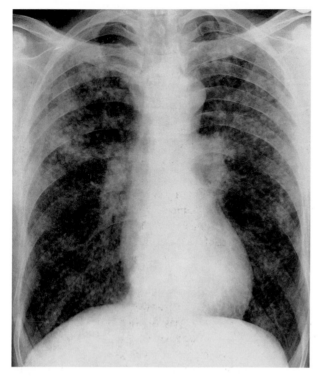

Fig. 2.92 Pneumoconiosis. There are many small nodules involving the whole of the lung fields. The patient was a coal miner.

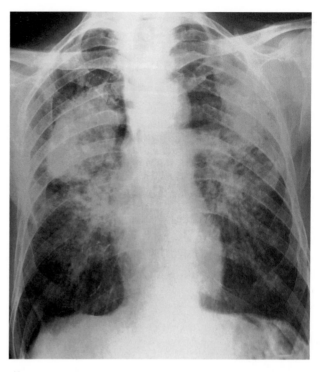

Fig. 2.93 Progressive massive fibrosis (PMF). Note the large oval shadows in the upper halves of both lungs. A nodular pattern is present elsewhere in the lung fields.

Simple pneumoconiosis does not give rise to symptoms and the diagnosis is made on the basis of the chest x-ray appearances.

For reasons that are not entirely clear, progressive massive fibrosis (PMF) may supervene. It causes homogeneous shadows, which are often ovoid in shape, in the upper halves of the lungs. The shadows may be unilateral or bilateral and there is usually nodular shadowing in the rest of the lungs (Fig. 2.93). Progressive massive fibrosis may be associated with breathlessness and it may result in cor pulmonale.

Asbestos-related disease

Inhalation of asbestos fibres may lead to:

1 *Pleural fibrosis and calcification.* Localized plaques of pleural thickening, some of which are calcified, are seen along the lateral chest wall and diaphragm (Fig. 2.90). The plaques in themselves are harmless, but they are a useful pointer to previous asbestos exposure.

The differential diagnosis from post-inflammatory and post-traumatic pleural thickening and calcification is made by noting the extent of the pleural disease: usually, it is bilateral in asbestos-related pleural disease whereas it is frequently unilateral in the other conditions. If the costophrenic angles are sharp, healed inflammatory disease or old haemothorax is very unlikely, whereas in asbestos-related pleural disease the costophrenic angles may be clear.

2 *Pulmonary fibrosis.* Unlike the pleural plaques, which may be seen following minor exposure to asbestos, pulmonary fibrosis only follows significant exposure. Pulmonary fibrosis in asbestosis is symmetrically bilateral and maximal at the bases, similar to cryptogenic fibrosing alveolitis.

3 *The development of malignant neoplasms.* Malignant mesothelioma (see Fig. 2.51, p. 54) and bronchial carcinoma are both seen with far higher frequency in asbestos-exposed patients than in the general population.

Diseases of the airways

Asthma

The chest film in asthma is usually normal or shows only a low flat diaphragm due to air trapping. Bronchial wall thickening may be seen. The main purpose of the chest x-ray in asthma is:

• to determine complications, e.g. atelectasis;
• to detect associated pneumonia;
• to exclude other causes of acute dyspnoea, e.g. pulmonary oedema, pneumothorax or, rarely, tracheal obstruction.

A chest x-ray should only be undertaken when one or more of the above is a realistic possibility.

Allergic bronchopulmonary aspergillosis results from hypersensitivity to *Aspergillus fumigatus*. Asthma is the cardinal clinical feature of this disease. The radiological signs are allergic consolidations in the lung and bronchiectasis, particularly in the mid and upper zones. The thickened walls of the dilated bronchi may be visible on a plain chest film.

Bronchiolitis

Severe bronchiolitis in young children, even when life-threatening, may show surprisingly little change on the chest film. The major sign is overinflation of the lungs leading to a low position of the diaphragm. Some children show widespread small ill-defined areas of consolidation, but in many the lungs are clear.

Acute bronchitis

Acute bronchitis in adults and older children does not produce any radiological abnormality unless complicated by pneumonia.

Chronic obstructive airway disease

Chronic obstructive airway disease is an imprecise but convenient term which includes several common diseases, including chronic bronchitis and emphysema, and bronchiectasis.

Chronic bronchitis and emphysema. Chronic bronchitis is a clinical diagnosis based on productive cough for at least three consecutive months in two successive years. Pathologically, there is hypertrophy of the mucous glands throughout the bronchial tree with a great increase in the number of goblet cells. Bronchopneumonia is a common complication.

Emphysema is defined pathologically as an increase beyond normal size of air spaces distal to the terminal bronchiole with destructive changes in their walls. Chronic bronchitis and emphysema often coexist though pure forms of each are seen.

The chest film in uncomplicated chronic bronchitis is normal. Indeed, patients may die from respiratory failure from chronic bronchitis and have a normal chest film. If the film is abnormal, a complication such as emphysema, pneumonia or cor pulmonale has occurred, and the radiological features are then those of the complication in question.

The signs of *emphysema* are (Fig. 2.94):

• Increased lung volume. The lungs increase in volume because of the combined effect of airways obstruction on abnormally compliant lungs. The diaphragm is pushed down and becomes low and flat. The heart is elongated and narrowed. The ribs are widely spaced and more lung lies in front of the heart and mediastinum. (Overinflation of the lungs can be said to be present if the hemidiaphragms at their midpoint are below the seventh rib anteriorly or the twelfth rib posteriorly.)

• Attenuation of the vessels. The reduction in size and number of the blood vessels can be generalized or localized. If severe, the involved area is called a bulla. The edge of a bulla may be indistinct or may be quite sharply limited by a line shadow. In some cases the normal lung adjacent to the bulla is compressed and appears opaque.

Bronchiectasis. Bronchiectasis is defined as irreversible dilatation of the bronchi often accompanied by impairment of drainage of bronchial secretions leading to persistent infection.

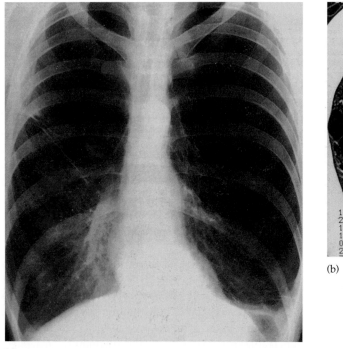

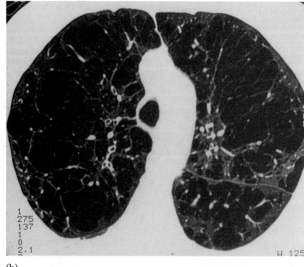

(b)

(a)

Fig. 2.94 Panacinar emphysema. (a) The diaphragm is low and flat and the ribs are widely spaced, indicating overinflation of the lungs. The peripheral vessels in most of the left lung and the upper half of the right lung are small and attenuated, indicating lung destruction. (b) CT scan showing innumerable bullae.

The conditions which cause bronchiectasis include pulmonary infection in childhood, cystic fibrosis and longstanding bronchial obstruction.

The radiological features are (Fig. 2.95):
• Visibly dilated bronchi. If these contain air, the thickened walls of the dilated bronchi may be seen as tubular or ring shadows. If filled with fluid, the dilated bronchi are either opaque or contain air-fluid levels. Since these fluid levels are very short they have to be looked for very carefully.
• Persistent consolidation, often containing dilated bronchi.
• Loss of volume of the affected lobe or lobes is almost invariable.

A proportion of patients with symptomatic bronchiectasis have normal plain chest films.

Computed tomography has now replaced bronchography as the method of determining the presence of bronchiecta-

sis, where this is in doubt, and the extent of disease. High resolution computed tomography (HRCT) is employed in order to obtain high resolution images (Fig. 2.96).

Cystic fibrosis

Cystic fibrosis is an inherited disorder of exocrine glands resulting in secretion of viscid mucus. In cystic fibrosis the small airways become blocked and secondary infections supervene. The finding of a high sodium chloride concentration in the sweat is diagnostic of the condition.

The radiological findings are (Fig. 2.97):
• Small ill-defined consolidations, maximal in the upper zones, some of which show cavitation.
• Bronchial wall thickening and the signs of bronchiectasis; both usually maximal in the upper zones.
• Evidence of airway obstruction. The diaphragm is

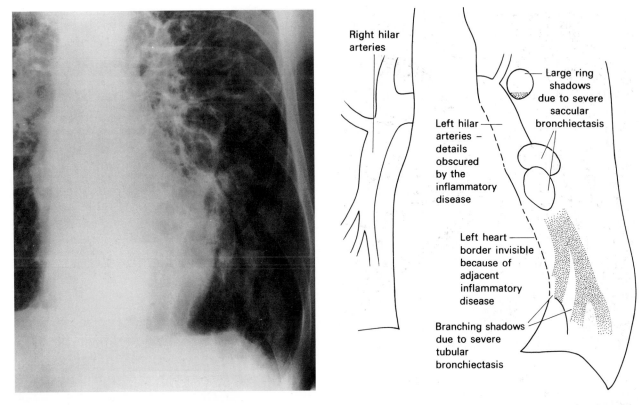

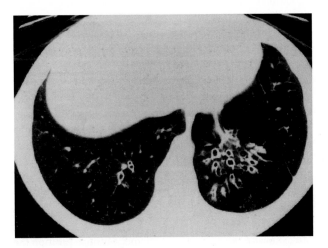

Fig. 2.95 Bronchiectasis. Plain film showing a mixture of saccular and tubular bronchiectasis. The branching ectatic bronchi resemble large blood vessels but should not be confused with them.

low and flat and the heart is narrow and vertical, until cor pulmonale develops when cardiac enlargement may occur.

Respiratory distress in the newborn

There are many causes of respiratory distress in the first few days of life. Abnormalities are visible on the chest x-ray in the majority; only two conditions are discussed here.

Hyaline membrane disease. This is one of the commonest abnormalities. It is a disease of the premature infant and is due to deficiency of surfactant in the lungs. Consequently the alveoli collapse, so preventing gas exchange. The chest radiographic appearance is one of the most important criteria in making the diagnosis.

The basic signs are widespread very small pulmonary

Fig. 2.96 Bronchiectasis. Thin-section high resolution CT scan showing thick walled, dilated bronchi crowded together in the left lower lobe. The normal appearance is seen in the right lower lobe.

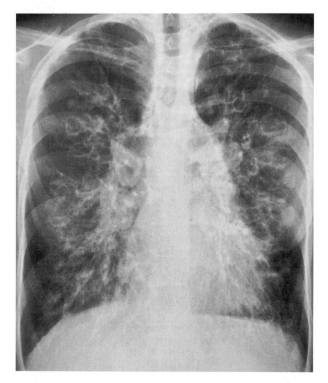

Fig. 2.97 Cystic fibrosis in a 14-year-old child. There is bronchial wall thickening, ring shadows of bronchiectasis and widespread ill-defined shadowing. All these phenomena tend to be maximal in the mid and upper zones. The diaphragm is somewhat low from obstructive airways disease.

opacities and visible air bronchograms (Fig. 2.98). The air bronchograms are visible because the bronchi are surrounded by airless alveoli. The changes are nearly always uniform in distribution. In the milder forms, the nodules are small and the air bronchograms may be the most obvious and easily recognized sign. In the more severe forms, the pulmonary opacities become more obvious and may be confluent; the lungs then appear almost opaque, except for air bronchograms.

Meconium aspiration (Fig. 2.99). In meconium aspiration the pulmonary shadowing is usually patchy and distinctly streaky. Air bronchograms are not an obvious feature. In meconium aspiration the diaphragm is often lower than

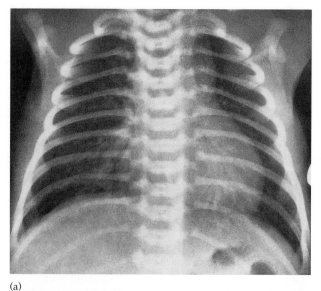

(a)

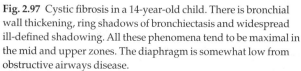

(b)

Fig. 2.98 The neonatal respiratory distress syndrome (hyaline membrane disease). (a) Normal premature neonatal chest film for comparison. (b) This film shows the general granular opacity of the lungs typical of hyaline membrane disease. The vessels, the heart borders and the diaphragm outlines are indistinct. (c) The air bronchogram sign in another baby with hyaline membrane disease. Note the uniformity of distribution of the changes in the lungs – an important diagnostic feature of hyaline membrane disease.

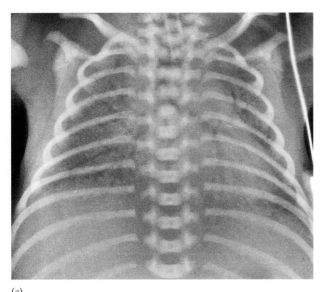

(c)

Fig. 2.98 *Continued*

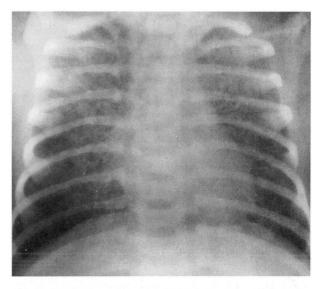

Fig. 2.99 Meconium aspiration. This baby born at term had fetal distress during delivery and was born through meconium-stained liquor. The film shows patchy consolidations rather than the uniform changes seen in hyaline membrane disease. The diaphragm is lower than normal in position, which is another differentiation from hyaline membrane disease.

normal due to airways obstruction associated with sticky meconium in the bronchi.

Complications of therapy. In addition to establishing the initial diagnosis in neonates with various causes of respiratory distress, the plain chest film is vital in detecting complications of therapy. These include lobar collapse, pneumomediastinum and pneumothorax.

Adult respiratory distress syndrome

Adult respiratory distress syndrome (ARDS) is the name given to a syndrome in which the pulmonary capillaries leak proteinaceous fluid from the vascular lumen into the surrounding pulmonary interstitium and alveoli. The condition is also known as 'non-cardiogenic pulmonary oedema'. There are many precipitating causes including severe trauma, significant hypotension, septicaemia and fat embolism. It is believed that these insults produce a cascade of events, the nature of which has yet to be fully elucidated, leading to capillary damage and hence to increased capillary permeability.

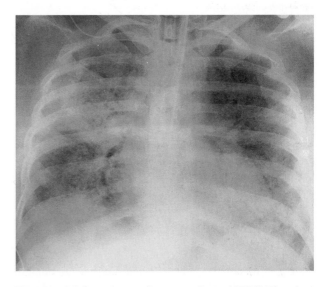

Fig. 2.100 Adult respiratory distress syndrome (ARDS). There is widespread consolidation of the lungs. This patient had suffered extensive trauma to the limbs.

The patients become increasingly short of breath and hypoxic, requiring mechanical ventilation to stay alive. The mortality, even with intense therapy and assisted ventilation, can be very high. There is no specific treatment.

Radiologically (Fig. 2.100), the chest x-ray shows widespread pulmonary shadowing resembling cardiogenic pulmonary oedema at first, but becoming more widespread and more uniform over the ensuing 24–48 hours. The radiological abnormality may only develop 12–24 hours after the onset of tachypnoea, dyspnoea or hypoxaemia. Since patients with ARDS require assisted ventilation, the chest film is used to detect the complications of ventilator therapy, notably pneumothorax and pneumomediastinum.

Pulmonary embolism and infarction

Pulmonary embolism from thrombi originating in the veins of the legs and pelvis is very common in patients confined to bed, particularly those with heart disease and those who have had major surgery. The clinical and radiological manifestations depend on the size and number of the emboli.

Plain film abnormalities

Massive embolism. In most cases the chest film in massive pulmonary embolism is unremarkable. There may be a visible reduction in the size of the arteries beyond any occlusion, but this is a very difficult sign to recognize and it is usually not possible to be sure that the smallness of the vessels is due to embolism rather than to pre-existing pulmonary disease, such as emphysema or old infection.

Large emboli. In many cases there is no infarction, even with large emboli, and therefore the chest film is normal. However, in some patients, particularly those with heart disease, infarction does occur. Radiologically, an infarct appears as an area of consolidation based on the pleura, indistinguishable from pneumonia. Infarcts often affect both lung bases and cause elevation of the diaphragm and/or pleural effusion. The differentiation between pneumonia and pulmonary infarction depends on clinical

factors and, if necessary, a radionuclide lung scan (see below).

Small emboli. Small emboli do not produce any radiological abnormality unless they occur over a long period of time and cause pulmonary hypertension. (See p. 120 for the signs of pulmonary hypertension.)

Radionuclide lung scans

The diagnosis of pulmonary embolism on radionuclide lung scanning depends on observing the distribution of radionuclide particles in the lungs following intravenous injection. The radionuclide particles do not reach the underperfused portions of the lungs and therefore one or more defects are seen in the perfusion scan. A normal perfusion scan for practical purposes excludes pulmonary embolism.

A ventilation scan is also required in patients with perfusion defects in order to differentiate between the various other causes of perfusion defects which include pneumonia, pulmonary oedema, tumours, bronchiectasis and emphysema.

The ventilation and perfusion scans are compared. If similar defects of the same size and position are present on both scans, they are regarded as matched; if not, the defects are mismatched.

The major patterns that may be seen when comparing the perfusion and ventilation scans with the chest radiographs are:

1 Mismatched ventilation/perfusion defects (Fig. 2.101).
   • Perfusion defects in areas with normal ventilation are highly suggestive of pulmonary embolism without infarction.
   • Perfusion defects which are larger than the corresponding ventilation defects suggest pulmonary infarction. Such cases will often show consolidation on plain chest radiograph.

2 Matched ventilation/perfusion defects (Fig. 2.102) are usually due to pneumonia, pulmonary oedema or airways disease. However, they may sometimes be seen with pulmonary infarction and are therefore classified as 'indeterminate'.

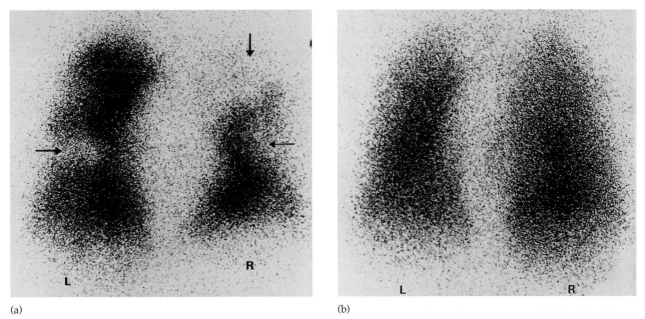

(a)   (b)

Fig. 2.101 Pulmonary emboli. (a) 99mTc macroaggregate perfusion scan showing multiple wedge-shaped defects. The more obvious ones have been arrowed. (b) The ventilation scan, using 81mKr, is normal.

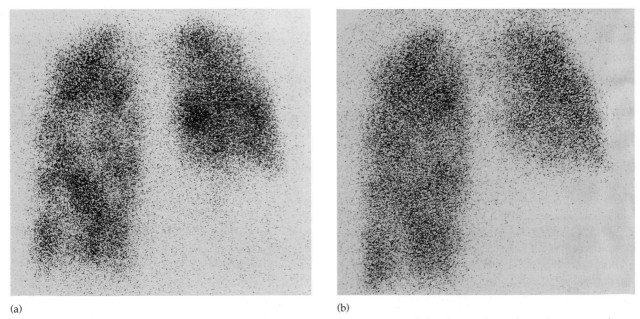

(a)   (b)

Fig. 2.102 Matched ventilation/perfusion defects. 99mTc macroaggregate perfusion scan (a) showing matched defects when compared to the 81mKr ventilation scan (b). Both are anterior scans. The patient had widespread emphysema.

Pulmonary angiography (Fig. 2.103)

Pulmonary angiography is the most accurate method of diagnosing pulmonary emboli. It requires definite indications: for example, to confirm massive embolism prior to surgical intervention, or when there is significant doubt about the presence or absence of pulmonary emboli after viewing the chest radiograph and radionuclide lung scans.

Computed tomography. Recently, spiral (helical) CT scanning has been used to detect larger pulmonary emboli (Fig. 2.104). The technique, known as CT angiography, involves imaging the central and larger branches of the pulmonary arteries during a rapid injection of a large bolus of intravenous contrast agent. CT angiography is currently used in a few centres only.

Trauma to the chest

Rib fracture can be diagnosed by noting a break or step in the cortex of a rib. Special views of the ribs may be necessary, since rib fractures are often invisible in the standard projections, particularly if the fracture lies below the diaphragm. Extrapleural soft tissue swelling from bruising, or frank haematoma may be visible and guide the observer toward the site of the fracture.

Rib fractures are frequently multiple and may result in a flail segment.

Pleural effusion often accompanies rib fractures, the fluid frequently being blood.

Pneumothorax. Pneumothorax may occur if the lung is punctured by direct injury or by the sharp edge of a rib fracture. An air–fluid level in the pleural cavity is common in such situations, from the associated haemorrhage.

Surgical emphysema of the chest wall may indicate the escape of air from the lungs. The presence of mediastinal emphysema in the absence of chest wall emphysema may indicate the unusual phenomenon of rupture of a bronchus.

Pulmonary contusion. Localized traumatic alveolar haemor-

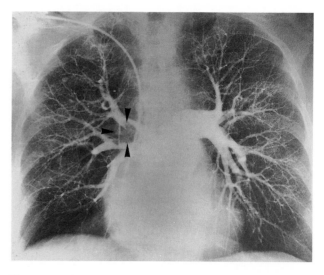

Fig. 2.103 Pulmonary arteriogram in pulmonary embolism. There is a large embolus causing a filling defect at the bifurcation of the right pulmonary artery (arrows). Note also the reduction in branches of the lower lobe arteries owing to obstruction by emboli. (The catheter can be seen passing from the right arm into the heart.)

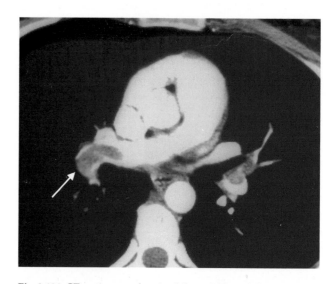

Fig. 2.104 CT angiogram showing bilateral filling defects owing to emboli in the central pulmonary arteries. The arrow points to the largest of these emboli.

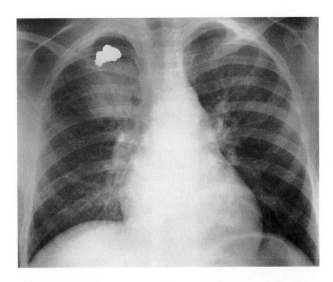

Fig. 2.105 Pulmonary contusion from a gunshot wound. The ill-defined consolidation represents haemorrhage and oedema in the right upper lobe. The deformed metallic fragments of the bullet are clearly visible.

rhage and oedema (Fig. 2.105) may be seen whether or not a rib fracture can be identified. The resulting pulmonary shadow is indistinguishable from other forms of pulmonary consolidation, the relationship to the injury being important in establishing the diagnosis.

Adult respiratory distress syndrome (ARDS). ARDS may follow severe trauma to any part of the body. *Fat embolism* is a specific subtype of ARDS, but its radiographic manifestations are identical to those of the other causes of ARDS (see p. 87).

Rupture of the diaphragm is due to penetrating injury or compression of the abdomen and may permit herniation of the stomach or intestines into the chest. Such herniation is much commoner on the left than the right. There is usually a pleural effusion and the 'diaphragm' outline becomes indistinct during the acute stage. Gas shadows of the stomach or intestines are seen above the presumed position of the diaphragm, the diaphragm itself often being invisible. Barium meal and follow-through may be indicated to establish the diagnosis. The only technique that can demonstrate the tear itself is ultrasound, but even when the ultrasound examination is performed by an expert it may be difficult to make the diagnosis.

Rupture of the aorta is a particularly serious consequence of rapid deceleration injuries. In patients that survive, the injury to the aorta is usually at the level of the ligamentum arteriosum. Bleeding into the mediastinum may cause visible mediastinal widening, and bleeding into the pleural cavity may occur.

Aortography is usually indicated in patients with unexplained mediastinal widening following trauma to establish the diagnosis of aortic rupture, because venous bleeding which does not require emergency surgery can cause similar signs. Widening of the mediastinum can be a very difficult sign to assess, particularly on the portable AP films that are often the only films that can be taken in these severely injured patients. Computed tomography scanning may be used to exclude blood in the mediastinum in those cases where the nature of mediastinal widening is uncertain from plain film observations. Spiral (helical) CT following a large intravenous bolus of contrast medium can demonstrate the aortic wall tear in some cases.

Although fractures of the ribs or sternum are usually present there are many cases of aortic rupture on record without visible damage to the thoracic cage.

In some patients the diagnosis of aortic rupture is only made several months or years after the injury when the development of an aneurysm is noted.

Rupture of the tracheobronchial tree only occurs with major chest trauma. The cardinal signs are pneumomediastinum, or pneumothorax that does not respond to chest tube suction. The main complication is subsequent bronchostenosis.

Neoplastic disease

Carcinoma of the bronchus

Carcinoma of the bronchus is one of the most common primary malignant tumours. It has a clear association with cigarette smoking. The majority of bronchial carcinomas arise in larger bronchi at, or close to, the hilum. It is convenient to consider the radiological features of central and peripheral tumours separately.

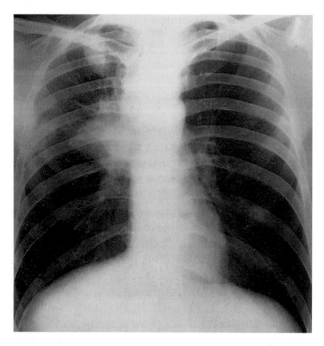

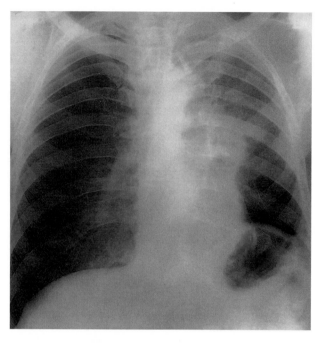

Fig. 2.106 Right hilar mass due to carcinoma of the bronchus. There is also a patch of consolidation in the right upper lobe laterally, from the central obstruction.

Fig. 2.107 Carcinoma of the bronchus at the left hilum causing collapse of the left upper lobe and paralysis of the left phrenic nerve. The elevated left hemidiaphragm is too high to be due to the lobar collapse; it is due to phrenic nerve involvement by the tumour at the left hilum.

Signs of a central tumour.
• The tumour itself may present as a hilar mass (Fig. 2.106) and/or narrowing of a major bronchus. The narrowing may be irregular or smooth.
• The effect of obstruction by the tumour (Fig. 2.107) is usually a combination of collapse and consolidation. The alveoli collapse because air is absorbed beyond the obstructed bronchus and cannot be replaced, whereas consolidation is the consequence of retained secretions and secondary infection.

Signs of a peripheral tumour. A peripheral tumour (Fig. 2.108) usually presents as a solitary pulmonary mass. There are several causes for such a mass and these are discussed on p. 38.
    The signs of a peripheral primary carcinoma are:
• A rounded shadow with an irregular border. Lobulation, notching and infiltrating edges are the common patterns.

• Cavitation within the mass. Peripheral squamous cell carcinomas show a particular tendency for cavitation. The walls of the cavity are classically thick and irregular, but thin-walled smooth cavities due to carcinoma do occur.

Spread of bronchial carcinoma. Evidence of spread of bronchial carcinoma may be visible on plain chest radiography, but CT and, in highly selected cases, MRI have made a major contribution to the staging of lung cancer. Both may show enlarged mediastinal lymph nodes suggesting involvement by tumour or direct invasion of the mediastinum that is either not visible or is questionable on the plain chest film – information that may save the patient unnecessary thoracotomy.
• *Hilar and mediastinal lymph node enlargement due to lymphatic spread of tumour.* Only greatly enlarged lymph nodes can be recognized on plain chest radiograph. The sites in which nodes are most readily identified are at the hilum and

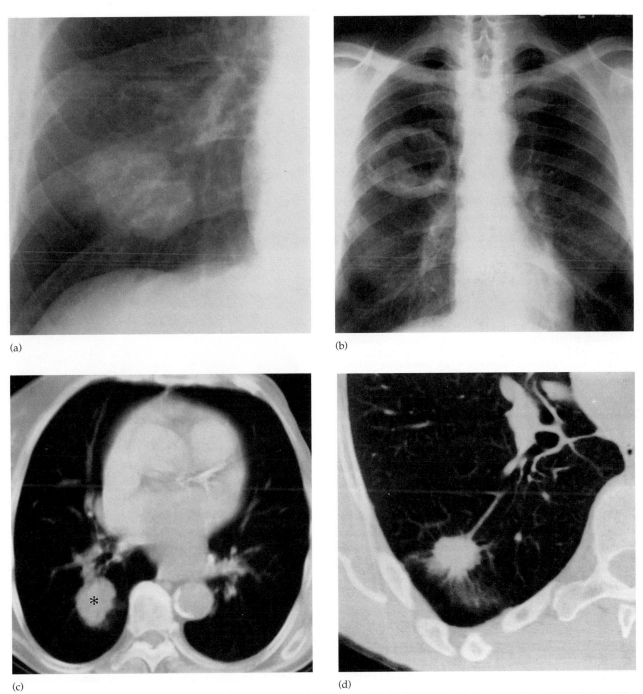

(a)

(b)

(c)

(d)

Fig. 2.108 Appearance of peripheral lung carcinoma. (a) A lobulated and (b) a cavitating mass are shown on plain films. (c) A lobulated (∗) and (d) a spiculated mass are shown on CT.

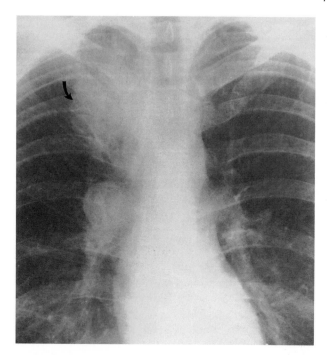

Fig. 2.109 Carcinoma of the right upper lobe (arrowed) with large lymph node metastases at the right hilum.

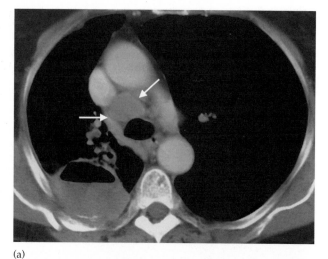

(a)

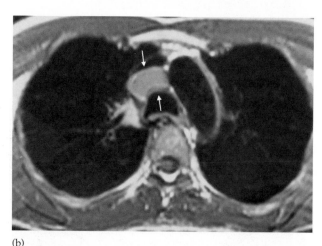

(b)

Fig. 2.110 Mediastinal adenopathy from metastatic lung cancer. (a) Computed tomography scan shows greatly enlarged node (arrows). Note that the primary tumour lying posteriorly in the right lung has invaded the chest wall and partially destroyed the adjacent rib. (b) Magnetic resonance imaging scan (T1-weighted) shows enlarged node (arrow) which stands out clearly against the background of no signal in lung, trachea or aorta.

in the right paratracheal area (Fig. 2.109). Nodes in the subcarinal region have to be massive if they are to be visible on a plain chest film. Computed tomography, on the other hand, has the ability to show even mildly enlarged nodes, nodes that are not identifiable on plain film. However, enlargement of lymph nodes does not necessarily mean metastatic involvement, because reactive hyperplasia to the tumour or associated infection can be responsible for nodal enlargement as can pre-existing disease such as previous granulomatous infection, sarcoidosis or coalworkers' pneumoconiosis. In practice, the role of CT is to decide which patients need preoperative lymph node biopsy, and to tell the surgeon which nodes to biopsy. Nodes below 1 cm in diameter can be considered as normal in size and need not be biopsied. Nodes above 1 cm in diameter should be biopsied prior to surgical resection of the primary tumour, although it should be borne in mind that nodes of 2 cm or

greater in short-axis diameter (Fig. 2.110) in a patient with a bronchial carcinoma almost invariably contain metastatic neoplasm.

• *Pleural effusion* in a patient with lung cancer is usually

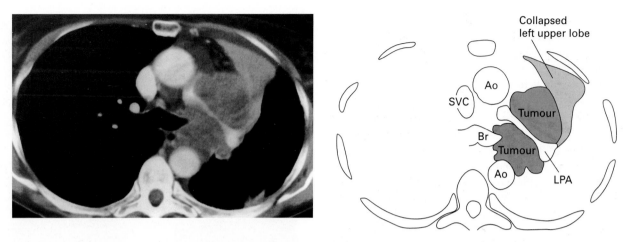

Fig. 2.111 Mediastinal invasion Computed tomography scan (contrast-enhanced) shows extensive tumour in mediastinum compressing the left pulmonary artery. Ao, aorta; Br, bronchus; LPA, left pulmonary artery; SVC, superior vena cava.

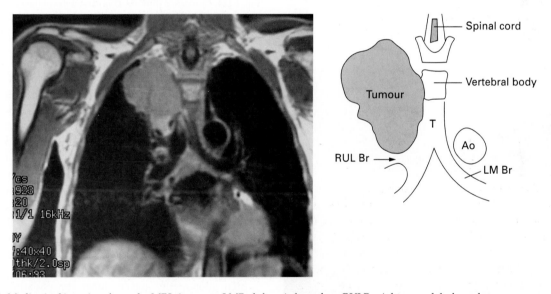

Fig. 2.112 Mediastinal invasion shown by MRI. Ao, aorta; LMBr, left main bronchus; RULBr, right upper lobe bronchus.

due to malignant involvement of the pleura, but it may be secondary to associated infection of the lung or coincidental, as in heart failure.

• *Invasion of the mediastinum*. On plain films, the signs are widening of the mediastinal shadow and elevation of a hemidiaphragm suggesting involvement of the phrenic nerve by tumour (Fig. 2.107). Mediastinal widening can be a difficult sign to evaluate, particularly in older people with aortic unfolding. Computed tomography and MRI are much more sensitive and accurate methods of assessing mediastinal invasion by tumour because the neoplasm can be directly visualized (Figs 2.111, 2.112).

• *Invasion of the chest wall* (Fig. 2.113). Destruction of a rib immediately adjacent to a pulmonary shadow is virtually diagnostic of bronchial carcinoma with chest wall invasion. Recognizing the rib destruction can be difficult. It is important therefore to make a conscious effort to look at the ribs directly. Oblique views may be helpful in detecting bone destruction. Computed tomography and MRI can demonstrate rib and soft tissue invasion when the bone is not visibly eroded on plain films. MRI is particularly useful for showing invasion of the apex of the chest, the so-called Pancoast's tumour (Fig. 2.114). Imaging techniques, even CT and MRI, may not always be reliable for determining chest wall invasion, and local chest wall pain remains the most important indication that the tumour has crossed the pleura.

• *Rib metastases*. Carcinoma of the lung frequently metastasizes to the ribs where it produces bone destruction. Sclerotic secondary deposits from lung carcinoma are rare.

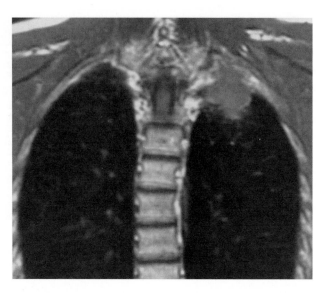

Fig. 2.114 Pancoast's tumour. This carcinoma of the lung can be seen invading the root of the neck on this coronal MRI scan (T1-weighted).

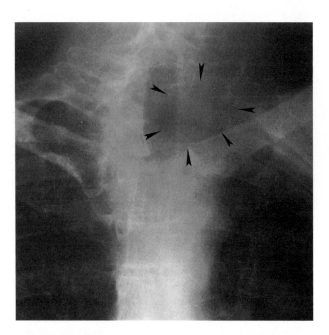

Fig. 2.113 Pancoast's tumour. The carcinoma arising at the apex of the left lung has invaded and destroyed the adjacent ribs and spine. Note that no bone is visible within the area indicated by the arrows.

• *Pulmonary metastases*. Primary lung carcinoma occasionally metastasizes to other parts of the lungs. The rounded shadows that result are similar to secondary deposits from other primary tumours.

• *Lymphangitis carcinomatosa* is the term applied to blockage of the pulmonary lymphatics by carcinomatous tissue. Lymphangitis carcinomatosa can be due to spread from abdominal and breast cancers as well as from carcinoma of the lung. The lymphatic vessels become grossly distended and the lungs become oedematous. The signs (Fig. 2.115) can be identical to those seen in interstitial pulmonary oedema (septal lines, loss of vessel clarity and peribronchial thickening), but if the heart is normal in size and there is hilar adenopathy and/or lobar consolidation, the diagnosis of lymphangitis carcinomatosa becomes more certain. The clinical story is very helpful, since if the changes are due to pulmonary oedema, the patient will usually complain of sudden onset of breathlessness, whereas the patient with lymphangitis carcinomatosa will give a story of slowly increasing dyspnoea over the preceding weeks or months.

Computed tomography particularly high resolution CT, has proved very valuable in demonstrating lymphangitis

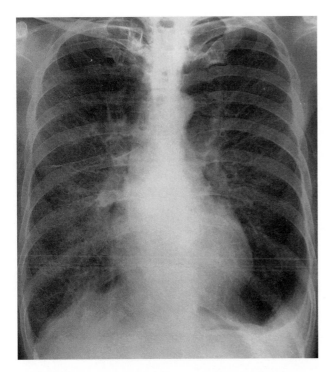

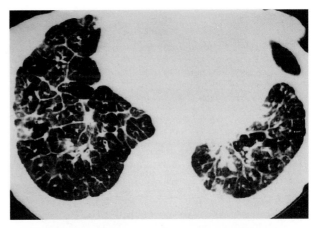

Fig. 2.116 Lymphangitis carcinomatosa. The widespread connecting lines representing irregularly thickened interlobular septa are very well shown by thin-section high resolution CT. This appearance is virtually pathognomonic of lymphangitis carcinomatosa.

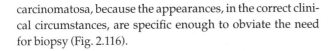

Fig. 2.115 Lymphangitis carcinomatosa. There is widespread ill-defined pulmonary shadowing with numerous septal lines. A small left pleural effusion is also present. The patient had a carcinoma of the stomach.

carcinomatosa, because the appearances, in the correct clinical circumstances, are specific enough to obviate the need for biopsy (Fig. 2.116).

Metastatic neoplasms

Metastases from extrathoracic primary tumours may be seen in the lungs, the pleura or the bones of the thoracic cage. Hilar and mediastinal lymph node enlargement from metastases is uncommon, other than from carcinoma of the bronchus.

Pulmonary metastases. Typically, metastases are spherical and well defined (Figs 2.117, 2.118), although irregular borders are occasionally seen. Usually, they are multiple

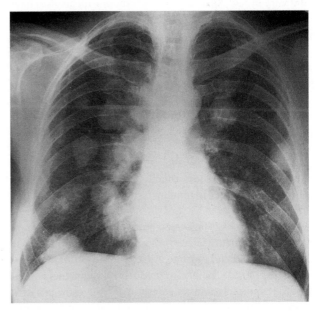

Fig. 2.117 Pulmonary metastases. There are numerous rounded shadows of varying sizes in both lungs.

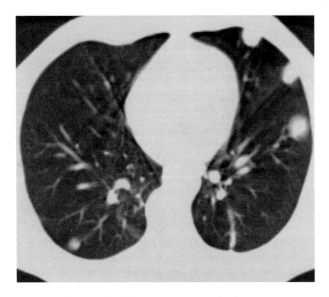

Fig. 2.118 CT scan of pulmonary metastases (malignant teratoma of testis). The peripheral location shown here is typical.

and vary in size. As with primary tumours, metastases have to be almost a centimetre in diameter or larger to be visible on plain chest radiographs. Computed tomography scanning can demonstrate metastases as small as 3–6 mm. There is, however, a disadvantage attached to the excellent sensitivity of CT. Some small nodules are not metastases, but benign processes such as tuberculomas or fungal granulomas. This is a major diagnostic problem in many parts of the United States where fungal granulomas are very common.

Pleural metastases. These usually give rise to pleural effusion. The individual pleural metastases are rarely seen.

Metastases to ribs. These are common with those primary tumours that metastasize to bone, namely bronchus, breast, kidney, thyroid and prostate. All except prostatic and breast cancers produce mainly or exclusively lytic metastases. Sclerotic metastases in an elderly man suggest a prostatic primary cancer. Sclerotic or mixed lytic and sclerotic deposits in a woman suggest that the primary carcinoma is in the breast.

With lytic metastases the best sign is destruction of the cortex, particularly of the upper border of the rib. One should be wary of diagnosing destruction of the lower borders of the posterior portions of the ribs, since these regions are indefinite even in the normal. When in doubt it is always wise to compare with the opposite side. Another pitfall in the diagnosis of rib metastases is that blood vessels in the lungs may cause confusing

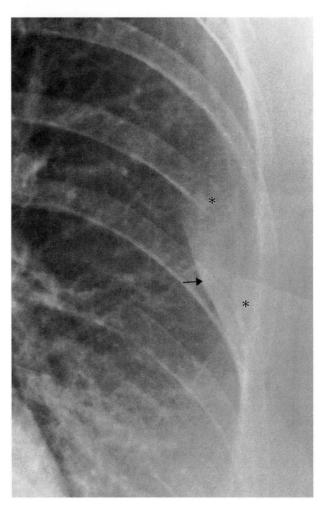

Fig. 2.119 Lytic metastasis. The soft tissue mass (arrow) is more obvious than the underlying bone destruction shown between the two asterisks.

shadows. This confusion cannot arise at the edges of the chest where there is no lung projected over the ribs, so that is a useful place to look for bone destruction. Soft tissue swelling is frequently seen adjacent to the rib deposit, so it is a good rule to look at the outer margin of the lung for soft tissue swelling as a clue to the presence of rib metastases (Fig. 2.119).

Lymphoma

The common manifestations of intrathoracic malignant lymphoma are mediastinal and hilar adenopathy and pleural effusion. These features can often be seen on plain films but CT scanning is much the best method of confirming or excluding intrathoracic lymph node enlargement. Pulmonary involvement by lymphoma is unusual (Fig. 2.120). It may take the form of large areas of infiltration of the lung parenchyma, resembling pulmonary consolidation, or occasionally it is seen as one or more mass lesions, which may cavitate. Pleural masses are a rare feature.

Since pulmonary infection is a common complication in patients with malignant lymphoma it may be impossible to decide on radiological grounds whether the pulmonary consolidation is due to lymphomatous tissue or to infection.

Mammography

X-ray examination of the breast is carried out with dedicated equipment designed to produce low kilovoltage x-rays in the range 28–32 kV which demonstrate the soft tissues of the breast to advantage. The normal breast tissue shows the glandular, ductal and connective tissue against a background of fat, the appearances changing with the age of the patient. With increasing age, involution of the breast occurs so that the glandular tissue atrophies. The mammographic appearances of the normal breast vary greatly from one patient to another.

The main purpose of mammography is to detect breast carcinoma. It is now used to screen women for breast cancer, and can also be helpful in patients presenting with a lump or lumpy areas in the breast.

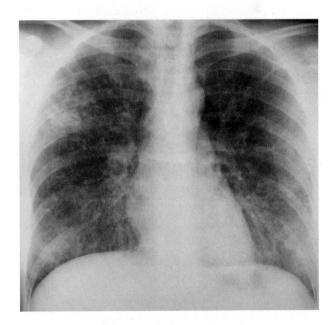

Fig. 2.120 Lymphoma involving the lung. The extensive pulmonary consolidations were due to neoplastic involvement. Pneumonia can give a similar appearance.

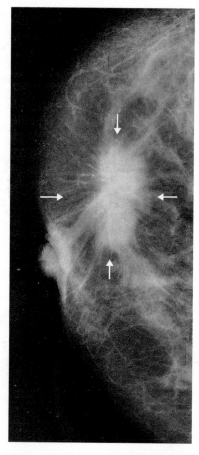

Fig. 2.121 Carcinoma of the breast. Mammogram showing irregular soft tissue mass (arrows) behind the nipple. Microcalcifications are present but difficult to see in reproduction.

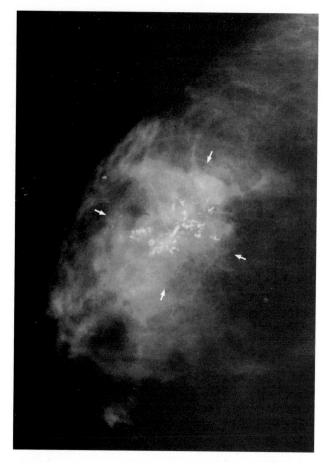

Fig. 2.122 Carcinoma of the breast. Mammogram showing ill-defined mass (arrows) containing numerous malignant linear and branching microcalcifications.

Mammographic signs

The cardinal mammographic signs of *carcinoma* are:
- a mass with ill-defined or spiculated borders (Fig. 2.121);
- clustered, fine linear or irregular calcifications – so-called malignant microcalcifications (Fig. 2.122), which can on occasion be the only sign of breast cancer even in the absence of a visible mass;
- Other signs that may point to the diagnosis of carcinoma are distortion of adjacent breast stroma and skin thickening. *Benign masses* tend to be spherical with well-defined borders (Fig. 2.123a) and not infrequently contain calcification. The calcifications differ from malignant microcalcification in that they are larger, coarser and often ring-like in configuration (Fig. 2.124).

Ultrasound can be very helpful in determining whether a mass is a simple cyst (Fig. 2.123b), and therefore benign, or solid and, therefore, possibly a carcinoma.

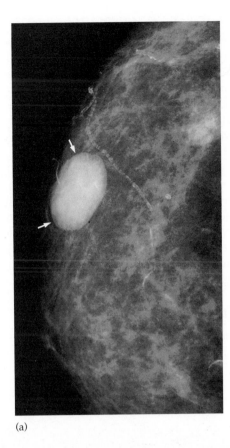

(a)

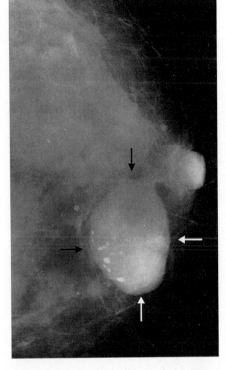

Fig. 2.124 Benign mass in breast (fibroadenoma). Mammogram showing mass (arrows) with very well defined borders and coarse structured calcification.

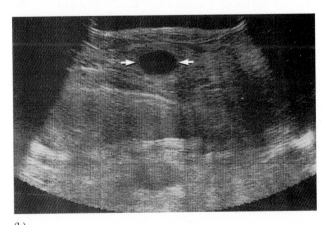

(b)

Fig. 2.123 Benign cyst of breast. (a) Mammogram showing oval, very well-defined mass without calcifications (arrows). (b) The mass (arrows) was shown to be cystic on ultrasound; cyst aspiration was undertaken.

Breast screening

Mammography can detect breast cancer in asymptomatic women even before the tumour is palpable (Fig. 2.125). There is evidence from large scale trials that early detection by mammography can reduce the mortality from breast cancer in women over the age of 50. Though the degree of improved survival varies from country to country, in some series reductions in mortality have been found to be as high as 30 % of those screened.

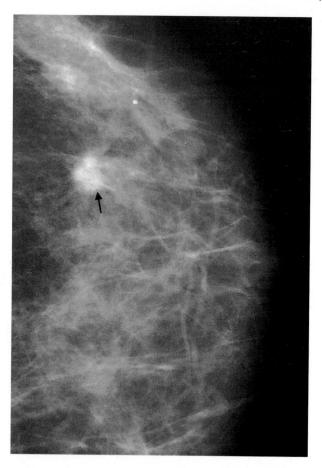

Fig. 2.125 Small (7 mm) primary breast carcinoma (arrow) detected by screening mammography. This tumour was asymptomatic and was not palpable.

Breast cancer is the most frequent cancer in women, affecting one woman in 12. In an attempt to reduce the mortality, the UK government has decided to invite all women aged 50–64 years to attend a regular screening programme, currently consisting of a mammogram every three years. It is expected that at least 50 cancers will be detected by mammography for every 10 000 women screened, but inevitably a number of breast carcinomas will escape detection.

Conversely, as with all screening tests, there are false–positive interpretations. For this reason, all patients with an abnormal mammogram are asked to attend an assessment clinic at which they undergo a physical examination, and further mammographic views, ultrasound, or needle biopsy as necessary. In some instances follow-up mammography after a short interval will be advised.

MRI of the breast

Magnetic resonance mammography is a developing subject with, at present, highly specific indications.

3

Cardiovascular System

Echocardiography, radionuclide examinations and plain films are the standard non-invasive imaging investigations used in cardiac disease. Echocardiography has now become a particularly important imaging technique that provides morphological as well as functional information. It is excellent for looking at the heart valves, assessing chamber morphology and volume, determining the thickness of the ventricular wall and diagnosing intraluminal masses. Doppler ultrasound is an extremely useful tool for determining the velocity and direction of blood flow through the heart valves and within cardiac chambers. Radionuclide examinations reflect physiological parameters such as myocardial blood flow and ventricular contractility but provide little anatomical detail, whereas plain radiographs are useful for looking at the effects of cardiac disease on the lungs and pleural cavities, but provide only limited information about the heart itself. MRI provides both functional and anatomical information but is only available in specialized centres and is used only for specific reasons.

Imaging techniques

Plain radiography

The standard plain films for the evaluation of cardiac disease are the posteroanterior (PA) view and a lateral chest film (Fig. 3.1). The PA view must be sufficiently penetrated to see the shadows within the heart, e.g. the double contour of the left atrium and valve calcification.

When plain films are examined from patients with possible cardiac disorders, the heart and great vessels should be assessed for size and shape. A potential pitfall is false diagnosis of heart disease in a patient with a severely *depressed*

sternum (pectus excavatum) in whom the cardiac outline appears altered from simple rotation and displacement (Fig. 3.2). Normally, there are no visible calcifications within the heart and, therefore, any cardiac or pericardial calcifications should be noted and their positions established. Before leaving the mediastinum, the aortic arch should also be examined to exclude signs of coarctation and to ensure that it is normally located to the left of the trachea. The lungs should then be examined for evidence of heart failure or alteration in blood flow.

Echocardiography

Three basic techniques are used in cardiac ultrasound: M-mode, two-dimensional sector scanning (sometimes called 'real time' echocardiography) and Doppler echocardiography. Because ultrasound is absorbed by the bones of the thorax and by air in the lungs, the views of the heart are necessarily limited.

M-mode

M-mode is a continuous scan recorded over a period of time with a pencil-beam of sound directed towards the structure of interest. The distance between the various structures and their movement towards and away from the transducer are recorded for short periods, usually 5–10s, allowing measurements of chamber dimensions and wall thickness to be made. Also, the pattern of movement of a structure, e.g. valve leaflets, may allow an abnormality to be diagnosed and may also provide an indication of its severity. The normal appearance of selected M-mode images is illustrated in Fig. 3.3. M-mode examinations have been largely

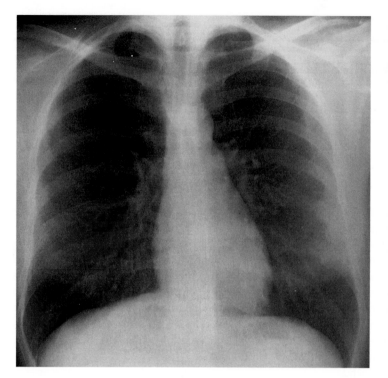

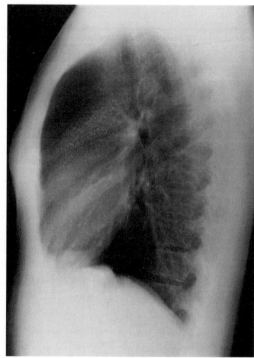

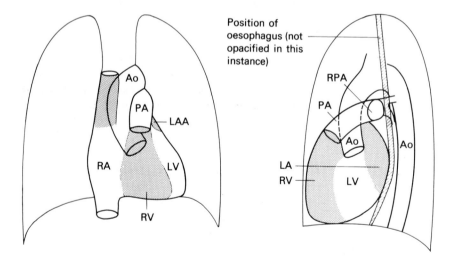

Position of oesophagus (not opacified in this instance)

Fig. 3.1 Outline of heart in PA and lateral views. Ao, aorta; LAA, left atrial appendage; LA, left atrium; LV, left ventricle; PA, pulmonary artery; RA, right atrium; RPA, right pulmonary artery; RV, right ventricle.

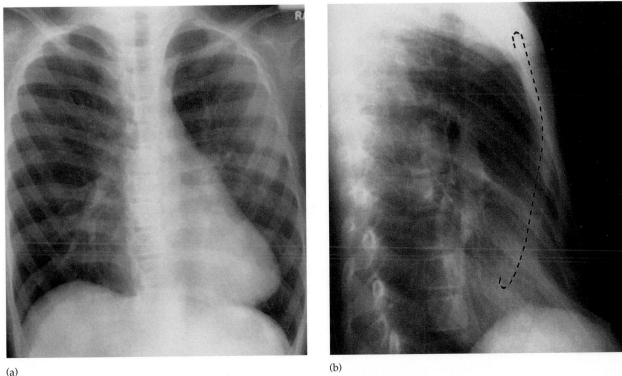

(a)   (b)

Fig. 3.2 Pectus excavatum. (a) PA view. Note how the heart is displaced and altered in shape by the depressed sternum. (b) Lateral film. The edge of the sternum has been traced in on this film. There was no cardiac disease in this patient.

replaced by two-dimensional sector scanning, but they are still used for certain specific measurements such as the dimensions of the left ventricle in systole and diastole.

Two-dimensional sector scanning

Two-dimensional echocardiography demonstrates a fan-shaped slice of the heart in motion that can be recorded on video tape; still photographs can also be made when necessary. If the transducer is angled, the 'slice' can be moved through the heart to allow the observer to build up a mental picture of a three-dimensional image. Since tiny bubbles of air accompany the injection of almost any liquid and because ultrasound reliably detects even tiny gas bubbles within the blood stream, injections of agitated saline can be used as a harmless intravascular 'contrast agent'.

The standard examination consists of a combination of short- and long-axis views, together with the so-called four

chamber view (Figs 3.4 and 3.5). The short- and long-axis views show a cross-section of the left ventricle and mitral and aortic valves. These views are obtained by placing the transducer in an intercostal space just to the left of the sternum (or, in some individuals, in a subcostal position). The four-chamber view, which shows both ventricles and both atria together with the mitral and tricuspid valves, is obtained by placing the transducer over the cardiac apex and aiming upward and medially. A newly introduced device is the oesophageal ultrasound probe, which looks at the cardiac structures from within the oesophagus from behind the heart.

Doppler echocardiography

As discussed on p. 8, when sound waves are reflected from a moving object, the frequency of the reflected waves is altered, depending on the velocity of the reflecting surface.

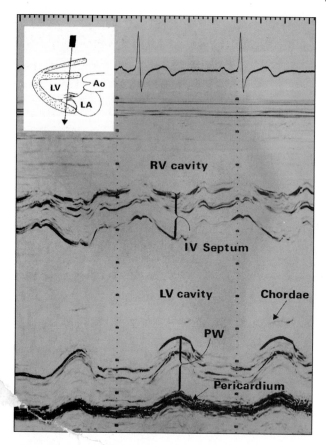

Fig. 3.3 M-mode scan. Parasternal long axis view through the mid left ventricular (LV) cavity. The thickness and movement of the interventricular septum (IV Septum) and the posterior wall (PW) of the left ventricle are well demonstrated and can be correlated with the ECG at the top of the trace. RV, right ventricular. Courtesy of Andrew A. McLeod and Mark J. Monaghan.

With the Doppler technique, red blood cells can be used as reflecting surfaces and the velocity of blood flow in a given direction can be calculated (Fig. 3.6). The accuracy of the technique depends on the angle of flow with respect to the ultrasound beam, flow directly in line with the beam being the most accurately measured.

Doppler flow measurements are used to:
• quantify pressure gradients across stenotic valves (using the Bernoulli equation: velocity squared × 4 estimates pressure difference between cardiac chambers);
• quantify flow;

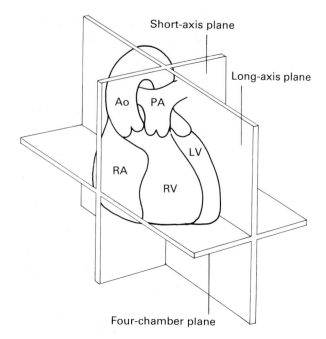

Fig. 3.4 Diagram illustrating the three orthogonal imaging planes used to demonstrate the heart with two-dimensional echocardiography. Ao, aorta; PA, pulmonary artery; RA, right atrium; RV, right ventricle; LV, left ventricle.

• measure cardiac output or left to right shunts;
• detect and quantify valvular regurgitation (see Plate 3, opposite p. 110).

Pressure gradients are derived mathematically from formulae that convert velocity across a valve into a pressure gradient. Flow measurements depend on measuring the velocity by Doppler methods and then using standard ultrasound techniques to calculate the cross-sectional areas of the structure through which the blood is flowing.

With colour Doppler the direction and velocity of flow are colour-coded to allow the observer to appreciate the direction and magnitude of flow in specific anatomical sites (see Plate 3, opposite p. 110). Colour Doppler is particularly useful in complex congenital heart disease, e.g. finding multiple or unusually situated ventricular septal defects.

Transoesophageal echocardiography

Good visualization of the heart and aorta may be obtained

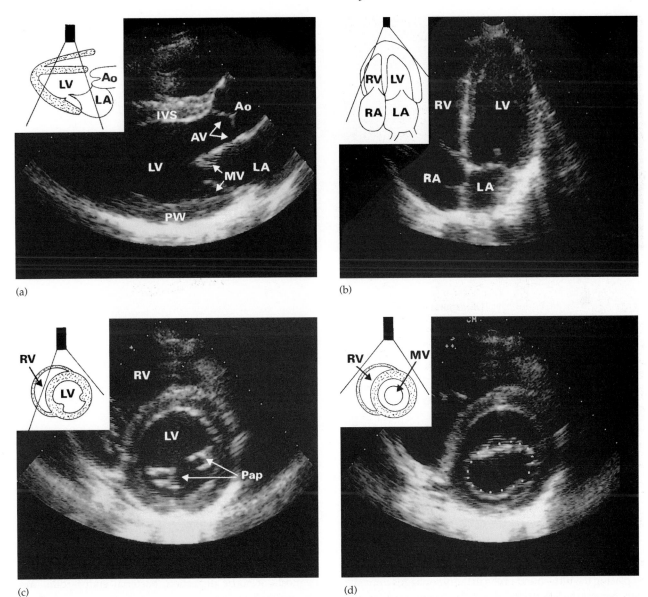

Fig. 3.5 Normal two-dimensional echocardiogram. (a) Parasternal long axis view. (b) Apical four chamber view. (c) Parasternal short axis view at the level of papillary muscles. (d) Similar view to (c) but at the level of the mitral valve. The dots indicate the area of the open valve. Ao, aorta; AV, aortic valve; IVS, interventricular septum; LA, left atrium; LV, left ventricle; MV, mitral valve; Pap, papillary muscles; PW, posterior wall of LV; RA, right atrium; RV, right ventricle. Courtesy of Andrew A. McLeod and Mark J. Monaghan.

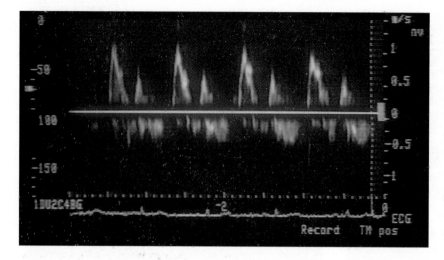

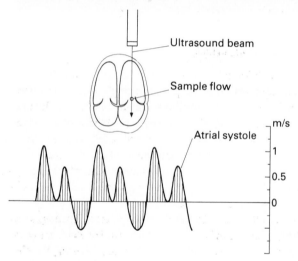

Fig. 3.6 Doppler ultrasound through a normal mitral valve in the four-chamber view. Note the rapid initial velocity at 1 m/s, the rapid decline and then a second smaller peak caused by atrial systole.

by placing the ultrasound probe in the oesophagus immediately behind the left atrium (Fig. 3.7). Patients are prepared for the endoscopy with sedation and local laryngeal lignocaine anaesthesia. Viewing the heart from behind the left atrium gives excellent views of the native or prosthetic mitral valve, the interatrial septum, and from the intragastric view an accurate estimate of blood velocity across the aortic valve (and therefore gradient) may be obtained. Transoesophageal echocardiography is very useful in the diagnosis of aortic dissection, bacterial endocarditis and intracardiac tumours.

Stress echocardiography

Echocardiography can be performed after exercise on a treadmill or bicycle or with a pharmacologically induced tachycardia with intravenous adenosine or dipyridamole. This procedure may allow the identification of dyskinetic

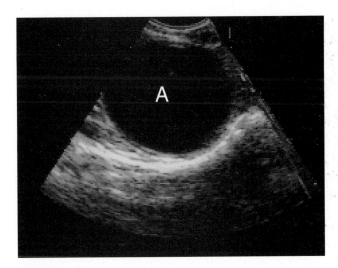

Fig. 3.7 Transoesophageal echocardiogram showing a normal descending thoracic aorta (A).

areas of ventricular muscle from underlying coronary artery disease.

Radionuclide studies

Nuclear medicine techniques are simpler to perform than angiocardiography, are non-invasive and can be readily repeated. They give information on cardiac function but provide only limited anatomical detail.

The two most frequently used radionuclide investigations in cardiology are myocardial perfusion scintigraphy and radionuclide angiocardiography. Myocardial infarct imaging is discussed on p. 129.

Myocardial perfusion scintigraphy

Myocardial perfusion scintigraphy makes use of the radionuclide thallium-201 (^{201}Tl) which is handled by the myocardial cells similarly to potassium. It is taken up in proportion to blood flow, so regions of reduced myocardial perfusion appear as areas of reduced uptake.

Thallium-201 myocardial imaging is used in the diagnosis of ischaemic heart disease and is particularly useful in patients with chest pain, in whom it is uncertain whether the pain is cardiac in origin. As many patients only show impaired myocardial perfusion on exercise, the patient exercises on a bicycle or on a treadmill. Just prior to maximal exercise, an intravenous injection of ^{201}Tl is given and the cardiac uptake of the radionuclide is then imaged in various projections using a gamma camera. If patients are unable to exercise for any reason it is possible to increase the heart rate pharmacologically with intravenous adenosine or dipyridamole and then inject the thallium at peak or symptomatic heart rate. The images are repeated after the patient has rested for 3–4 hours. The sites and sizes of ischaemic areas can be assessed and a distinction between ischaemic and infarcted regions can be made by comparing peak exercise and resting images (see p. 128 and Plate 4, opposite p. 110). The investigation should only be performed under medical supervision with full resuscitation equipment available.

Radionuclide angiography

Radionuclide angiocardiography is also known as 'multiple gated equilibrium blood pool imaging', sometimes abbreviated to MUGA (multiple gated) scanning. It uses technetium-99m (^{99m}Tc) attached to red blood cells to image the blood pool. A convenient method of labelling is to inject stannous pyrophosphate intravenously, which acts as a reducing agent. Fifteen minutes later ^{99m}Tc-pertechnetate is injected intravenously, which enters and binds to the red blood cells for several hours.

As an alternative to this so called *in vivo* labelling, an *in vitro* technique can be used whereby 10 ml of blood are withdrawn; the red cells are separated by centrifuging, labelled with ^{99m}Tc, resuspended and then injected into the patient. After about 15 minutes to allow for complete mixing of the radionuclide tagged cells with the remainder of the patient's blood, the heart is imaged using a gamma camera.

Because insufficient radioactive counts are collected from each cardiac cycle, images from successive cardiac cycles are combined with the use of electronic gating. Starting from the R wave of the ECG, each cardiac cycle is divided into a number of equal intervals. Data from each interval in each successive cardiac cycle are summed to give a representative cycle which is then displayed as a moving image on a TV monitor or cine loop. It is usually necessary to record data from about 400–500 cardiac cycles to obtain an adequate image.

Radionuclide angiograms are used to calculate the *ventricular ejection fraction* in patients with valvular disease and myocardial disorders, and for *wall motion analysis* in patients with ischaemic heart disease.

Since there is uniform mixing of the radionuclide with the blood, the radioactivity is proportional to the amount of blood in the ventricles. Individual frames from the summed cardiac cycles can be displayed on a television monitor. The boundaries of either ventricle in systole and diastole are drawn in by light pen or other electronic device and the computer can then construct curves of ventricular volume against time (Fig. 3.8).

After correction for background activity, the values of the maximum (end diastole) and minimum (end systole) counts can be obtained and the ejection fraction can then be calculated:

$$\text{ejection fraction} = \frac{\text{end diastolic vol} - \text{end systolic vol}}{\text{end diastolic vol}}$$

Normally, the left ventricular ejection fraction should be greater than 50 % and all parts of the ventricular outline should show equal movement. Segments of the wall with reduced movement or aneurysm formation can be demonstrated.

Computed tomography

Computed tomography with conventional equipment, plays little or no part in the management of intracardiac disorders, mainly because of the long scanning times required to image the heart. Pericardial effusions (see Fig. 3.16b, p. 117) and cardiac tumours are recognizable, but they are usually equally well or better seen at ultrasound. Specialised ultrafast CT scanners suitable for cardiac imaging are available in a few centres.

Magnetic resonance imaging

Electronic gating of the standard MRI sequences using an electrocardiogram provides separate images of the heart at various times in the cardiac cycle. With this particular technique, fast flowing blood produces no signal and therefore provides a natural contrast medium (Fig. 3.9). An alternative and more recently introduced technique is so-called 'fast imaging', a technique in which the images are obtained in much shorter times than with the standard techniques. The images are viewed as cine-images and are the equivalent of a tomographic cine-angiogram, usually displayed with the blood white and the heart muscle as darker signal.

Magnetic resonance imaging is capable of providing an immense amount of information, but currently its role is relatively limited because the technique is expensive and the specialised equipment and expertise to obtain high-quality cardiac images are only available in a few centres. Also, the other non-invasive diagnostic techniques, notably ultrasound and radionuclide imaging, provide so much information. MRI does, however, provide unique information. It can show:
- details of complex congenital heart disease;
- details of myocardial thickness and disease;
- details of the great vessels, e.g. dissecting aneurysm;
- pericardial disease;
- intracardiac tumours, which can be shown with great precision, better in many cases than with ultrasound.

Cardiac catheterization and angiography

Catheters can be introduced under fluoroscopic control into the various chambers of the heart and into vessels that lead in and out of these chambers. Contrast injected through such catheters will provide images of the heart and great vessels. Cardiac angiography is a specialized topic which will not be discussed further.

Coronary angiography, which provides detailed information about coronary artery stenoses, occlusions and collateral or anomalous vessels, is widely practised in patients being considered for cardiac surgery, particularly

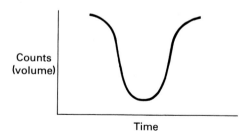

Fig. 3.8 Radionuclide angiocardiography. Graph of counts (ventricular volume) against time.

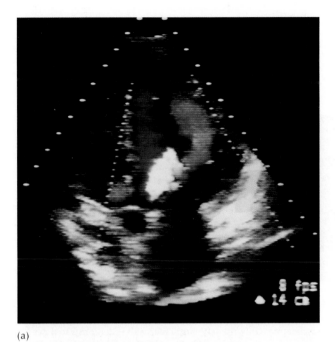

(a)

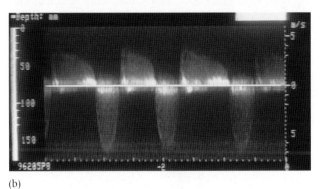

(b)

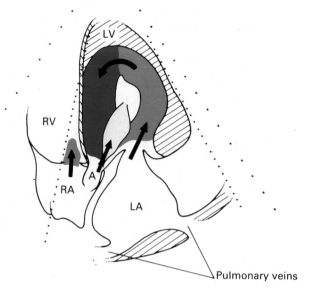

LV

RV

RA

A

LA

Pulmonary veins

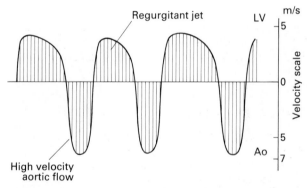

Regurgitant jet

LV

m/s

5

0

Velocity scale

5

Ao

7

High velocity
aortic flow

Plate 3 Aortic valve disease. (a) Colour flow Doppler in a patient with aortic regurgitation. Apical four-chamber view showing turbulent jet (white) of regurgitant blood impinging on anterior leaflet of mitral valve to mix with the stream (red) passing from left atrium to left ventricle. Note change in colour to blue as the stream is directed by the ventricular apex towards the aortic valve. A small portion of right atrial to right ventricular flow is depicted in red. (b) Continuous wave Doppler from the apical position in a patient with aortic stenosis and regurgitation showing a high velocity (7m/s) jet into the aorta. There is immediate diastolic flow back into the left ventricle representing aortic regurgitation.

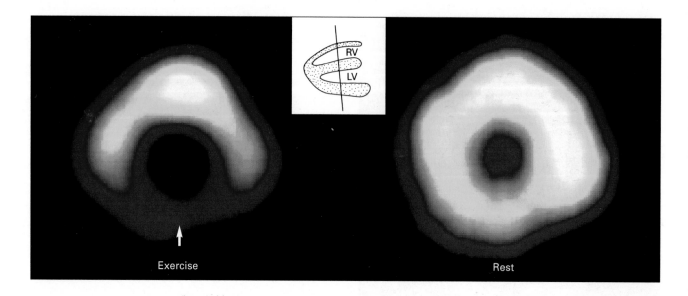

Exercise

Rest

Plate 4 Thallium-201 myocardial perfusion scans. On the exercise scan there is a large area of very reduced uptake in the inferior wall of the left ventricle (arrow) with normal redistribution of the thallium on the rest scan indicating an area of ischaemia. Only the left ventricular wall is demonstrated as there is too little uptake of thallium by the normal right ventricle.

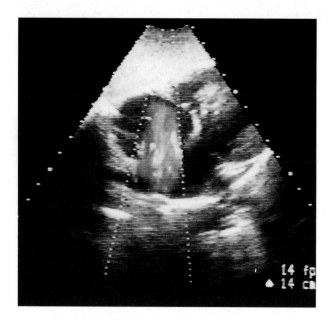

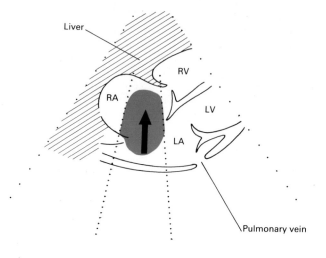

Plate 5 Atrial septal defect. Colour flow Doppler in the subcostal four-chamber view showing substantial flow (red) passing from left to right atrium.

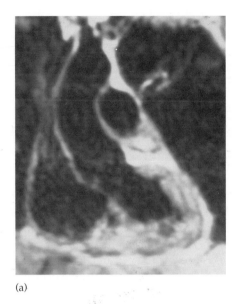

(a)

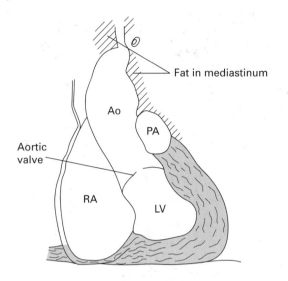

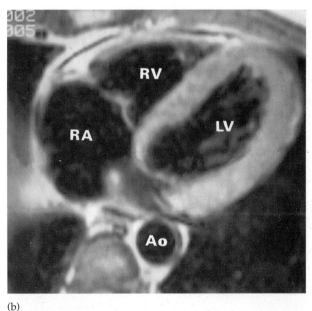

(b)

Fig. 3.9 Magnetic resonance imaging of the normal heart. Note that flowing blood has no signal and appears black. (a) Coronal plane showing the ascending aorta and left ventricle to advantage. (b) Transaxial plane (similar to that used for CT). Ao, aorta; LV, left ventricle; PA, pulmonary artery; RA, right atrium; RV, right ventricle.

for coronary artery revascularization. Catheters are introduced into the femoral artery by the Seldinger technique (see p. 431), or into the brachial artery, usually by cut down, and passed selectively into the orifices of each coronary artery. With transfemoral techniques, separate catheters are usually needed for the left and right sides; 4–7 ml of contrast medium are injected and observed fluoro-scopically with video and cine recordings being made simultaneously.

HEART DISEASE

Evidence of heart disease is given by:
• the size and shape of the heart;

• the pulmonary vessels which provide information on blood flow;

• the lungs, which may show pulmonary oedema.

Heart

Heart size

Overall heart size is most easily assessed on plain chest radiographs. The cardiothoracic ratio (CTR) is a widely used but crude method of measurement; in normal people the transverse diameter of the heart is usually less than half the internal diameter of the chest (Fig. 3.10). Knowing whether or not the heart has increased in size compared with previous films is often more useful than the CTR in isolation. It should, however, be realized that the transverse cardiac diameter varies with the phase of respiration and, to some extent, with the cardiac cycle. Thus changes in trans-

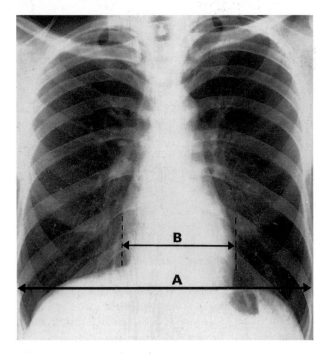

Fig. 3.10 Measurement of heart size. The transverse diameter of the heart is the distance between the two vertical tangents to the heart outline. When the cardiothoracic ratio (CTR) is calculated, the transverse diameter of the heart (B) is divided by the maximum internal diameter of the chest (A).

verse diameter of less than 1.5 cm should be interpreted with caution. An overall increase in heart size may be due to dilatation of one or more cardiac chambers and/or to pericardial effusion.

Chamber hypertrophy and dilatation

The causes of chamber enlargement are given in Table 3.1.

Echocardiography

Echocardiography is the most widely used method of diagnosing dilatation and hypertrophy of individual cardiac chambers. The dimensions of each chamber can be readily assessed. For example, the internal diameter of the left ventricle should not exceed 5.7 cm, and that of the left atrium in the parasternal view should be less than 4.0 cm. Echocardiography also provides accurate estimates of wall thickness; for example, the left ventricular wall and interventricular septum should be between 0.6 and 1.1 cm.

Table 3.1 Common causes of chamber enlargement.

Left atrial enlargement
• mitral stenosis
• mitral incompetence
• left atrial tumour, e.g. myxoma

Right atrial enlargement
• right ventricular failure
• tricuspid stenosis
• tricuspid incompetence

Left ventricular enlargement
• aortic and mitral incompetence
• aortic stenosis and systemic hypertension only *after* left ventricular decompensation has occurred
• ischaemic heart disease and cardiomyopathy of many types, once substantial muscle damage has occurred
• patent ductus arteriosus and ventricular septal defect in cases with large left to right shunts

Right ventricular enlargement
• atrial septal defect
• tricuspid regurgitation
• pulmonary stenosis and pulmonary hypertension only *after* right ventricular decompensation has occurred

Plain films

Diagnosing ventricular enlargement on plain films is fraught with problems. Only one, or at most two, of the borders of either ventricle are visible (Fig. 3.1, p. 104). Also, it is difficult to distinguish ventricular hypertrophy from dilatation when looking at the external contours of the heart. In 'pressure overload' conditions such as systemic hypertension and aortic or pulmonary stenosis, the hypertrophied wall encroaches on the ventricular cavity and there is little change in the external contour of the heart until the ventricle fails. 'Volume overload' conditions such as valvular incompetence, left to right shunts, and damaged heart muscle result in dilatation of the relevant ventricles, which is recognized only as an overall increase in transverse cardiac diameter. A further problem is that enlargement of

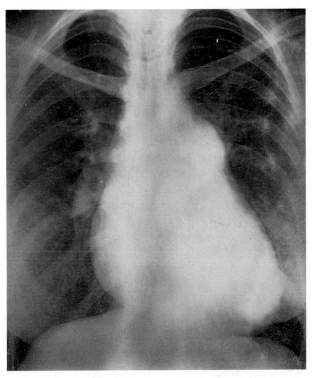

Fig. 3.12 Right ventricular enlargement in an adult with primary pulmonary hypertension. The heart is enlarged with the apex of the heart somewhat lifted off the diaphragm. Note also the features of pulmonary arterial hypertension – enlargement of the main pulmonary artery and hilar arteries with normal vessels within the lungs.

one ventricle affects the shape of the other and it is therefore only occasionally possible to recognize the classic features of left or right ventricular enlargement (Figs 3.11 and 3.12).

Assessment of atrial size on the plain chest radiographs, particularly left atrial enlargement, is easier: the right border of an enlarged left atrium is visible as a double contour adjacent to the right heart border, usually within the main cardiac shadow (Fig. 3.13). The left border is rarely visible although the left atrial appendage, when dilated, is seen as a bulge below the main pulmonary artery on the PA view. With massive enlargement, the left main bronchus is pushed upwards. The posterior margin of the left atrium is best evaluated on the lateral view. Right atrial enlargement causes an increase in the curvature of the right heart border

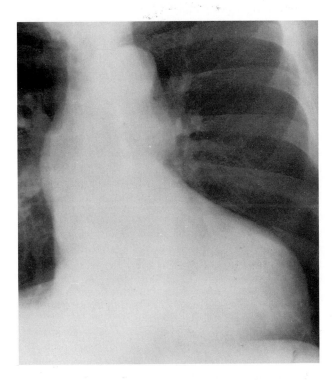

Fig. 3.11 Left ventricular enlargment in a patient with aortic incompetence. The cardiac apex is displaced downwards and to the left. Note also that the ascending aorta causes a bulge of the right mediastinal border – a feature that is almost always seen in significant aortic valve disease.

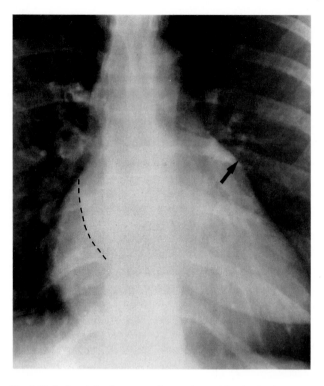

Fig. 3.13 Left atrial enlargement in a patient with mitral valve disease showing the 'double contour sign' (the left atrial border has been drawn in) and dilatation of the left atrial appendage (LAA) (arrow). The enlarged LAA should not be confused with dilatation of the main pulmonary artery. The main pulmonary artery is the segment immediately below the aortic knuckle. The LAA is separated from the aortic knuckle by the main pulmonary artery (compare with Fig. 3.19).

and is often accompanied by enlargement of the superior vena cava.

Valve movement, deformity and calcification

Information regarding valve movement and deformity is best obtained by echocardiography. The mitral valve is particularly well demonstrated. Normally, the leaflets of all the valves are thin and give rise to clearly defined echoes. The anterior leaflet of the mitral valve moves rapidly towards the transducer as it opens at the beginning of diastole. It then wafts backwards to a half-closed position before being pushed forward again by atrial contraction. With the com-

mencement of systole it closes rapidly. The movements of the posterior leaflet mirror those of the anterior leaflet, but the amplitude is less.

The motion of the aortic valve leaflets is less complex. They open abruptly, stay maximally open during the remainder of systole and then close abruptly. The pulmonary and tricuspid valves are more difficult to image – their movements resemble those of the aortic and mitral valves respectively.

Echocardiography is especially valuable in evaluating mitral (Fig. 3.14) and aortic valve disease. Valve stenosis causes thickening of the valve leaflets, restriction of movement and narrowing of the orifice. Calcification, which is often present, is seen as a multiplicity of bright echoes arising within the leaflets (Fig. 3.14a). Valve gradients can be calculated using Doppler estimates for blood velocity and Doppler techniques can also be used to grade the severity of any regurgitation.

The only plain film information directly relating to the morphology of the valves is calcification. Calcification is better seen at fluoroscopy than on plain films. It occurs in the mitral and/or aortic valves in rheumatic heart disease and in the aortic valve alone in adults with congenital aortic stenosis. Valve calcification is easiest to identify on the lateral view. A line at approximately 45° to the horizontal can be drawn from the junction of the diaphragm and sternum obliquely upwards and backwards to the left main bronchus (Fig. 3.15). Calcification in the mitral valve lies behind and below the line, whereas aortic valve calcification lies in front of and above it. Should the line pass through the calcification the smaller portion is ignored, but should it bisect the calcification, serious consideration should be given to the possibility that both valves are calcified. Calcification of the mitral valve ring is occasionally seen in the elderly, and is often associated with mild mitral regurgitation.

Ventricular contractility

Real time echocardiography, radionuclide angiocardiography and cine-MRI are all good non-invasive methods of assessing ventricular wall motion. Two major patterns of *decreased* contractility (hypokinesis) are seen:
• Generalized uniform reduction in contractility, which is usually due to valvular disorder or congestive cardiomy-

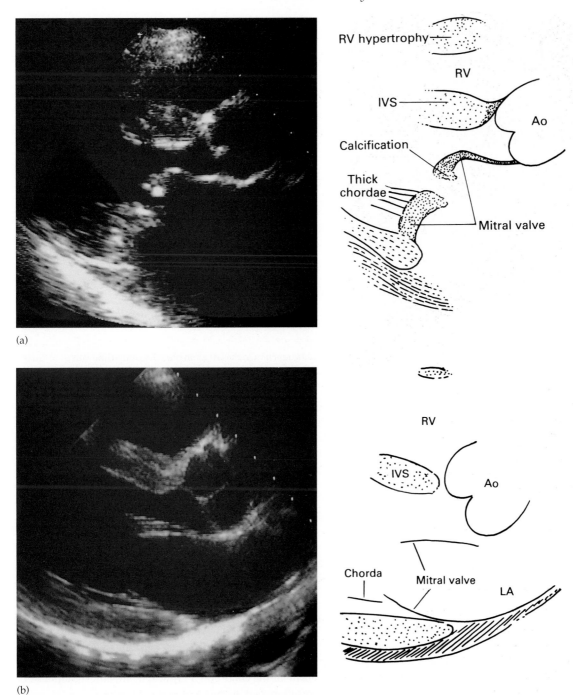

(a)

(b)

Fig. 3.14 Mitral stenosis. Two-dimensional echocardiogram – parasternal long axis view. (a) The mitral valve is markedly thickened and shows calcification. The image is during diastole when the valve should be open, but in this case the orifice is narrowed and opening is impaired. (b) Normal image for comparison. Ao, aorta; IVS, interventricular septum; LA, left atrium; RV, right ventricle. Courtesy of Andrew A. McLeod and Mark J. Managhan.

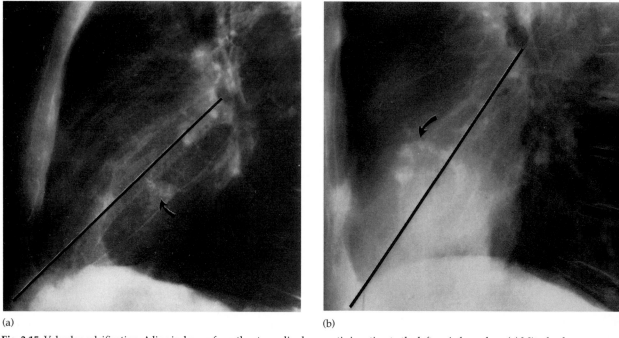

(a) (b)

Fig. 3.15 Valvular calcification. A line is drawn from the sternodiaphragmatic junction to the left main bronchus. (a) Mitral valve calcification. The calcification lies below this line. (b) Aortic valve calcification. The calcification lies above this line.

opathy. The ventricles in these conditions are usually dilated. Occasionally, multivessel coronary artery disease can cause a similar pattern.

• Focal reduction in contractility, which may or may not be accompanied by dilatation, is seen with ischaemic heart disease.

Increased contractility of the left ventricle indicates hypertrophy, which can be primary (hypertrophic cardiomyopathy) or secondary to other conditions such as aortic stenosis or systemic hypertension.

Pericardial disease

Echocardiography is ideally suited to detect pericardial fluid (Fig. 3.16a). Since patients are examined supine, fluid in the pericardial space tends to flow behind the left ventricle and is recognized as an echo-free space between the wall of the left ventricle and the pericardium. A smaller amount of fluid can usually be seen anterior to the right ventricle. Even quantities as small as 20–50 ml of pericardial fluid can be diagnosed by ultrasound. The nature of the fluid cannot usually be ascertained, and needle aspiration of the fluid may be necessary; such aspiration is best performed under ultrasound control. Pericardial effusion can also be recognized at CT (Fig. 3.16b) and MRI, although they are rarely performed primarily for this purpose. Computed tomography and MRI are particularly useful for assessing thickening of the pericardium, whereas echocardiography is poor in this regard.

It is unusual to be able to diagnose a pericardial effusion from the plain chest radiograph. Indeed, a patient may have sufficient pericardial fluid to cause life-threatening tamponade, but only have mild cardiac enlargement with an otherwise normal contour. A marked increase or decrease in the transverse cardiac diameter within a week or two, particularly if no pulmonary oedema occurs, is virtually diagnostic of the condition. Pericardial effusion should also be considered when the heart is greatly enlarged and there are no features to suggest specific chamber enlargement (Fig. 3.17).

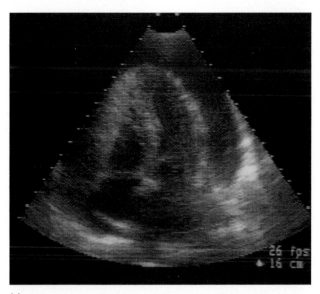

(a)

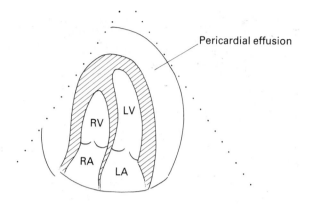

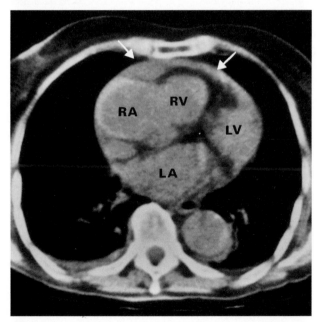

(b)

Fig. 3.16 (a) Large pericardial effusion on an apical four-chamber view echocardiogram. (b) CT scan showing fluid density (arrows) in pericardium. LA, left atrium; LV, left ventricle; RA, right atrium; RV, right ventricle.

Pericardial calcification is seen in up to 50 % of patients with constrictive pericarditis (Fig. 3.18). Calcific constrictive pericarditis is usually postinfective in aetiology, tuberculosis and Coxsackie infections being the common known causes. In many cases no infecting agent can be identified. The calcification occurs patchily in the pericardium, even though the pericardium is thickened and rigid all over the heart. It may be difficult or even impossible to see the calcification on the frontal view. On the lateral film, it is usually maximal along the anterior and inferior pericardial borders. Widespread pericardial calcification is an important sign, because it makes the diagnosis of constrictive pericarditis certain.

Pulmonary vessels

The plain chest film provides a simple method of assessing the pulmonary vasculature. Even though it is not possible to measure the true diameter of the main pulmonary artery on plain film, there are degrees of bulging that permit one to say that it is indeed enlarged (Fig. 3.19). Conversely, the pulmonary artery may be recognizably small. The assessment of the hilar vessels can be more objective since the diameter of the right lower lobe artery can be measured: the diameter at its midpoint is normally between 9 and 16 mm. The size of the vessels within the lungs reflects pulmonary blood flow.

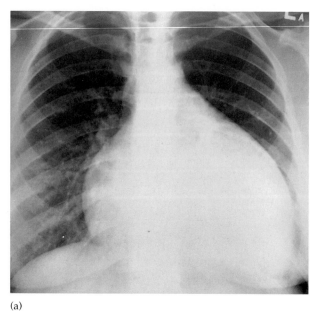

(a)

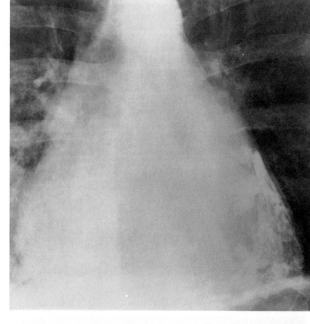

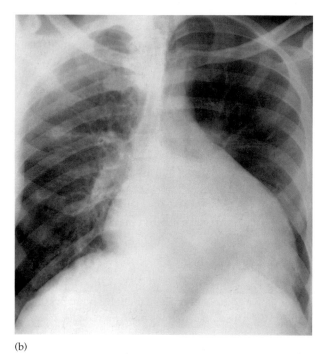

(b)

Fig. 3.17 (a) Pericardial effusion. The heart is greatly enlarged. (Three weeks before, the heart had been normal in shape and size.) The outline is well defined and the shape globular. The lungs are normal. The cause in this case was a viral pericarditis. This appearance of the heart, though highly suggestive of, is not specific to pericardial effusion. (Compare with (b).) (b) Congestive cardiomyopathy causing generalized cardiac dilatation. This appearance can easily be confused radiologically with a pericardial effusion.

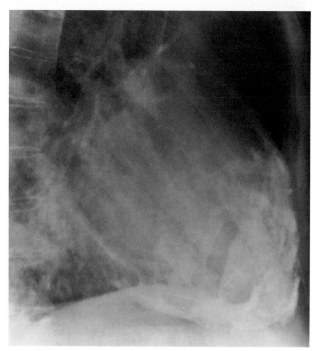

Fig. 3.18 Pericardial calcification in a patient with severe constrictive pericarditis. The distribution of the calcification is typical. It follows the contour of the heart and is maximal anteriorly and inferiorly. As always, it is more difficult to see the calcification on the PA film. (This patient also had pneumonia in the right lower lobe.)

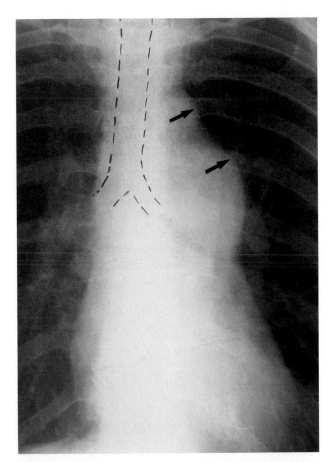

Fig. 3.19 Enlarged main pulmonary artery in a patient with
pulmonary valve stenosis. The bulge of the main pulmonary artery
(lower arrow) is clearly greater than normal and at first glance one
might be deceived into diagnosing enlargement of the aorta.
However, the aortic knuckle is the first 'bump' on the left
mediastinal border (upper arrow). It projects 2.5–3 cm lateral to the
trachea. The pulmonary artery forms the segment immediately
below the aortic knuckle.

There are no generally accepted measurements of normal-
ity, so the diagnosis is based on experience with normal
films.

By observing the size of these various vessels it may be
possible to diagnose one of the following haemodynamic
patterns.

Increased pulmonary blood flow (Fig. 3.20)

Atrial septal defect, ventricular septal defect and patent
ductus arteriosus are the common anomalies in which there
is shunting of blood from the systemic to the pulmonary cir-
cuits (so-called left to right shunts), thereby increasing pulmonary blood flow. The severity of the shunt varies greatly.
In patients with a haemodynamically significant left to right
shunt (2:1 or more), all the vessels from the main pulmonary artery to the periphery of the lungs are large. This
radiographic appearance is sometimes called *pulmonary
plethora*. There is reasonably good correlation between the
size of the vessels on the chest film and the degree of
shunting.

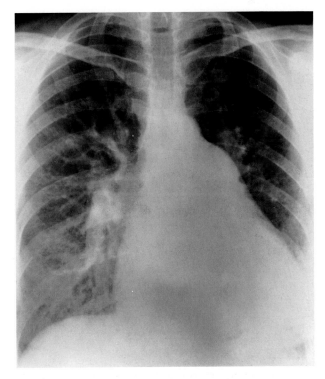

Fig. 3.20 Increased pulmonary blood flow in an atrial septal
defect. Note the large heart and enlargement of the pulmonary
vessels from the main pulmonary artery to the periphery of the
lungs.

Decreased pulmonary blood flow

To be recognizable radiologically, the reduction in pulmonary blood flow must be substantial. The pulmonary vessels are all small, an appearance known as *pulmonary oligaemia*. The commonest cause is the tetralogy of Fallot (see Fig. 3.36, p. 133), where there is obstruction to the right ventricular outflow and a ventricular septal defect which allows right to left shunting of the blood.

Pulmonary valve stenosis only causes oligaemia in extremely severe cases in babies and very young children.

Pulmonary arterial hypertension (Figs 3.12 and 3.21)

The pressure in the pulmonary artery is dependent on cardiac output and pulmonary vascular resistance. The con-ditions that cause significant pulmonary arterial hypertension all increase the resistance of blood flow through the lungs. There are many such conditions including:

• various lung diseases (cor pulmonale);
• pulmonary emboli;
• pulmonary arterial narrowing in response to mitral valve disease or left to right shunts;
• idiopathic pulmonary hypertension.

Pulmonary arterial hypertension has to be severe before it can be diagnosed on plain films and it is difficult to quantify in most cases. The plain chest film features are enlargement of the pulmonary artery and hilar arteries, the vessels within the lung being normal or small. When the pulmonary hypertension is part of Eisenmenger's syndrome (greatly raised pulmonary arterial resistance in association with atrial septal defect, ventricular septal defect or patent

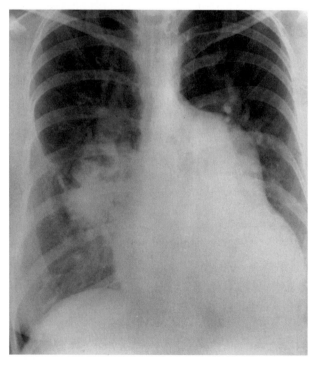

Fig. 3.21 Pulmonary arterial hypertension due, in this case, to an atrial septal defect with Eisenmenger's syndrome. The main pulmonary artery and hilar arteries are massive with an abrupt change in calibre of the vessels at the level of the segmental arteries. Note that the heart is also large.

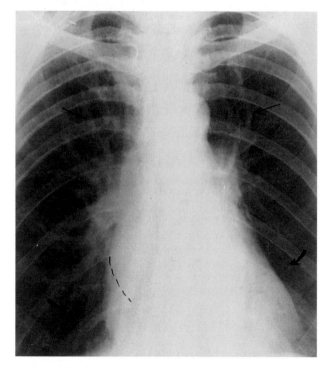

Fig. 3.22 Pulmonary venous hypertension in a patient with mitral valve disease. The upper zone vessels (straight arrows) are larger than the equivalent vessels in the lower zones (curved arrows). This is the reverse of the normal situation. (The left atrial border has been drawn in.)

ductus arteriosus, leading to reversal of the shunt so that it becomes right to left), the vessels within the lungs may also be large, but there is still disproportionate enlargement of the central vessels (Fig. 3.21).

The reason for pulmonary arterial hypertension may be visible on the chest film; in cor pulmonale the lung disease is often radiologically obvious, and in mitral valve disease the other features described on p. 124 will be seen.

Pulmonary venous hypertension (Fig. 3.22)

Mitral valve disease and left ventricular failure are the common causes of elevated pulmonary venous pressure. In the normal upright person, the lower zone vessels are larger than those in the upper zones. In raised pulmonary venous pressure, the upper zone vessels enlarge and in severe cases become larger than those in the lower zones. Eventually, pulmonary oedema will supervene and may obscure the blood vessels.

Pulmonary oedema

The common cardiac conditions causing pulmonary oedema are left ventricular failure and mitral stenosis. Cardiogenic pulmonary oedema occurs when the pulmonary venous pressure rises above 24–25 mmHg (the osmotic

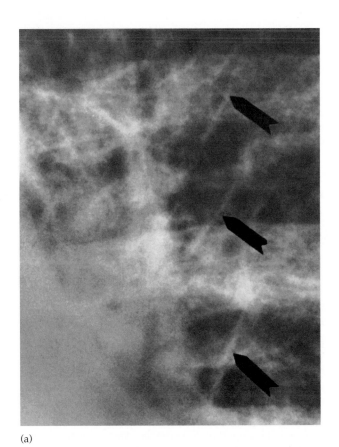

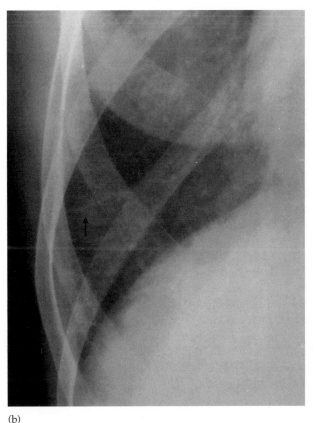

(a)   (b)

Fig. 3.23 Septal lines in interstitial pulmonary oedema. (a) Left upper zone showing the septal lines known as Kerley A lines (arrowed) in a patient with acute left ventricular failure following a myocardial infarction. Note that these lines are narrower and sharper than the adjacent blood vessels. (b) Right costophrenic angle showing the septal lines known as Kerley B lines in a patient with mitral stenosis. Note that these oedematous septa are horizontal non-branching lines which reach the pleura. One such line is arrowed.

pressure of plasma). Initially, the oedema is confined to the interstitial tissues of the lung, but if it becomes more severe fluid will also collect in the alveoli. Both interstitial and alveolar pulmonary oedema are recognizable on plain chest films.

Interstitial oedema (Fig. 3.23)

There are many septa in the lungs which are invisible on the normal chest film because they consist of little more than a sheet of connective tissue containing very small blood and lymph vessels. When thickened by oedema, the peripherally located septa may be seen as line shadows. These lines, known as Kerley B lines, named after the radiologist who first described them, are horizontal lines never more than 2 cm long seen laterally in the lower zones. They reach the lung edge and are therefore readily distinguished from blood vessels, which never extend into the outer centimetre of the lung. Other septa radiate towards the hila in the mid and upper zones (Kerley A lines). These are much thinner than the adjacent blood vessels and are 3–4 cm in length. Another sign of interstitial oedema is that the outline of the blood vessels may become indistinct owing to oedema collecting around them. This loss of clarity is a difficult sign to evaluate and it may only be recognized by looking at follow-up films after the oedema has cleared. Fissures may appear thickened because oedema may collect against them.

Alveolar oedema (Fig. 3.24)

Alveolar oedema is a more severe form of oedema in which the fluid collects in the alveoli. It is almost always bilateral, involving all the lobes. The pulmonary shadowing is usually maximal close to the hila and fades out peripherally leaving a relatively clear zone that may contain septal lines, around the edge of the lobes. This pattern of oedema is sometimes referred to as the 'butterfly' or 'bat's wing' pattern.

Aorta

With increasing age the aorta elongates. Elongation necessarily involves unfolding, because the aorta is fixed at the aortic valve and at the diaphragm. This unfolding results in the ascending aorta deviating to the right and the descend-

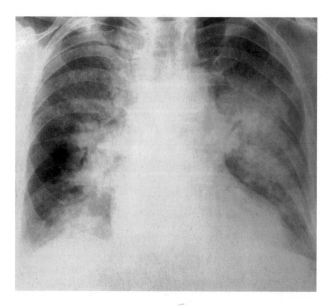

Fig. 3.24 Alveolar oedema in a patient with acute left ventricular failure following a myocardial infarction. The oedema fluid is concentrated in the more central portion of the lungs leaving a relatively clear zone peripherally. Note that all the lobes are fairly equally involved.

ing aorta to the left. Aortic unfolding can easily be confused with aortic dilatation.

True dilatation of the ascending aorta may be due to aneurysm formation or secondary to aortic regurgitation, (Fig. 3.11, p. 113) aortic stenosis or systemic hypertension.

The two common causes of *aneurysm* of the descending aorta are atheroma and aortic dissection. A rarer cause is previous trauma, usually following a severe deceleration injury. The diagnosis of aortic aneurysm may be obvious on plain film but substantial dilatation is needed before a bulge of the right mediastinal border can be recognized. Atheromatous aneurysms invariably show calcification in their walls and this calcification is usually recognizable on plain film. Computed tomography with intravenous contrast enhancement is very useful when aortic aneurysms are assessed. It is important to know the extent of aortic dissections (Fig. 3.25) as those involving the ascending aorta are treated surgically while those confined to the descending aorta are usually treated conservatively with hypotensive drugs. Standard echocardiography shows dissection of the aortic root but transoesophageal echocardiography shows

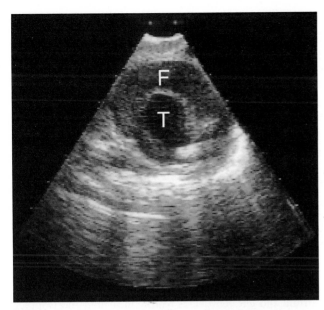

(a)

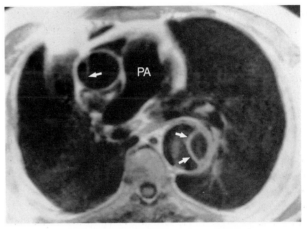

(c)

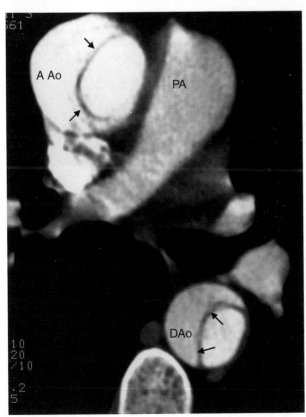

(b)

Fig. 3.25 Aortic dissection. (a) Transoesophageal echocardiogram showing the true (T) and false (F) lumina in the descending aorta. (b) CT scan showing the displaced intima (arrows) separating the true and false lumina in the ascending and descending aorta. (c) MRI scan showing the displaced intima in the ascending and descending aorta (arrows). AAo, ascending aorta; DAo, descending aorta; PA, pulmonary artery.

dissections distal to the aortic root and in the descending aorta as well. Dissecting aneurysms can also be shown with CT and MRI and these non-invasive techniques have largely replaced aortography, which is only performed in selected cases.

Two *congenital anomalies* of the aorta may be visible on plain films of the chest: coarctation (see p. 133) and right-sided aortic arch, a condition that is sometimes seen in association with intracardiac malformations, notably tetralogy of Fallot, pulmonary atresia and truncus arteriosus. It can also be an isolated and clinically insignificant abnormality. In right aortic arch, the soft tissue shadow of the arch is seen to the right, instead of to the left, of the lower trachea.

Specific cardiac disorders

Heart failure

Signs of heart failure may be seen on plain chest radiographs (Fig. 3.26). (These may coexist with the specific disorders described in the remainder of the chapter). One or more of the following signs may be seen:

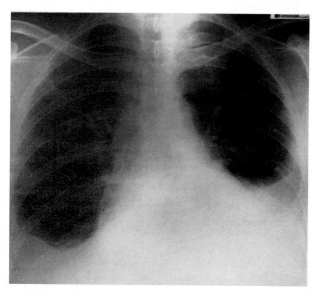

Fig. 3.26 Congestive cardiac failure. There are large bilateral pleural effusions. The heart is enlarged although it is difficult to measure it precisely because the pleural fluid obscures its borders.

• cardiac enlargement, with or without specific chamber enlargement;
• evidence of raised pulmonary venous pressure, namely enlargement of the vessels in the upper zones of the lung;
• evidence of pulmonary oedema;
• pleural effusions, which are usually bilateral, often larger on the right than the left, and if unilateral are almost always right sided. (In acute left ventricular failure small effusions are seen in the costophrenic angles running up the lateral chest wall. This fluid may, in fact, be oedema in the lungs rather than true pleural effusions.)

Valvular heart disease

Valve stenosis and incompetence often coexist. It is, however, convenient to describe each separately.

Mitral stenosis. At *echocardiography*, the important features of mitral stenosis are enlargement of the left atrium, thickening of the valve leaflets and restriction of valve movement (Fig. 3.27a). The left atrial cavity should be routinely examined for thrombi. Calcifications of the valve appear as intensely echoreflective areas. The ability to measure the orifice of the mitral valve during diastole is a major advantage of two-dimensional echocardiography; a valve area of less than 1 cm² is classified as 'severe stenosis'. Right ventricular hypertrophy and dilatation may be present in patients whose mitral stenosis has resulted in pulmonary arterial hypertension. With Doppler techniques it is possible to measure the blood flow through the valve and so predict the gradient across the mitral valve. Left atrial myxoma, which can mimic mitral stenosis clinically, can be readily excluded by echocardiography.

The *plain chest radiograph* (Fig. 3.27b) reveals left atrial enlargement, possibly calcification of the mitral valve and evidence of raised pulmonary venous pressure and pulmonary oedema. Unless pulmonary hypertension develops, the transverse cardiac diameter is often normal.

Mitral regurgitation. At *echocardiography*, the size of the left atrium and left ventricle is readily measured and Doppler techniques can be used to grade the severity of regurgitation. The appearance of a regurgitant valve depends on the cause. In cases of rheumatic valvular regurgitation, there is thickening of the valve cusps, whereas in conditions such as regurgitation secondary to left ventricular dilatation or rupture of the papilla, the valve cusps show no thickening. The abnormal motion seen in mitral valve prolapse, a condition in which there is myxomatous degeneration of the mitral valve, is readily detected with two-dimensional echocardiography and any associated regurgitation can be graded with Doppler techniques.

As with mitral stenosis, left atrial enlargement and evidence of raised pulmonary venous pressure are the important signs of mitral regurgitation on the *plain chest radiograph*. An important difference from mitral stenosis is the presence of left ventricular enlargement.

Aortic stenosis. The *echocardiographic* hallmark of aortic stenosis is thickening of the aortic valve leaflets with narrowing of the orifice. The orifice can be measured; a valve area of less than 1 cm² indicates 'severe' stenosis. Again, Doppler ultrasound can be used to quantify the gradient.

The major features of aortic stenosis on *plain chest radiograph* are aortic valve calcification and poststenotic dilatation of the ascending aorta (Fig. 3.28). It is rare for an adult patient to have a severe gradient across the aortic valve

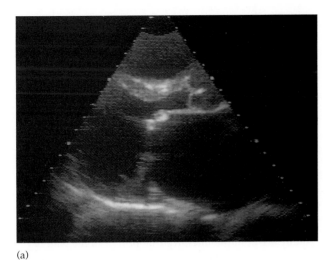

(a)

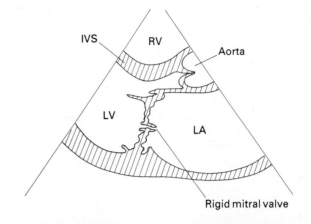

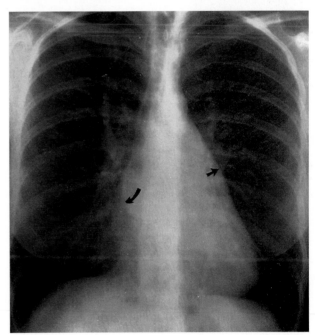

(b)

Fig. 3.27 Mitral stenosis. (a) Parasternal long axis view echocardiogram. Note the thickened mitral valve, which has hardly opened during diastole. (b) Plain film showing enlarged left atrium as a double contour at the right heart border (curved arrow). The left atrial appendage is also enlarged (straight arrow). Note how the upper zone vessels are larger than those in the lower zones. The overall size of the heart is not increased. IVS, interventricular septum; LA, left atrium; LV, left ventricle; RV, right ventricle.

unless aortic valve calcification is present. Recognizable left ventricular enlargement and raised pulmonary venous, pressure are late signs indicating left ventricular failure.

Aortic regurgitation. Echocardiography can demonstrate the regurgitant jet (Plate 3a) and it is possible to grade the severity of regurgitation using Doppler techniques (Plate 3b, opposite p. 110). Diastolic fluttering of the mitral valve secondary to the regurgitant jet can be seen and is an indirect sign of the condition. Another major use of echocardiography in aortic regurgitation is to show left ventricular volume and contraction.

On *plain film* the ascending aorta is dilated and aortic regurgitation, when severe, leads to enlargement of the left

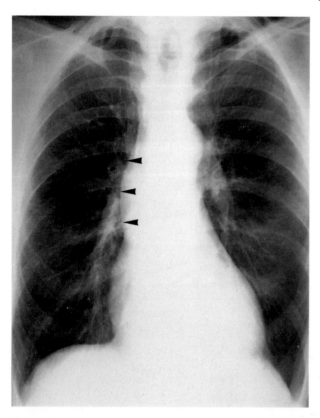

Fig. 3.28 Aortic stenosis showing poststenotic dilatation of the aorta (arrows). Despite the presence of a severe gradient there is little if any, cardiac enlargement. The lateral view (see Fig. 3.15b) showed heavy calcification of the aortic valve – a feature not visible on the frontal view in this instance.

ventricle which can be recognised early in the course of the disease (Fig. 3.11, p. 113).

Pulmonary stenosis. This condition is discussed under congenital heart disease on p. 131.

Tricuspid stenosis and regurgitation. Both of these conditions give rise to enlargement of the right atrium and superior vena cava. They are almost never seen as isolated abnormalities and the features of coexistent mitral valve disease or pulmonary hypertension often dominate the picture. The echocardiographic features are similar in principle to those seen in mitral valve disease.

Subacute bacterial endocarditis

The only imaging techniques that are capable of diagnosing the infection itself, as opposed to the accompanying valvular regurgitation, are echocardiography and MRI. They can demonstrate the infective vegetations of the endocardial surfaces, particularly on the valves, as well as any adjacent abscess formation (Fig. 3.29). Vegetations on prosthetic valves are extremely difficult to identify.

Left atrial myxoma and other intracardiac masses

Intracardiac tumours are rare: left atrial myxoma is the most frequently encountered. It is a benign tumour which usually arises in the interatrial septum or in the wall of the left atrium. As it enlarges, it becomes pedunculated to float in the left atrial cavity. The myxoma may therefore interfere with the function of the mitral valve and mimic mitral stenosis or regurgitation both clinically and on plain chest radiographs. Echocardiography has proved to be an excellent tool for its diagnosis. A mass of echoes is seen in the cavity of the left atrium just behind the mitral valve (Fig. 3.30). The mass usually prolapses into the mitral valve orifice during diastole. The only differential diagnosis is left atrial thrombus in patients with rheumatic mitral stenosis. MRI has also proved to be an excellent method of demonstrating left atrial myxoma and other intracardiac tumours.

Ischaemic heart disease

Most patients with angina or myocardial infarction have a normal plain chest film and a normal echocardiogram. The signs which may be present on *plain chest radiograph* include:
• Signs of raised pulmonary venous pressure and pulmonary oedema. The chest radiograph is a sensitive method of detecting these phenomena; indeed it is often more reliable than the physical examination.
• Cardiac enlargement and aneurysm formation. It is only when there is substantial muscle damage that cardiac enlargement occurs. Usually, there are no specific features to the cardiac contour, but an aneurysm may occasionally be recognised on plain film (Fig. 3.31a). Myocardial infarcts occasionally calcify, usually in association with aneurysm formation.

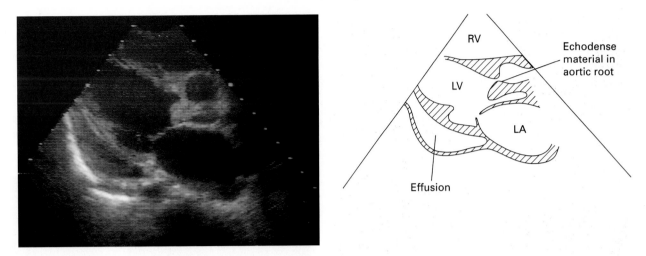

Fig. 3.29 Aortic root abscess and pericardial effusion: parasternal long axis view echocardiogram. Note the echodense material in the aortic root. LA, left atrium; LV, left ventricle; RV, right ventricle.

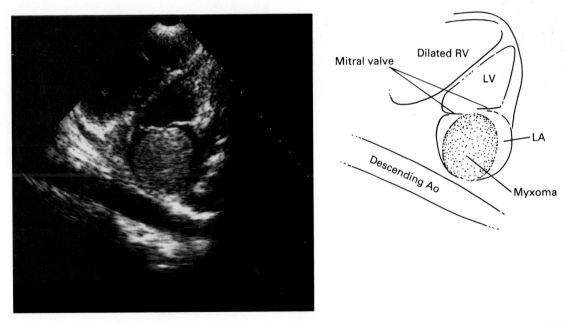

Fig. 3.30 Left atrial myxoma shown by two-dimensional echocardiography – modified apical four-chamber view. Ao, aorta; LA, left atrium; LV, left ventricle. Courtesy of Andrew A. McLeod and Mark J. Monaghan.

• Atheromatous calcification may be seen in the coronary arteries but, as elsewhere in the body, arterial calcification, though indicating the presence of atheroma, is a poor indicator of its severity.

Two-dimensional *echocardiography* allows one to observe the volume of the left ventricle and the motion of the various segments of its wall. Areas of diminished movement from infarction can be demonstrated. A major use of echocardiography is to show aneurysms which appear as outwardly bulging thin areas of the myocardium (Fig. 3.31b). They most commonly involve the anterior wall and upper septum of the left ventricle. Blood clot contained within an aneurysm can be recognized as numerous constant echoes in the cavity of the aneurysm.

Thallium-201 *myocardial scintigraphy* allows one to determine areas of myocardial ischaemia and from their location

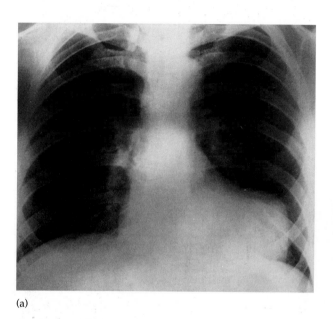

(a)

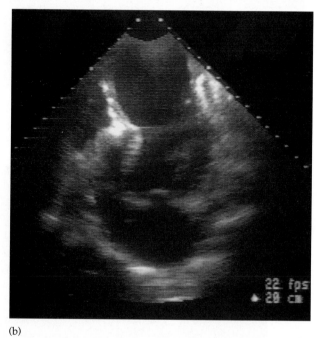

(b)

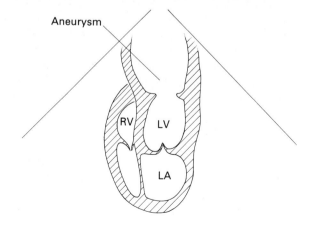

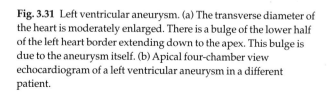

Fig. 3.31 Left ventricular aneurysm. (a) The transverse diameter of the heart is moderately enlarged. There is a bulge of the lower half of the left heart border extending down to the apex. This bulge is due to the aneurysm itself. (b) Apical four-chamber view echocardiogram of a left ventricular aneurysm in a different patient.

it is sometimes possible to predict which of the coronary arteries is compromised. Thallium scanning not only enables a diagnosis of ischaemia to be made but it can also help distinguish ischaemic muscle from scar due to infarction. Ischaemic areas seen on the exercise scan as regions of reduced uptake show normal activity on the resting scan (Plate 4, opposite p. 110). Infarcted areas in which there is little, if any, remaining viable myocardium will show a persisting defect on the resting scan. This ability to distinguish ischaemia and infarction may be useful when planning cardiac surgery.

Radionuclide gated blood pool studies are sometimes performed as an alternative to ^{201}Tl scintigraphy in order to diagnose myocardial ischaemia. Ischaemic but viable areas may move normally at rest but not on exercise, whereas infarcted areas move poorly both at rest and on exercise. Alternatively, changes in ejection fraction between rest and exercise can be used. A fall of greater than 5% on exercise indicates ischaemia, provided valvular disease or cardiomyopathy are excluded. A ventricular aneurysm can be readily recognized by viewing the gated blood pool studies. It appears as an area of paradoxical movement which bulges outward when the remainder of the ventricle contracts.

Acute myocardial infarcts can be imaged by radionuclide techniques. In practice, however, these tests are rarely performed. Technetium-99 m pyrophosphate – the bone scanning agent – may concentrate in necrotic tissue, including myocardial infarcts, producing a 'hot spot'.

Magnetic resonance imaging has been used to show areas of myocardial thinning following infarction and even to show altered signal in subacute infarction, but there is little clinical utility as yet for MRI in ischaemic heart disease.

The state of the coronary arteries can be determined by coronary angiography. Each artery is examined separately by multiple views to determine the extent of coronary artery occlusions and stenoses (Fig. 3.32). From this information the appropriate treatment can be decided; this may be bypass surgery or balloon dilatation of the artery.

Coronary arteriography is usually combined with a left ventricular angiogram when a cine film is taken of contrast injected directly into the left ventricle. Left ventricular angiography shows the contractility of the left ventricle and gives an indication of left ventricular function as well as showing abnormalities of wall movement and any left

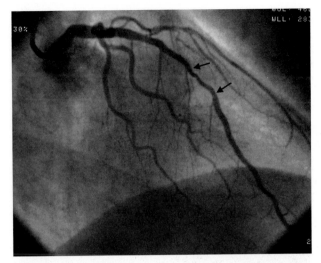

(a)

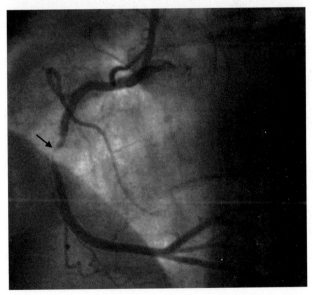

(b)

Fig. 3.32 Coronary artery disease. (a) Left coronary artery injection showing a moderate stenosis between the arrows in the mid left anterior descending artery. (b) Right coronary artery injection showing tight stenosis (arrow) of the mid right coronary artery.

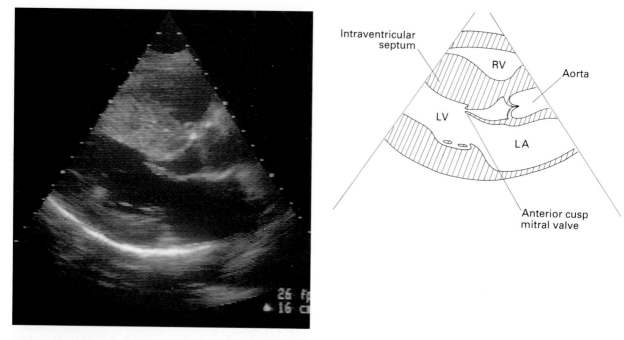

Fig. 3.33 Hypertrophic cardiomyopathy, parasternal long axis view echocardiogram. Note very thickened septum (almost 3 cm) and thickened ventricular walls. The anterior cusp of the mitral valve contacts the septum during diastole – a diagnostic feature of this condition. LA, left atrium; LV, left ventricle; RV, right ventricle.

ventricular aneurysm. Concomitant mitral incompetence, which may occur after myocardial infarction, will be shown and is important information if surgery is planned.

Hypertensive heart disease and other myocardial problems

As discussed previously, ventricular hypertrophy without dilatation does not cause recognizable abnormality on plain chest films. Therefore, in systemic hypertension and various forms of cardiomyopathy the chest x-ray only becomes abnormal once ventricular dilatation has taken place. If there is a rise in left ventricular end-diastolic pressure, moderate left atrial enlargement and the signs of elevation of the pulmonary venous pressure may be seen. The shape of the heart is the same regardless of the cause of the myocardial disorder. The aorta is, however, large only in systemic hypertension.

Echocardiography in systemic hypertension shows symmetrical increase in the thickness of the left ventricular wall with a normal aortic valve. Once decompensation occurs, the cavity will enlarge. The pattern of hypertrophy is different in idiopathic hypertrophic cardiomyopathy (also known as idiopathic hypertrophic subaortic stenosis or IHSS), in which the hypertrophy is much greater in the ventricular septum than in the free wall. This asymmetrical septal hypertrophy is diagnostic of the condition (Fig. 3.33).

Congenital heart disease

There are a large number of congenital malformations of the heart and great vessels. Frequently they are multiple. Some conditions may be detected antenatally (p. 280). Echocardiography, MRI or angiocardiography are usually necessary for their elucidation, topics which are beyond the scope of this book. Only the plain film findings in a few selected disorders are discussed here. A major role of the

	Plethora	Normal vascularity	Oligaemia
Table 3.2 Commoner congenital heart disease: diagnosis based on blood vessel pattern.	*Not cyanosed* ASD ⎤ VSD ⎬ shunt > 2:1 PDA ⎦	ASD ⎤ VSD ⎬ shunt < 2:1 PDA ⎦ Pulmonary stenosis Coarctation of aorta	Severe pulmonary stenosis
	Cyanosed Transposition of great arteries Total anomalous pulmonary venous drainage Truncus arteriosus Eisenmenger ASD, VSD, PDA	Fallot's tetralogy Pulmonary atresia	Fallot's tetralogy Pulmonary atresia Tricuspid atresia

ASD, atrial septal defect; VSD, ventricular septal defect; PDA, patent ductus arteriosus.

chest radiograph is to assess pulmonary vascularity (Table 3.2).

Atrial septal defect, ventricular septal defect and patent ductus arteriosus. All these conditions give rise to cardiac enlargement and enlargement of the main pulmonary artery, large hilar arteries and pulmonary plethora (Fig. 3.34). These signs are usually only visible when the shunt through the defect is 2:1 or more. The value of plain film radiology is that it provides a simple method of estimating the degree of shunting in a patient known to have a left to right shunt. It is, however, of limited value in making a diagnostic distinction between the three major causes of left to right shunt. In cases of clinical diagnostic doubt (notably pulmonary stenosis which can be confused with atrial septal defect, and mitral regurgitation which can be confused with a ventricular septal defect), the presence of plethora indicates that the patient has a left to right shunt.

Echocardiography shows the size of the various cardiac chambers and a defect in the atrial or ventricular septum can be visualized directly. Even if the defect is not seen it may be possible to make the correct diagnosis by knowing which chambers are enlarged, e.g. absence of left ventricular enlargement in the presence of substantially increased pulmonary flow suggests an atrial septal defect. Colour Doppler is particularly useful in demonstrating septal defects (see Plate 5, opposite p. 326).

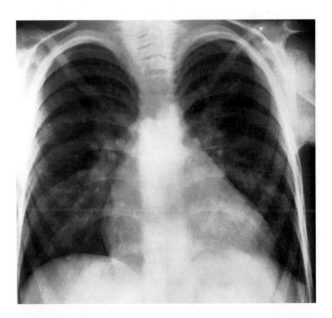

Fig. 3.34 Ventricular septal defect in a child. The heart is enlarged and there is obvious enlargement of the pulmonary vessels. The left to right shunt in this case was 3:1.

Pulmonary valve stenosis. Stenosis of the pulmonary valve can give rise to a specific appearance on plain chest radiography, namely enlargement of the main pulmonary artery and enlargement of the left pulmonary artery, the remain-

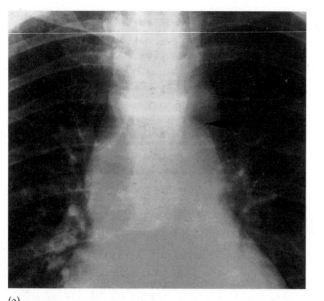

(a)

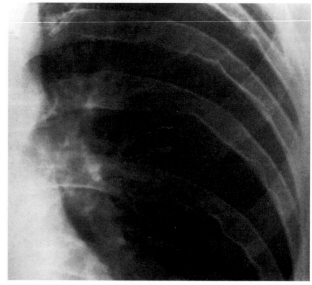

(b)

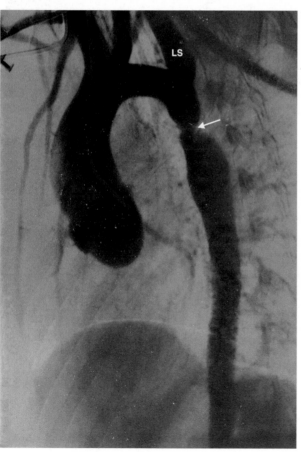

(c)

Fig. 3.35 Coarctation of the aorta. (a) Abnormal aortic knuckle: the lower arrow points to the poststenotic dilatation of the aorta immediately below the coarctation. The upper arrow indicates the dilated left subclavian artery above the coarctation. (b) Rib notching: portion of the ribs showing notching on the under surfaces. (c) Aortogram showing a coarctation (arrow) as a narrowing of the aorta just distal to the left subclavian artery (LS).

der of the lung vasculature being normal. The dilatation of these vessels is due to the phenomenon of poststenotic dilatation. Usually, the heart is not enlarged.

Coarctation of the aorta (Fig. 3.35). An abnormal aortic arch is the commonest finding in coarctation of the aorta. The site of narrowing, which most commonly occurs just distal to the left subclavian artery, may be seen on a plain film as an indentation and there is sometimes a bulge above the coarctation from dilatation of the left subclavian artery, as well as bulge below, due to poststenotic dilatation of the aorta. The heart is often enlarged, as is the ascending aorta, due to the long-standing hypertension.

Rib notching is a frequent sign in older childhood and in adults. It is due to the enlargement of intercostal arteries which act as collateral vessels, and which produce one or more small corticated indentations on the inferior margins of the posterior halves of the ribs from the third or fourth ribs downwards. The coarctation itself can be shown by angiography or MRI.

Tetralogy of Fallot. Fallot's tetralogy consists essentially of a ventricular septal defect and right ventricular outflow obstruction, usually subvalvar or valvar stenosis. Right ventricular hypertrophy and the aorta overriding the ventricular septal defect are the other features that make up the tetralogy.

Approximately half the cases have a normal chest film. The abnormal radiological signs, when present, are an upturned cardiac apex and a bay in the region of the main pulmonary artery (Fig. 3.36), a shape sometimes referred to as a 'boot-shaped heart'. An important diagnostic feature is oligaemia of the lungs. The aorta is right-sided in 25% of patients.

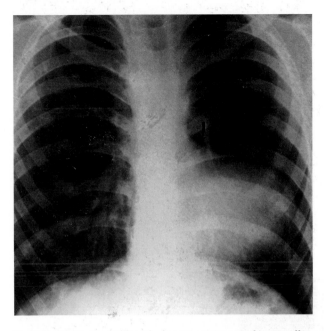

Fig. 3.36 Tetralogy of Fallot. The heart is not increased in overall size but shows a very abnormal outline. The apex is lifted up and there is a bay in the region of the main pulmonary artery (arrow). This combination is known as 'coeur en sabot' (boot-shaped heart). The aorta is right-sided as it is in 25% of cases. The hilar vessels are very small and the vessels in the lungs are also small.

4

Plain Abdomen

The standard plain films of the abdomen are the supine and erect AP views. An alternative to the erect AP view in patients unable to sit or stand is to take a lateral decubitus view (i.e. an AP film with the patient lying on his or her side). This view, like the erect view, uses a horizontal x-ray beam. The main purpose of horizontal beam films is to detect air–fluid levels and free intraperitoneal air.

How to look at a plain abdominal film (Fig. 4.1)

- Relatively large amounts of gas are usually present in the stomach and colon in a normal patient. The stomach can be readily identified by its location above the transverse colon, by the band-like shadows of the gastric rugae in the supine view, and by the air–fluid level beneath the left hemidiaphragm in the erect view. The duodenum often contains air and shows a fluid level. There may be some gas in the normal small bowel, but it is rarely sufficient to outline the whole of a loop. Short fluid levels in the small and large bowel are normal. Fluid levels become abnormal when they are seen in dilated loops of bowel or when they are very numerous. If the bowel is dilated it is important to try and decide which portion is involved.
- Look for any gas outside the lumen of the bowel. Its location and pattern often give valuable diagnostic information.
- Look for ascites and any soft tissue masses in the abdomen and pelvis.
- If there is any calcification try to locate exactly where it lies.
- Identify the liver and spleen. The liver is seen as a homogeneous opacity in the right upper quadrant, usually extending into the left upper quadrant. Occasionally, there is a tongue-like extension of the right lobe into the right iliac fossa. This is a normal variant known as a *Reidl's lobe* and should not be confused with generalized liver enlargement. The lower border of the liver is often difficult to see but its position can be predicted by the position of the gas in the hepatic flexure and transverse colon.
- Identify the borders of the kidneys, bladder and psoas muscles.

Dilatation of the bowel

The distinction between dilatation of the large and small bowel can be difficult. It depends on the appearance of the dilated bowel, the position and number of the bowel loops, and the presence of solid faeces. The presence of solid faeces is a useful and reliable indication of the position of the colon.

The colon can be recognized by its haustra, which usually form incomplete bands across the colonic gas shadows. They are always present in the ascending and transverse colon but may be absent distal to the splenic flexure. When the jejunum is dilated the valvulae conniventes can be identified. They are always closer together than the colonic haustra and cross the width of the bowel, often giving rise to the appearance known as 'a stack of coins' (Fig. 4.2). Problems may be encountered in distinguishing the lower ileum from the sigmoid colon because both may be smooth in outline. The radius of curvature of the loops is sometimes helpful in this respect: the tighter the curve the more likely it is to be a dilated loop of small bowel.

The small bowel usually lies in the centre of the abdomen within the 'frame' of the large bowel, but the sigmoid and transverse colon are frequently very redundant and may

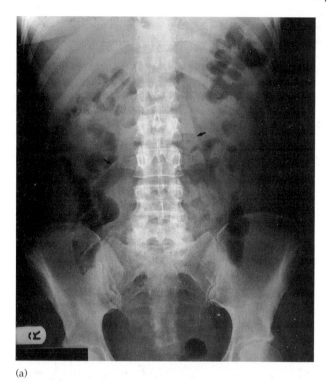

(a)

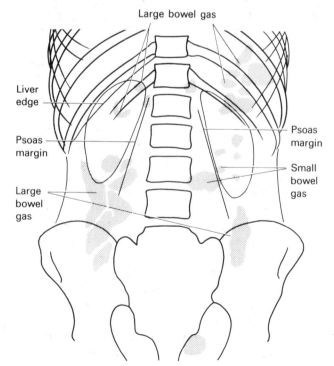

Large bowel gas

Liver edge

Psoas margin

Large bowel gas

Psoas margin

Small bowel gas

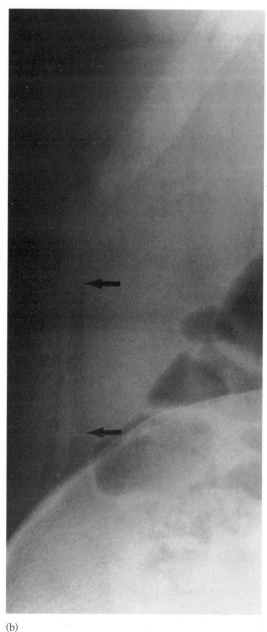

(b)

Fig. 4.1 Normal plain abdominal film. (a) Normal abdomen. The arrows point to the lateral borders of the psoas muscles. The renal outlines are obscured by the overlying colon; (b) Normal extraperitoneal fat stripe. Part of the right flank showing the layer of extraperitoneal fat (arrows) which indicates the position of the peritoneum.

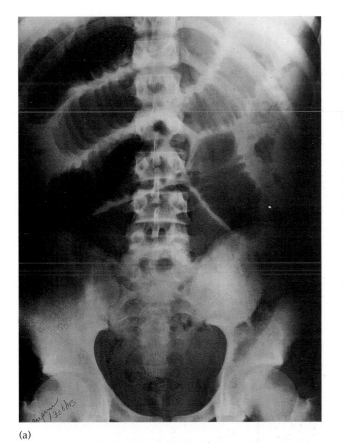

(a)

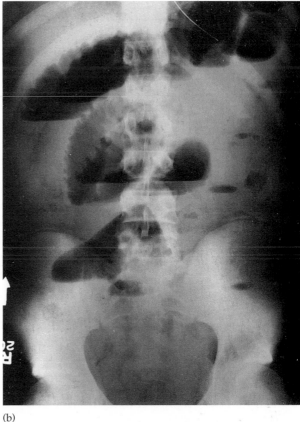

(b)

Fig. 4.2 Small bowel obstruction due to adhesions. (a) Supine. (b) Erect. The jejunal loops are markedly dilated and show air–fluid levels in the erect film. The jejunum is recognized by the presence of valvulae conniventes. The 'stack of coins' appearance is well demonstrated in the supine film. Note the large bowel contains less gas than normal.

also lie in the centre of the abdomen, particularly when dilated.

The number of dilated loops is a valuable distinguishing feature between small and large bowel dilatation, because even with a very redundant colon the numerous layered loops that are so often seen with small bowel dilatation are not present.

Dilatation of the bowel occurs in mechanical obstruction, paralytic ileus, acute ischaemia and inflammatory bowel disease. The radiological diagnosis of these phenomena depends mainly on the distribution of the dilated loops. The following patterns can be recognized:

• *Mechanical obstruction of the small bowel* (Fig. 4.2) causes small bowel dilatation with a normal or reduced calibre to the large bowel.

• *Obstruction of the large bowel* (Fig. 4.3) causes dilatation of the colon down to the point of obstruction, and may be accompanied by small bowel dilatation if the ileocaecal valve becomes incompetent.

• In *generalized paralytic ileus* (Fig. 4.4) both the large and the small bowel are dilated. The dilatation often extends down into the sigmoid colon and gas may be present in the rectum. It may be difficult to differentiate such cases from low large bowel obstruction.

• *Local peritonitis* often results in dilatation of the loops adjacent to the inflammatory process, giving rise to the so-called 'sentinel loops' which may be seen, for example, in appendicitis and pancreatitis.

• Patients with *gastroenteritis* may show a number of patterns: some patients have a normal film and some show

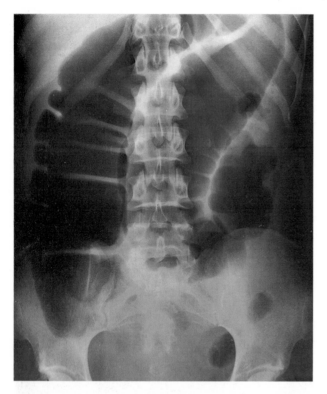

Fig. 4.3 Large bowel obstruction due to carcinoma at the splenic flexure. There is marked dilatation of the large bowel from the caecum to the splenic flexure.

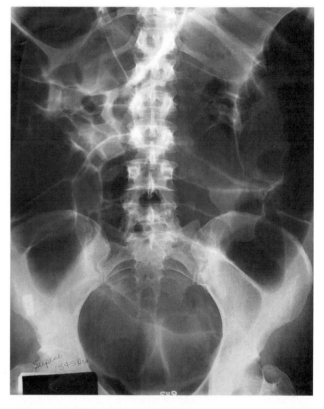

Fig. 4.4 Paralytic ileus. There is considerable dilatation of the whole of the large bowel extending well down into the pelvis. Small bowel dilatation is also seen.

excess fluid levels without dilatation, whereas some mimic paralytic ileus and others small bowel obstruction.

• *Small bowel infarction* may mimic both obstruction of the small bowel and obstruction of the large bowel.

• *Closed loop obstruction.* The diagnosis depends on whether the loop in question contains air. If it does, as for example in a caecal or sigmoid volvulus, the dilated loop is seen filled with gas in a characteristic shape (Fig. 4.5). If the closed loop is filled with fluid it may not be visible – the common situation in most obstructed hernias.

• *Toxic dilatation of the colon.* Should this occur in patients with ulcerative colitis, or more rarely Crohn's disease, the large bowel becomes distended (Fig. 4.6). Usually, the dilatation is maximal in the transverse colon; indeed, the descending colon may be narrower than normal. The haustra are lost or grossly abnormal and the swollen islands of mucosa between the ulcers can be recognized as poly-

poid shadows. If the transverse colon is more than 6 cm in diameter in a patient with colitis, toxic dilatation should be strongly suspected.

Gas outside the lumen of the bowel

Gas outside the lumen of the bowel is abnormal. Its location can usually be assessed by plain films.

Gas in the peritoneal cavity (Fig. 4.7)

Gas is almost always due to perforation of the gastrointestinal tract, or follows surgical intervention in the abdomen. The most common cause of spontaneous pneumoperitoneum is a perforated peptic ulcer and two-thirds of such

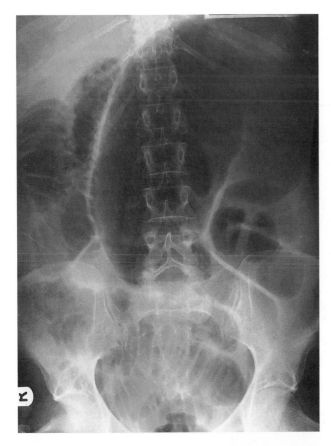

Fig. 4.5 Volvulus of the caecum. The twisted obstructed caecum and ascending colon now lie on the left side of the abdomen and appear as a large gas shadow. There is also extensive small bowel dilatation from obstruction by the volvulus.

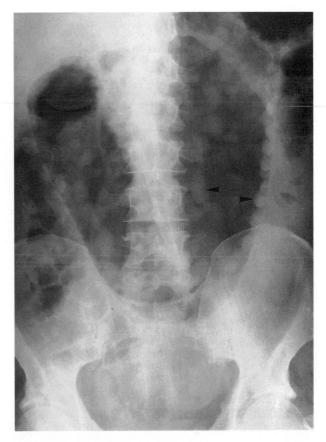

Fig. 4.6 Toxic dilatation of the large bowel from ulcerative colitis. The dilatation is maximal in the transverse colon. Note the loss of haustra and islands of hypertrophied mucosa. Two of these pseudopolyps are arrowed.

cases are recognizable radiologically. The largest quantities of free gas are seen after colonic perforation and the smallest amounts with leakage from the small bowel. A pneumoperitoneum is very rare in acute appendicitis even if the appendix is perforated.

Free intraperitoneal air is a normal finding after a laparotomy. In adults, all the air is usually absorbed within seven days. In children, the air absorbs much faster, usually within 24 hours. An increase in the amount of air on successive films indicates continuing leakage of air.

Air under the right hemidiaphragm is usually easy to recognize on an erect abdominal or chest film as a curvilinear collection of gas between the line of the diaphragm and the opacity of the liver. Free gas under the left hemidiaphragm is more difficult to identify because of the overlapping gas shadows of the stomach and splenic flexure of colon. Gas in these organs may mimic free intraperitoneal air when none is present.

Gas under the diaphragm is much easier to diagnose on an erect chest film than on an upright abdominal film. If there is doubt about the presence of a pneumoperitoneum, a lateral decubitus film will show the air collected beneath the flank. It is important to realize that when the patient is lying flat the free gas collects centrally beneath the abdominal wall and is very difficult to identify on the conventional supine film.

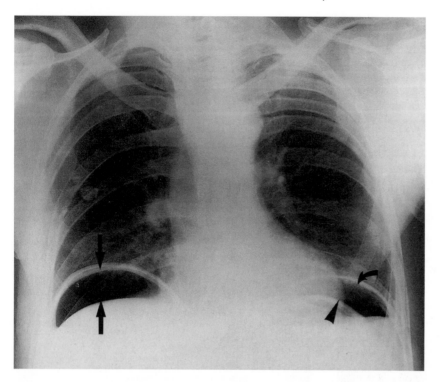

Fig. 4.7 Free gas in the peritoneal cavity. On this chest radiograph air can be seen under the domes of both hemidiaphragms. The curved arrow points to the left hemidiaphragm and the arrow head to the wall of the stomach. The two vertical arrows on the right point to the diaphragm and upper border of the liver.

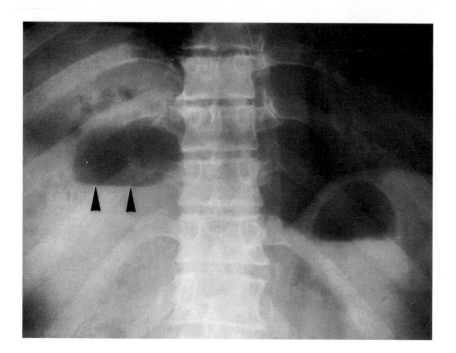

Fig. 4.8 Gas in a right subphrenic abscess. There are several collections of gas within the abscess. The largest of these contains a fluid level (arrows). The air–fluid level under the left hemidiaphragm is normal. It is in the stomach.

Gas in an abscess (Fig. 4.8)

This produces a very variable pattern on plain films. It may form either small bubbles or larger collections of air, both of which could be confused with gas within the bowel. Fluid levels in abscesses may be seen on a horizontal ray film. Since abscesses are mass lesions they displace the adjacent structures; for example, the diaphragm is elevated with a subphrenic abscess, and the bowel is displaced by pericolic and pancreatic abscesses. Pleural or pulmonary shadows are very common in association with subphrenic abscess. Ultrasound, radionuclide examinations and CT are extensively used to evaluate abdominal abscesses (see p. 286).

Gas in the wall of the bowel

Numerous spherical or oval bubbles of gas are seen in the wall of the large bowel in adults in the benign condition known as *pneumatosis coli*. Linear streaks of intramural gas have a more sinister significance as they usually indicate infarction of the bowel wall. Gas in the wall of the bowel in the neonatal period, whatever its shape, is diagnostic of *necrotizing enterocolitis* (Fig. 4.9), a disease that is fairly common in premature babies with respiratory problems.

Gas in the biliary system

This is seen on plain films following sphincterotomy or anastomosis of the common bile duct to the bowel (Fig. 4.10). It is also seen with a fistula from erosion of a gall stone into the duodenum or colon, or following penetration of a duodenal ulcer into the common bile duct.

Gas may be seen, very occasionally, in the wall or lumen of the gall bladder in acute cholecystitis from gas-forming organisms.

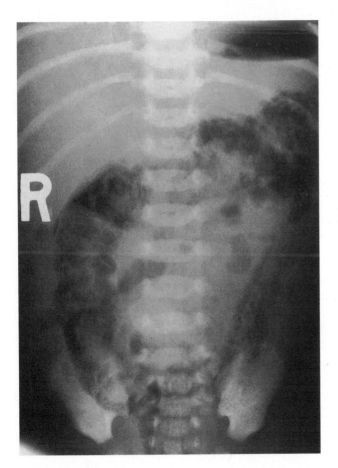

Fig. 4.9 Necrotizing enterocolitis in a neonate. There is intramural gas throughout the colon.

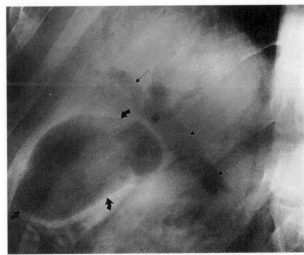

Fig. 4.10 Gas in the biliary tree. The gall bladder (curved arrows) and the duct system (straight arrows) have been outlined with air. The patient had an anastomosis of the common bile duct to the bowel.

Ascites

Small amounts of ascites cannot be detected on plain films. Larger quantities separate the loops of bowel from one another and displace the ascending and descending colon from the fat stripes which indicate the position of the peritoneum along the lateral abdominal walls (see Fig. 4.1, p. 136). The loops of small bowel float to the centre of the abdomen (Fig. 4.11).

In practice, plain films are of very limited value in the diagnosis of ascites, since the signs are so difficult to interpret confidently except when large amounts of ascites are present. Ascites is readily recognized at ultrasound or CT (see p. 285).

Abdominal calcifications

An attempt should always be made to determine the nature of any abdominal calcification. The first essential is to localize the calcification; for this, a lateral or oblique view may be

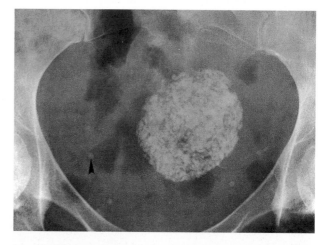

Fig. 4.12 Calcification in a large uterine fibroid. There are also several phleboliths, one of which is arrowed.

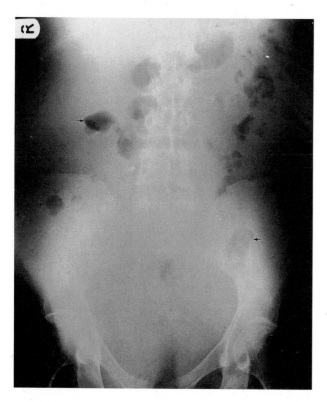

Fig. 4.11 Ascites. Note how the gas in the ascending and descending colon (arrows) is displaced by the fluid away from the side walls of the abdomen.

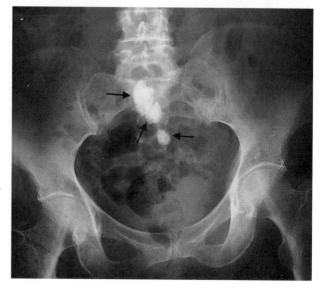

Fig. 4.13 Calcified mesenteric lymph nodes from old tuberculosis (arrows).

necessary. Once the organ of origin is known, the pattern or shape of the calcification will usually limit the diagnosis to just one or two choices.

The most common calcifications are of little or no significance to the patient. These include phleboliths, calcified lymph nodes, costal cartilages and arterial calcification.

Calcifications in the abdomen are likely to be one of the following:

• *Pelvic vein phleboliths* (Fig. 4.12) are very common; they may cause diagnostic confusion in that they may be mistaken for urinary calculi and faecoliths. *Calcified mesenteric lymph nodes* (Fig. 4.13) caused by old tuberculosis, are important only in that they may be difficult to differentiate from other calcifications. Their pattern is often specific: they are irregular in outline and very dense and because they lie

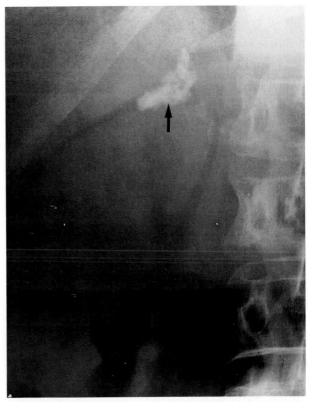

Fig. 4.15 Adrenal calcification (arrow).

in the mesentery they are often mobile. It is usually possible to see that they are composed of a conglomeration of smaller rounded calcifications.

• *Vascular calcification* occurs in association with atheroma, but there is no useful correlation with the haemodynamic severity of the vascular disease. Calcification is frequently present in the walls of *abdominal aortic aneurysms* (Fig. 4.14). It is usually easier to assess the size of such aneurysms on the lateral projection.

• *Uterine fibroids* (Fig. 4.12) may contain numerous irregularly shaped well-defined calcifications conforming to the spherical outline of fibroids. Again, the calcification is by itself of no significance to the patient.

• *Malignant ovarian masses* occasionally contain visible calcium. The only benign ovarian lesion that is visibly calcified is the *dermoid cyst*, which may contain various calcified

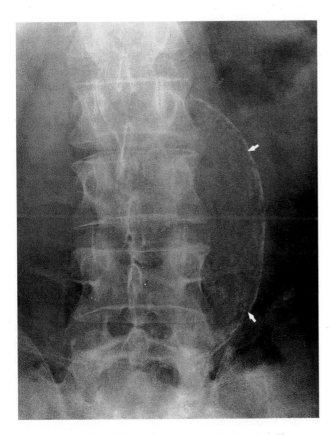

Fig. 4.14 Calcified abdominal aortic aneurysm (arrows). The aneurysm measured 8 cm in diameter on the lateral view.

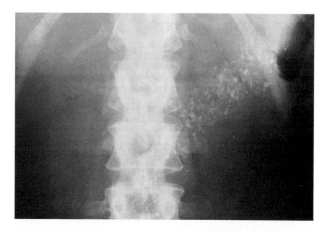

Fig. 4.16 Pancreatic calcification.

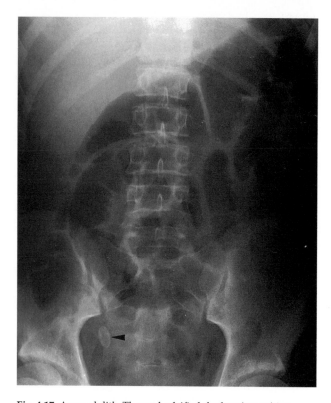

Fig. 4.17 Appendolith. The oval calcified shadow (arrow) is a faecalith in the appendix. The patient had perforated appendicitis. Note the dilated loops of small bowel in the centre of the abdomen due to peritonitis – the so-called 'sentinel loops'.

components, of which teeth are the commonest (Fig. 8.7, p. 268).

• *Adrenal calcification* (Fig. 4.15) occurs after adrenal haemorrhage, after tuberculosis and occasionally in adrenal tumours. However, the majority of patients with adrenal calcification are asymptomatic healthy people in whom the cause of the calcification is unclear. Only a minority of patients with Addison's disease have adrenal calcification.

• *Liver calcification* occurs in hepatomas and rarely in other tumours. Hydatid cysts, old abscesses and tuberculosis may also calcify. Gall stones, renal stones and costal cartilage are common causes of calcification projected over the liver shadow.

• *Splenic calcification* is rarely of clinical significance. It is seen in cysts, infarcts, old haematomas and following tuberculosis.

• *Pancreatic calcification* occurs in chronic pancreatitis. The calcifications are mainly small calculi within the pancreas. The position of the calcification usually enables the diagnosis to be made without difficulty (Fig. 4.16).

• *Faecoliths.* Calcified faecoliths may be seen in diverticula of the colon or in the appendix (Fig. 4.17). Appendiceal faecoliths are an important radiological observation since the presence of an appendolith is a strong indication that the patient has acute appendicitis, often with gangrene and perforation. However, only a small proportion of patients with appendicitis have a radiologically visible appendolith.

• *Soft tissue calcification* in the buttocks may be seen following injection of certain medicines. These shadows can at times be confused with intraabdominal calcifications.

• *Calcification of the urinary tract* is discussed on page 231.

Plain films of the liver and spleen

Substantial enlargement of the liver has to occur before it can be recognized on a plain abdominal film. As the liver enlarges it extends well below the costal margin displacing the hepatic flexure, transverse colon and right kidney downwards and displacing the stomach to the left. The diaphragm may also be elevated.

As the spleen enlarges the tip becomes visible in the left upper quadrant below the lower ribs. Eventually, it may fill the left side of the abdomen and even extend across the midline into the right lower quadrant. The splenic flexure of

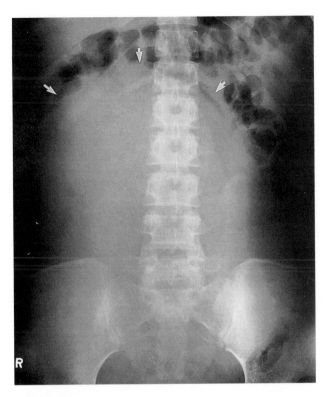

Fig. 4.18 Mass arising out of pelvis (arrows) displacing bowel to the sides of the abdomen. The mass was a large cystadeno-carcinoma of the ovary.

the colon and the left kidney are displaced downwards and medially, and the stomach is displaced to the right.

Following trauma, rupture of the spleen occurs more frequently than of the liver. As a haematoma forms, the plain films may show a mass in the upper abdomen displacing adjacent structures. There may be paralytic ileus and fractures of the lower ribs may also be present. These signs, although helpful if present, are often not seen even with significant lacerations of the liver and spleen. For this reason, ultrasound or, preferably, CT is usually carried out in cases of suspected internal abdominal injury (see Chapter 6).

Abdominal and pelvic masses

Attempting to diagnose the nature of an abdominal mass on a plain film is notoriously difficult, and ultrasound or CT is invariably necessary. The site of the mass, displacement of adjacent structures and presence of calcification are important diagnostic signs but plain films are unable to distinguish between solid and cystic masses.

An enlarged bladder can be seen as a mass arising from the pelvis displacing loops of bowel. In females, uterine and ovarian enlargement also appear as masses arising from the pelvis. Ovarian cysts can become very large, almost filling the abdomen and displacing the bowel to the sides of the abdomen (Fig. 4.18).

Retroperitoneal tumours and lymph nodes, when large, become visible on plain films. Renal masses, especially cysts and hydronephrosis, can become large and appear as masses in the flank. With retroperitoneal masses the outline of the psoas muscle may become invisible.

5

Gastrointestinal Tract

Imaging techniques

Contrast examinations

The previous chapter showed that the plain film can be very informative in patients with an acute abdomen, but for most other intestinal disorders some form of contrast examination is necessary. Barium sulphate is the best contrast medium for the gastrointestinal tract. It produces excellent opacification, good coating of the mucosa and is completely inert. Its only major disadvantange is that when water is reabsorbed in the colon the barium may solidify and impact proximal to a colonic or rectal stricture. The other available contrast is water-soluble medium, Gastrografin. It has several disadvantages: it is hypertonic and soon becomes diluted; it is irritant should it inadvertently enter the lungs; and it is less radio-opaque than barium. Its major use is for opacifying the bowel prior to CT scanning of the abdomen.

Gastrointestinal contrast examinations are carried out under fluoroscopic control so that the passage of contrast can be observed on a television monitor. By watching the television screen the radiologist is able to position the patient so that any abnormality is shown clearly. Films are taken to show fine detail and to serve as a permanent record. One of the values of fluoroscopy is to ensure that an abnormality has a constant appearance. Peristaltic waves are transitory and so can be easily distinguished from a true narrowing, which is constant.

The double-contrast examination of the stomach and colon is now widely practised. In the single-contrast method the bowel is filled only with barium. In the double-contrast technique the mucosa is coated with barium and the stomach or colon distended by introducing gas, often in combination with an injection of a short-acting smooth muscle relaxant to paralyse the bowel. The double-contrast method is a little more time consuming but shows the mucosa to advantage and demonstrates small abnormalities which would be obscured by a large volume of barium.

It is important to understand some basic terms applicable to barium examinations of the gastrointestinal tract.

The wall of the bowel is never seen as such. What is seen is the outline of the lumen and conclusions have to be drawn about the state of the wall. Usually, the most reliable information is obtained when the bowel is fully distended.

Mucosal folds are seen when the bowel is in a contracted state so that the mucosa becomes folded (see Fig. 5.6b, p. 150). When the bowel is distended these mucosal folds disappear. The normal mucosal fold pattern may be altered by smoothing out or by abnormal irregularity.

Filling defect is a term used to describe something occupying space within the bowel thereby preventing the normal filling of the lumen with barium. This creates an area of total or relative radiolucency within the barium column. There are three types of filling defects, each having distinct radiological signs:

1 An intraluminal filling defect is entirely within the lumen of the bowel (e.g. food), and has barium all around it (Fig. 5.1a).

2 An intramural filling defect arises from the wall of the bowel (e.g. a carcinoma or leiomyoma). It causes an indentation from one side only, making a sharp angle with the wall of the bowel and is not completely surrounded by barium (Fig. 5.1b).

3 An extramural filling defect arises outside the bowel but compresses it, e.g. enlarged pancreas or lymph nodes. It also gives a narrowing from one side only but makes a

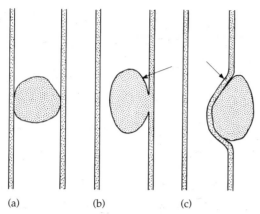

(a)   (b)   (c)

Fig. 5.1 Filling defects in the bowel. (a) Intraluminal.
(b) Intramural. Note the sharp angle (arrow) made with the wall.
(c) Extramural. There is a shallow angle (arrow) with the wall of
the bowel.

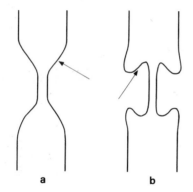

a   b

Fig. 5.2 Stricture. (a) Tapering ends (arrow). (b) Overhanging
edges or shouldering (arrow).

shallow angle with the wall of the bowel. The mucosa is preserved but stretched over the filling defect (Fig. 5.1c).

A *stricture* is a circumferential or annular narrowing. A
stricture must be differentiated from the transient narrowing which occurs with normal peristalsis. A stricture may
have tapering ends (Fig. 5.2a) or it may end abruptly
and have overhanging edges giving an appearance known
as 'shouldering' (Fig. 5.2b). Shouldering is a feature of
malignancy.

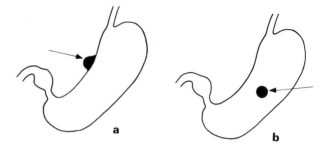

a   b

Fig. 5.3 Ulceration. (a) In profile the ulcer is seen as an outward
projection (arrow); (b) *en face* the ulcer appears rounded (arrow).

Ulceration. An ulcer is a breach of a mucosal surface which
becomes visible when the crater contains barium. When
viewed in profile it appears as an outward projection from
the barium-filled lumen (Fig. 5.3a). When viewed *en face* the
ulcer crater appears as a rounded collection of barium (Fig.
5.3b).

Other imaging modalities

Although the barium study is the mainstay for examining
the gastrointestinal tract, other modalities now have an
increasing role to play.

Ultrasound can assess the bowel wall and detect intra-
abdominal fluid but gives little useful information on the
mucosa. Ultrasound is used for the diagnosis of intussusception and in cases of suspected appendicitis when the
diagnosis is not obvious clinically.

For *CT* it is necessary to opacify and distend the bowel
with a dilute water-soluble contrast agent or dilute barium,
otherwise unopacified loops of bowel may be misdiagnosed
as an abscess, lymphadenopathy or tumour. The barium
used for barium enemas cannot be used to opacify the
bowel as it is too dense and causes artefacts on the scan. Like
the barium examination, CT can show mucosal folds, filling
defects, strictures and ulcers but CT can also assess the full
width of the bowel wall. However, a barium study is
usually an easier way to examine the bowel as satisfactory
opacification and distension of the bowel may be difficult to
achieve for CT. Computed tomography is useful for diagnosing and staging tumours, the assessment of inflammatory bowel disease and the complications of gastrointestinal
disease and surgery (Fig. 5.4). Magnetic resonance imaging

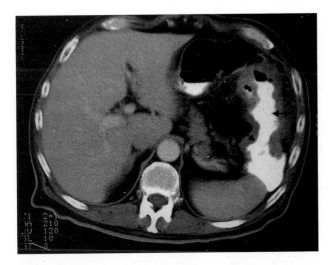

Fig. 5.4 Computed tomography showing a carcinoma of the splenic flexure of the colon. The bowel wall is thickened (arrows) and the tumour is indenting the contrast-filled lumen.

has a limited role in gastrointestinal disease because peristalsis degrades the images and there is as yet no satisfactory means of opacifying the bowel although agents for this purpose are being developed.

Oesophagus

Plain films do not normally show the oesophagus unless it is very dilated (e.g. achalasia), but they are of use in demonstrating an opaque foreign body such as a bone lodged in the oesophagus (Fig. 5.5).

The barium swallow is the contrast examination employed to visualize the oesophagus. The patient drinks some barium and its passage down the oesophagus is observed on a television monitor. Films are taken in an oblique position to project the oesophagus clear of the spine, with the oesophagus both full of barium to show the outline, and empty to show the mucosal pattern.

Normal barium swallow

The oesophagus when full of barium should have a smooth outline. When empty and contracted, barium normally lies in between the folds of mucosa which appear as three or four long, straight parallel lines (Fig. 5.6).

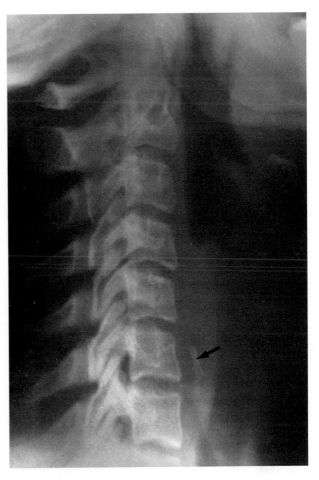

Fig. 5.5 Foreign body in the oesophagus. Lateral view of the neck showing a chicken bone (arrow) lodged in the upper end of the oesophagus.

The aortic arch gives a clearly visible impression on the left side of the oesophagus, which is more pronounced in the elderly as the aorta becomes tortuous and elongated. Below the aortic impression there is often a smaller impression made by the left main bronchus. The lower part of the oesophagus sweeps gently forward closely applied to the back of the left atrium and left ventricle.

Peristaltic waves can be observed during fluoroscopy. They move smoothly along the oesophagus to propel the barium rapidly into the stomach even if the patient swallows when lying flat. It is important not to confuse a con-

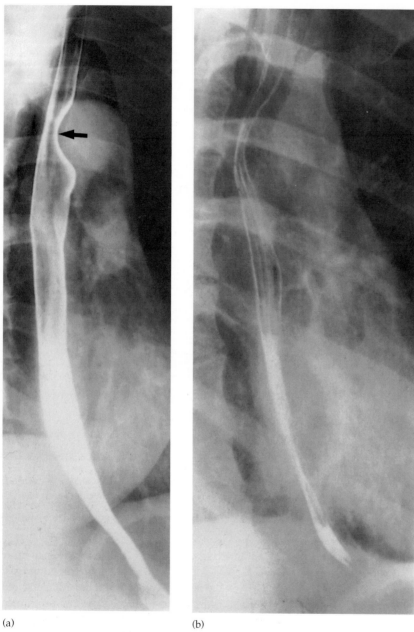

(a)   (b)

Fig. 5.6 Normal oesophagus. (a) Full of barium to show the smooth outline and indentation made by the aortic arch (arrow). (b) Film taken after the main volume of barium has passed, to show the parallel mucosal folds.

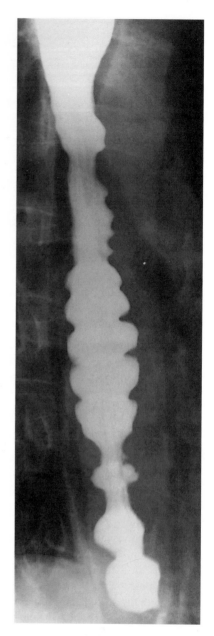

Fig. 5.7 Tertiary contractions (corkscrew oesophagus) giving the oesophagus an undulated appearance.

traction wave with a true narrowing: a narrowing is constant whereas a contraction wave is transitory. Sometimes the contraction waves do not occur in an orderly fashion but are pronounced and prolonged to give the oesophagus an undulated appearance (Fig. 5.7). These so-called tertiary contractions usually occur in the elderly and in most instances they do not give rise to symptoms. Occasionally, these contractions give rise to dysphagia and the condition is known as diffuse oesophageal spasm.

Abnormal barium swallow

Strictures

Strictures are an important cause of dysphagia. There are four main causes; carcinoma, peptic, achalasia and corrosive. In order to distinguish between these possibilities it is useful to answer the following questions:

- Where is the stricture?
- What is its shape?
- How long is it?
- Is there a soft tissue mass?

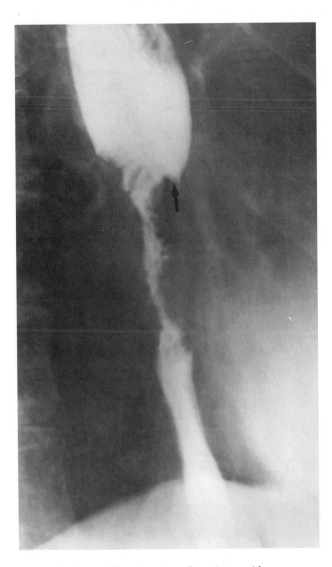

Fig. 5.8 Carcinoma. There is an irregular stricture with shouldering (arrow) at the upper end.

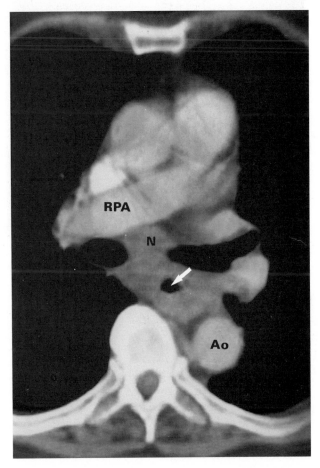

Fig. 5.9 Carcinoma of the oesophagus. The carcinoma is shown as a mass around the lumen of the oesophagus (arrow). Subcarinal nodes (N) are also present. Ao, descending aorta; RPA, right pulmonary artery.

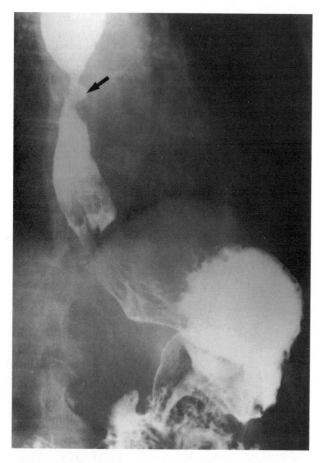

Fig. 5.10 Peptic stricture due to gastro-oesophageal reflux in a patient with a hiatus hernia. There is a short smooth stricture at the oesophagogastric junction with an ulcer crater within the stricture (arrow).

the tumour causing thickening of the oesophageal wall. In addition it may show invasion of adjacent structures, evidence of spread to draining lymph nodes and any liver or lung metastases (Fig. 5.9).

Peptic strictures are found at the lower end of the oesophagus and are almost invariably associated with a hiatus hernia and gastro-oesophageal reflux and, therefore, the stricture may be some distance above the diaphragm. Peptic strictures are characteristically short and have smooth outlines with tapering ends (Fig. 5.10). An ulcer may be seen in close proximity to the stricture.

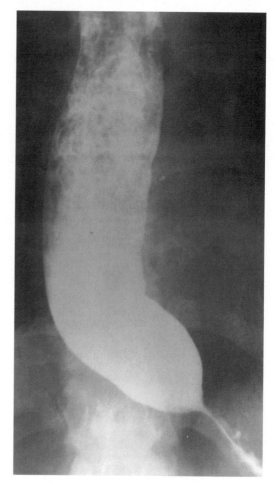

Fig. 5.11 Achalasia. The very dilated oesophagus containing food residues shows a smooth narrowing at its lower end.

Carcinomas rarely arise from only one wall but usually involve the full circumference to form strictures. The stricture, which may occur anywhere in the oesophagus, shows an irregular lumen with shouldered edges and is normally several centimetres in length (Fig. 5.8). A soft tissue mass may be visible.

Computed tomography may be carried out, particularly if surgery is contemplated. Computed tomography shows

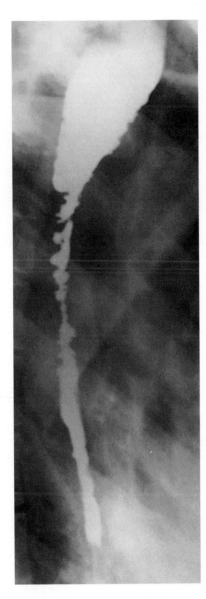

Fig. 5.12 Corrosive stricture.

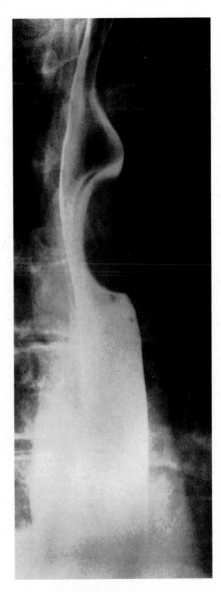

Fig. 5.13 Leiomyoma. There is an intramural filling defect in the eosophagus below the aortic arch (arrows). The sharp angle this makes with the wall of the oesophagus indicates that the filling defect is due to a mass arising in the wall of the oesophagus.

Achalasia is a neuromuscular abnormality resulting in failure of relaxation at the cardiac sphincter which presents radiologically as a smooth, tapered narrowing which is always at the lower end of the oesophagus (Fig. 5.11). There is associated dilatation of the oesophagus, which often shows absent peristalsis. The dilated oesophagus

usually contains food residues and may be visible on the plain chest radiograph. The lungs may show consolidation and bronchiectasis from aspiration of the oesophageal contents. The stomach gas bubble is usually absent because

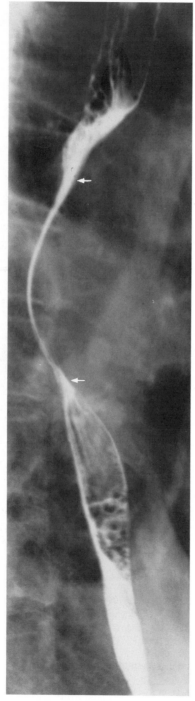

(a)

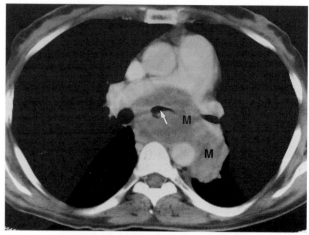

(b)

Fig. 5.14 Extraluminal compression of oesophagus by carcinoma of the bronchus. (a) Barium swallow shows extraluminal compression (arrows) making a shallow angle with the wall of the oesophagus. (b) CT of the same patient shows a very large mass (M) surrounding and indenting the oesophagus (arrow).

the oesophageal contents act as a water seal, but this sign is not diagnostic of achalasia as it is seen in other causes of oesophageal obstruction and can occasionally be observed in healthy people.

Corrosive strictures are the result of swallowing corrosives such as acids or alkalis. They are long strictures which begin at the level of the aortic arch. As with the other benign strictures they are usually smooth with tapered ends, but may be irregular (Fig. 5.12).

Filling defects on barium swallow

Filling defects may be caused by a tumour arising in the wall of the oesophagus, by a lesion arising from outside the oesophagus or by objects in the lumen of the oesophagus.

An intramural filling defect is likely to be a *leiomyoma* (Fig. 5.13). A leiomyoma causes a smooth, rounded indentation into the lumen of the oesophagus. A soft tissue mass may be seen in the mediastinum indicating extraluminal extension.

A carcinoma may cause an irregular filling defect, but as mentioned above, carcinomas usually present as strictures.

Extramural lesions compressing the oesophagus include carcinoma of the bronchus (Fig. 5.14), enlarged mediastinal lymph nodes and an aneurysm of the aorta. In all these conditions the chest film or CT will usually show the underlying pathology.

An anomalous right subclavian artery, which instead of coming from the innominate artery, arises as the last major branch from the aortic arch, gives rise to a characteristic short, smooth narrowing as it crosses behind the upper oesophagus (Fig. 5.15).

Intraluminal filling defects. A lump of food may impact in the oesophagus and may cause a complete obstruction (Fig. 5.16). This is usually associated with a stricture.

Dilatation of the oesophagus

There are two main types of oesophageal dilatation – obstructive and non-obstructive.

• Dilatation due to obstruction is associated with a visible stricture. The patient with a carcinoma usually presents with dysphagia before the oesophagus becomes very dilated. On the other hand, a markedly dilated oesophagus indicates a very long-standing condition, usually achalasia or occasionally a benign stricture.

• Dilatation without obstruction occurs in scleroderma. The disease involves the oesophageal muscle resulting in dilatation of the oesophagus, which resembles an inert tube with no peristaltic movement so that barium does not flow from the oesophagus into the stomach unless the patient stands upright.

Varices

Oesophageal varices appear as lucent, tortuous, wormlike filling defects which distort the mucosal pattern so that the folds are no longer parallel (Fig. 5.17). The primary diagnostic test to confirm or exclude varices is endoscopy.

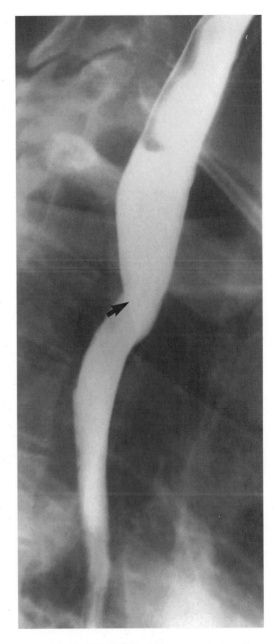

Fig. 5.15 Anomalous right subclavian artery. There is a localized indentation caused by the anomalous artery as it passes behind the oesophagus (arrow).

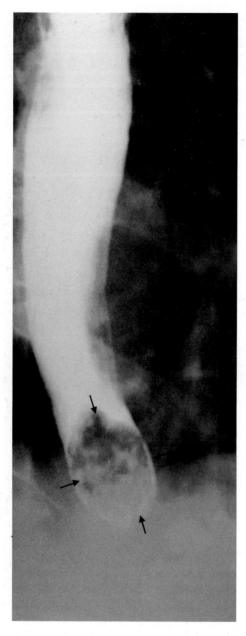

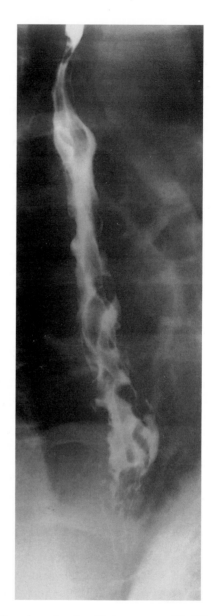

Fig. 5.17 Oesophageal varices. Tortuous, worm-like filling defects are seen in the lower half of the oesophagus.

Fig. 5.16 Impacted food. A piece of meat is lodged at the lower end of the oesophagus and appears as a filling defect (arrows) surrounded by barium.

Oesophageal web

A web is a thin, shelf-like projection arising from the anterior wall of the cervical portion of the oesophagus. To demonstrate it, that part of the oesophagus must be full of barium (Fig. 5.18). A web may be an isolated finding but the combination of a web, dysphagia and iron deficiency anaemia is known as the Plummer–Vinson syndrome.

Diverticula

Diverticula are saccular outpouchings, which are often seen as chance findings, in the intrathoracic portion of the oesophagus. One type of diverticulum, the pharyngeal pouch or Zenker's diverticulum (Fig. 5.19), is important as it may give rise to symptoms caused by retention of food and pressure upon the oesophagus. A pharyngeal pouch arises through a congenital weakness in the inferior constrictor muscle of the pharynx and comes to lie behind the oesophagus near the midline. It may reach a very large size and can cause displacement and compression of the oesophagus.

Oesophageal atresia

In oesophageal atresia, the oesophagus ends as a blind pouch in the upper mediastinum. Several different types exist (Fig. 5.20) but the most frequent is for the upper part of the oesophagus to be a blind sac with a fistula between the lower segment of the oesophagus and the tracheobronchial tree. A plain abdominal film will show air in the bowel if a fistula is present between the tracheobronchial tree and the oesophagus distal to the atretic segment.

To confirm the diagnosis of oesophageal atresia it is usually sufficient to pass a soft tube into the oesophagus and show that the tube holds up or coils in the blindly ending pouch. Oily contrast, such as the bronchographic medium Dionosil (0.5–1.0 ml), injected through the tube has been used to outline the oesophagus (Fig. 5.20b), but is a hazardous procedure because the viscous contrast may cause respiratory obstruction if it spills over into the trachea.

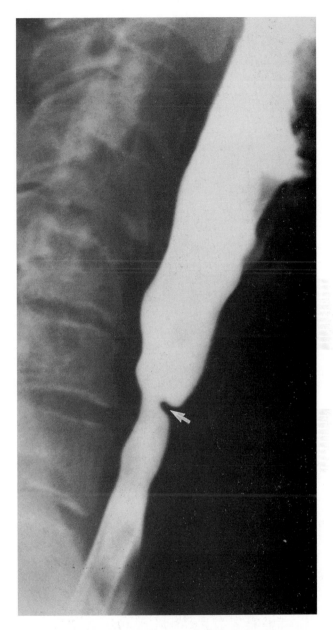

Fig. 5.18 Oesophageal web. There is a shelf-like indentation (arrow) from the anterior wall of the upper oesophagus.

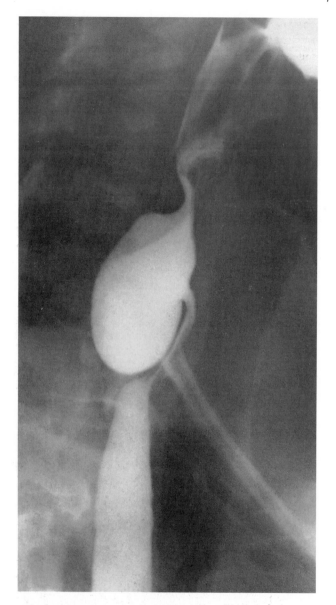

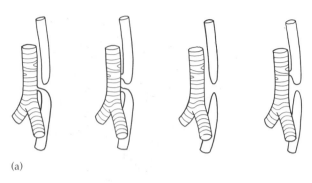

(a)

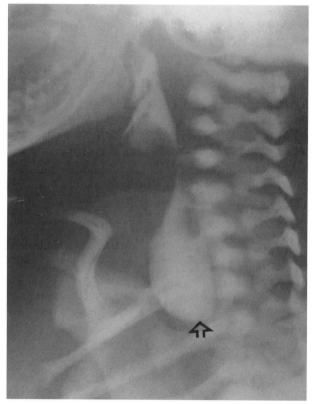

(b)

Fig. 5.19 Pharyngeal pouch (Zenker's diverticulum). The pouch is lying behind the oesophagus which is displaced forward.

Candidiasis

Involvement of the oesophagus with the fungus Candida (monilia) fungus occurs in severely ill or immunocompromised patients. It causes mucosal ulceration which is seen

Fig. 5.20 Oesophageal atresia. (a) Diagram of the various types. The first two types also have an oesophagotracheal fistula distal to the atretic segment and will show air in the stomach. (b) The dilated oesophagus ends blindly at the thoracic inlet (arrow). There was a fistula from the oesophagus below the atretic segment to the trachea. This is the commonest type of oesophageal atresia.

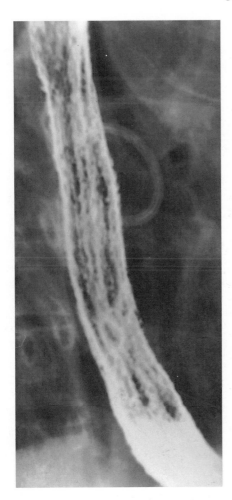

Fig. 5.21 Candidiasis. Mucosal ulceration has caused a shaggy appearance of the oesophagus in this patient with lymphoma undergoing chemotherapy.

as fine irregularities projecting from the lumen of the oesophagus on barium swallow (Fig. 5.21).

Stomach and duodenum

The barium meal is the standard contrast study to examine the stomach and duodenum. The patient drinks about 200 ml of barium. Each radiologist has his own routine but the aim is to take films in various positions with the patient both erect and lying flat, so that each part of the stomach

and duodenum is shown distended by barium and also distended with air but coated with barium to show the mucosal pattern (Fig. 5.22). To provide better mucosal detail, the stomach is distended with a gas-producing agent, and an intravenous injection of a short-acting smooth muscle relaxant is often given (Fig. 5.23).

Food residues in the stomach produce pictures which are very difficult to interpret. For this reason it is most important that the patient fasts for at least 6 hours prior to the examination.

Normal barium meal

Each part of the stomach and duodenum should be checked to ensure that no abnormal narrowing is present. A transient

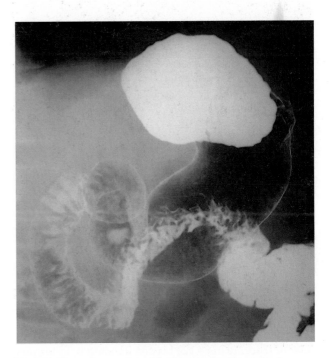

Fig. 5.22 Normal stomach and duodenum: double-contrast barium meal. On this supine view barium collects in the fundus of the stomach. The body and the antrum of the stomach together with the duodenal cap and loop are coated with barium and distended with gas. Note how the fourth part of the duodenum and duodenojejunal flexure are superimposed on the body of the stomach.

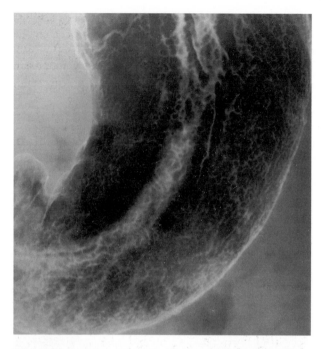

Fig. 5.23 Normal stomach. With a double-contrast technique the mucosa is coated with barium and the stomach distended with gas to show the fine mucosal detail, in this case in the body of the stomach.

contraction wave must not be confused with a constant pathological narrowing. The outline of the lesser curve of the stomach is smooth with no filling defects or projections visible but the greater curve is nearly always irregular due to prominent mucosal folds. In the stomach the mucosa is thrown up into a number of smooth folds and barium collects in the troughs between the folds. There should be no effacement of the folds or rounded collections of barium.

The duodenal cap or bulb should be approximately triangular in shape. It arises just beyond the short pyloric canal and may be difficult to recognize if deformed from chronic ulceration.

The duodenum forms a loop around the head of the pancreas to reach the duodenojejunal flexure. Diverticula arising beyond the first part of the duodenum are a common finding (Fig. 5.24) and are usually without significance.

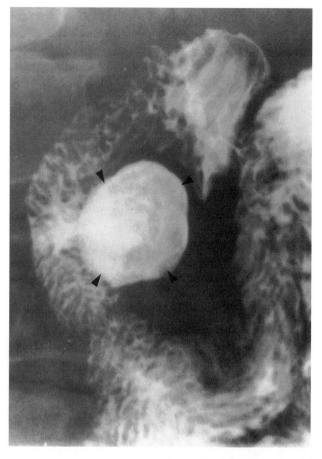

Fig. 5.24 Duodenal diverticulum arising from the second part of the duodenum (arrows).

Gastroscopy

Gastroscopy enables the mucosa of the stomach and duodenum to be directly inspected and biopsied. Gastroscopy and barium meal are complementary investigations and nowadays gastroscopy is widely used as the initial investigation in patients with dyspepsia or suspected carcinoma.

Although gastroscopy will not be discussed in detail the main indications for its use are:
• demonstrating mucosal lesions such as gastritis which cannot be reliably visualized on a barium examination;
• making a histological diagnosis of an abnormality shown on a barium meal;

- investigating persistent dyspepsia in a patient with a normal barium meal;
- assessing healing of an ulcer;
- examining patients after gastric surgery when the radiological appearances may be difficult to interpret;
- diagnosing the cause of acute bleeding from the upper gastrointestinal tract.

Abnormal barium meal

Filling defects in the stomach

Filling defects may arise from the wall of the stomach or be due to masses that press in from outside the stomach. A few are entirely intraluminal. It should be remembered that carcinoma is by far the commonest cause of a filling defect in an adult.

Carcinoma usually produces an irregular filling defect with alteration of the normal mucosal pattern (Fig. 5.25). The tumour is often larger than is readily appreciated from the barium meal. Overhanging edges or shouldering may be seen at the junction of the tumour and the stomach wall. A carcinoma at the fundus may obstruct the oesophagus while one in the antrum may cause gastric outlet obstruction (see Fig. 5.31, p. 164). Carcinoma diffusely involving the stomach is known as *linitis plastica* and is discussed below.

Because of the much better prognosis, emphasis has been placed on the diagnosis of early gastric cancer which is confined to the mucosa. It may be flat or appear as a shallow ulcer indistinguishable from a benign ulcer. This stage of cancer is difficult to detect and is usually only diagnosed with a double contrast barium meal.

Leiomyoma. A smooth, round filling defect arising from the wall of the stomach may be caused by a benign tumour such as a leiomyoma (Fig. 5.26). A leiomyoma is a submucosal tumour which, as well as projecting into the lumen of the stomach, may show a large extraluminal extension. One of

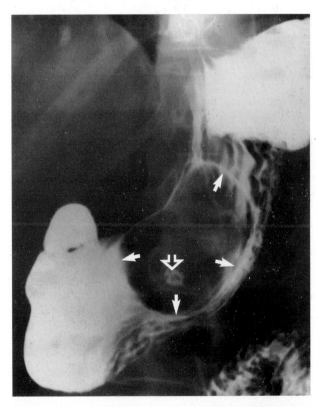

Fig. 5.26 Leiomyoma. There is a large filling defect in the stomach with smooth borders (outer arrows). An ulcer crater (central arrow) is present within the filling defect – a characteristic feature of a leiomyoma.

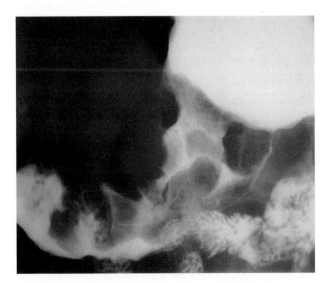

Fig. 5.25 Carcinoma. There are a number of large filling defects in the antrum and body of the stomach.

the characteristic features of a leiomyoma is that it may have an ulcer on its surface.

Polyps. Polyps may be single or multiple. They may be sessile or have a stalk. Even with high quality radiographs it is often impossible to distinguish benign from malignant polyps. For this reason gastroscopy with biopsy or operative removal is invariably carried out on all suspected polyps.

Intraluminal defects. These are completely surrounded by barium and are often mobile in the stomach. Examples are food or blood following a haematemesis. Sometimes ingested fibrous material such as hair may intertwine forming a ball or bezoar (Fig. 5.27).

Gastric ulcers

Endoscopy with biopsy, when necessary, is the primary method of diagnosing gastric ulcers in many centres. On a barium meal an ulcer may be seen either *en face* as a collection of barium occupying the ulcer crater or in profile as a projection from the lumen of the stomach depending on the view obtained (Fig. 5.28).

Gastric ulcers may be benign or malignant. Features on barium studies which favour a benign state are an ulcer on the lesser curve projecting beyond the lumen of the stomach with radiating mucosal folds reaching the edge of the ulcer crater. Although it may be possible to diagnose an ulcerative carcinoma with confidence (Fig. 5.29) it is never possible to be sure a gastric ulcer is benign until it has healed.

Narrowing of the stomach

If constant, narrowing is an important feature as it may herald malignancy.

When the whole stomach is involved, the narrowing is due to a carcinoma. This is the so-called 'leather bottle stomach' or 'linitis plastica' (Fig. 5.30). The stomach behaves as a thick rigid tube lacking peristalsis with obliteration of the mucosal folds. Rapid gastric emptying takes place because the cardia and pylorus are held open by the rigid stomach wall.

It is when the narrowing is localized that diagnostic difficulties arise as it may be due to either an infiltrating carcinoma, an active ulcer causing spasm or an ulcer which has healed with scarring and fibrosis.

Thick gastric mucosal folds

Enlarged mucosal folds are associated with a high acid secretion. They are seen in patients with duodenal ulcers and also in the Zollinger–Ellison syndrome which comprises a high acid secretion, gastrin secreting tumour in the pancreas and multiple peptic ulcers. Thickened folds are also seen with gastritis due to *Helicobacter pylori*.

Occasionally, diffuse infiltration of the stomach with malignant lymphoma can produce generalized thickening of the mucosal folds.

Gastric outlet obstruction

Emptying of the stomach can be a difficult feature to assess on a barium meal. In most patients barium rapidly leaves the stomach to enter the duodenum, but in others this only

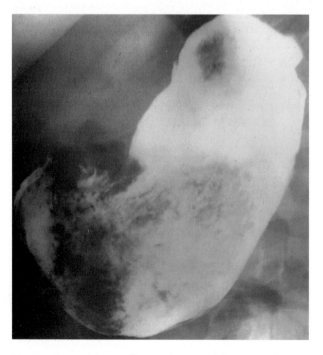

Fig. 5.27 Bezoar. Masses of hair in the stomach have caused irregular filling of the stomach with barium.

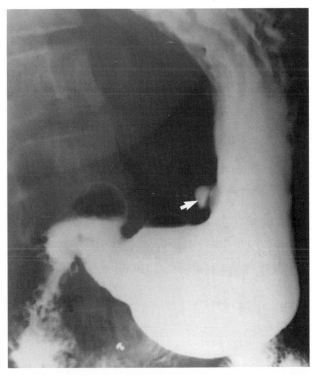

(a)

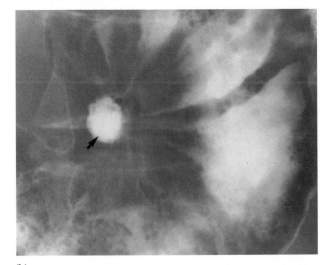

(b)

Fig. 5.28 Benign ulcer. (a) In profile the ulcer (arrow) projects from the lesser curve of the stomach. (b) *En face* the ulcer (arrow) is seen as a rounded collection of barium.

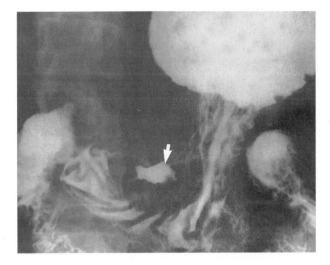

Fig. 5.29 Malignant ulcer. The ulcer (arrow) does not project from the lumen of the stomach. Note how the mucosal folds do not reach the ulcer crater.

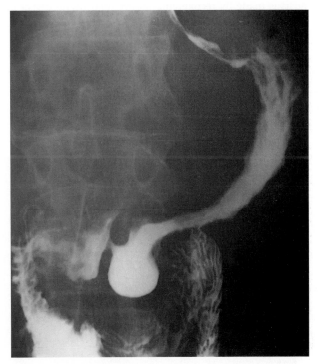

Fig. 5.30 Linitis plastica. The stomach is narrowed by an extensive carcinoma converting it to a rigid tube with obliteration of mucosal folds.

occurs after the patient has been lying on the right side for several minutes. In gastric outlet obstruction less than 50% of the barium leaves the stomach after 4 hours and some may still be present after 24 hours. The stomach will be large and contain food residues.

Gastric emptying can be assessed by giving a radioactive test meal and measuring the disappearance of radioactivity from the stomach, with the patient positioned under a gamma camera. By making corrections for radioactive decay, the half-emptying time for the stomach can be calculated.

It is not sufficient merely to diagnose gastric outlet obstruction; an attempt must be made to find the underlying cause, which may be situated in the duodenum, pylorus or antrum.

In adults the causes of gastric outlet obstruction are:
• *Chronic duodenal ulceration.* The diagnosis depends on demonstrating a very deformed, stenosed duodenal cap. It may or may not be possible to identify an actual ulcer crater.
• *Carcinoma of the antrum* may cause narrowing. The diagnosis is made by recognizing an irregular filling defect in the antrum of the stomach (Fig. 5.31).

In infants, pyloric stenosis is by far the commonest cause of gastric outlet obstruction. Often, the diagnosis is made clinically and can be confirmed with ultrasound, which has superseded the barium meal. Ultrasound shows a thickened, elongated pyloric canal (Fig. 5.32).

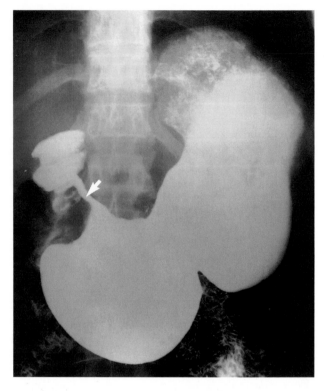

Fig. 5.31 Gastric outlet obstruction. A carcinoma is causing narrowing of the antrum (arrow). The speckled appearance in the fundus of the enlarged stomach is due to food residues.

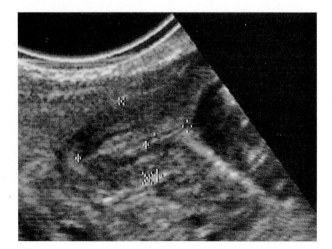

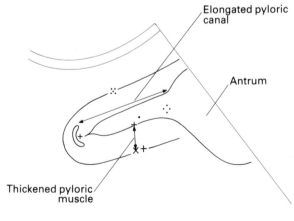

Fig. 5.32 Pyloric stenosis. Ultrasound scan in a neonate showing a thickened elongated pyloric canal.

Gastritis

Often, gastritis may only be diagnosed endoscopically, as the mucosal changes are too slight to be detected on a barium meal. However, erosive gastritis, which is associated with taking alcohol or aspirin, may be seen on a double contrast barium meal. The erosions appear as small, shallow collections of barium surrounded by a radiolucent halo due to oedema (Fig. 5.33).

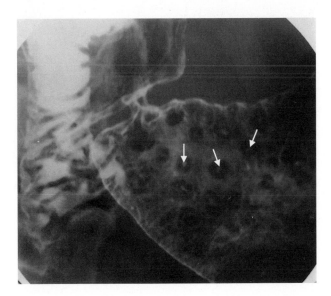

Fig. 5.33 Erosive gastritis. The erosions appear on this double-contrast barium meal as many small collections of barium, some of which are arrowed, surrounded by a radiolucent halo of oedema.

Hiatus hernia

A hiatus hernia is a herniation of the stomach into the mediastinum through the oesophageal hiatus in the diaphragm. It is a common finding. Two main types of hiatus hernia exist: sliding and rolling. An alternative name for a rolling hernia is 'para-oesophageal' (Fig. 5.34).

The commoner type is the sliding hiatus hernia where the gastro-oesophageal junction and a portion of the stomach are situated above the diaphragm (Fig. 5.35a). The cardiac sphincter is usually incompetent, so reflux from the stomach to the oesophagus occurs readily and this may cause oesophagitis, ulceration or peptic stricture. A small sliding hernia may be demonstrated in most people during a barium meal examination, provided that enough manoeuvres have been undertaken to increase intra-abdominal pressure. It is, therefore, difficult to assess the significance of a small hernia with little or no reflux.

In a rolling or para-oesophageal hernia (Fig. 5.35b), the fundus of the stomach herniates through the diaphragm but the oesophagogastric junction often remains competent below the diaphragm.

A large hernia, particularly one of the para-oesophageal type, may not be reduced when the patient is in the erect position. In these instances the hiatus hernia will be seen on chest films.

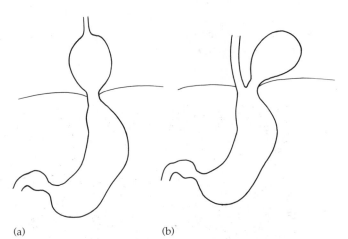

(a) (b)

Fig. 5.34 Hiatus hernia. (a) Sliding: a portion of the stomach and the gastro-oesophageal junction are situated above the diaphragm. (b) Rolling or para-oesophageal: the gastro-oesophageal junction is below the diaphragm.

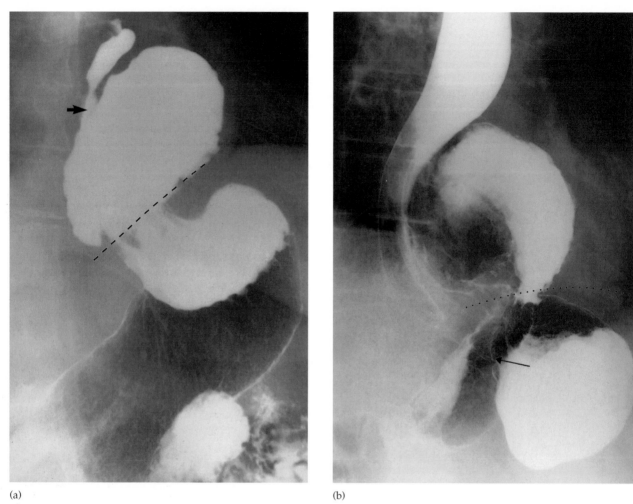

(a)   (b)

Fig. 5.35 Hiatus hernia. (a) Sliding: the fundus of the stomach and the gastro-oesophageal junction (arrow) have herniated through the oesophageal hiatus and lie above the diaphragm (dotted line). (b) Rolling: the gastro-oesophageal junction (arrow) is below the diaphragm (dotted line) and the fundus of the stomach has herniated into the chest.

Duodenal ulcer

The great majority of duodenal ulcers occur in the duodenal cap (duodenal bulb) but a few are found just beyond the cap and are known as postbulbar ulcers. The ulcer crater (Fig. 5.36a) may have a surrounding lucent zone from oedema and mucosal folds are often seen radiating towards the ulcer (Fig. 5.36b). With chronic ulceration the cap becomes deformed from scarring. In a grossly scarred cap it is often impossible to be certain of the presence of an ulcer.

It is not worthwhile carrying out repeat barium meal examinations to assess healing of duodenal ulcers for the following reasons:

• It is often not possible to comment on the presence or absence of an ulcer in a deformed cap.

• Follow-up for malignant change is unnecessary as duodenal ulcers are almost invariably benign and do not undergo malignant degeneration.

Radiology in acute upper gastrointestinal bleeding

The patient presenting with haematemasis and melaena is a common medical emergency. The main causes of bleeding are:

• peptic ulcer
• gastric erosions
• varices
• carcinoma.

Gastroscopy is the key investigation which has the advantage of actually demonstrating the site of bleeding and it can show gastric erosions that may be too shallow to be seen on a barium meal.

Small intestine

The standard contrast examination for the small intestine is the barium small bowel follow-through. The patient drinks about 200–300 ml of barium and its passage through the small intestine is observed by taking films at regular intervals until the barium reaches the colon. This can be a time-consuming procedure and usually takes 2–3 hours, but the transit time is very variable.

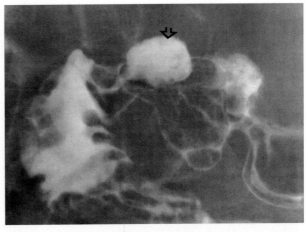

(a)

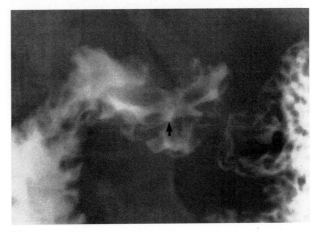

(b)

Fig. 5.36 Duodenal ulcer (two patients). (a) Ulcer seen as a large collection of barium in the duodenal cap (arrow); (b) mucosal folds radiating to a central ulcer crater (arrow).

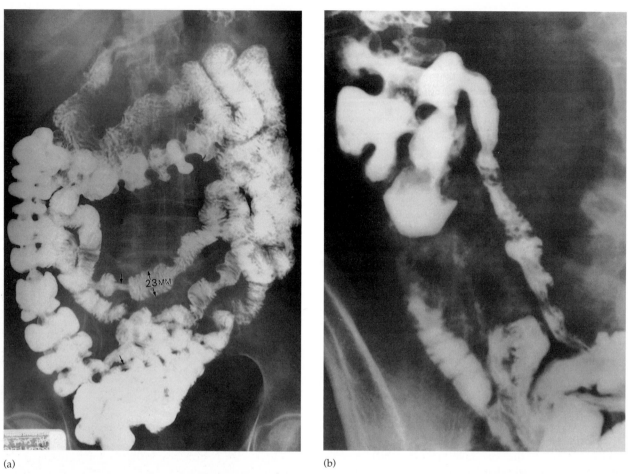

(a)   (b)

Fig. 5.37 (a) Normal barium follow-through. The small intestine, ascending and transverse colon are filled with barium. The jejunum in the left side of the abdomen has a much more marked mucosal fold pattern than the ileum which is lying in the pelvis. When a peristaltic wave contracts the bowel the mucosal folds lie longitudinally (arrows). Note the way of measuring the diameter of the bowel. In the pelvis the loops overlap and details of the bowel become hidden. (b) Normal terminal ileum.

Normal barium follow-through

The normal small intestine (Fig. 5.37) occupies the central and lower abdomen, usually framed by the colon. The terminal portion of the ileum enters the medial aspect of the caecum through the ileocaecal valve. As the terminal ileum may be the first site of disease this region is often fluoroscoped and observed on a television monitor so that peristalsis can be seen and films can be taken with the terminal ileum unobscured by other loops of small intestine.

The barium forms a continuous column defining the diameter of the small bowel which is normally not more than 25 mm. Transverse folds of mucous membrane project into the lumen of the bowel and barium lies between these folds which appear as lucent filling defects of about 2–3 mm in width. The appearance of the mucosal folds depends upon the diameter of the bowel. When distended, the folds are seen as lines traversing the barium column known as valvulae conniventes. When the small bowel is contracted, the folds lie longitudinally and when it is relaxed the folds assume an appearance described as feathery. The mucosal folds are largest and most numerous in the jejunum and tend to disappear in the lower part of the ileum.

An alternative method of examining the small bowel is the so-called small bowel enema (enteroclysis) which distends the bowel and gives excellent mucosal detail (Fig. 5.38). The disadvantage is that it requires intubation with a nasoduodenal tube, which is passed to the duodenojejunal flexure. Barium is injected through the tube followed by water or methyl cellulose to propel the barium through the small bowel.

This technique is appropriate for structural deformities, e.g. Crohn's disease or tumours, but is not used in cases with the malabsorption syndrome.

Abnormal barium follow-through

There are a number of signs to look for.

Dilatation

Dilatation usually indicates either malabsorption, paralytic ileus or small bowel obstruction (Fig. 5.39). If necessary, measure the diameter of the bowel; a value over 30 mm is definitely abnormal but make sure that two overlapping loops are not being measured. As the bowel dilates the normal mucosal pattern becomes largely effaced and the valvulae conniventes become clearly visible.

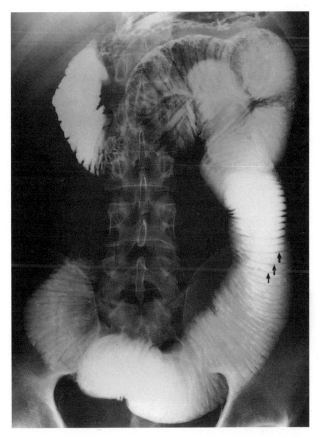

Fig. 5.39 Dilatation from small bowel obstruction. The diameter of the bowel is greatly increased. The feathery mucosal pattern is lost and the folds appear as thin lines traversing the bowel, known as valvulae conniventes (arrows).

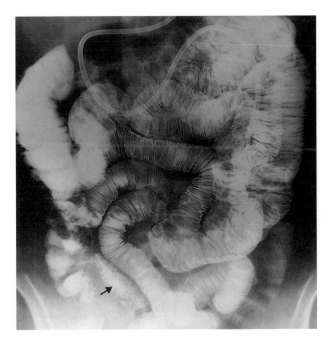

Fig. 5.38 Normal small bowel enema. This technique gives good mucosal detail. The arrow points to the terminal ileum. Note that a tube has been passed through the stomach into the jejunum.

Mucosal abnormality

The mucosal folds become thickened in many conditions, e.g. malabsorption states, oedema or haemorrhage in the bowel wall, and when inflamed or infiltrated (Fig. 5.40). Since mucosal fold thickening occurs in many diseases it is not possible to make a particular diagnosis unless other more specific features are present.

Narrowing

The only normal narrowings are those caused by peristaltic waves. They are smooth, concentric and transient with normal mucosal folds traversing them and normal bowel proximally. The common causes of strictures are Crohn's disease (Fig. 5.41), tuberculosis and lymphoma. Strictures do not contain normal mucosal folds and usually result in dilatation of the bowel proximally.

Ulceration

The outline of the small bowel should be smooth apart from the indentation caused by normal mucosal folds. Ulcers appear as spikes projecting outwards, which may be shallow or deep (Fig. 5.42). Ulceration is seen in Crohn's disease, tuberculosis and lymphoma. When there is a combination of fine ulceration and mucosal oedema, a 'cobblestone' appearance may be seen.

Alteration in position

(a) Congenital malrotation. During intrauterine life the bowel undergoes a series of rotations. Failure of the normal rotation may result in the small bowel being situated in the right side of the abdomen and the colon on the left side (Fig. 5.43). However, this state of affairs only occasionally gives rise to problems, mainly volvulus associated with abnormal mesenteric attachments.
(b) Displacement by a mass. Because of its mesentery the small intestine is freely mobile and will be displaced by an abdominal or pelvic mass (Fig. 5.44). The bowel appears stretched around any mass but the mucosal pattern is usually preserved.

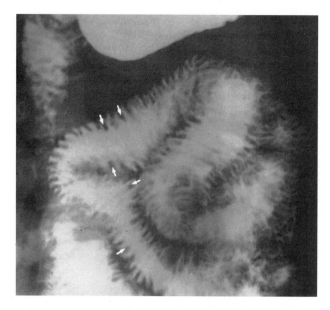

Fig. 5.40 Mucosal abnormality with infiltration of the bowel, in this case from oedema. The mucosal folds become thickened. Some of the thickened folds are arrowed.

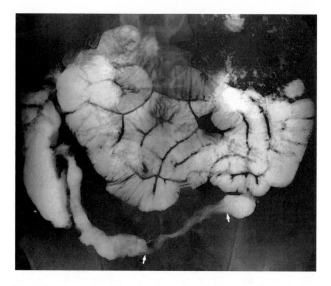

Fig. 5.41 Narrowing. There is a long irregular stricture (arrows) in the terminal ileum due to Crohn's disease. There is an abnormal mucosal pattern in the remainder of the terminal ileum. Note the contracted caecum – another feature of the disease.

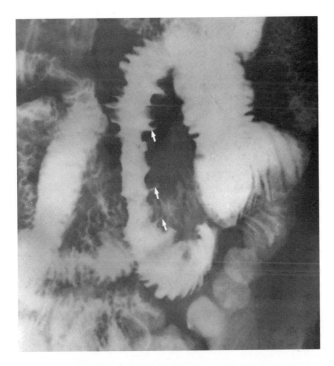

Fig. 5.42 Ulceration. Abnormal loops of bowel in Crohn's disease showing the ulcers as outward projections (arrows).

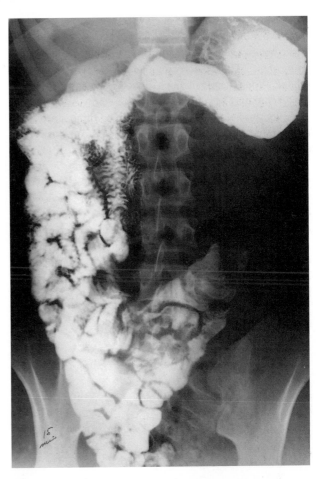

Fig. 5.43 Malrotation. The small bowel is situated in the right side of the abdomen. Later films showed the colon on the left side.

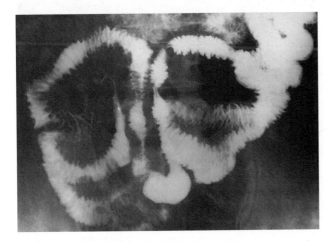

Fig. 5.44 Displacement. The small bowel is displaced around enlarged abdominal lymph nodes from a metastatic teratoma of the testis.

Crohn's disease

Crohn's disease is a disease of unknown aetiology characterized by localized areas of non-specific chronic granulomatous inflammation, which nearly always affects the terminal ileum. In addition, it may cause disease in several different parts of the small and large intestine, often leaving normal intervening bowel, the affected parts being known as skip lesions. The major signs on the barium follow-through are strictures and mucosal abnormality (Fig. 5.45).

The strictures are extremely variable in length. Sometimes a loop of bowel is so narrow, either from spasm in an extensively ulcerated loop of bowel or oedema and fibrosis in the bowel wall, that its appearance has been called 'the string sign'. The bowel proximal to a stricture is often dilated. When there is obvious disease in the terminal ileum the caecum may be contracted.

Ulcers are seen which are sometimes quite deep. Fine ulceration combined with mucosal oedema gives rise to the so-called 'cobblestone' appearance.

Owing to thickening of the bowel wall the mucosal folds may become thickened, distorted or even disappear. When this thickening of the bowel wall is severe then the loops of bowel become separated; the presence of an inflammatory mass will cause even greater displacement of the loops.

Fistulae may occur to other small bowel loops, colon, bladder or vagina. When the fistula is between adjacent loops of small intestine it can be difficult to detect on the barium follow-through.

Crohn's disease may cause malabsorption so the radiological features of this condition may be present as well.

Tuberculosis

Tuberculosis is indistinguishable from Crohn's disease on barium examination. It commonly affects the ileocaecal region and also causes contraction of the caecum.

Lymphoma

The infiltration in the wall of the bowel with lymphoma gives an appearance that is often extremely difficult to distinguish from Crohn's disease. Additional features to look for that may help differentiate the two conditions are small mucosal filling defects due to tumour nodules (Fig. 5.46), and displacement of loops caused by enlarged lymph nodes. Enlargement of the liver and spleen may also be present.

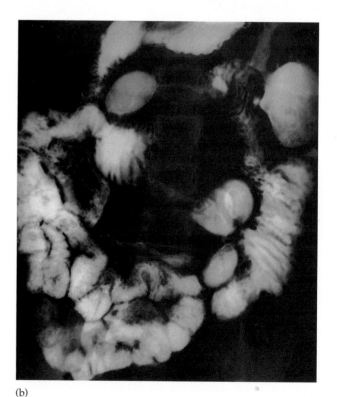

(a)

(b)

Fig. 5.45 Crohn's disease. (a) Many of the features are illustrated in this film. There are long strictures affecting different loops of ileum. The outlines of the strictures are irregular due to ulceration. Note how the affected loops lie separately, displaced from other loops because of the presence of inflammatory masses. (b) In this patient there are several strictures with dilatation of the bowel proximal to the strictures.

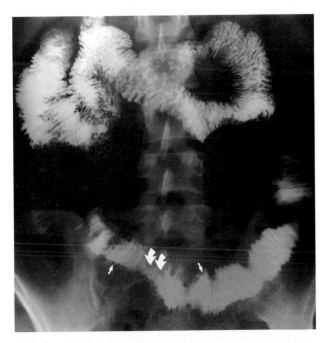

Fig. 5.46 Lymphoma. Lymphomatous infiltration has occurred in the lower loops of bowel causing thickening of the mucosal folds (small arrows) and discrete filling defects due to tumour nodules (curved arrows).

Malabsorption

A number of disorders result in defective absorption of foodstuffs, minerals or vitamins. The definitive test for malabsorption is the jejunal biopsy. Radiology is no substitute for a jejunal biopsy but along with biochemical tests is an important complementary investigation. The use of the barium follow-through in malabsorption is twofold:

1 It may show a structural abnormality causing the malabsorption.

2 It may help to make the diagnosis in doubtful cases where the biochemical tests are equivocal or normal.

The signs of malabsorption in the small bowel follow-through are (Fig. 5.47):

• small bowel dilatation, the jejunum being affected more than the ileum;

• thickening of mucosal folds;

• flocculation and dilution of the barium in advanced disease. Instead of the barium forming a continuous

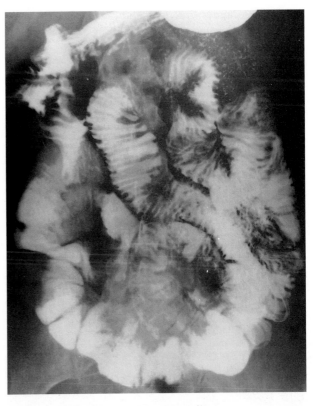

Fig. 5.47 Malabsorption. The bowel is dilated and the mucosal folds thickened. In the lower loops the barium appears less dense due to it becoming diluted. No specific cause for the malabsorption can be detected, which in this case was due to gluten enteropathy.

column there may be clumping or flocculation so that the barium column is broken up into a number of segments. The barium may become diluted by the excessive fluid in the small bowel and so appears less dense.

The above signs occur with any of the causes of malabsorption.

In the following conditions no clue to the cause can be obtained from a study of the barium follow-through:

1 Diffuse mucosal lesions.

• gluten enteropathy (coeliac disease and idiopathic steatorrhoea);

• tropical sprue.

2 Deficiency of absorptive factors, e.g. bile or pancreatic enzymes.

3 Postgastrectomy, due to rapid emptying of gastric remnant and insufficient mixing with bile and pancreatic juice.

Those conditions where the cause of malabsorption may be seen include:

1 Crohn's disease (see p. 171).

2 Lymphoma (see p. 172).

3 Anatomical abnormalities.

• decreased length of small bowel available for absorption, e.g. surgical resection or a fistula short-circuiting a length of small bowel;

• stagnation of bowel contents, allowing bacterial overgrowth, which utilizes nutrients from the bowel lumen, caused by:

(a) multiple small bowel diverticula (Fig. 5.48);

(b) a dilated loop cut off from the main stream of the bowel in which there is delayed filling and emptying (blind loop);

(c) a dilated loop proximal to a stricture (stagnant loop).

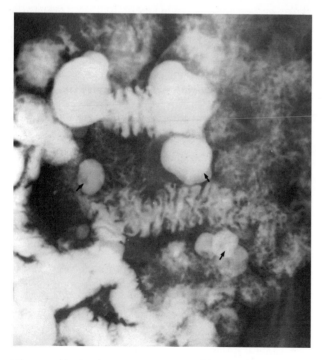

Fig. 5.48 Diverticulosis. A number of diverticula of varying size are arising from the small bowel. Some of these are arrowed.

Disaccharidase deficiency

Patients suffering from milk intolerance from a deficiency of the enzyme lactase in the small bowel mucosa have an abnormal appearance on a barium follow-through if lactose is added to the barium. The small bowel becomes dilated, the barium diluted and the barium rapidly reaches the colon.

Acute small bowel obstruction

A barium examination is not carried out in most cases of obstruction as the diagnosis is usually made on clinical examination with the help of plain abdominal films (p. 137). When barium is given by mouth it shows that the small bowel proximal to an obstruction is dilated, often markedly, and the barium becomes diluted by the excess fluid in the bowel (Fig. 5.39, p. 169).

Although a barium follow-through must be avoided in a colonic obstruction because the barium may become solid and impact proximal to the obstruction, this danger is not present in a small bowel obstruction because the fluid in the bowel prevents the barium solidifying. However, because of the dilution of the barium it is often difficult to diagnose the nature or site of the obstruction.

Worm infestation

Roundworms (Ascaris) are the commonly encountered worms large enough to be seen as filling defects in the lumen of the bowel (they may grow up to 35 cm long) (Fig. 5.49). The worms themselves may ingest the barium to have their own barium meal and barium may be seen in their digestive tracts.

Large intestine

The standard examination of the large intestine is the barium enema. Barium is run into the colon under gravity through a tube inserted into the rectum. Films are taken in various projections so that all the loops of colon are unravelled. In the 'single-contrast method' the whole colon is distended with barium. When a 'double-contrast technique' is used only part of the colon is filled with barium and air is then blown in to push the barium around the

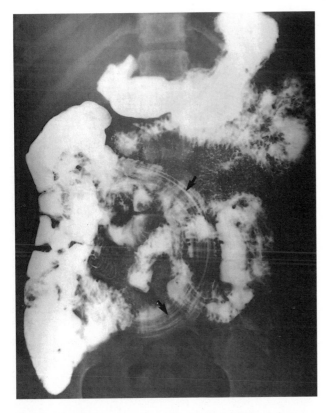

Fig. 5.49 Worm infestation. Several long tubular filling defects (arrows) due to roundworms (Ascaris) in the small bowel.

colon with the result that the colon is distended with air and the mucosa coated with barium.

Prior bowel preparation by means of aperients or washout is most important to rid the colon of faecal material, which might otherwise mask small lesions and cause confusion by simulating polyps.

Endoscopy

Sigmoidoscopy should be performed in every patient in whom a barium enema is requested because lesions in the rectum, especially mucosal abnormalities, may be missed by barium examinations.

Colonoscopy is becoming more widely practised with the advent of flexible endoscopes. Colonoscopy is complementary to a barium enema examination and requires specific indications:

- inspecting and biopsying abnormalities demonstrated on barium enema;
- investigating patients with persistent symptoms with a normal barium enema – this applies particularly to rectal bleeding when an undiagnosed polyp may be discovered;
- screening patients with a strong family history of colonic carcinoma;
- performing polypectomy;
- assessing the extent of ulcerative colitis and Crohn's disease.

Normal barium enema

The radiological anatomy of the normal colon is shown in Fig. 5.50. Certain features are worth emphasizing.

The length of the colon is very variable and sometimes there are redundant loops, particularly in the sigmoid and transverse colon. The calibre decreases from the caecum to the sigmoid colon.

The caecum is usually situated in the right iliac fossa but it may be seen under the right lobe of the liver or even in the centre of the abdomen if it possesses a long mesentery. The lips of the ileocaecal valve may project into the caecum and cause a filling defect which must not be mistaken for a tumour. Filling of the terminal ileum and appendix may occur but if they do not fill no significance can be attached to this.

Haustra can usually be recognized in the whole of the colon although they may be absent in the descending and sigmoid regions. The outline of the distended colon, apart from the haustra, is smooth.

Abnormal barium enema

Narrowing of the lumen

Narrowing of the colon may be due to spasm, stricture formation or compression by an extrinsic mass.

Spasm is often seen in normal patients and providing it is an isolated finding it can be ignored. Spasm is also seen in conjunction with diverticular disease and various inflammatory disorders.

Spasm gives rise to a smooth concentric narrowing which usually varies in severity during the period under observa-

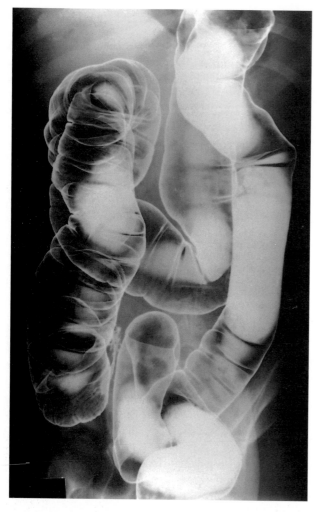

Fig. 5.50 Normal double contrast barium enema.

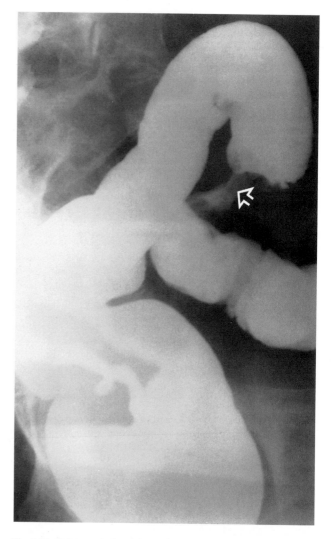

Fig. 5.51 Stricture. A short circumferential narrowing is seen in the sigmoid colon (arrow) from a carcinoma.

tion. It can often be abolished by the intravenous administration of a smooth muscle relaxant, e.g. Buscopan or glucagon.

Strictures. The main causes of stricture formation are:

- carcinoma
- diverticular disease
- Crohn's disease
- ischaemic colitis.

Rarer causes include tuberculosis, lymphogranuloma venereum, amoebiasis and radiation fibrosis.

When attempting to diagnose the nature of a stricture in the colon the following points should be borne in mind:

- *Neoplastic strictures* have shouldered edges, an irregular lumen and are rarely more than 6 cm in length (Fig. 5.51), whereas benign strictures classically have tapered ends, a relatively smooth outline and may be of any length.
- *Ulceration* may be seen in strictures due to Crohn's disease and sacculation of the colon is a feature of ischaemic strictures.

• *Narrowing due to diverticular disease* is usually accompanied by other signs of diverticular disease. It is sometimes impossible to distinguish a stricture owing to a carcinoma in an area of diverticular disease from a stricture owing to diverticular disease.

• The *site* of the stricture can help in limiting the differential diagnosis. Strictures due to diverticular disease are almost always confined to the sigmoid colon. Ischaemic strictures are usually centred somewhere between the splenic flexure and the sigmoid colon. Crohn's disease and tuberculosis have a predilection for the caecum.

Extrinsic compression by a mass arising outside the wall of the bowel causes a smooth narrowing of the colon frequently from one side only and often displaces the colon, e.g. ovarian and uterine masses (Fig. 5.52). Extrinsic compression causing a smooth indentation on the caecum may be seen with a mucocele of the appendix, appendix abscess (Fig. 5.53) or an inflammatory mass in Crohn's disease.

Dilatation

Dilatation of the colon is difficult to assess. The barium enema, particularly the double-contrast examination, involves distending the colon, so that its diameter is partly dependent on the amount of barium and air introduced.

The causes of dilatation of the colon are:

• *Obstruction.* Here the important consideration is not the dilatation itself but the nature of the obstructing lesion. In complete obstruction the barium enema may only show one end of the stricture, so some of the valuable signs described above are lost.

• *Paralytic ileus.* This diagnosis is usually made on clinical grounds with the help of plain films of the abdomen (p. 137). In those few cases where it proves difficult to distin-

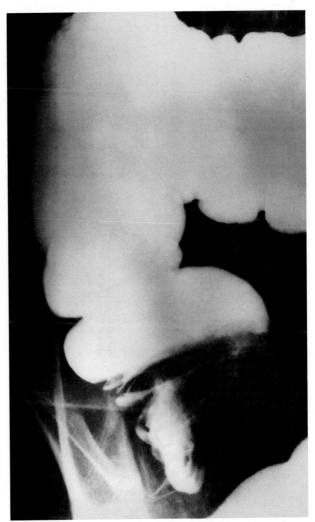

Fig. 5.53 Extrinsic compression. An appendix abscess is compressing and narrowing the caecum.

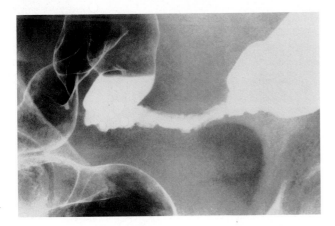

Fig. 5.52 Extrinsic compression. A narrowed length of sigmoid colon is seen caused by compression by an adjacent ovarian carcinoma.

guish paralytic ileus which in this context is sometimes called pseudo-obstructing from mechanical obstruction to the distal colon, a barium enema can be undertaken. This will show a dilated but otherwise normal colon.

- *Volvulus.*
- *Ulcerative colitis* with toxic dilatation (see Fig. 4.6, p. 139).
- *Hirschsprung's disease* and *megacolon.*

Filling defects

Filling defects in the colon, as elsewhere in the gastrointestinal tract, may be intraluminal, arise from the wall or be due to pressure from an extrinsic mass.

In a clean colon, a localized filling defect is likely to be a polyp or a neoplasm. Faeces will cause a filling defect and can be very difficult to distinguish from a polyp or tumour (Fig. 5.54). Faeces have no attachment to the wall of the bowel, are completely surrounded by barium or air, and move freely, varying with the position of the patient. All barium enema examinations should be made with a clean colon in order to avoid misdiagnosing polyps that are in fact faeces.

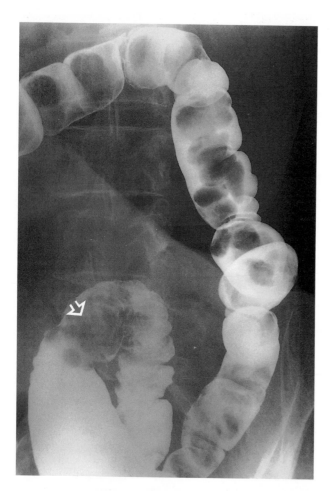

Fig. 5.54. Filling defects. Lumps of faeces have caused smooth filling defects surrounded by barium. However, in the sigmoid colon there is a large filling defect with ill-defined edges (arrow). This is a carcinoma. A clean colon is essential for a satisfactory barium enema.

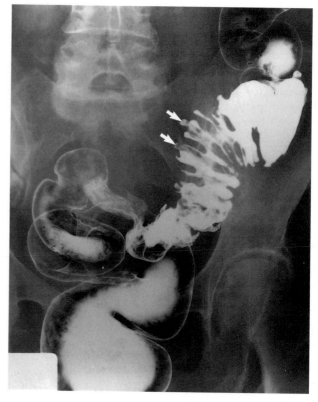

Fig. 5.55 Muscle hypertrophy and diverticula. Muscle hypertrophy gives the sigmoid colon a serrated appearance. Two small diverticula are arrowed.

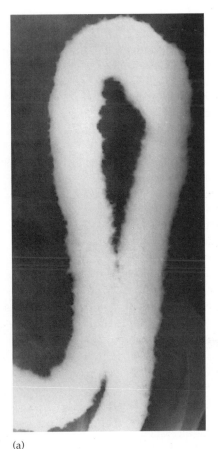 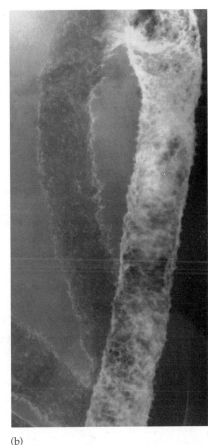

Fig. 5.56 Ulceration. (a) Single contrast. (b) Double contrast. In this case of ulcerative colitis the ulceration causes the normally smooth outline of the colon to be irregular.

(a)　　　　　　　　　　　　　　(b)

Intramural haemorrhage, oedema or air in the wall of the colon (pneumatosis coli) all cause multiple smooth filling defects arising from the wall of the bowel.

A unique type of filling defect is seen in intussusception (p. 186).

Diverticula and muscle hypertrophy

These are seen with diverticular disease (Fig. 5.55) and are discussed on p. 182.

Ulceration

Ulcers of the colonic mucosa can be recognized as small projections from the lumen into the wall of the bowel. This results in the normally smooth outline of the colon having a fuzzy or shaggy appearance (Fig. 5.56). The two major causes of ulceration are ulcerative colitis and Crohn's disease. Rarer causes include tuberculosis, and amoebic and bacillary dysentery.

Displacement of the colon

Displacement of the colon from its normal position may be caused by a variety of abdominal or pelvic masses, e.g. enlargement of the liver and spleen, or ovarian cyst. These masses may also compress the colon. Scrutiny of the plain abdominal films should be made as these may show further details of the mass but ultrasound or CT is usually necessary.

Displacement of the colon is also seen in malrotation.

Ulcerative colitis and Crohn's disease of the colon

Although classical changes are described for both ulcerative colitis and Crohn's disease it is sometimes difficult to distinguish between them. Radiology is important not only to diagnose these conditions but also to assess the extent and severity of the disease and to detect complications.

Ulcerative colitis

Ulcerative colitis is a disease of unknown aetiology characterized by inflammation and ulceration of the colon. The disease always involves the rectum. When more extensive it extends in continuity around the colon, sometimes affecting the whole colon. The cardinal radiological sign is widespread ulceration (Fig. 5.56). The ulcers are usually shallow but in severe cases may be quite deep. In all but the milder cases, there is loss of the normal colonic haustra in the affected portions of the colon. Oedema of the perirectal tissues causes widening of the space between the sacrum and the rectum. Narrowing and shortening of the colon, giving the appearance of a rigid tube (Fig. 5.57), and pseudopolyps are seen in advanced disease. Pseudopolyps are small filling defects projecting into the lumen of the bowel formed by swollen mucosa in between the areas of ulceration. The swelling of these islands of inflamed mucosa makes it difficult to assess the true depth of the ulceration.

Strictures are rare and when present are likely to be due to carcinoma: the incidence of colonic carcinoma in long-standing ulcerative colitis is significantly increased.

When the whole colon is involved, the terminal ileum may become dilated. Since the ileocaecal valve in this situation is incompetent, the abnormal terminal ileum is usually demonstrated at barium enema.

Toxic dilatation (toxic megacolon) is a serious complication. The diagnosis is made on clinical grounds and on examination of the plain abdominal film. A barium enema should never be performed in the presence of toxic dilatation owing to the risk of perforating the colon.

Crohn's disease of the colon

Crohn's disease is a chronic granulomatous condition of unknown aetiology which may affect any part of the gas-

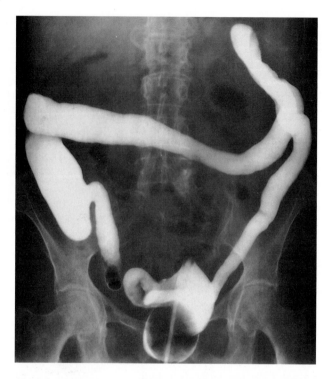

Fig. 5.57 Ulcerative colitis. With long-standing disease the haustra are lost and the colon becomes narrowed and shortened coming to resemble a rigid tube. Reflux into the ileum through an incompetent ileocaecal valve has occurred.

trointestinal tract, but most frequently involves the lower ileum and the colon. The colon may be the only part of the alimentary tract to be involved, but usually the disease affects the small bowel if the colon is involved.

At an early stage in the disease, the findings at barium enema are: loss of haustration, narrowing of the lumen of the bowel and shallow ulceration. This criss-crossing ulceration combined with mucosal oedema may give rise to a 'cobblestone' appearance of the mucosa (Fig. 5.58). Later, the ulcers become deeper and may track in the submucosa (Fig. 5.59). The ulcers may be very deep, penetrating into the muscle layer, when they are described as 'rose-thorn' ulcers or deep fissures. The deep ulceration in Crohn's disease may lead to the formation of intra- and extramural abscesses. Fistulae are an important complication.

Strictures are a common finding in Crohn's disease (Fig. 5.60). The strictures are smooth and have tapered ends.

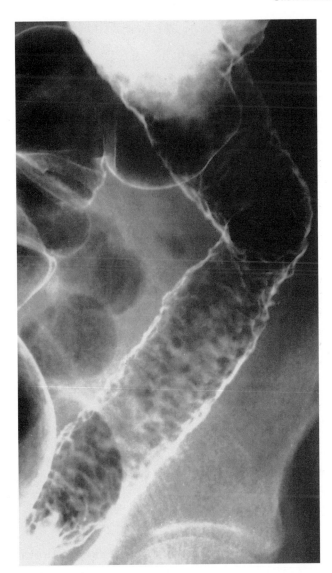

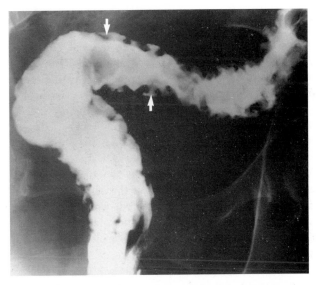

Fig. 5.59 Crohn's disease. Very deep ulcers are present. Two examples of an ulcer tracking in the submucosa are arrowed.

Fig. 5.58 Crohn's disease. The mucosal pattern has a 'cobblestone' appearance due to criss-crossing fine ulceration.

Fig. 5.60 Crohn's disease – strictures. A long stricture is present in the transverse colon (between curved arrows) and a shorter one in the sigmoid colon (between small arrows). In this case the outline of the strictures are irregular, due to ulceration. These two abnormal segments with normal intervening bowel are an example of 'skip lesions' – an important diagnostic feature of Crohn's disease.

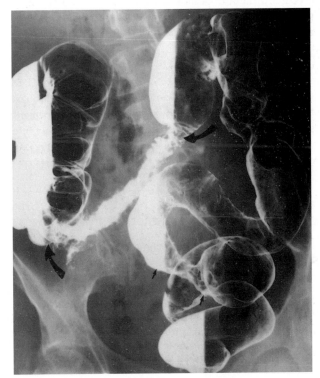

When the caecum is involved it is usually markedly contracted. Ulcers may or may not be present in the strictured area. The disease is not always circumferential; one of the features that distinguishes it from ulcerative colitis is that it may involve only one portion of the circumference of the bowel.

Another important diagnostic feature is the presence of the so-called 'skip lesion' (Fig. 5.60), namely areas of disease with intervening normal bowel. Skip lesions are virtually diagnostic of Crohn's disease. However, the entire colon may be involved or the disease may be limited to just one segment. There is a predilection for the caecum and terminal ileum. The rectum is often spared – another important differentiating feature from ulcerative colitis. Fistulae may also occur between the colon and the small bowel, bladder or vagina (Fig. 5.61).

Differences between ulcerative colitis and Crohn's disease

The only specific features are the presence of skip lesions and a normal rectum providing this is confirmed sigmoidoscopically. If either of these are seen then the diagnosis of Crohn's disease can be confidently made. Other differences are listed in Table 5.1.

Diverticular disease

Diverticula are sac-like out-pouchings of mucosa through the muscular layer of the bowel wall. They are associated with hypertrophy of the muscle layer and are probably due

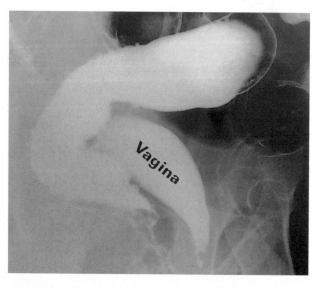

Fig. 5.61 Crohn's disease – rectovaginal fistula. During the barium enema filling of the vagina with barium occurred. Note the ulceration in the rectum.

to herniation of mucosa through areas of weakness where blood vessels penetrate the muscle. Diverticula are very common, particularly in the elderly. They are seen in all parts of the colon but are commonest in the sigmoid colon. At one time, the term 'diverticulitis' was applied when infection was thought to be causing symptoms and diverticulosis when the diverticula were considered asymptomatic. As no radiological distinction can be made between these

Table 5.1 Differences between Crohn's disease and ulcerative colitis.

Crohn's disease	Ulcerative colitis
1 Rectum involved in half the cases	1 Rectum involved in all the cases
2 Colon may be affected segmentally	2 Colon always affected continuously
3 Ulcers deep	3 Ulcers shallow
4 Some cases show asymmetrical loss of haustra	4 Symmetrical loss of haustra is the rule
5 Fistulae are a feature	5 Fistulae very rarely occur
6 Anal or perianal lesions frequent	6 Anal or perianal lesions uncommon
7 Small bowel involvement common – particularly of the terminal ileum with narrowing in the region of the ileocaecal valve.	7 Small bowel normal – dilatation of the terminal ileum may be seen

two entities the term 'diverticular disease' is nowadays used to cover both situations.

The diverticula when filled with barium are seen as spherical out-pouchings with a narrow neck (Fig. 5.62). The colon may also show a 'saw tooth' serrated appearance from hypertrophy of the muscle coats (see Fig. 5.55, p. 178). Sometimes, the signs of muscle hypertrophy are seen in isolation. Some diverticula may not fill; this is particularly true when inflammation occludes the necks of the diverticula.

A diverticulum may perforate, resulting in a pericolic abscess or fistula into the bladder, small bowel or vagina. This is recognized by noting barium outside the colon, either in the pericolic region (Fig. 5.63) or within the structure to which the fistula has occurred. An abscess can be most readily diagnosed with CT. Occasionally, diverticula perforate directly into the peritoneal cavity giving rise to peritonitis, and free intraperitoneal air should be looked for on a plain abdominal film. A stricture with or without local abscess formation (Fig. 5.64) may occur. Usually, this is clearly within an area of recognizable diverticular disease. It is, however, often impossible to differentiate such a stricture from a carcinoma occurring coincidentally in a patient with diverticular disease.

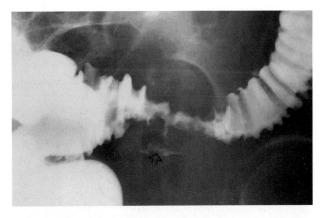

Fig. 5.63 Diverticular disease. Barium is seen outside the lumen of the bowel in a pericolic abscess (arrow). Muscle hypertrophy gives the bowel a serrated appearance.

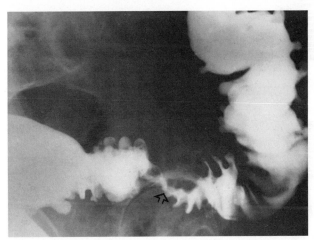

Fig. 5.64 Diverticular disease. A stricture is present (arrow). Although there is recognizable diverticular disease at both ends of the stricture, it is impossible to exclude definitely a carcinoma.

Appendicitis

In most cases the diagnosis of appendicitis is obvious clinically and imaging is unnecessary. In cases of doubt the diagnosis can be made with ultrasound which shows a distended non-compressible appendix with a thickened oedematous wall (Fig. 5.65). An appendolith may be visible within the appendix as a hyperechoic area casting an acoustic shadow. An appendix abscess can be diagnosed

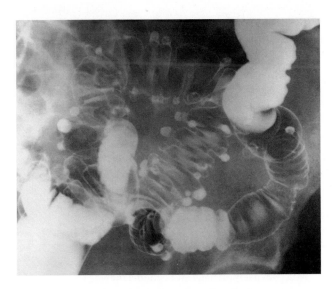

Fig. 5.62 Diverticular disease. Numerous diverticula are seen as out-pouchings from the sigmoid colon.

with CT (Fig. 5.66) or ultrasound as a mass in the right iliac fossa.

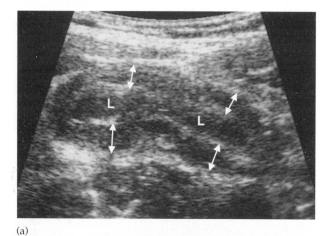

(a)

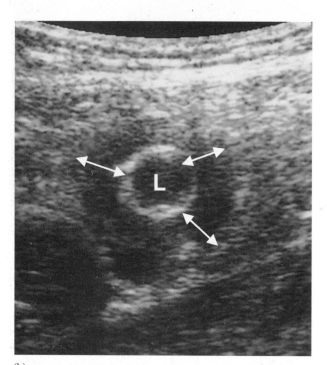

(b)

Fig. 5.65 Appendicitis. (a) Longitudinal scan. (b) Transverse ultrasound of the right iliac fossa showing marked thickening of the wall of the appendix (arrows) and distension of its lumen (L).

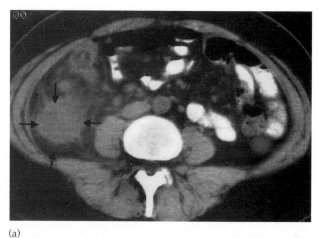

(a)

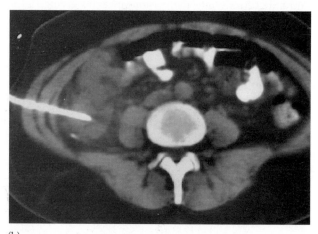

(b)

Fig. 5.66 Appendix abscess. (a) Computed tomography scan shows a mass (arrows) in the right iliac fossa. (b) The abscess was drained under CT guidance.

Ischaemic colitis

Acute infarction of the large bowel is very rare. Ischaemia is usually a more chronic process giving rise, initially, to mucosal oedema and haemorrhage which may resolve. In the later stages a stricture may form. The findings on barium enema depend on the stage at which the examination is performed.

Mucosal haemorrhage and oedema may be recognized by observing multiple smooth indentations into the lumen of the bowel, resembling thumb prints (Fig. 5.67a). If stricture formation occurs, the stricture will be smooth and have tapered ends. The site is usually centred between the splenic flexure and the sigmoid colon because these are the regions of the colon with the most vulnerable blood supply (Fig.

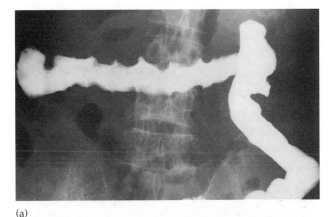

(a)

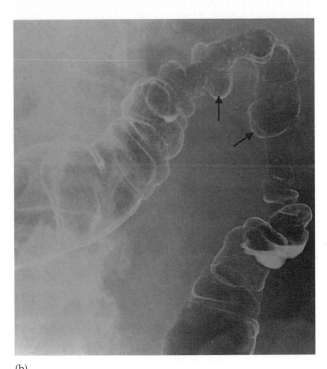

(b)

Fig. 5.67 Ischaemic colitis. (a) Mucosal haemorrhage and oedema have caused indentations resembling thumb prints in the transverse colon. (b) A long smooth stricture involving the splenic flexure with sacculations arising from the colon (arrows) in another patient.

5.67b). Sacculations may be seen arising from one side of the strictured area.

Pneumatosis coli

In this unusual condition gas-filled spaces are present in the wall of the bowel. These cyst-like spaces do not communicate with the lumen. They can be identified on a plain film of the abdomen but the diagnosis is much easier with a barium enema where the cysts cause smooth translucent filling defects projecting from the wall of the bowel (Fig. 5.68). The appearance could be confused with intramural haemor-

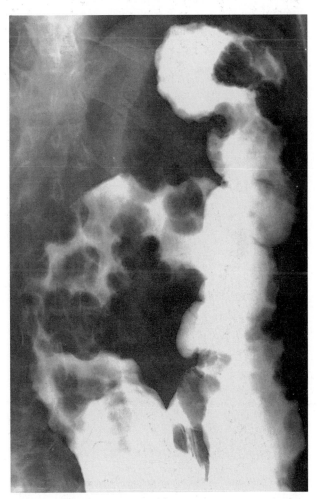

Fig. 5.68 Pneumatosis coli. Part of the colon showing numerous translucencies in the wall of the colon owing to many gas-filled cysts.

rhage and oedema, or with colitis if the presence of air within the cysts is not appreciated.

Volvulus

In a volvulus a loop of bowel twists on its mesentery. This happens most frequently in the sigmoid colon, particularly when it is redundant, and less often in the caecum. The twisted loop becomes greatly distended and the bowel proximal to the volvulus is obstructed by the twist and may therefore also be dilated.

The diagnosis is usually made on the plain abdominal films (see p. 138) but a barium enema may be helpful in doubtful cases so that if confirmed, non-operative reduction of the volvulus may be attempted. This will show a smooth, tapered narrowing (Fig. 5.69) from twisting of the colon, with marked dilatation of the bowel proximal to the twist.

Intussusception

An intussusception is the invagination of one segment of the bowel into another. Infants are much more liable to intussusception than adults.

By far the commonest type is the ileum invaginating into the colon; this is known as an *ileocolic intussusception*. Other types are *colocolic*, when the colon invaginates into another part of the colon, and *ileo-ileal* when the ileum invaginates into a more distal segment of ileum.

Nowadays the diagnosis of intussusception is based on

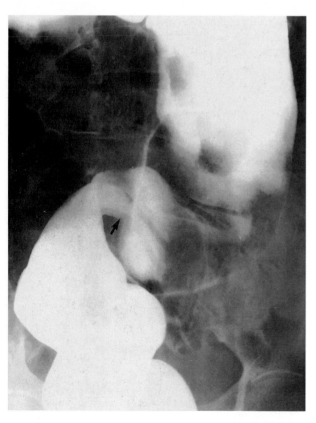

Fig. 5.69 Volvulus. A smooth narrowing is seen in the sigmoid colon where the colon has twisted (arrow). Note the dilated colon proximal to this.

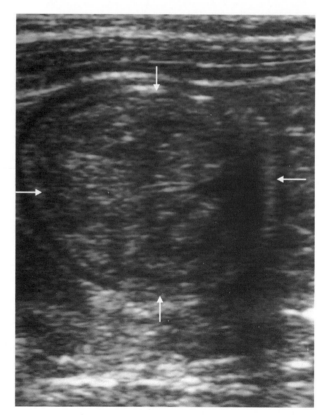

Fig. 5.70 Intussusception. Ultrasound of upper abdomen showing the intussusception as a mass (arrows).

diagnosing an abdominal mass often with a hyperechoic centre on ultrasound (Fig. 5.70). The diagnosis is confirmed by an enema with air or carbon dioxide as the contrast agent. When gas is insufflated *per rectum* under fluoroscopic or ultrasound control, the flow of gas will be obstructed by the leading edge of the intussusception and an attempt at pneumatic reduction can be made in order to avoid a laparotomy (Fig. 5.71). If such a reduction is to be safely carried out, the child should have no clinical signs of peritonitis. The longer the symptoms have been present, the greater the risk of perforating gangrenous bowel. Alternatively, though less commonly employed nowadays, a barium enema can confirm the diagnosis and be used to reduce the intussusception.

In adults, surgical treatment is invariable as an intussusception is normally caused by a tumour.

Tumours

Polyps

The word 'polyp' means a small mass of tissue arising from the wall of the bowel projecting into the lumen. Polyps may be sessile or on a stalk, single or multiple. They are best demonstrated with a double-contrast barium enema. Polyps may be neoplastic, inflammatory or occasionally developmental in origin. It is often impossible on radiologi-

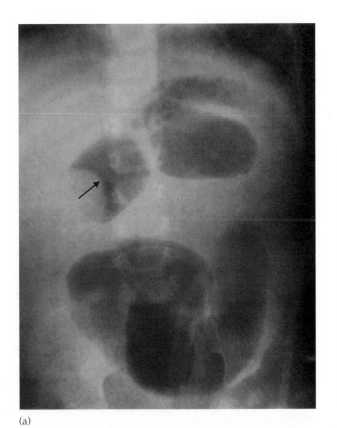

(a)

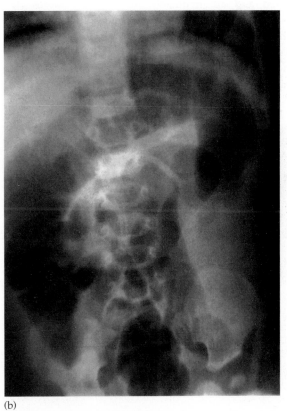

(b)

Fig. 5.71 Intussusception. (a) Film taken during reduction of the intussusception with air insufflated *per rectum* showing a filling defect in the transverse colon (arrow) owing to ileum invaginated into the colon. (b) Later film showing that the intussusception has been reduced with air filling the caecum and entering the small bowel.

cal grounds to exclude malignancy in a polyp. However, only a tiny minority of polyps less than 1 cm in size and very few less than 2 cm are cancers.

The features that suggest malignancy are: a diameter of more than 2 cm; a short thick stalk; irregular surface; rapid rate of growth as judged by serial barium enema examinations.

The common polyps are:

• *Adenomatous polyps* (Fig. 5.72). These are benign neoplasms. They may be single or multiple and are found most frequently in the rectosigmoid region. In *familial polyposis* they are numerous and one or more will, in time, undergo malignant change (Fig. 5.73).

• *Villous adenomas* are benign sessile tumours showing a sponge-like appearance owing to barium trapped between the villous strands. They are usually large when first discovered and are frequently mistaken for faeces. The common sites are the rectum and the caecum. There is a high incidence of malignant change.

• *Polypoid adenocarcinomas.*

• *Juvenile polyps.* Almost all isolated polyps in children are benign. They are probably developmental in origin.

• *Inflammatory polyps (pseudopolyps)* are seen in ulcerative colitis.

• *Hyperplastic or metaplastic polyps.*

Carcinoma

Carcinomas may arise anywhere in the colon but they are commonest in the rectosigmoid region and the caecum. The appearance and behaviour of a carcinoma in these two sites are usually quite different. The patient with a rectosigmoid carcinoma often has an annular stricture and presents with alteration in bowel habit and obstruction, whereas with a caecal carcinoma the tumour can become very large without obstructing the bowel, so anaemia and weight loss are the common presenting features.

A barium enema shows the annular carcinoma as an irregular stricture with shouldered edges (see Fig. 5.51, p. 176). Such strictures are rarely more than 6 cm in length. The polypoid or fungating carcinoma (Fig. 5.74) causes an irregular filling defect projecting into the lumen of the bowel.

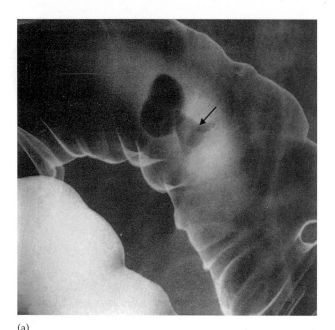

(a)

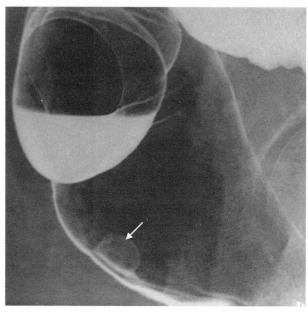

(b)

Fig. 5.72 Polyps. (a) Pedunculated polyp (arrow) outlined by barium in the sigmoid colon. (b) Sessile polyp (arrow) in the rectum.

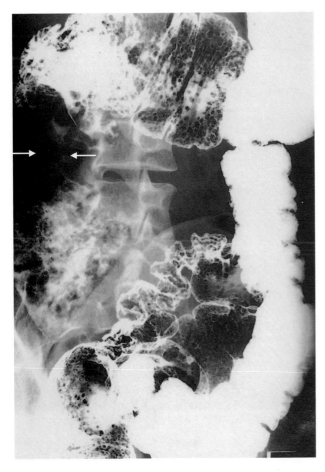

Fig. 5.73 Familial polyposis. Numerous small polyps are present throughout the colon. An annular carcinoma has developed in the ascending colon (arrows).

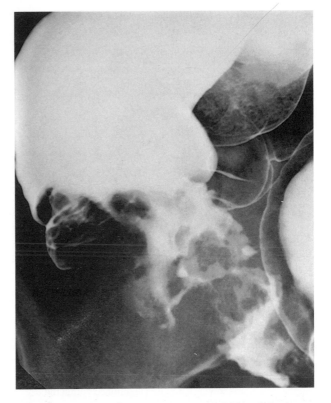

Fig. 5.74 Polypoid carcinoma. A large irregular filling defect is present in the caecum.

Multiple primary tumours must be excluded, as a patient with one carcinoma of the colon has a higher than normal risk of developing a second colonic cancer. This may be present at the time of the diagnosis or may present after the first tumour has been removed.

In very elderly or frail patients a CT scan is an alternative examination to a barium enema for the diagnosis of a colonic carcinoma. The colon has to be opacified with contrast or distended with air. A carcinoma can be recognized as thickening of the bowel wall and an irregular narrowing of the lumen of the colon (Fig. 5.4, p. 149).

CT/MRI of rectal carcinoma (Fig. 5.75)

The main value of CT and MRI is to demonstrate any tumour that has spread through the wall of the rectum and also to diagnose postoperative recurrence. Pelvic fat surrounds the rectum, and tumour infiltrating this fat can be readily recognized. Invasion into adjacent organs, the pelvic side walls, sacrum and lymph node metastases may also be demonstrated. Often, images of the abdomen are also taken in order to detect any para-aortic adenopathy or liver metastases.

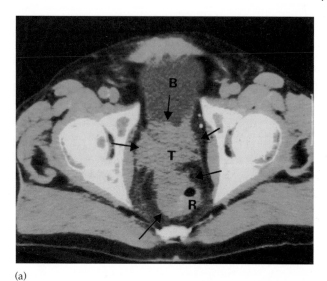

(a)

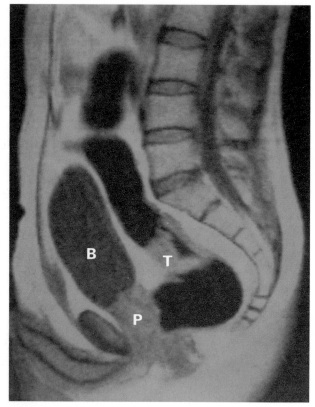

(b)

Fig. 5.75 Carcinoma of the rectum. (a) CT scan showing the tumour (T) invading the peripelvic fat and the bladder (B). The extent of the tumour is indicated by the arrows. R, rectum. (b) Sagittal MRI scan showing a tumour (T) confined within the rectum (R). B, bladder; P, prostate.

Hirschsprung's disease (congenital aganglionosis)

Hirschsprung's disease is due to absence of ganglion cells beyond a certain level in the colon, usually in the sigmoid or rectosigmoid region. In time, the colon proximal to the aganglionic segment becomes grossly distended, but in those patients who present soon after birth the dilatation may not be obvious.

The aganglionic segment, usually the rectum, is either normal or small at barium enema and the diagnosis depends on recognizing the transition from the normal or reduced calibre colon to the dilated colon (Fig. 5.76). To prevent the danger of water intoxication from the dilated colon, the colon is not washed out before the barium enema. The barium introduced is usually limited to the amount required to show the zone of transition from aganglionic to dilated bowel.

Idiopathic megacolon (functional megacolon)

The cause of idiopathic megacolon believed to be chronic constipation. At barium enema both the rectum and colon are dilated and contain large amount of faeces. The large-sized rectum serves as a differentiating feature from Hirschsprung's disease.

Radiology in acute bleeding from the small and large bowel

A Meckel's diverticulum, if it contains ectopic gastric

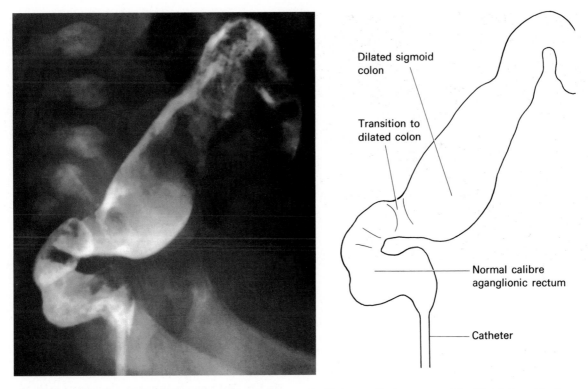

Dilated sigmoid
colon

Transition to
dilated colon

Normal calibre
aganglionic rectum

Catheter

Fig. 5.76 Hirschsprung's disease. Note the transition between the normal calibre aganglionic rectum and the dilated sigmoid colon.

mucosa, may be responsible for unexplained bleeding, particularly in children. A Meckel's diverticulum is very difficult to demonstrate on a barium follow-through but may be visualized with radionuclide techniques. An intravenous injection of technetium-99m (^{99m}Tc-pertechnetate) is given, which localizes in gastric mucosa. High uptake is seen in the stomach and in any gastric mucosa within a Meckel's diverticulum (Fig. 5.77).

Acute bleeding may occur in large and small bowel tumours. The condition angiodysplasia, a disorder comprising dilated vessels in the caecum, is a fairly common cause of bleeding in elderly patients. A barium enema should be avoided as the first examination because the presence of barium in the colon may preclude other investigations. Colonoscopy is usually performed but may be unrewarding as it is sometimes not possible to reach the right side of the colon. Even when the caecum is reached, angiodysplasia may not be visible through the colonoscope.

Arteriography may demonstrate the bleeding site, provided the patient is actively bleeding, by showing contrast in the lumen of the bowel. Sometimes arteriography also permits a diagnosis to be made, e.g. angiodysplasia or small bowel tumour. Embolization of the feeding vessel can be carried out to arrest bleeding at the time of arteriography when appropriate.

If the patient is actively bleeding at a rate of more than 0.5 ml/min then nuclear medicine techniques can be employed to localize the bleeding. Two different methods are available.

• The patient's red blood cells are labelled with ^{99m}Tc and the patient is then imaged under a gamma camera, so that any blood collecting in the bowel will be visualized (Fig. 5.78).

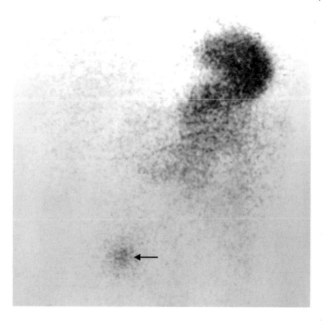

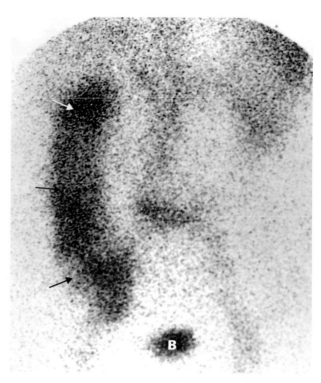

Fig. 5.77 Meckel's diverticulum. 99mTc-pertechnetate scan showing an isolated area of uptake in ectopic gastric mucosa in a Meckel's diverticulum (arrow). Normal uptake of radionuclide is seen in the stomach.

Fig. 5.78 Gastrointestinal bleeding. The patient's red blood cells have been labelled with 99mTc. Blood has collected in the ascending colon (arrows) from an active bleeding site in the caecum. B, bladder.

• The patient can be given an intravenous injection of 99mTc labelled colloid, the agent used for liver scanning. This is rapidly cleared from the circulation by the reticuloendothelial system. Any bleeding into the bowel can readily be demonstrated.

Radionuclide imaging techniques are simpler but almost as accurate as arteriography in localizing active haemorrhage and will assist in planning possible surgery or subsequent arteriography.

6

Hepatobiliary System, Pancreas and Spleen

Many different methods of imaging the hepatobiliary system and pancreas are available, including plain films, contrast examinations of the biliary system, ultrasound, computed tomography (CT), radionuclide imaging and magnetic resonance imaging (MRI). Invasive studies such as percutaneous or operative cholangiography and endoscopic retrograde cholangiopancreatography (ERCP) may be indicated, as may selective arteriography. Each of these tests has its own advantages and disadvantages. Ultrasound, for example, is particularly useful for diagnosing gall bladder disease, recognizing dilated bile ducts, diagnosing cysts and abscesses, and defining perihepatic fluid collections, whereas CT and MRI are particularly sensitive for detecting mass lesions such as metastases and abscesses. Often the various methods complement each other. Since the roles of the individual procedures are not clear cut, practice will vary from one centre to another.

In order to simplify the presentation, we will discuss the liver parenchyma separately from the biliary tract, although in clinical practice they usually need to be considered together.

Interventional techniques designed to treat or remove gall stones and to drain the biliary system are described on p. 440.

LIVER

Imaging techniques

Ultrasound of the liver

The *normal hepatic parenchyma* (Fig. 6.1) is of uniform echoreflectivity, composed of low and medium amplitude echoes, interspersed with the bright echoes of the portal triads and echo-free areas corresponding to large hepatic veins.

The normal liver displays considerable variation in size and shape. The right hepatic lobe is much larger than the left, which may be diminutive. The falciform ligament, which contains the ligamentum teres, lies between the medial and lateral segments of the left lobe. The ligamentum teres is often surrounded by fat; the resulting echo pattern should not be confused with a mass (Fig. 6.2).

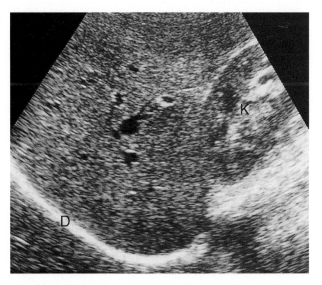

Fig. 6.1 Ultrasound of normal liver. Longitudinal scan showing uniform echo pattern interspersed with bright echoes of portal triads and echo-free areas of hepatic and portal veins. D, diaphragm; K, right kidney.

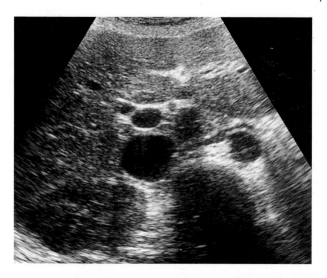

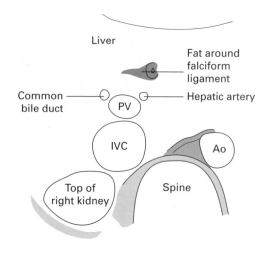

Fig. 6.2 Ultrasound of normal liver. Transverse scan across the porta hepatis. Ao, aorta; IVC, inferior vena cava; PV, portal vein.

The portal vein within the liver divides into right and left branches. Running alongside the portal veins are the hepatic arteries and bile ducts, both of which are usually too small to be visualized within the liver. Surrounding these portal triads is an echo-reflective sheath of fibrous and fatty tissue. The hepatic veins run separately, increasing in diameter as they drain towards the inferior vena cava at the level of the diaphragm (Fig. 6.3).

Focal masses are recognized sonographically as alterations of the normal echo pattern. They can be divided into cysts, solid masses, or complex combinations of the two. Cysts which are echo free and have thin or invisible walls can be assumed to be non-neoplastic (Fig. 6.4). Solid and complex masses (Figs 6.5 and 6.6) within the liver may be either benign or malignant in nature. Theoretically, most benign solid masses are encapsulated and should demonstrate a relatively sharp margin with the adjacent hepatic parenchyma, whereas malignant lesions should demonstrate a more irregular border. However, in practice it is often difficult to distinguish benign from malignant lesions unless the mass is clearly a simple cyst.

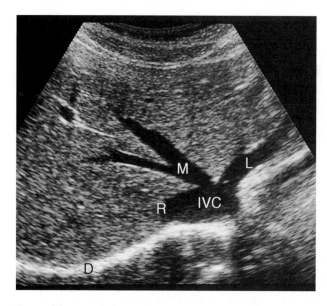

Fig. 6.3 Ultrasound of normal liver. Transverse scan through the superior portion of the liver showing the right (R), middle (M) and left (L) hepatic veins draining into the inferior vena cava (IVC) as it penetrates the diaphragm (D).

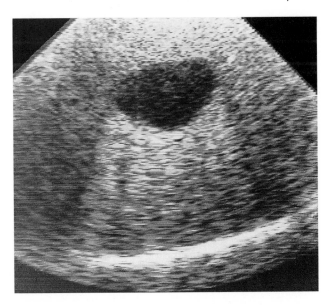

Fig. 6.4 Ultrasound of benign cyst. Note the imperceptible walls and acoustic enhancement behind the cyst. (CT scan of same case is shown in Fig. 6.14a.)

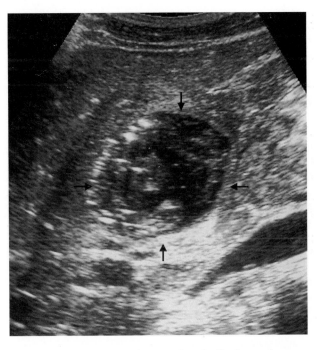

Fig. 6.6 Ultrasound of complex mass. Longitudinal scan of an abscess showing spherical mass (arrows) with areas of echogenicity both greater and less than normal liver.

When multiple solid or complex masses are seen within the liver, metastatic disease is the likely diagnosis, especially in patients with a known primary tumour. The prime differential diagnoses of multiple masses are multiple abscesses, regenerating nodules in cirrhosis of the liver and multiple haemangiomas.

Diffuse parenchymal diseases such as diffuse chronic inflammation and diffuse neoplastic infiltration can cause a generalized increase in the intensity of echoes from the liver parenchyma, and are difficult to distinguish from one another.

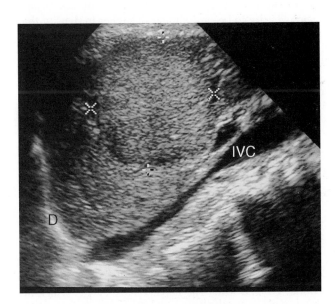

Fig. 6.5 Ultrasound of solid mass. Longitudinal scan. The cursors indicate an echogenic mass which proved to be a metastasis. D, diaphragm; IVC, inferior vena cava.

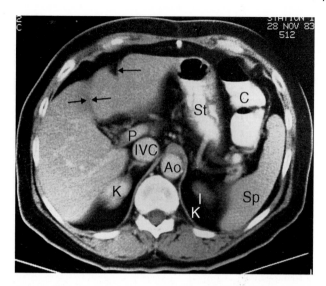

Fig. 6.7 CT scan of normal liver through porta hepatis (enhanced scan). A, aorta; C, colon; IVC, inferior vena cava; K, kidney; P, portal vein; Sp, spleen; St, stomach; single arrow = fissure for falciform ligament, Double arrow = fissure for gall bladder which divides liver into right and left lobes.

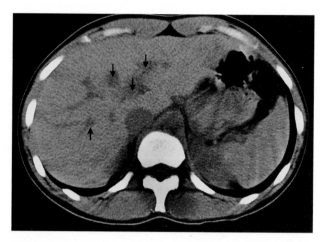

Fig. 6.8 CT scan showing unopacified hepatic veins (arrows) which should not be confused with metastases.

CT of the liver (Fig. 6.7)

The usual technique is to perform contiguous 10 mm sections through the liver. Intravenous contrast medium is often given in order to increase the density of normal liver parenchyma and to emphasize the density difference between the normal parenchyma and lesions that enhance poorly, such as tumours, abscesses or haematomas. Occasionally, very vascular lesions such as haemangiomas and a few neoplasms show greater enhancement than the surrounding parenchyma.

The lobar anatomy of the liver is defined by the fissure of the gall bladder, which divides the right and left lobes. The fissure for the falciform ligament is also clearly shown dividing the left lobe into medial and lateral segments.

The normal hepatic parenchyma has a relatively high density prior to contrast enhancement; higher than that of muscle and higher or equal in density to the spleen. On images taken without intravenous contrast medium, the hepatic veins are seen as branching, low density structures coursing through the liver. Since CT is a sectional technique, some of these branches may be seen as round or oval low-density areas which should not be confused with metastases (Fig. 6.8). After contrast enhancement, the hepatic veins opacify to become similar or higher in density than the surrounding parenchyma. Because the normal intrahepatic bile ducts are not visible and hepatic vessels opacify with contrast medium, the normal hepatic parenchyma after contrast shows either uniform density, or shows the hepatic veins clearly opacified against a background of uniform density. The region of the porta hepatis is recognizable as the entrance and exit points of the major vessels and bile ducts. The biliary system distal to the right and the left hepatic ducts can be identified on good quality images, but the smaller intrahepatic bile ducts are not visible in the normal patient.

Radionuclide liver imaging

Radionuclide liver scanning (^{99m}Tc-labelled sulphur or tin colloid) has been almost completely replaced by ultrasound, CT and MRI. The hepatobiliary agents which are discussed on p. 205 also show the liver parenchyma, but their primary indication is to show disease of the extrahepatic biliary system.

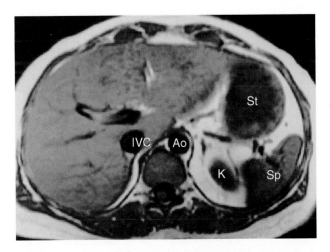

Fig. 6.9 Normal MRI scan of liver (T1-weighted image). The liver parenchyma shows intermediate signal. The blood vessels within the liver (predominantly the portal and hepatic veins) show no signal. Ao, aorta; IVC, inferior vena cava; K, kidney; Sp, spleen; St, stomach.

MRI of the liver (Fig. 6.9)

Magnetic resonance imaging is used as a problem-solving technique to give additional information to ultrasound and CT. Axial sections give images akin to CT but images can also be obtained in the coronal and sagittal planes. By using special sequences information can also be obtained on the arterial and venous circulation of the liver which is particularly well demonstrated on coronal sections.

Liver masses

Ultrasound, CT and MRI are all good methods of deciding whether a mass is present. It may be possible to predict the nature of the mass, as for example with cysts or haemangiomas. Sometimes, the diagnosis can be suggested, as in the case of multiple metastases, but frequently the definitive diagnosis depends on biopsy.

Liver neoplasms

Metastases, notably from carcinoma of the stomach, colon, pancreas, lung and breast are much more common than primary tumours (hepatoma and malignant lymphoma, both of which can be multifocal).

Metastases are often multiple, situated peripherally and of variable size. At ultrasound, they may show increased echogenicity (Fig. 6.10a) or, more usually, decreased echogenicity compared with the surrounding parenchyma (Fig. 6.10b). At times, they show a complex echo pattern and when they undergo central necrosis they may even resemble cysts. A metastasis may have an echogenic centre giving an appearance described as a target lesion (Fig. 6.10c). Some metastases have an echo pattern virtually identical to that of the surrounding parenchyma, which means they cannot be identified at sonography. At CT, metastases are seen as rounded areas, usually lower in density than the contrast enhanced surrounding parenchyma (Fig. 6.11). Most are well demarcated from the adjacent parenchyma. Intense contrast enhancement is sometimes seen within the tumour, or immediately surrounding it – a useful differentiating feature, which is not seen with cysts. MRI is an excellent method of demonstrating metastases (Fig. 6.12) that have a signal lower than normal liver on a T1-weighted scan and a high signal on a T2-weighted scan.

Primary carcinomas of the liver, which include hepatocellular carcinoma and cholangiocarcinoma, are often large and usually solitary but they may be multifocal. Their CT, ultrasound and MRI features are similar to metastatic neoplasms (Fig. 6.13).

Liver cysts

Simple cysts of the liver, both single and multiple, are usually congenital in origin; some are due to infection. Multiple hepatic cysts occur in adult polycystic disease, which not only affects the kidneys but may also involve the liver and other organs. These cysts are variable in size and are scattered through the liver.

At ultrasound, liver cysts show the typical features of cysts elsewhere in the body, namely sharp margin, no echoes within the lesion, and intense echoes from the front and back walls with acoustic enhancement deep to the larger cysts (see Fig. 6.4, p. 195).

At CT, cysts show very well-defined margins and have attenuation values similar to that of water (Fig. 6.14a). Lesions below 2 cm in diameter may be difficult to distinguish from solid neoplasms because portions of the normal

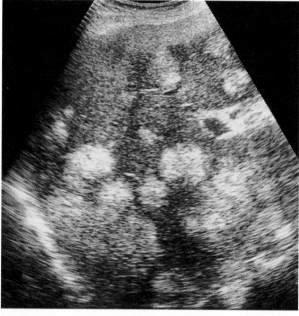

(a)

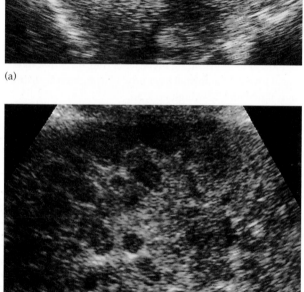

(b)

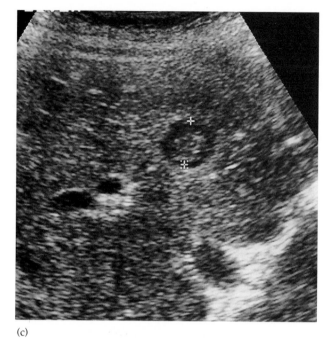

(c)

Fig. 6.10 Ultrasound of liver metastases. (a) Multiple hyperechoic metastases scattered throughout the liver. (b) Multiple metastases appearing as well-defined round hypoechoic lesions scattered throughout the liver. (c) The cursors indicate a metastasis showing reduced echogenicity but with an echogenic centre known as a target lesion.

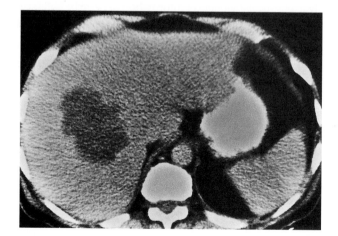

Fig. 6.11 CT scan of metastasis. This large low density mass is situated deeply in the right lobe of the liver.

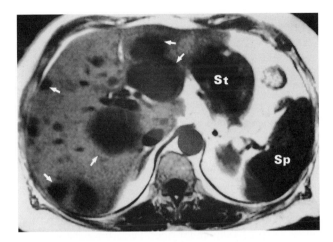

Fig. 6.12 Metastases. MRI scan showing multiple rounded low signal areas in the liver (arrows) on this T1-weighted image. Compare with the normal image shown in Fig. 6.9. Sp, spleen; St, stomach.

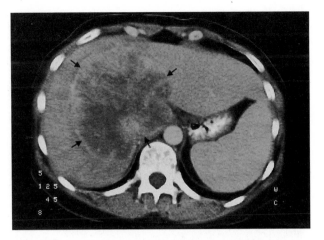

Fig. 6.13 Hepatoma. The CT scan shows a large, well-defined mass of variable density (arrows).

liver may be present on a particular CT section, and partial volume averaging may then result in a CT number close to that of soft tissues. Below 1 cm in diameter it is almost never possible to distinguish cyst from neoplasm.

At MRI, the features are similar to those found at CT. Cysts have the expected signal intensity of water, namely low signal on a T1-weighted scan and high signal on a T2-weighted scan.

Cysts due to echinococcus (hydatid) disease may be single or multiple; a few show calcified walls. Daughter cysts may be seen within a main cyst at both ultrasound and CT (Fig. 6.14b). Unless these features are present, hydatid cysts may prove indistinguishable from simple cysts at both ultrasound and CT.

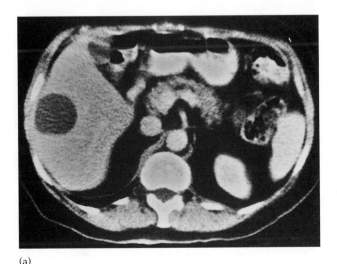

(a)

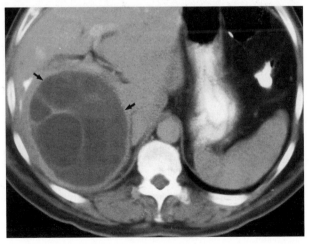

(b)

Fig. 6.14 Liver cysts. (a) Simple cyst of liver. CT scan shows a well-defined lesion of water density. (The ultrasound scan of this patient is shown in Fig. 6.4.) (b) CT scan showing a multilocular hydatid cyst in the right lobe of the liver (arrows).

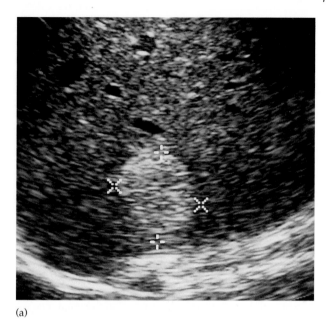

(a)

Haemangiomas of the liver (Figs 6.15 and 6.16)

One or more haemangiomas of the liver are common incidental findings and rarely require surgical resection. Occasionally they can cause significant haemorrhage, especially following trauma, and therefore percutaneous biopsy should be avoided if possible. Haemangiomas of the liver resemble neoplasms and other masses at ultrasound. At CT, there is one feature that permits a differentiation to be made. Initially, a haemangioma appears as a rounded, low density lesion but when sections are repeated after contrast, at intervals of a few minutes, the density increases to become similar with that of the surrounding liver.

Magnetic resonance imaging shows uniform very high intensity on T2-weighted images (Fig. 6.16), a characteristic that is shared with benign cysts, but which is very unusual with malignant neoplastic lesions.

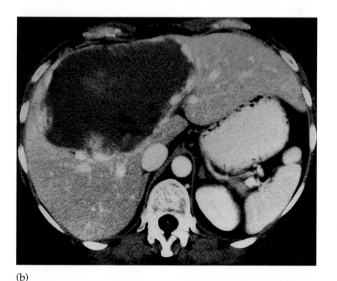

(b)

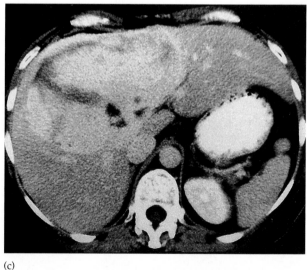

(c)

Fig. 6.15 Haemangioma (incidental finding). (a) Ultrasound scan shows a reflective mass in the right lobe of the liver (cursors). (b) CT scan, in another patient, immediately after intravenous contrast enhancement shows a large, low density lesion in the right lobe of the liver with appearances similar to a tumour. (c) A scan taken 10 minutes later shows that almost the entire lesion enhances to the same or to a greater degree than the normal liver.

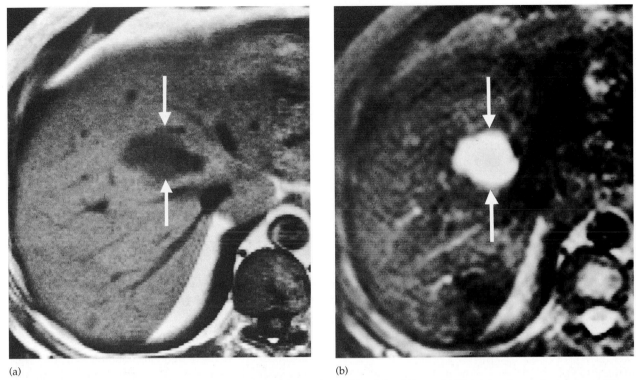

(a)   (b)

Fig. 6.16 MRI scan of a haemangioma. (a) Low intensity area (arrows) on a T1-weighted image. (b) High intensity area (arrows) on a T2-weighted image. This haemangioma was an incidental finding.

Liver abscess (Fig. 6.17)

Abscesses appear somewhat similar to cysts but usually they can be distinguished. Hepatic abscesses tend to have fluid centres, with walls that are thicker, more irregular and more obvious than those of simple cysts. Although the CT attenuation values in the centre of an abscess may be the same as water, usually they are higher. At ultrasound, a layer of necrotic debris may be seen within the abscess. (It should be noted that even simple cysts may demonstrate some fine low-level echoes within them, believed to be due to cholesterol crystals which are the remnants of old haemorrhages into the cysts.) Occasionally, chronic abscesses calcify.

Abscesses cannot usually be distinguished from necrotic tumours at either ultrasound, CT or MRI, but the clinical situation should aid in making the distinction. Aspiration is invariably undertaken in any case of suspected abscess; this is conveniently performed under ultrasound guidance.

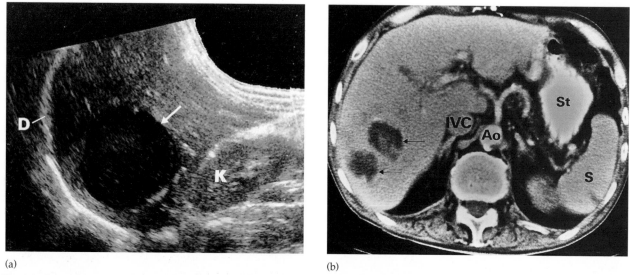

(a)   (b)

Fig. 6.17 Liver abscess. (a) Ultrasound showing a large transonic area (arrow) with echoes arising within it. (b) CT scan in another patient showing bilocular area of low attenuation in the right lobe of the liver (arrows). Ao, aorta; D, diaphragm; IVC, inferior vena cava; K, kidney; S, spleen; St, stomach.

Liver trauma

Trauma to the liver is the commonest abdominal injury that leads to death. Parenchymal lacerations are the most frequent injury and they are often accompanied by subcapsular haematomas (Fig. 6.18). Both are recognized as low density areas on CT; occasionally isodense or high density blood clots are seen. The major differential diagnoses are artefacts from surrounding structures, and pre-existing mass lesions. Although ultrasound and MRI can demonstrate liver injuries, CT is the best technique because it also surveys other injured organs (e.g. kidneys and spleen) and can identify small quantities of fluid in the peritoneal cavity.

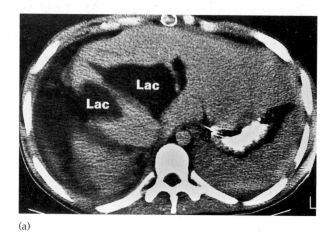

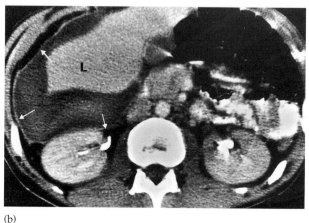

(a)   (b)

Fig. 6.18 Liver trauma. CT scan. (a) Two large lacerations (Lac.) are shown in the right lobe of the liver. These contained a mixture of bile and blood. (b) A lower section. Between the liver capsule (arrows) and the liver (L) is an area of soft tissue density representing haematoma.

Cirrhosis of the liver and portal hypertension

In portal hypertension the pressure in the portal venous system is elevated due to obstruction to the flow of blood in the portal or hepatic venous systems. Cirrhosis of the liver is by far the most frequent cause. Other causes include occlusion of the hepatic veins (Budd–Chiari syndrome) and thrombosis of the portal vein, particularly following infection of the umbilical vein in the neonatal period.

Because the portal venous pressure is raised, blood flows through anastomotic channels, known as portosystemic anastomoses, to enter the vena cavae by-passing the liver. These collateral channels may be found in various sites, but the most important are varices at the lower end of the oesophagus (see Fig. 5.17, p. 156). The collateral channels can sometimes be shown with colour-flow Doppler ultrasound.

The signs of cirrhosis of the liver at CT and ultrasound are reduction in size of the right lobe of the liver together with splenomegaly. The texture of the liver at ultrasound may be diffusely abnormal; at CT, the parenchyma appears normal until late in the disease.

Portal venography may be undertaken to assess the patency of the portal vein but only when portosystemic shunts are under consideration. Contrast is injected into the coeliac axis, splenic artery or superior mesenteric artery; films are then taken during the venous phase to show the portal venous system.

Nowadays, surgical portocaval anastamoses are being replaced by the percutaneous procedure known as TIPS (transjugular intrahepatic portosystemic shunt). In this procedure a connection between the portal and systemic venous system is created by placing a stent connecting a large hepatic and portal vein within the liver (see p. 443).

Fatty degeneration of the liver

Fatty degeneration of the liver, whilst not normal, is a relatively frequent finding, particularly in those who take alcohol to excess and those who are malnourished or debilitated for any reason. Fatty degeneration may involve the whole liver, or it may just involve individual subsections.

Fatty degeneration leads to a reduction in the attenuation of the affected parenchyma causing low density on CT scans (Fig. 6.19). The vessels are then seen as relatively high attenuation structures against a background of low density parenchyma, even on images taken without intravenous contrast medium. On ultrasound, the liver parenchyma shows increased echogenicity, the so-called 'bright liver', in which the echogenicity of the liver is similar to that of the central echo-complex of the kidney. Magnetic resonance imaging can be very helpful in problem cases because fat gives a characteristic set of signals.

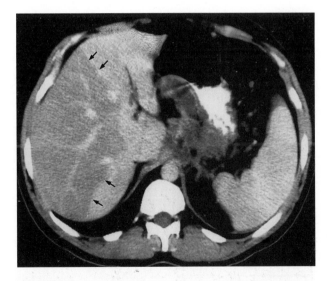

Fig. 6.19 Fatty degeneration of the liver shown by CT as a large focal area of reduced attenuation in the right lobe of the liver (arrows).

BILIARY SYSTEM

The gall bladder and bile duct system can be demonstrated by a variety of imaging techniques. Ultrasound is the best all-purpose method of investigation because it is the simplest and best test for showing gall stones and diseases of the gall bladder and is also an excellent test for confirming or excluding bile duct dilatation. Oral cholecystography has a very limited role nowadays and has been largely abandoned as a diagnostic test. Radionuclide imaging using hepatobiliary agents has an important role in excluding obstruction to the cystic duct.

Gall stones, gall bladder wall thickening and dilatation of the common bile duct are all recognizable at CT, but since ultrasound provides better information at less cost, ultrasound is used as the primary method of examination for these problems.

Imaging techniques

Ultrasound of the gall bladder and bile ducts

As the gall bladder is a fluid-filled structure, it is particularly amenable to sonographic examination. Because it is important that the gall bladder should be full of bile, the

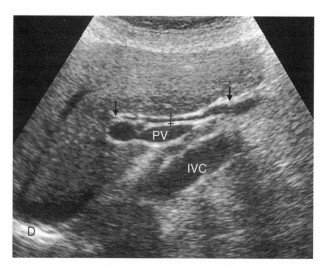

Fig. 6.21 Normal common bile duct. Longitudinal ultrasound scan showing the common bile duct, situated between the arrows, lying anterior to the portal vein. The common bile duct measures 4 mm in diameter (crosses). D, diaphragm; PV, portal vein; IVC, inferior vena cava.

patient is asked to fast in order to prevent gall bladder contraction, but no other preparation is necessary. The normal gall bladder wall is so thin that it is sometimes barely perceptible (Fig. 6.20). *Gall bladder wall thickening* suggests either acute or chronic cholecystitis. *Gall stones* greater than 1 or 2 mm in size can usually be identified at ultrasound examination. It is usually impossible to diagnose cystic duct obstruction with ultrasound; the cystic duct is too small to identify and the stones that impact in it are often too small to see.

Ultrasonography is also the best test for demonstrating the *bile ducts*. The common hepatic or common bile duct can be visualized in almost all patients; it is seen as a small tubular structure lying anterior to the portal vein in the porta hepatis and should not measure more than 7 mm in diameter (Fig. 6.21). The lower end of the common bile duct is often obscured by gas in the duodenum, which lies just anterior to it.

The normal intrahepatic biliary tree is of such small calibre that only small portions a few millimetres long may be seen at ultrasound.

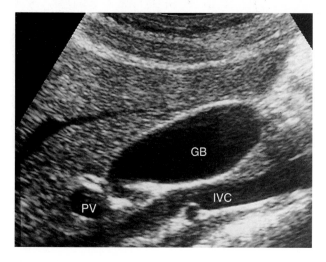

Fig. 6.20 (a) Ultrasound of normal gall bladder. Note the thin wall and absence of echoes from within the gall bladder. GB, gall bladder; IVC, inferior vena cava; PV, portal vein.

Hepatobiliary radionuclide scanning

Iminodiacetic acid (IDA) pharmaceuticals labelled with ^{99m}Tc are excreted by the liver following intravenous injection and may be used for imaging the bile duct system. Their main use is in patients with suspected acute cholecystitis. Hepatic excretion occurs despite relatively high serum bilirubin levels and therefore these agents can be used when the patient is jaundiced, even with serum bilirubin levels of up to 250 μmol/l (15 mg%). All that is required is that the patient fasts for 4 hours prior to the injection of the radionuclide. Normally, the gall bladder, common bile duct, duodenum and small bowel are all seen within the first hour, confirming the patency of both the cystic duct and the common bile duct (Fig. 6.22a). If the common bile duct and duodenum or small bowel are seen within the first hour, but the gall bladder is not visualized, the cystic duct is considered to be obstructed (Fig. 6.22b).

Endoscopic retrograde cholangiopancreatography (ERCP)

ERCP consists of injecting contrast material directly into the common bile duct through a catheter inserted into the papilla of Vater via an endoscope positioned in the duodenum (Fig. 6.23).

The indications are:
- To determine the cause of jaundice, notably in patients with large duct obstruction (Figs 6.23b and c), and to undertake endoscopic treatment (see p. 440).
- To investigate unexplained abdominal pain thought to be biliary in origin, when other investigations have been equivocal. An added advantage is that the pancreatic duct system can be demonstrated.
- To demonstrate the common bile duct in patients undergoing laparoscopic cholecystectomy, particularly in those where the history or biochemical investigations suggest stones in the common bile duct. Such stones are treated by sphincterotomy and endoscopic basket or balloon extraction.

Other diagnostic procedures

Oral cholecystography

The widespread use of ultrasound has replaced oral

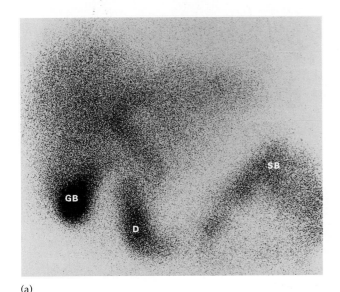

(a)

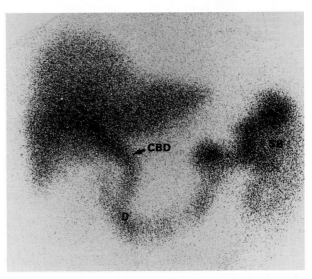

(b)

Fig. 6.22 Hepatobiliary scan. (a) Normal IDA scan. There is obvious filling of the gall bladder. Activity is also present in the duodenum and small bowel. (b) Cystic duct obstruction. The IDA scan in this patient with acute right upper quadrant pain shows the duct system but no filling of the gall bladder. CBD, common bile duct; D, duodenum; GB, gall bladder; SB, small bowel.

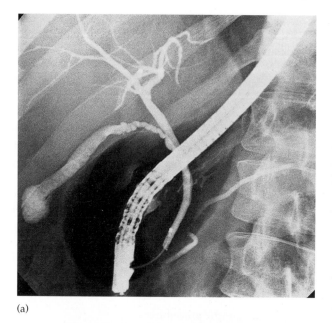

(a)

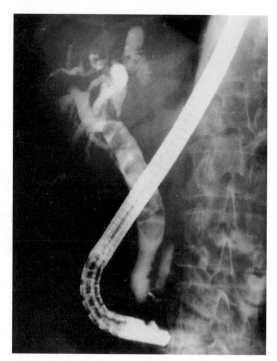

(b)

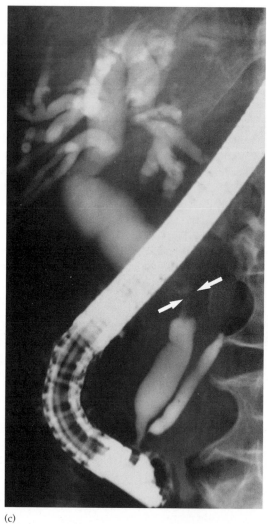

(c)

Fig. 6.23 Endoscopic retrograde cholangiopancreatography (ERCP). (a) A normal biliary system has been shown by injecting contrast through a catheter passed from the endoscope into the common bile duct. The pancreatic duct has also been filled. (b) A dilated ductal system with numerous large calculi in the hepatic and common bile ducts. (c) A localized stricture in the common bile duct from cholangiocarcinoma (arrows).

cholecystography, a technique which opacified the gall bladder by taking an iodine containing oral contrast agent (Fig. 6.24).

Percutaneous transhepatic cholangiogram (PTC)

PTC is an alternative to ERCP for demonstrating the bile duct system in order to show the site and cause of obstruction and is usually only performed if an ERCP is unsuccessful. The procedure is carried out under local anaesthesia and because it is far easier and safer to perform if the intrahepatic bile ducts are dilated, the patient is usually jaundiced at the time of examination. The examination consists of passing a fine needle (usually 22 or 23 gauge) through the abdominal wall into the liver and injecting contrast directly into an intrahepatic bile duct. Haemorrhage is an occasional problem, as are septicaemia and biliary peritonitis.

Magnetic resonance cholangiopancreatography (MRCP)

Special sequences enable the biliary duct system to be visualized directly without the need for any contrast agent.

Gall stones and chronic cholecystitis

Gall stones are a frequent finding in adults, particularly middle-aged females. Together with accompanying chronic cholecystitis they are a major cause of recurrent upper abdominal pain. The presence of stones within the gall bladder does not necessarily mean the patient's pain is due to gall stones. In the appropriate clinical setting, however, identification of gall stones may be sufficient for many surgeons to take action.

Some 20–30 % of gall stones contain sufficient calcium to be visible on plain film (Fig. 6.25). They vary greatly in size and shape and, typically, have a dense outer rim with a

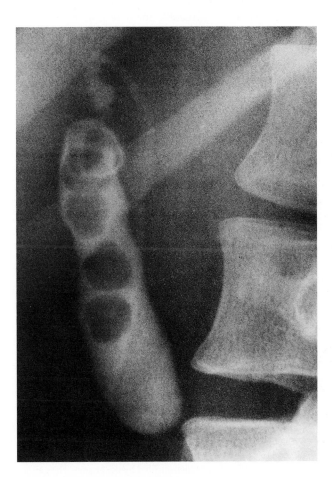

Fig. 6.24 Oral cholecystogram showing multiple gall stones as filling defects in the opacified gall bladder.

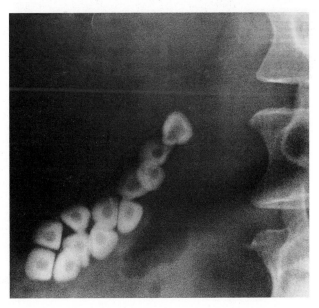

Fig. 6.25 Radio-opaque gall stones. Plain film showing multiple faceted stones with lucent centres.

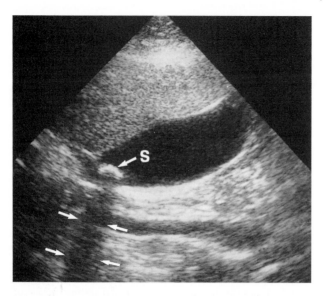

Fig. 6.26 Gall stone. Ultrasound shows a stone (S) in the gall bladder. The arrows point to the acoustic shadow behind the stone.

more lucent centre. Calcified sludge within the gall bladder is known as 'milk of calcium' bile.

At ultrasound, gall stones are seen as strongly echogenic foci within the dependent portion of the gall bladder. Acoustic shadows are usually seen behind stones, because most of the ultrasound beam is reflected by the stones and only a little passes on through the patient (Fig. 6.26). The presence of an acoustic shadowing is an important diagnostic feature for diagnosing stones in the gall bladder or common bile ducts. Acoustic shadowing is not seen with polyps. The vast majority of polyps are small (Fig. 6.27), measuring only a few millimetres and are not neoplasms but aggregations of cholesterol.

Although ultrasound is very accurate at diagnosing gall stones it is much less reliable for detecting stones in the common bile duct.

In *adenomyomatosis* the gall bladder wall is thickened and may show altered echogenicity due to small projections of

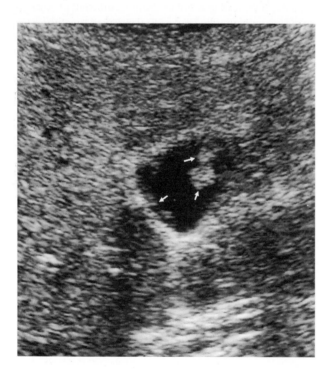

Fig. 6.27 Polyps. These tiny polyps (arrows) in the gall bladder are aggregations of cholesterol and do not cause acoustic shadowing.

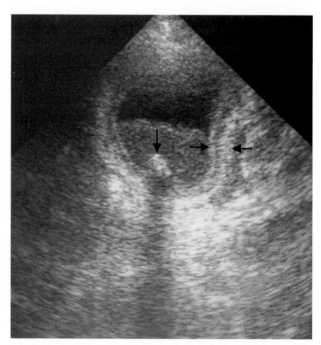

Fig. 6.28 Acute cholecystitis. Ultrasound showing a thick oedematous gall bladder wall indicated by the arrows. The gall bladder contains a gall stone (arrow head) and inflammatory debris.

the lumen into the wall, known as Rokitansky–Aschoff sinuses. There is dispute as to whether this condition causes symptoms.

Acute cholecystitis

In acute cholecystitis, sonography will usually detect gall stones, inflammatory debris and gall bladder wall thickening (Fig. 6.28), but unless there is visible oedema adjacent to the wall of the gall bladder, ultrasound cannot distinguish acute from chronic cholecystitis. In patients with abdominal pain and tenderness, ultrasound is sometimes used primarily to locate the gall bladder to determine whether it is truly the gall bladder that is tender.

A hepatobiliary radionuclide scan actually answers the question 'Is the cystic duct patent'? No available test is very good at diagnosing the gall bladder inflammation itself, but since the cystic duct is always obstructed in acute cholecystitis, a normal hepatobiliary scan excludes the diagnosis. Conversely, a diagnosis of cystic duct obstruction in the correct clinical setting strongly indicates acute cholecystitis (see Fig. 6.22b).

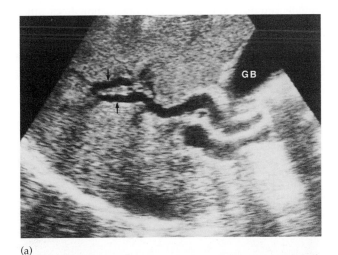

(a)

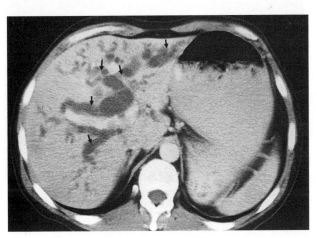

(c)

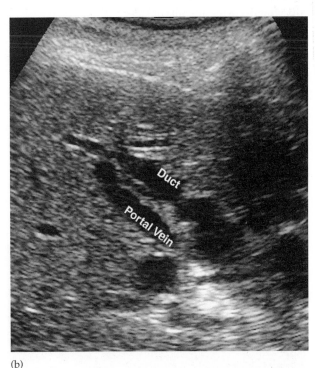

(b)

Fig. 6.29 Dilated intrahepatic ducts. (a) Longitudinal scan through the liver showing dilatation of the biliary system. Dilated intrahepatic ducts are arrowed. GB, gall bladder. (b) Double-channel sign. A dilated biliary duct lies in front of a portal vein. Normally the duct is much smaller than the accompanying portal vein. (c) CT scan showing dilated intrahepatic ducts (arrows) in the liver.

Jaundice

Clinical examination and biochemical tests often permit the cause of jaundice to be diagnosed. Imaging tests may, however, be required when there is doubt as to the nature of the jaundice. The basis of this distinction is that dilated biliary ducts are a feature of jaundice from biliary obstruction. More often, imaging is used to determine the site and, if possible, the cause of obstruction in those patients with known large duct obstruction, the common causes of which are:

- impacted stone in the common bile duct;
- carcinoma of the head of the pancreas;
- carcinoma of the ampulla of Vater.

Dilatation of the intra- and extrahepatic biliary system can be identified at both ultrasound and CT (Fig. 6.29). Ultrasound is the more sensitive test and is usually the first test to be performed.

Dilated intrahepatic biliary ducts are seen at ultrasound as serpentine structures paralleling the portal veins, a finding known as 'the double-channel sign'. The common bile duct lies just in front of the portal vein and is dilated when more than 7 mm in diameter.

If there is large duct obstruction, the biliary tree will be dilated down to the level of obstruction. Ultrasound is good for demonstrating the level of obstruction and sometimes the specific cause for biliary obstruction can be seen, e.g. a stone impacted within the common bile duct (Fig. 6.30) or a mass in the pancreatic head. More often, the cause cannot be seen, mainly because associated inflammation causes localized ileus of the duodenum and bowel gas then obscures the common bile duct. Computed tomography may provide useful information about the cause of obstruction. Two points should be appreciated: substantial dilatation of the common hepatic and common bile ducts may be present with only minimal dilatation of the intrahepatic ducts; and secondly, the intrahepatic biliary tree may not dilate at all within the first 48 hours following obstruction. An ERCP or percutaneous cholangiogram may be needed both to differentiate jaundice from large duct obstruction from other causes of jaundice, and to establish the site and determine the cause of any obstruction that may be present (Figs 6.23 and 6.31) and, if possible, to treat the condition.

Some centres use a radionuclide hepatobiliary agent to

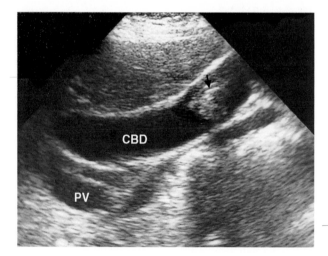

Fig. 6.30 Stones in the common bile duct (CBD). The common bile duct is dilated measuring 2 cm in diameter and a large stone (arrow) is seen in its lower portion. PV, section through portal vein.

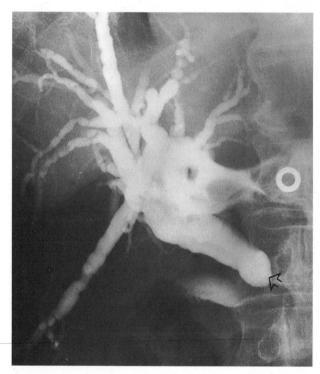

Fig. 6.31 Percutaneous cholangiogram. Carcinoma of the pancreas. There is complete obstruction of the common bile duct (arrow). Note the dilated intrahepatic ducts.

confirm or exclude biliary obstruction. The problem with this approach is that with severe jaundice there may be insufficient excretion of the radionuclide to distinguish bile duct obstruction from hepatocellular disease.

SPLEEN

Imaging the spleen is in many respects similar to imaging the liver. At ultrasound, the spleen has a homogeneous appearance with the same echo density as the liver. Computed tomography and MRI are excellent ways to examine the spleen; normal CT images are shown in the appendix. Because the spleen contains reticuloendothelial cells, it is well demonstrated on a ^{99m}Tc-sulphur or tin colloid scan, but the technique has been largely superseded by ultrasound and CT.

The commonly encountered splenic masses are cysts, including hydatid cysts (Fig. 6.32), abscesses and tumours; lymphoma (Fig. 6.33) is much commoner than metastases, which are rare in the spleen.

Many conditions cause enlargement of the spleen but cause no change in splenic texture on ultrasound, or any change in density on a computed tomography scan. These conditions include lymphoma, portal hypertension, chronic infection and various blood disorders, e.g. haemolytic anaemias and leukaemia. As the appearance of the enlarged spleen in all these conditions is similar, imaging does little except confirm the presence of splenomegaly.

The spleen is the most commonly injured organ in blunt abdominal trauma and lacerations, contusions or haematomas may result. *Splenic injury* may be detected by ultrasound, but CT is a superior method of investigation, since not only does it demonstrate well the damage to the spleen, but it can show intraperitoneal blood and visualize injuries to other abdominal organs, particularly the adjacent liver and left kidney.

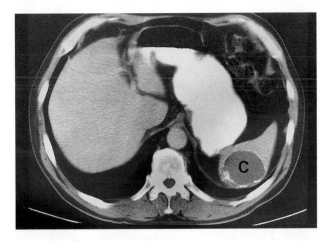

Fig. 6.32 Hydatid cyst. Computed tomography showing a cyst (C) in the spleen with calcification in its walls.

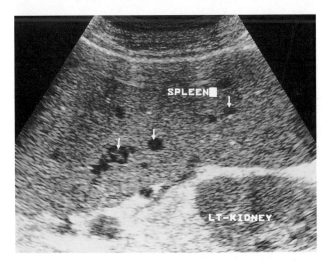

Fig. 6.33 Lymphoma. Ultrasound showing an enlarged spleen with several hypoechoic areas within it. Some of these are arrowed.

PANCREAS

CT and ultrasound have now become the mainstays for imaging the pancreas. A major advantage of CT over ultrasound is that it can image the pancreas regardless of the amount of bowel adjacent to it, whereas the ultrasound beam is absorbed by gas in the gastrointestinal tract. Arteriography, ERCP (Fig. 6.34) and MRI are used in selected cases.

The normal pancreas is an elongated retroperitoneal organ surrounded by a variable amount of fat (Fig. 6.35). The head nestles in the duodenal loop (for CT scanning the duodenum is opacified by an oral contrast agent) and the uncinate process folds behind the superior mesenteric artery and vein; these vessels form a useful landmark to help identify the head of the pancreas. The body of the pan-

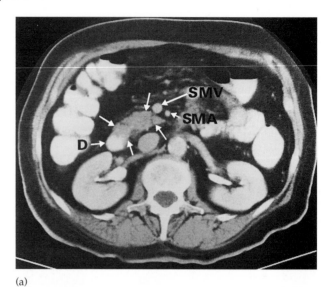

(a)

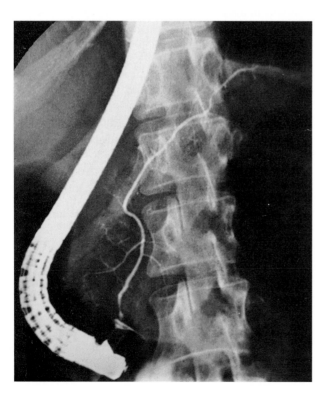

Fig. 6.34 Endoscopic retrograde pancreatography. The pancreatic duct has been cannulated from the endoscope in the duodenum. Contrast has been injected to demonstrate a normal duct system.

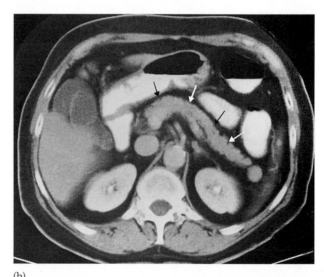

(b)

Fig. 6.35 CT of normal pancreas. Note that several sections are needed to display the pancreas. (a) The head (arrows) nestling between the second part of the opacified duodenum (D) and the superior mesenteric vessels (SMA and SMV). (b) CT taken 3 cm higher, showing the body and part of the tail (arrows). Note the feathery texture of the pancreas. *Continued opposite.*

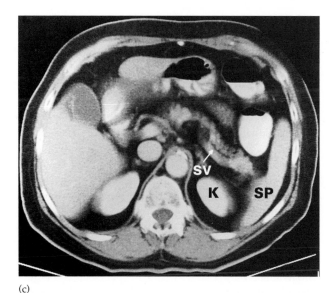

(c)

Fig. 6.35 *Continued.* (c) CT taken 1 cm higher, showing the tail of the pancreas nestling against the spleen. In this patient the splenic vein is particularly well seen and is almost the same diameter as the pancreas. K, kidney; SP, spleen; SV, splenic vein.

creas lies in front of the superior mesenteric artery and vein, and passes behind the stomach, with the tail situated near the hilum of the spleen. The splenic vein, which can be a surprisingly large structure, is another very useful landmark. Lying behind the pancreas, it joins the superior mesenteric vein posterior to the neck of the pancreas to form the portal vein.

In most people the pancreas runs obliquely across the retroperitoneum, being higher at the splenic end. Because of this oblique orientation, CT shows different portions of the pancreas on the various sections. The normal pancreas shows a feathery texture, corresponding to pancreatic lobules interspersed with fat. At ultrasound, the pancreas gives reasonably uniform echoes of medium to high level compared to the adjacent liver (Fig. 6.36). The pancreatic duct may be seen over short segments as a linear echo in the centre of the pancreas, the normal lumen being no more than 2 mm in diameter. The normal pancreatic duct is not visible on CT.

The shape and size of the pancreas is so variable that normal measurements have not proved very useful. Atrophy is a common feature with ageing.

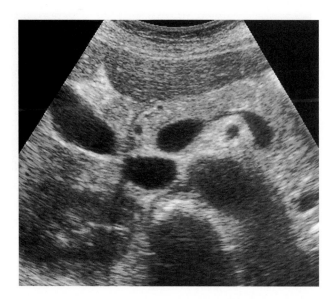

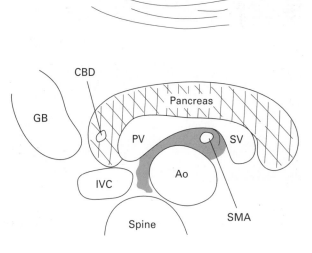

Fig. 6.36 Ultrasound of normal pancreas (transverse scan). Ao, aorta; CBD, common bile duct; GB, gall bladder; IVC, inferior vena cava; PV, portal vein; SMA, superior mesenteric artery; SV, splenic vein.

Pancreatic masses

The usual causes of masses in, or immediately adjacent to, the pancreas are: carcinoma of the pancreas, neoplasm of the adjacent lymph nodes, focal pancreatitis, pancreatic abscess and pseudocyst formation. Occasionally, congenital cysts may be seen.

Most neoplasms of the pancreas are *adenocarcinomas*, two-thirds of which occur in the head of the pancreas. Tumours arising in the head may obstruct the common bile duct giving rise to jaundice and are therefore sometimes diagnosed when relatively small. Tumours arising in the body and tail have to be fairly large to give rise to signs or symptoms, pain being the cardinal symptom. Since the pancreas is so variable, measurements have not proved useful in diagnosing masses. The important sign of carcinoma of the pancreas at both CT and ultrasound is therefore a focal mass deforming the outline of the gland (Fig. 6.37). These neoplasms have frequently already invaded the retroperitoneum at the time of presentation, causing irregular obliteration of the fat around the pancreas, a feature which is readily recognized at CT. If CT is used with intravenous contrast enhancement, it is sometimes possible to differentiate the relatively lower density of the tumour from the enhancing normal pancreatic tissue.

Obstructive dilatation of the pancreatic duct can be seen at CT but is more readily apparent at sonography. With obstruction of the common bile duct, it is often possible to recognize dilatation of the duct down to the level of the tumour. The liver, which should always be included in any examination of the pancreas, should routinely be examined carefully for signs of spread of tumour.

The presence of *endocrine secreting tumours*, of which insulinoma is the commonest example, is suggested by biochemical investigations. These tumours are difficult to detect as they are usually small and do not deform the pancreatic contour. They may be seen on ultrasound, CT or MRI as small round masses within the pancreas. Sometimes selective angiography is required, where they stand out from the rest of the pancreas by virtue of their hypervascularity (Fig. 6.38).

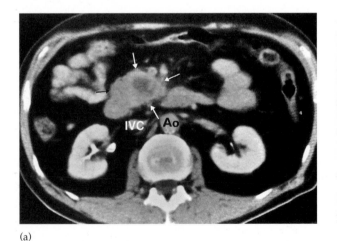
(a)

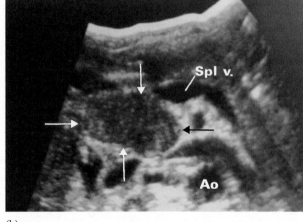
(b)

Fig. 6.37 Carcinoma of pancreas. (a) CT scan showing focal mass in head of pancreas (arrows). Ao, aorta; IVC, inferior vena cava. (b) Ultrasound, transverse scan (different patient), showing a similarly situated mass (arrows). Ao, aorta; Spl v., splenic vein.

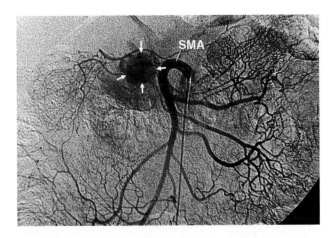

Fig. 6.38 Insulinoma. Selective superior mesenteric angiogram showing the tumour as a vascular blush (arrows). SMA, superior mesenteric artery.

Acute pancreatitis

Acute pancreatitis causes abdominal pain, fever, vomiting and leucocytosis, together with elevation of the serum amylase. The findings at CT and ultrasound vary with the amount of necrosis, haemorrhage and suppuration (Fig. 6.39). The pancreas is usually enlarged, often diffusely and may show irregularity of its outline, caused by extension of the inflammatory process into the surrounding retroperitoneal fat: features that are well seen at CT. There may be low density areas at CT and echo-poor areas at sonography,

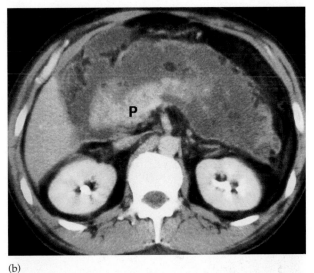

(b)

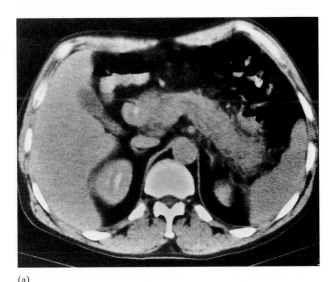

(a)

Fig. 6.39 Acute pancreatitis. (a) CT scan showing diffuse enlargement of the pancreas with ill-defined edges. (b) CT scan showing considerable inflammation around the pancreas (P). (c) Ultrasound. Transverse scan showing a swollen pancreas (P) with some fluid around the pancreas (arrows).

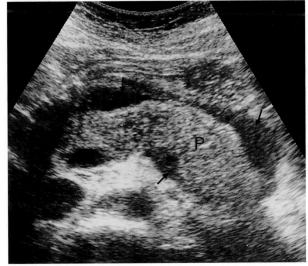

(c)

representing oedema and focal necrosis within or adjacent to the pancreas. With very severe disease, large fluid-filled areas representing abscess formation may be seen. Such abscesses occasionally contain gas bubbles.

The diagnosis of pancreatitis is usually made on clinical and biochemical grounds, the purpose of imaging being to demonstrate complications such as abscesses and pseudo-cysts. Occasionally, CT is used to exclude an underlying carcinoma.

Pseudocysts are a complication of acute pancreatitis in which tissue necrosis leads to a leak of pancreatic secretions, which are then contained in a cyst-like manner within and adjacent to the pancreas. They can be well demonstrated by either CT or ultrasound as thin or thick walled cysts

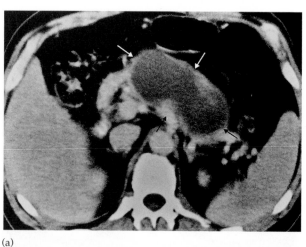

(a)

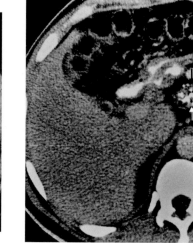

(a)

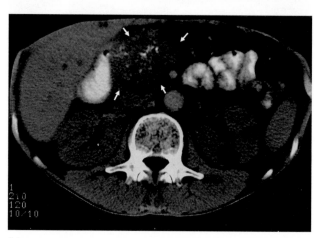

(b)

(b)

Fig. 6.40 Pancreatic pseudocyst. (a) CT scan showing large cyst arising within the pancreas (arrows). (b) Ultrasound (transverse scan). The arrows indicate a pseudocyst arising from the body of the pancreas. P, pancreas. Same patient as Fig. 6.39c, 6 weeks later.

Fig. 6.41 Chronic pancreatitis. (a) CT scan showing numerous small areas of calcification within the pancreas (arrows). (b) Focal chronic pancreatitis presenting as a mass (arrows) which could be confused for a carcinoma were it not for the presence of calcification within it.

containing fluid, arising within or adjacent to the pancreas (Fig. 6.40). They vary in size from very small to many centimetres in diameter and may even be seen on a barium meal causing anterior displacement and compression of the stomach and/or duodenum. Many pseudocysts resolve in the weeks following an attack of acute pancreatitis. Some persist and may need surgical or percutaneous drainage. Both CT and ultrasound are excellent methods of following such cysts and determining the best approach to treatment.

Chronic pancreatitis

Chronic pancreatitis results in fibrosis, calcifications, and ductal stenoses and dilatations. Pseudocysts are seen with chronic pancreatitis just as they are in the acute form. The calcification in chronic pancreatitis is mainly due to small calculi within the pancreas; they are often recognizable on plain films (see Fig. 4.16, p. 144) and ultrasound, but are particularly obvious at CT (Fig. 6.41a). The gland may enlarge generally or focally. Focal enlargement is rare and is then often indistinguishable from carcinoma (Fig. 6.41b). Con-versely, the pancreas may atrophy focally or generally. Atrophy is a non-specific sign; it is frequently seen in normal elderly people and also occurs distal to a carcinoma. The pancreatic duct may be enlarged and irregular, a feature that is visible at CT, and particularly striking at ultrasound.

Endoscopic retrograde cholangiopancreatography (ERCP) is occasionally used to try and document chronic pancreatitis and exclude carcinoma. The generalized irregular dilatation of the duct system seen with chronic pancreatitis is very well demonstrated with this method.

Pancreatic trauma

Trauma to the pancreas is uncommon but serious. Injuries to other structures are frequent, so CT is the best method of investigation. In addition to lacerations and haematomas, the release of pancreatic enzymes into the surrounding tissues leads to traumatic pancreatitis and tissue necrosis. The features here are similar to other forms of acute pancre-atitis (see above), including the subsequent development of pseudocysts.

7

Urinary Tract

The four basic examinations of the urinary tract are intravenous urography (IVU), computed tomography (CT), ultrasound and radionuclide examinations. Magnetic resonance imaging (MRI), arteriography and studies requiring catheterization or direct puncture of the collecting systems are limited to highly selected patients.

The IVU provides both functional and anatomical information. CT, MRI and ultrasound are essentially used for anatomical information; the functional information they provide is limited. The converse is true of radionuclide examinations where functional information is paramount.

Ultrasound is the first-line investigation to demonstrate or exclude hydronephrosis, particularly in patients with renal failure, and to diagnose renal tumours, cysts and abscesses.

Computed tomography is pre-eminent for staging renal tumours, for diagnosing or excluding trauma to the urinary tract and for showing pathology in the retroperitoneum.

IMAGING TECHNIQUES

Intravenous urogram

The IVU previously dominated as the all-purpose examination, but now the newer modalities offer advantages in many areas and often replace the IVU. The IVU provides an excellent overview of the urinary tract. It shows more detail of pelvicalyceal and ureteric anatomy than other imaging modalities and is an ideal method for investigating calculi.

Contrast medium and its excretion

Urographic media are highly concentrated solutions of organically bound iodine. A large volume, e.g. 50–100 ml, is injected intravenously and is carried in the blood to the kidneys, where it passes into the glomerular filtrate. Contrast is not absorbed by the tubules, so substantial concentration is achieved in the urine, particularly after fluid restriction. The visualization of the renal substance (the nephrogram) is dependent on the amount of contrast reaching the kidneys, whereas the visualization of the collecting systems (the pyelogram) depends mainly on the ability of the kidneys to concentrate the urine.

Adverse reactions to intravenous contrast media are discussed on p. 6.

Preparation of the patient

Fluid restriction is an advantage in patients with normal renal function, as it increases the concentration of the urine and produces a dense pyelogram. This does *not* apply to patients in renal failure, since they could be harmed by the withholding of fluids and there would in any event be no advantage, because many are unable to increase their urinary concentration.

Routine IVU

One or more plain films are taken to show the whole of the urinary tract. The precise timing of the films following the injection of contrast medium varies in different hospitals but each film should be assessed at the time it is taken, so that appropriate extra views, such as tomography or

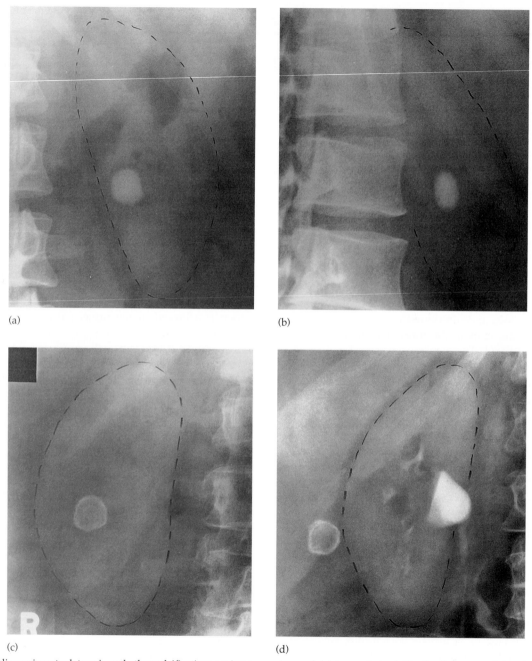

(a)

(b)

(c)

(d)

Fig.7.1 Oblique views to determine whether calcifications are intra- or extrarenal. (a) A rounded calcification is seen overlying the left kidney in the AP plain film. (b) In the oblique plain film, the calcification is in the same position within the renal shadow and is, therefore, a renal calculus. (c) A rounded calcification is seen over the right renal shadow. (d) An oblique film after contrast shows that the calcification lies outside the kidney. It was later confirmed to be a gall stone.

oblique views (Fig. 7.1), can be obtained. A film taken 1 min after the injection is designed to show the renal parenchyma, particularly the renal outlines. Further films are then taken to show the kidneys, ureters and bladder (Fig. 7.2).

The following routine is useful when interpreting an IVU.

The plain film

1 *Identify all calcifications*. Decide if they are in the urinary tract by relating them to the renal outlines or the expected position of the ureters, bladder, prostate and urethra with oblique views or tomograms where necessary. The major causes of urinary tract calcification are:

- urinary calculi;
- nephrocalcinosis;
- localized calcification due to conditions such as tuberculosis or tumours;
- prostatic calcification.

Note that calcification can be obscured by contrast medium. Stones would often be missed if no plain film were taken (Fig. 7.3).

2 *Look at the other structures on the film*. Include the bones, just as you would on any plain abdominal film. Do not waste time drawing conclusions about the renal outlines on plain films; they are always better seen after contrast has been given.

Films taken after injection of contrast medium

Kidneys

1 *Check that the kidneys are in their normal positions* (Fig. 7.2) and that their axes are parallel to the outer margins of the psoas muscles. The left kidney is usually higher than the right.

There are two basic reasons why the position or axis of a kidney might be abnormal: congenital malposition or displacement by a retroperitoneal mass.

2 *Identify the whole of both renal outlines*. (They are usually better seen on tomography.) If any indentations or bulges are present they must be explained.

- *Local indentations* (Fig. 7.4). The renal parenchymal width should be uniform and symmetrical: between 1.5 and 2 cm, except at the poles where there is an extra

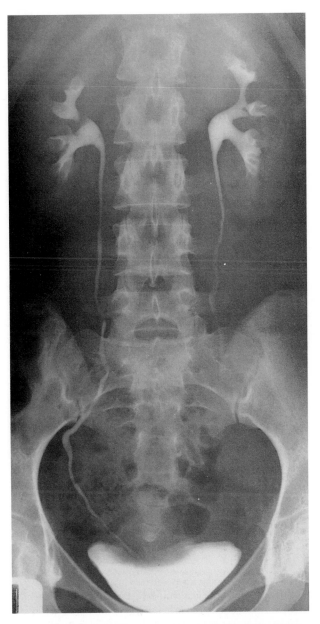

Fig. 7.2 Normal IVU. Full length 15 min film. Note that the bladder is well opacified. The whole of the right ureter and part of the left ureter are seen. Often, only a portion of the ureter is visualized owing to peristalsis emptying certain sections. The bladder outline is reasonably smooth. The roof of the bladder shows a shallow indentation from the uterus.

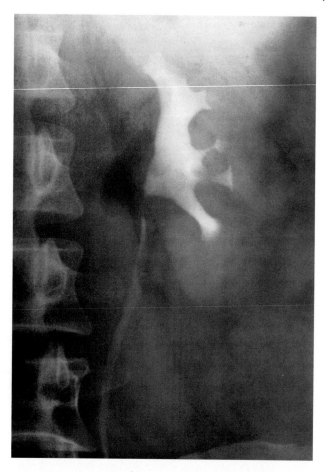

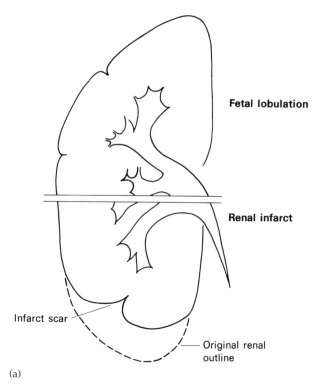

(a)

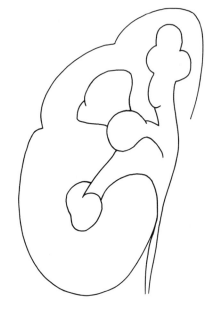

(b)

Fig. 7.3 Large calcified calculus in the pelvis of the kidney obscured by contrast medium. This is the same patient as illustrated in Fig. 7.1a and b. Since the contrast medium and the calculus have the same radiographic density, the calculus is hidden by the contrast medium.

Fig. 7.4 (a) The distinction between fetal lobulation and renal infarction. With fetal lobulation, indentations in the renal outline are shallow and correspond to the lobules of the kidney, i.e. the indentations are between calices. With renal infarction, the maximal indentation is opposite a calix and there is usually extensive loss of renal parenchyma. (b) Scars in chronic pyelonephritis (drawing of Fig. 7.7b) The reductions in renal parenchymal width are opposite calices, and these calices are dilated. The overall kidney size is reduced, as is usual. Scars in tuberculosis have much the same appearance but are usually associated with other signs of tuberculosis.

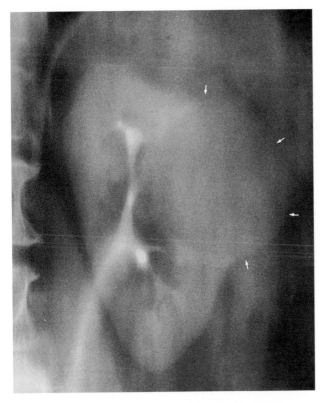

Fig. 7.5 Renal mass. A renal cyst (arrows) has caused a bulge on the lateral aspect of the kidney with splaying of the calices.

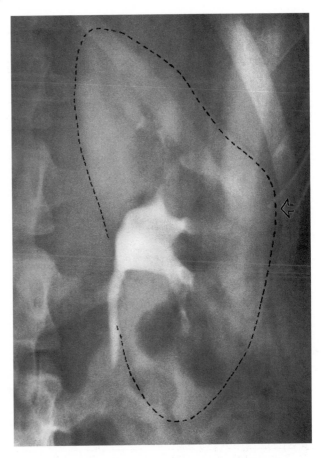

Fig. 7.6 The 'splenic hump'. A bulge is present on the lateral aspect of the left kidney (arrow) but there is no displacement of the calices. This 'splenic hump' is a normal variant.

centimetre of thickness. Minor indentations between normal calices are due to persistent fetal lobulations. All other local indentations are scars. Visible scars occur with chronic pyelonephritis, tuberculosis and renal infarction.

• *Local bulges of the renal outline.* A bulge of the renal outline usually means a mass. Most masses large enough to deform the renal outline displace and deform the adjacent calices (Fig. 7.5). An important normal variant causing a bulge of the outline is the so-called 'splenic hump' (Fig. 7.6).

3 *Measure the renal lengths.* The normal adult kidney at IVU is between 10 and 16 cm from top to bottom; the length varies with age, being maximal in the young adult. There

may be a difference between the two kidneys, normally less than 1.5 cm. A kidney with a bifid collecting system is usually 1–2 cm larger than expected. Minor changes in size occur in many conditions. Diseases where the increase or decrease in size is sufficient to be recognizable, even without comparison with previous examinations, are listed in Tables 7.1 and 7.2. It will be noted that it is usually possible to diagnose the cause of a unilateral small kidney and bilaterally enlarged kidneys but, except for bilateral chronic pyelonephritis, it is often not possible to distinguish between the various causes of bilaterally small kidneys.

Table 7.1 Small kidneys.

Diagnosis		Comments
Unilateral but may be bilateral	Chronic pyelonephritis	Focal scars and dilated calices
	Tuberculosis	See p. 245
	Following acute infection	Very rare
	Obstructive atrophy	Dilatation of all calices with uniform loss of renal parenchyma
	Renal artery stenosis or occlusion	Outline may be smooth or scarred, but the calices appear normal. In severe unilateral cases the density of the pyelogram on the affected side may be increased. If very severe the pyelogram may be delayed by a minute or two.
	Hypoplasia	Very rare; kidneys may be smooth or irregular in outline. Calices may be clubbed.
	Radiation nephritis	
Always bilateral	Chronic glomerulonephritis of many types Hypertensive nephropathy Diabetes mellitus Collagen vascular diseases	Usually no distinguishing features. In all these conditions the kidneys may be small with smooth outlines and normal pelvicaliceal systems
	Analgesic nephropathy	Calices often abnormal (p. 246)

Table 7.2 Enlarged kidneys*.

Diagnosis		Intravenous urogram (IVU)
Always unilateral	Compensatory hypertrophy	Opposite kidney small or absent
May be unilateral or bilateral	Bifid collecting system	Diagnosis obvious from abnormalities of collecting systems
	Renal mass	
	Hydronephrosis	
	Lymphomatous infiltration	May show obvious masses; the kidneys may, however, be large but otherwise unremarkable
	Renal vein thrombosis	
Always bilateral	Polycystic disease	Characteristic IVU (Fig. 7.44, p. 253)
	Acute glomerulonephritis	Non-specific enlargement
	Amyloidosis	Non-specific enlargement (rare)
	Diabetic nephropathy	Slight non-specific enlargement (a rare cause of enlarged kidney)

* Minor degrees of enlargement occur in many conditions. Only those conditions that give rise to easily recognized enlargement are listed here.

Calices

The calices should be evenly distributed and reasonably symmetrical. The term often used to describe the shape of a normal calix is 'cupped' and that to describe the dilated calix 'clubbed' (Fig. 7.7). The normal 'cup' is due to the indentation of the papilla into the calix. Caliceal dilatation has two basic causes:

1 obstruction;
2 destruction of the papilla, the causes of which include:
   - chronic pyelonephritis
   - tuberculosis
   - obstructive atrophy
   - papillary necrosis.

The first step therefore, when faced with dilated calices, is to try and decide whether or not there is obstruction, i.e. dilatation of the collecting system down to a specific point (Fig. 7.7c). If there is no evidence of obstruction, the conditions causing papillary destruction will have to be considered.

Renal pelvis

The position of the normal renal pelvis varies: it may be almost totally intrarenal or it may be entirely outside the kidney. It varies in size and shape. Usually, the inferior border of the pelvis is concave but even normal pelves may show a downward bulge. The pelvi-ureteric junction is usually funnel-shaped, but an abrupt change from pelvis to ureter may be normal. True dilatation of the pelvis suggests obstruction.

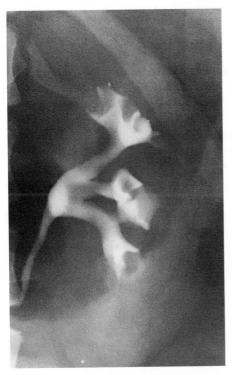
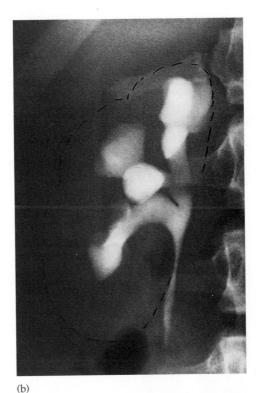
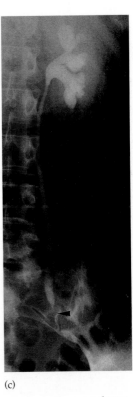

(a) (b) (c)

Fig. 7.7 The calices. (a) Normal calices. Each calix is 'cup-shaped'. (b) Many of the calices are clubbed. There is scarring of the parenchyma of the upper half of the kidney indicating that the diagnosis is chronic pyelonephritis. (c) All the calices are dilated, the dilatation of the collecting system extending down to the point of obstruction (arrow), in this case owing to a malignant retroperitoneal lymph node.

Filling defects within the renal pelvis should be looked for. The three common causes of a filling defect in the collecting systems are tumours, calculi and blood clot.

Nearly all urinary stones contain visible calcification and virtually all calcified filling defects are stones. Therefore, provided the preliminary film is reviewed, filling defects due to stones very rarely present a diagnostic problem.

The diagnosis of blood clot as the cause of a filling defect rests on knowing that the patient has severe haematuria and noting the smooth outline of the filling defect (Fig. 7.8). Sometimes the distinction between tumour and clot is difficult. A repeat examination after some days will usually show change or clearing if the filling defect is due to blood clot.

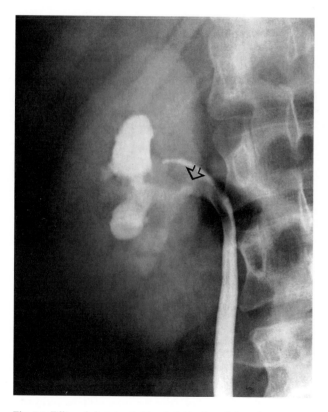

Fig. 7.8 Filling defect due to blood clot in the pelvis and upper ureter (arrow).

Ureters

The ureters are usually seen in only part of their length on any one film owing to obliteration of the lumen by peristalsis. No portion of either ureter should be more than 7 mm in diameter, but the normal effects of pregnancy and the contraceptive pill can cause moderate dilatation. Dilatation is usually due to obstruction. Occasionally, it is due to vesicoureteric reflux without obstruction. Displacement of a ureter may, on rare occasions, be recognizable.

Bladder

The bladder is a centrally located structure that should have a smooth outline. It often shows normal smooth indentations from above owing to the uterus or the sigmoid colon, and from below by muscles of the pelvic floor. After micturition the bladder should be empty, apart from a little contrast trapped in the folded mucosa.

Ultrasound

The main indications for ultrasound are to:
• demonstrate or exclude hydronephrosis, particularly in patients with renal failure or a non-functioning kidney at IVU;
• evaluate renal tumours, cysts and abscesses, including polycystic disease;
• measure renal size in renal failure;
• follow up transplant kidneys and various chronic renal diseases;
• assess and follow up with serial ultrasound renal size and scarring in children with urinary tract infections;
• guide percutaneous interventional techniques;
• assess renal blood flow using Doppler techniques;
• assess the prostate and bladder.

Normal renal ultrasound (Fig. 7.9)

At ultrasound, the kidneys should be smooth in outline. The parenchyma surrounds a central echodense region, known as the central echo complex (also called the renal sinus), consisting of the pelvicaliceal system, together with surrounding fat and renal blood vessels. In most instances, the normal pelvicaliceal system is not separately visualized.

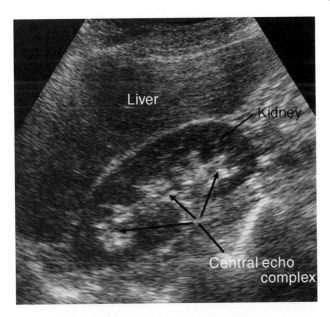

Fig. 7.9 Normal ultrasound of the right kidney.

The renal cortex generates homogeneous echoes which are less intense than those of the adjacent liver or spleen and the renal pyramids are seen as triangular sonolucent areas adjacent to the renal sinus. During the first two months of life, cortical echoes are relatively more prominent and the renal pyramids are strikingly sonolucent.

The normal adult renal length, measured by ultrasound, is 9–12 cm. These figures are lower than those for renal size measured by IVU, because there is no swelling from the action of contrast medium and there is no magnification of the image.

Normal ureters are not usually visualized. The urinary bladder should be examined in the distended state: the walls should be sharply defined and barely perceptible.

CT and MRI

Computed tomography is used for specific indications, often after IVU or ultrasound have identified a problem. Like ultrasound, CT can characterize masses and it shows the retroperitoneal space particularly well (see Chapter 10). It is an extremely sensitive method of detecting calculi and is also useful when assessing trauma or infarction.

The technique is virtually the same as for standard abdominal and pelvic CT, except that sections of the kidneys are usually performed both before and after intravenous contrast medium has been given.

Magnetic resonance imaging gives similar information to CT, with a few specific advantages, but it has several disadvantages and is only used in selected circumstances, e.g. demonstrating renal artery stenosis and inferior vena caval extension of renal tumours.

Normal CT (Fig. 7.10)

The basic principles of interpretation are the same as for IVU. The renal parenchyma should have a smooth outline and opacify uniformly after intravenous contrast administration, although early images may show opacification of the cortex before medullary opacification has had time to occur. The pelvicaliceal system should show cupped calices with uniform width of renal parenchyma from calix to renal edge, and the fat that surrounds the pelvicaliceal system should be clearly visualized. The ureters are seen in cross-section as dots lying on the psoas muscles. They will not necessarily be seen at all levels because peristalsis obliterates the lumen intermittently. The bladder has a smooth outline contrasted against the pelvic fat; its wall is thin and of reasonably uniform diameter. Contrast opacification of the urine in the bladder is variable depending on how much contrast has reached the bladder. The contrast medium is heavier than urine and therefore, the dependent portion is usually more densely opacified (Fig. 7.10).

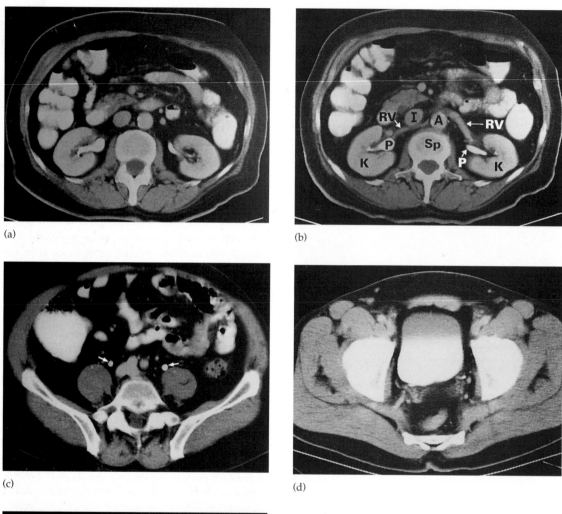

(a)

(b)

(c)

(d)

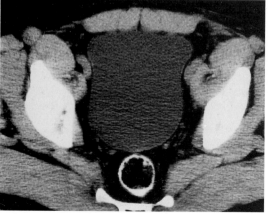

(e)

Fig. 7.10 Normal CT of kidneys and bladder. (a), (b) Adjacent
sections, (b) 1 cm higher than (a), showing uniform opacification of
parenchyma with well-defined cortical edge. The pelvicaliceal
system, which is densely opacified, is surrounded by fat. The renal
veins are well shown on the higher section. (c) Section through
the level of the ureters (arrows) after contrast has been given.
(d) Section through opacified bladder in a male patient shows that
the bladder wall is too thin to be seen. Note the layering of contrast
medium. (e) Section through bladder without contrast
opacification. The bladder wall can be identified as a thin line.
A, aorta; I, inferior vena cava; K, kidney; P, pelvis; RV, renal vein;
Sp, spine.

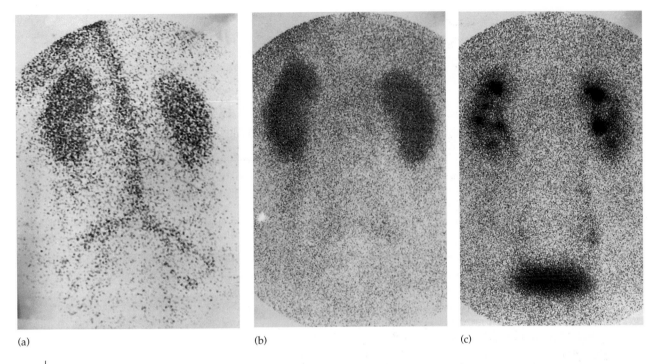

(a)   (b)   (c)

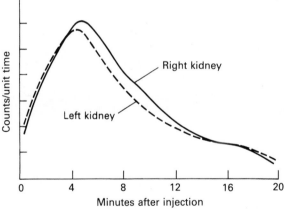

(d)

Fig. 7.11 ^{99m}Tc DTPA renogram, serial images. (a) Vascular phase. (b) Filtration phase. (c) Excretion phase. (d) The renogram curve.

Radionuclide examination

There are two main radionuclide techniques for studying the kidneys:

1 The renogram which measures renal function.
2 Scans of renal morphology (DMSA scan). The advent of

CT and ultrasound has reduced the need for such scans. They are now used mainly for evaluating renal scarring (see Fig. 7.34c, p. 247).

Renogram (Fig. 7.11)

If substances which pass into the urine are labelled with a radionuclide and injected intravenously, their passage through the kidney can be observed with a gamma camera.

The two agents of choice are ^{99m}Tc DTPA (diethylene triamine pentacetic acid) and ^{99m}Tc MAG-3 (mercaptoacetyl triglycine). DTPA is filtered by the glomeruli and not absorbed or secreted by the tubules, whereas MAG-3 is both filtered by the glomeruli and secreted by the tubules.

The gamma camera is positioned posteriorly over the kidneys and a rapid injection of the radiopharmaceutical is given. Early images show the major blood vessels and both kidneys. Subsequently, activity is seen in the renal parenchyma and by 5 min the collecting systems should be visible. Serial images over 20 min show progressive excretion and clearance of activity from the kidneys. Quantitative assessment with a computer enables a renogram curve to be produced and the relative function of each kidney calculated.

The main indications for a renogram are:

• measurement of relative renal function in each kidney – this may help the surgeon decide between nephrectomy or more conservative surgery;

• investigation of urinary tract obstruction, particularly pelvi-ureteric junction obstruction;

• investigation of renal transplants.

Special techniques

Retrograde and antegrade pyelography

The techniques of retrograde and antegrade pyelography (the term pyelography means demonstrating the pelvicaliceal system and ureters) involve direct injection of contrast material into the pelvicaliceal system or ureters through catheters placed via cystoscopy (retrograde pyelography) or percutaneously into the kidney via the loin (antegrade pyelography). The indications are limited to those situations where the information cannot be achieved by less invasive means, for example in those few cases of hydronephrosis where further information about the level and nature of obstruction is required.

Voiding cystourethrogram (micturating cystogram) and videourodynamics (see Fig. 7.56, p. 259)

In voiding cystourethrography, contrast medium is run into the empty bladder through a catheter. The bladder is filled to capacity and films are taken during voiding. The entire process is observed fluoroscopically to identify and quantify vesicoureteric reflux. The bladder, bladder neck and urethra can be assessed in order to show obstructions such as strictures or urethral valves.

In patients with a suspected functional disorder of bladder emptying, a videourodynamic examination can be of value. This requires bladder and rectal transducer lines to monitor pressures and simultaneous video images of contrast in the bladder and urethra during voiding. Videourodynamic examination is a specialized procedure and is particularly useful in the investigation of incontinence to distinguish detrusor instability from sphincter weakness. The test is also helpful in patients with obstructive symp-

toms, mainly elderly men, to differentiate true obstruction from bladder instability, and in those patients with a neurogenic bladder.

Urethrography (see Fig. 7.55, p. 259)

Urethrography can be part of voiding cystourethrography or it can be performed by retrograde injection (the retrograde technique is rarely performed in females). The usual indications for the examination are the identification of urethral strictures and to demonstrate extravasation from the urethra or bladder neck following trauma.

Renal arteriography

Renal arteriography is performed via a catheter introduced into the femoral artery by the Seldinger technique (see p. 431). Selective injections are made into one or both renal arteries (Fig. 7.12). It is mainly used to demonstrate the details of vascular anatomy prior to renal surgery and to assess renal artery stenosis. Renal arteriography is an inte-

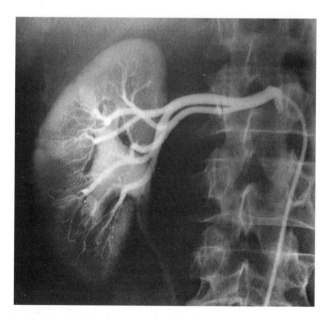

Fig. 7.12 Normal selective right renal arteriogram. Note, that not only are the arteries well shown but there is also an excellent nephrogram. The renal pelvis and ureter are opacified because of a previous injection of contrast.

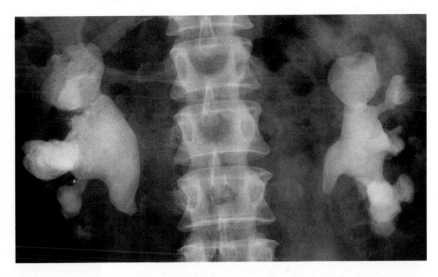

Fig. 7.13 Plain film showing a calcified staghorn calculus in each kidney.

gral part of therapeutic embolization of the renal artery and percutaneous balloon angioplasty (see p. 434).

URINARY TRACT DISORDERS

Urinary calculi

Nearly all urinary calculi are calcified and appear partly or totally opaque on plain x-ray examinations. Many are uniformly calcified but some, particularly bladder stones may be laminated. Only pure uric acid and xanthine stones are radiolucent on plain radiography, but they can be identified at CT or ultrasound.

Small renal calculi are often round or oval; the larger ones frequently assume the shape of the pelvicaliceal system and are known as staghorn calculi (Fig. 7.13).

Plain film examination of the urinary tract is more sensitive than ultrasound and is the easiest method of identifying calculi. It is essential to examine the preliminary film of an IVU carefully, because even large calculi can be completely hidden within the opacified collecting system once contrast has been given (see Fig. 7.3, p. 222).

Stones may cause obstruction to the collecting system. Ultrasound and IVU are equally good at assessing the resulting dilatation of the collecting system. The IVU is the best method of showing the precise site of obstruction – information that can be vital if surgical treatment is required.

Most renal calculi of more than 5 mm in size are readily seen at ultrasound but smaller calculi may be missed. Stones, regardless of their composition, produce intense echoes and cast acoustic shadows (Fig. 7.14). Sometimes the acoustic shadowing is more evident than the echo. Staghorn calculi, filling the caliceal system, cast very large acoustic

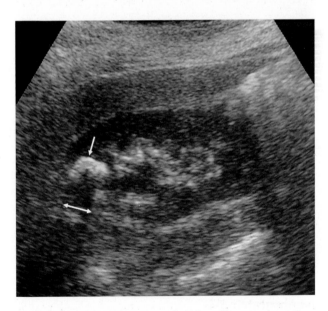

Fig. 7.14 Ultrasound of stone in right kidney. The stone (arrow) appears as a bright echo. Note the acoustic shadow behind the stone (double headed arrow).

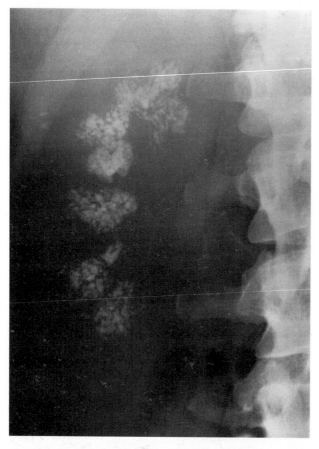

Fig. 7.15 Nephrocalcinosis. There are numerous calcifications in the pyramids of both kidneys (the left kidney is not illustrated).

shadows which may even mask an associated hydronephrosis.

Calculi located within the renal sinus may be obscured by echoes from surrounding fat. Also, ultrasound fails to demonstrate a significant proportion of ureteric calculi.

Computed tomography, when performed without intravenous contrast, is exquisitely sensitive for the detection of calculi but is not indicated solely for this purpose.

Nephrocalcinosis

Nephrocalcinosis is the term used to describe widespread numerous irregular spots of calcium in the parenchyma

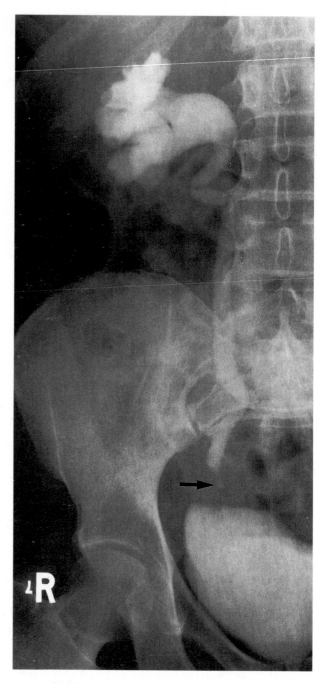

Fig. 7.16 Ureteric obstruction. The pelvicaliceal system and ureter are dilated down to the level of the obstructing pathology (arrow), in this instance a small calculus.

of both kidneys (Fig. 7.15). The causes fall into two main categories:

• nephrocalcinosis associated with hypercalcaemia and/or hypercalcuria, notably hyperparathyroidism and renal tubular acidosis;
• nephrocalcinosis *not* associated with disordered calcium metabolism, namely widespread papillary necrosis and medullary sponge kidney, a congenital condition with dilated collecting tubules in which small calculi can form.

Urinary tract obstruction

The principal feature of obstruction is dilatation of the collecting system. All the affected calices are dilated to approximately the same degree, the degree depending on the chronicity as well as the severity of the obstruction. The obstructed collecting system is dilated down to the level of the obstructing pathology and demonstrating this level is a prime objective of imaging (Fig. 7.16). The IVU and ultra-sound examination play major roles when urinary tract obstruction is being evaluated. Computed tomography and radionuclide studies show typical changes, but are rarely the primary imaging procedures.

Intravenous urogram in urinary tract obstruction

Opacification of the urine in an obstructed system usually takes a long time. Delayed films are therefore an essential part of any IVU where the level of obstruction is not shown on the routine films. Even if the flow of urine has stopped completely, provided glomerular filtration is still occurring, the collecting system will opacify at IVU even though it may take many hours. In acute obstruction – usually from a stone in the ureter – contrast accumulates and is concentrated in the tubules producing a very dense nephrogram. The pyelogram phase is greatly delayed, but in time the collecting system and the level of obstruction can be demonstrated (Fig. 7.17). Once the site of obstruction is established, the

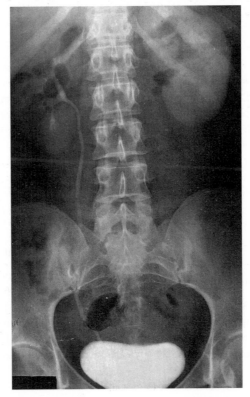 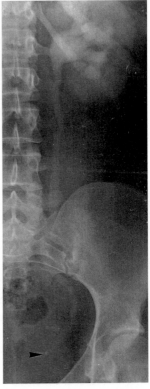

(a) (b)

Fig. 7.17 Acute ureteric obstruction from a stone in the lower end of the left ureter. (a) A film taken 30 min after the injection of contrast medium. There is obvious delay in the appearance of the pyelogram on the left. The left kidney shows a very dense nephrogram which is characteristic of acute ureteric obstruction. (b) A film taken 23 h later shows opacification of the obstructed collecting system down to the obstructing calculus (arrow).

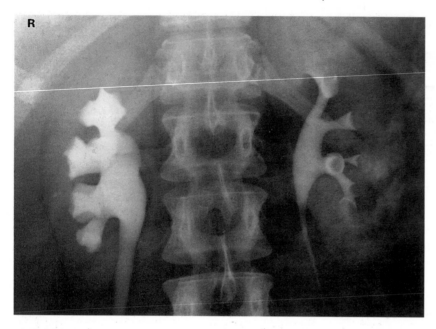

R

Fig. 7.18 Obstructive atrophy. The right kidney is small with a smooth outline from reduction in renal parenchyma and shows dilatation of the collecting system. This loss of renal tissue was due to obstruction by a stone in the ureter.

plain film should be looked at again to confirm or exclude an opaque calculus responsible for the obstruction.

Prolonged obstruction causes atrophy of the kidney substance; this is recognized by observing the reduction in renal parenchymal width (Fig. 7.18).

Obstruction can be intermittent and between attacks the IVU may be normal. If, however, the urogram is performed during an attack of colic (the so-called 'emergency urogram') the level of obstruction is nearly always demonstrated. Conversely, a normal urogram taken during an episode of acute pain effectively excludes ureteric colic as the cause of pain.

Ultrasound in urinary tract obstruction

Dilatation of the pelvicaliceal system is demonstrated sonographically as a spreading apart of the central echo complex, caused by pooling of urine within the pelvis and calices. Initially, these are seen as fluid collections in the centre of the kidney (Fig. 7.19a). As the distension becomes more severe, the dilated calices can resemble multiple renal cysts, but dilated calices, unlike cysts, show continuity with the renal pelvis (Fig. 7.19b,c). With prolonged obstruction, thinning of the cortex due to atrophy will be seen.

Proximal ureteric dilatation can frequently be identified, but dilatation of the distal ureter is often obscured by overlying bowel. It follows therefore that while some causes of obstruction are identifiable, e.g. carcinoma of the bladder, it is often not possible to determine the cause of urinary tract obstruction at ultrasound examination. Plain films are useful in this context to demonstrate calculi that may be responsible for the obstruction.

Computed tomography in urinary tract obstruction

Dilated portions of the collecting systems can be identified on CT both before and after intravenous contrast administration (Fig. 7.19d). The dilated system can frequently be traced down to the site of the obstruction. An advantage over the IVU is that tumours responsible for obstruction may be visualized directly.

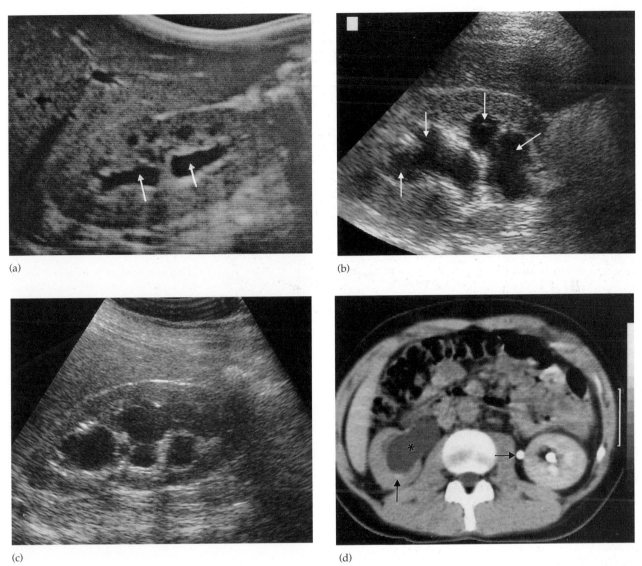

(a)

(b)

(c)

(d)

Fig. 7.19 Dilatation of the pelvicaliceal system. (a) Longitudinal ultrasound scan of right kidney showing spreading of the central echo complex of the dilated collecting system (arrows). (b) Here the dilatation of the calices is greater (arrows). (c) In this image from a patient with pelviureteric obstruction, the dilated calices resemble cysts. (d) CT scan after contrast showing a dilated renal pelvis (asterisk). The vertical arrow points to a small amount of contrast pooling in a dependent calix. Note the normal left ureter (horizontal arrow).

Causes of obstruction to the ureters and pelvicaliceal systems

There are many causes of obstruction to the ureters and pelvicaliceal systems. Calculi, tumours or strictures may be responsible for obstruction at any level. When obstruction is seen at the pelvi-ureteric junction, an additional cause to consider is the congenital disorder 'intrinsic pelvi-ureteric junction obstruction'. Aberrant renal artery, retroperitoneal fibrosis and retroperitoneal tumours are further causes of ureteric obstruction.

Calculi

Calculi are by far the commonest cause of obstruction of the urinary tract. A calcified opacity will usually be visible on the plain film, but since parts of the ureter overlie the transverse processes of the vertebrae and the wings of the sacrum, the calculus may be impossible to see on plain film.

Sloughed papilla

A sloughed papilla in papillary necrosis is a rare cause of ureteric obstruction. The diagnosis can be suspected when other papillae still within the kidney show signs of papillary necrosis (see p. 248).

Tumours

Transitional cell carcinomas of the calices or pelvis usually produce a recognizable filling defect at IVU, but if the tumour is in the ureter it may not be visible. The best test to demonstrate the tumour in such cases is pyelography, either retrograde or antegrade. Carcinoma of the bladder causing ureteric obstruction can usually be easily identified on IVU, CT or ultrasound, though cystoscopy is the best method of establishing the diagnosis.

Renal parenchymal masses may narrow and obstruct a calix or the pelvis but the explanation is usually obvious because of other signs due to the mass.

Infective strictures

Infective strictures are mostly due to tuberculosis or schistosomiasis. In the case of tuberculosis there is usually other imaging evidence to suggest the diagnosis (p. 245).

Congenital intrinsic pelviureteric junction obstruction

In this disorder peristalsis is not transmitted across the pelviureteric junction, i.e. a functional obstruction exists, but there is no naked-eye evidence of the cause. The disease may present at any age but it is usually discovered in children or young adults. The diagnosis depends on identifying

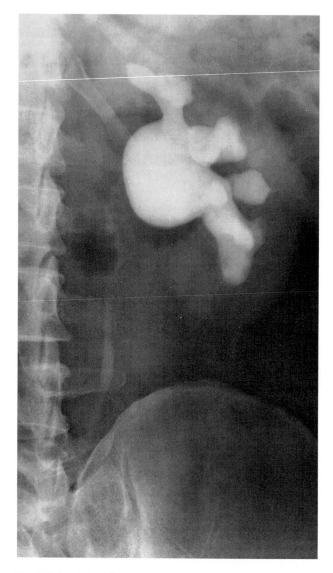

Fig. 7.20 Intrinsic pelviureteric junction obstruction. The pelvicaliceal system is considerably dilated, but the ureter from the pelviureteric junction onward is normal in calibre.

dilatation of the pelvis and calices, with an abrupt change in calibre at the pelvi-ureteric junction (Fig. 7.20). Often, the ureter cannot be identified at all. If it is seen, it will be either narrow or normal in size.

Pelviureteric junction obstruction can be difficult to distinguish on IVU from an otherwise normal, unobstructed

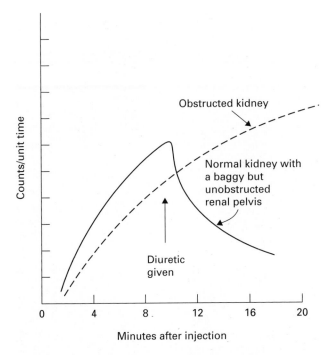

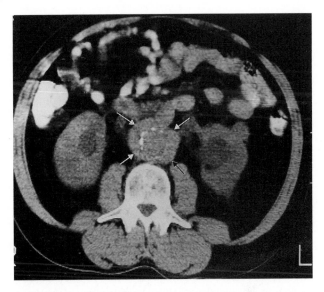

Fig. 7.22 Retroperitoneal fibrosis. CT scan showing bilateral hydronephrosis. The aorta is surrounded by a mass of fibrous tissue (arrows). The position of the aortic wall is shown by its atheromatous calcification. The retroperitoneal fibrosis extended down to the level of aortic bifurcation.

Fig. 7.21 Diuretic renogram comparing pelviureteric junction obstruction (dotted line) with a 'baggy' but otherwise normal renal pelvis (continuous line). Frusemide was given at 10 min and in the case of the 'baggy' pelvis resulted in rapid wash-out of radioactivity from the kidney.

dilated renal pelvis – the so-called 'baggy' pelvis. This distinction can be made by giving a diuretic intravenously. In pelviureteric junction obstruction the induced diuresis causes dilatation of the pelvicaliceal system and the patient develops loin pain. Similarly, a diuretic can be given during a renogram (Fig. 7.21). If there is obstruction, the radionuclide accumulates within the kidney and renal pelvis, whereas with a 'baggy' pelvis there is rapid washout of the radionuclide from the suspect kidney.

Retroperitoneal disease

Tumours. Carcinoma of the cervix and rectosigmoid junction, and malignant lymph node enlargement are frequent causes in this category of ureteric obstruction. The ureters may be visibly deviated by the tumour but frequently the ureteric course is normal. Because some of these tumours originate in the midline or are bilateral, both ureters may be obstructed. Computed tomography, or ultrasound in some cases, is the ideal method of diagnosis because it shows the tumour mass, whereas the IVU only shows the site of obstruction.

Retroperitoneal fibrosis. In most cases, no cause can be found for this benign fibrotic condition which encases the ureters and causes obstruction. When first seen, only one side may be obstructed but eventually the condition becomes bilateral. The obstruction is usually at the L4/5 level. Here again, CT has become the diagnostic method of choice, because it shows the retroperitoneum so well (Fig. 7.22).

Ureteric dilatation in pregnancy

Pronounced unilateral or bilateral ureteric dilatation together with dilatation of the pelvicaliceal systems occurs during the second half of pregnancy, or in women taking the contraceptive pill. It may take three months or more to return to normal.

Unilateral 'non-functioning' kidney at IVU

The phrase unilateral 'non-functioning' kidney implies non-visualization of the pyelogram of one kidney at IVU not, as the term would suggest, a total absence of function by that kidney. Total non-visualization is rare; a nephrogram is often seen.

The common cause of a 'non-functioning' kidney, other than previous nephrectomy, is *ureteric obstruction*. Other causes include renal agenesis, renal artery occlusion and renal vein thrombosis.

It is worth noting that renal parenchymal tumours (renal cell carcinoma and Wilms' tumour) are very rare causes of 'non-function'. When they do result in absence of a pyelogram, the usual mechanism is obstruction of the ureter by tumour or blood clot. On the other hand, transitional cell carcinomas of the pelvis, ureter and bladder readily obstruct the drainage of a kidney.

Most cases of unilateral non-visualization at IVU require further investigation. It is here that ultrasound is so valuable, since it does not rely on renal function. Ultrasound can demonstrate the renal size, the thickness of the parenchyma and can determine whether there is hydronephrosis.

In patients with *renal artery occlusion* the kidney is visible on plain film or CT but no nephrogram is seen after contrast is given. Renography will confirm absence of blood flow and function. Ultrasound shows a normal pelvicaliceal pattern, but Doppler images show absence of blood flow.

Acute renal vein thrombosis is a rare cause of non-visualization. With time, collateral venous channels open up and a visible pyelogram usually returns. The thrombus in the renal veins or inferior vena cava may be detectable with ultrasound or CT.

Renal parenchymal masses

Almost all solitary masses arising within the renal parenchyma are either *malignant tumours* or *simple cysts*. In adults, the malignant tumour is almost certain to be a renal cell carcinoma, whereas in young children the common neoplasm is Wilms' tumour.

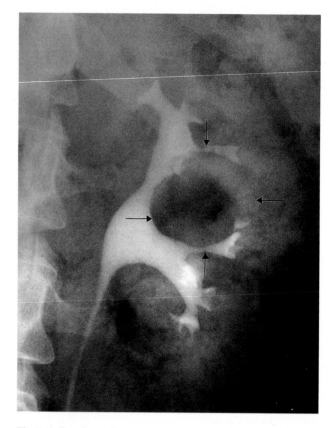

Fig. 7.23 Renal pseudotumour (arrows) which was subsequently shown to be normal renal cortical tissue.

Unusual causes of a renal mass include: renal abscess, hydatid cyst, benign tumour, notably angiomyolipoma, and metastasis.

Occasionally, invagination of normal cortical tissue into the renal medulla (sometimes called a 'renal pseudotumour') may produce the signs of a localized mass at IVU (Fig. 7.23). Here the distinguishing feature is uniform opacification of the 'mass'. Ultrasound or CT can be used to exclude a true tumour.

Multiple renal masses usually indicate multiple simple cysts, polycystic disease or malignant lymphoma.

Intravenous urography

The basic signs of a renal parenchymal mass on an IVU are (Fig. 7.24):

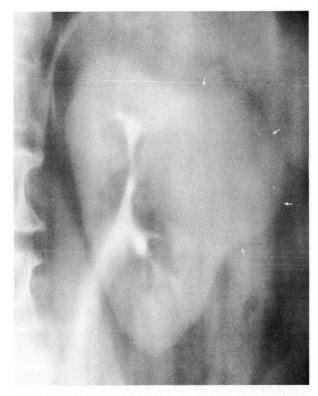

Fig. 7.24 Signs of a renal mass. The renal outline is bulged (arrows) and there is a corresponding displacement of the calices. In this patient the mass is a cyst. Note the lower density of the mass compared with the opacified renal parenchyma and its clear-cut border.

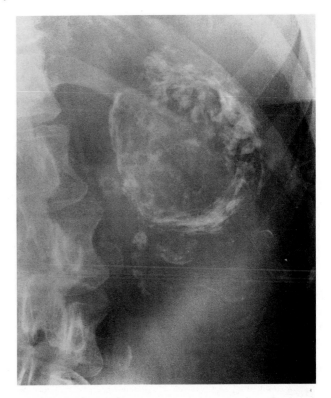

Fig. 7.25 Partially calcified renal cell carcinoma.

• Bulging of the renal outline. Sometimes, the outline is so indistinct that the bulge cannot be appreciated.
• Displacement of major and minor calices.
• Increase in renal size, particularly if the mass is at the upper or lower pole where its bulk adds to the renal length.
• Calcification in a small proportion of renal carcinomas (Fig. 7.25). Calcification in the wall of a benign cyst is exceedingly uncommon.

Once a mass is seen or suspected at IVU, the next step is to diagnose its nature using ultrasound or CT. It should be noted that any solitary mass in a young child, or any mass that contains visible calcification, particularly if the calcification is more than just a thin line at the periphery, is likely to be a malignant tumour.

Ultrasound (Fig. 7.26)

Ultrasound is used to establish whether a mass is a simple cyst, and can therefore be ignored, or whether the lesion is solid and, therefore, is likely to be a carcinoma. A mass with mixed cystic and solid features falls into the indeterminate category and could be a renal tumour, a renal abscess, or possibly a complex benign cyst or other benign condition.

Simple cysts are very common. Being filled with clear fluid, they show obvious echoes from the front and back wall but no echoes from within the cyst itself. They also show a column of increased echoes behind the cyst, owing to increased through-transmission of the sound, known as 'acoustic enhancement'. Most cysts are spherical in shape. They may be solitary or multiple, unilocular or have septations. Some cysts contain low level echoes in their dependent portions, presumably due to previous

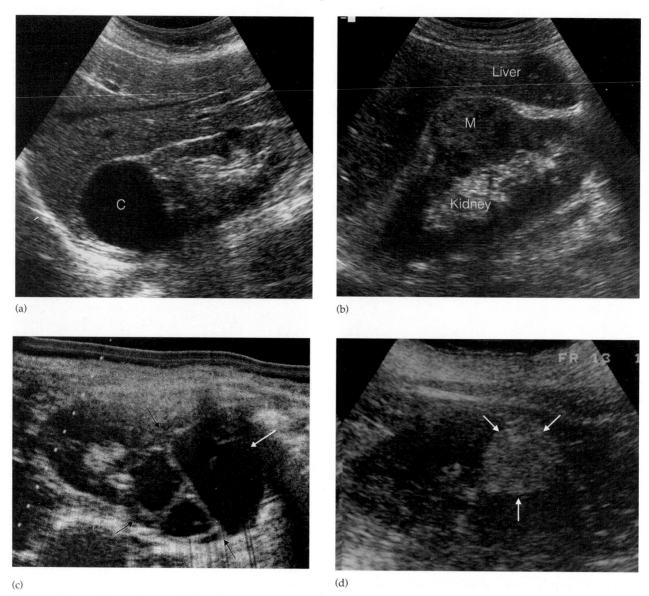

Fig. 7.26 Ultrasound in renal masses. (a) Cyst (C) showing sharp walls and no echoes arising within the cyst. Note the acoustic enhancement behind the cyst. (b) Tumour showing echoes within a solid mass (M). (c) Complex mass due to cystic renal cell carcinoma. The arrows point to the edge of the mass. Note the thick septa within the mass. (d) Angiomyolipoma. This incidental finding shows the typical appearance of a small echogenic mass (arrow). Same patient as in Fig. 7.27(c).

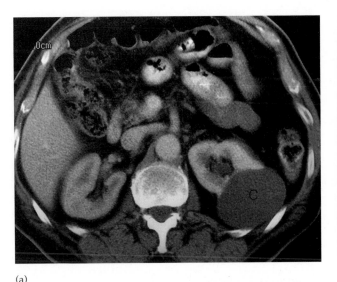

(a)

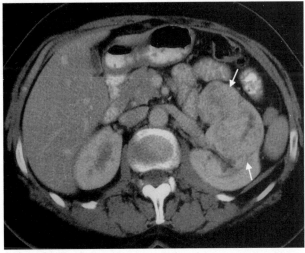

(b)

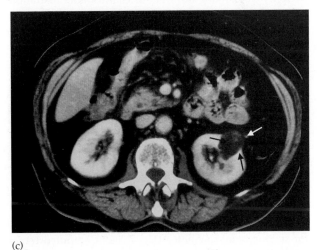

(c)

Fig. 7.27 Computed tomography (contrast-enhanced) in renal masses. (a) Cyst in left kidney (C) showing a well-defined edge, imperceptible wall and uniform water density. The cyst shows no enhancement. It was an incidental finding. (b) Renal cell carcinoma. The mass (arrows) is not clearly demarcated from the adjacent kidney and shows substantial enhancement. (c) Angiomyolipoma (same patient as in Fig. 7.26(d)) with a small mass (arrow) of fat density.

haemorrhage. When the ultrasonographer is sure that the diagnosis is a simple cyst, no further investigation is needed.

Solid renal masses have numerous internal echoes of varying intensity. Because sound is attenuated during its passage through a solid lesion, the back wall is not as sharp as that seen with a cyst, and there is often little or no 'acoustic enhancement' deep to the mass. Solid masses may be irregular in outline.

When a tumour is demonstrated, the ultrasonographer will also look for extension into the renal vein and inferior vena cava, check for liver and retroperitoneal metastases, and examine the opposite kidney.

Angiomyolipomas are a fairly frequent incidental finding at ultrasound, appearing as small echogenic masses. CT is the usual method of definitive diagnosis (see below).

Computed tomography of renal masses

Computed tomography has proved very useful for differentiating cysts from tumours, diagnosing angiomyolipomas, and staging known renal carcinoma (Fig. 7.27).

At CT, a typical *simple renal cyst* is a spherical mass with an imperceptible wall. The interior of the cyst is homogeneous with attenuation values similar to those of water. The margins between the cyst and the normal renal parenchyma are sharp. When all of these criteria are met the diagnosis of simple cyst is certain and there is no need to proceed further. An important diagnostic feature is that simple cysts do not enhance following intravenous contrast injection.

Renal cell carcinomas are approximately spherical, usually lobulated and frequently have poorly defined margins. The attenuation value of renal tumours on scans without intravenous contrast enhancement is often fairly close to that of normal renal parenchyma, but focal necrotic areas may result in areas of low density, and stippled calcification may be present in the interior of the mass as well as around the periphery. Following intravenous contrast administration, renal cell carcinomas enhance but not to the same degree as the normal parenchyma and they are inhomogeneous in their enhancement pattern. The CT diagnosis of renal carcinoma is usually sufficiently accurate that preoperative biopsy is rarely performed.

Angiomyolipomas are usually incidental findings. They are benign tumours which rarely cause problems, although on occasion they cause significant retroperitoneal haemorrhage. At CT their fatty nature allows a confident diagnosis (Fig. 7.27c).

Staging of renal carcinoma

Computed tomography is currently the method of choice for staging renal carcinoma (Fig. 7.28a). Computed tomography shows local direct spread, can demonstrate enlargement of draining lymph nodes in the retroperitoneum, diagnose liver metastases and show tumour growing along the renal vein into the inferior vena cava. MRI may in future be as good or better for demonstrating these features (Fig. 7.28b).

Urothelial tumours

Almost all tumours that arise within the collecting systems of the kidneys are *transitional cell carcinomas*. The tumours sometimes occur in multiple sites. In the pelvicaliceal system they are seen as lobulated or, very occasionally, as fronded filling defects either projecting into the lumen or completely surrounded by contrast (Fig. 7.29). It is easy to confuse such tumours with overlying gas shadows on an IVU and tomography may be required during an IVU to solve the problem.

At ultrasound, transitional cell carcinomas can be difficult to see because they blend with the renal sinus fat.

Urothelial tumours may obstruct the ureter in which they are growing, in which case it is usually only possible to determine the site of obstruction from the IVU or ultrasound. The tumour itself may be visible on antegrade or retrograde pyelography or at CT.

Acute infections of the upper urinary tracts

Acute pyelonephritis

Acute pyelonephritis is usually due to bacterial infection from organisms that enter the urinary system via the urethra. Anatomical abnormalities such as stones, duplex systems, obstructive lesions and conditions such as diabetes mellitus all predispose to infection. Only a few adults with urinary tract infection require imaging: repetitive infection and severe ureteric colic are the common indications. Urinary tract infection in young children often leads to imaging after the first infection in boys and second infection in girls.

In most cases, the IVU is normal even during the acute attack. In severe cases with suppuration of the kidney, the caliceal system is compressed by the swelling of the renal substance and the concentration of contrast on the affected side is reduced or not visible. At ultrasound, one or both kidneys may appear significantly enlarged and show diminished echoes due to cortical oedema.

Renal and perinephric abscesses

Renal and perinephric abscesses are usually difficult to see on IVU, since in many cases there is poor visualization of the kidneys owing to pre-existing hydronephrosis or calculous disease. Ultrasound and CT are the best methods of diagnosis.

Most *intrarenal abscesses* (Fig. 7.30) have thick walls and show both cystic and solid components recognizable at both

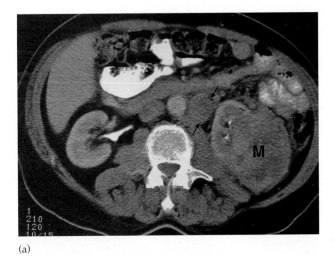

(a)

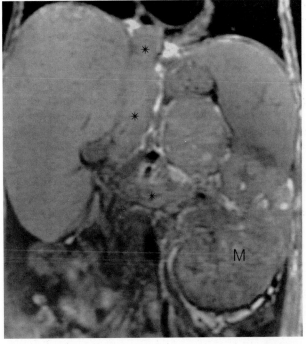

(b)

Fig. 7.28 Staging renal carcinoma. (a) CT scan showing a large mass (M) in the left kidney from renal cell carcinoma and a greatly enlarged lymph node (arrows) in the left para-aortic area. This node contained metastatic tumour cells. (b) Coronal MRI scan showing a huge left renal carcinoma (M) with tumour extending into the inferior vena cava (IVC) via the left renal vein. The caval extension of tumour (*) extends to the top of the IVC. (c) Axial MRI scan showing the IVC extension of tumour (arrows). Normally, the IVC is seen as a signal void.

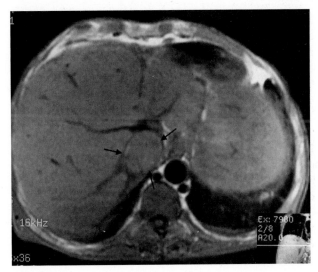

(c)

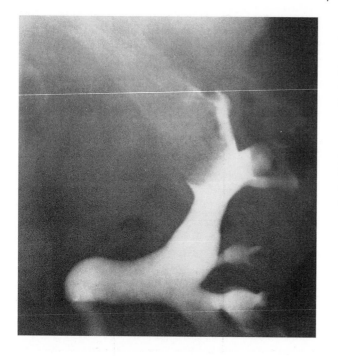

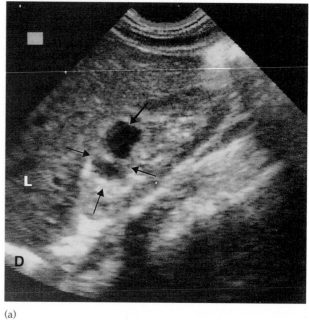

(a)

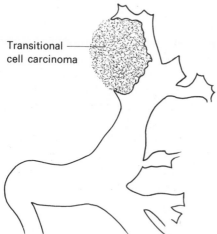

Transitional cell carcinoma

Fig. 7.29 Filling defect in an upper calix due to transitional cell carcinoma.

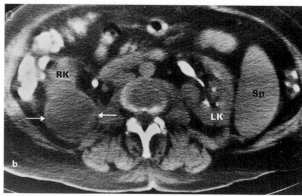

(b)

Fig. 7.30 Renal abscess. (a) Ultrasound scan showing a complex mass (arrows) in the right kidney. (b) CT scan in a different patient showing encapsulated fluid collection in the lower pole of the right kidney (arrows). D, diaphragm; L, liver; LK, left kidney; RK, right kidney; Sp, spleen.

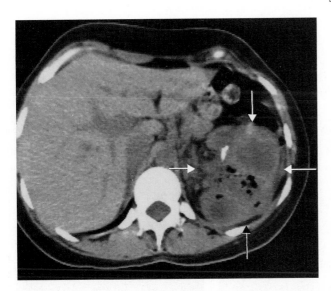

Fig. 7.31 Perinephric abscess. CT scan showing a rounded loculation of fluid and gas in the left perinephric space (arrows).

ultrasound and CT. With CT, it is possible to see enhancement of the wall of the abscess following intravenous contrast injection.

Simple cysts may become secondarily infected, in which case the ultrasound and CT features resemble those of a simple cyst, but the wall may be a little thicker and there will frequently be a layer of echogenic debris in the dependent portion of the cyst.

Perinephric abscesses (Fig. 7.31) frequently conform to the shape of the underlying kidney. The CT and sonographic characteristics are variable, usually showing both solid and cystic elements. The cystic portions frequently contain internal echoes at ultrasound owing to debris. Since most perinephric abscesses are secondary to an infective focus within the kidney, an underlying renal abnormality is often demonstrable.

Pyonephrosis

Pyonephrosis only occurs in collecting systems that are obstructed. At IVU, it may occasionally be possible to identify hydronephrosis, but usually no opacification of the affected side can be seen. Ultrasound is the most useful imaging modality for pyonephrosis. In addition to showing the hydronephrosis, it may demonstrate multiple echoes within the collecting system from infected debris.

Tuberculosis

Urinary tuberculosis follows blood-borne spread of *Mycobacterium tuberculosis*, usually from a focus of infection in the lung.

The tubercle bacilli infect the cortex of the kidneys and may cause cortical abscesses which can ulcerate into the renal pelvis. The infection may then spread to involve other portions of the urinary and genital systems.

In the early stages of the disease, even though tubercle bacilli can be recovered from the urine, the IVU may be normal. There are various signs that develop in the later stages:

- Calcification is common (Fig. 7.32). Usually, there are one or more patches of irregular calcification, but in advanced cases with long-standing tuberculous pyonephrosis the majority of the kidney and hydronephrotic collecting system may be calcified, leading to a so-called 'autonephrectomy'. Calcification implies healing but does not mean that the disease is inactive.
- The earliest change on the post-contrast films is irregularity of a calix. Later, a definite contrast-filled cavity may be seen adjacent to the calix (Fig. 7.33).
- Strictures of any portion of the pelvicaliceal system or ureter may occur, producing dilatation of one or more calices. The multiplicity of strictures is an important diagnostic feature.
- If the bladder is involved, the wall is irregular because of inflammatory oedema; advanced disease causes fibrosis resulting in a thick-walled small volume bladder. Multiple strictures may be seen in the urethra.

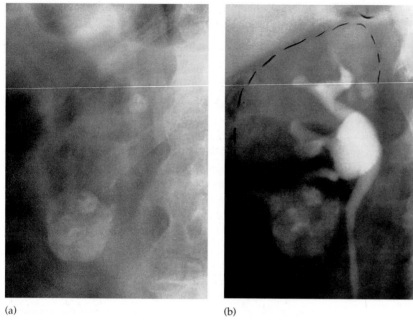

(a)   (b)

Fig. 7.32 Renal parenchymal calcification from tuberculosis. (a) Plain film. (b) After contrast.

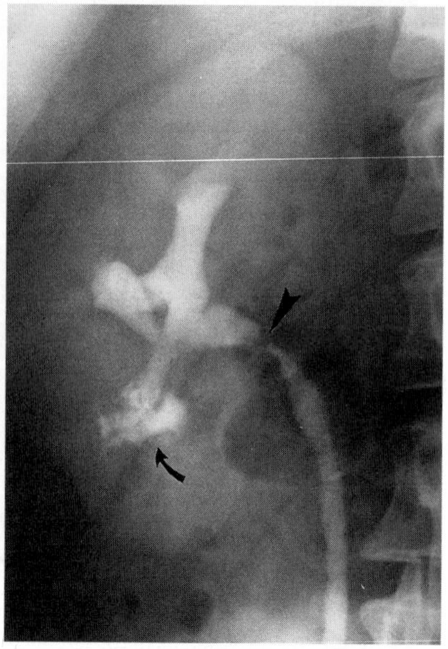

Fig. 7.33 Tuberculosis, showing irregularity of the calices (curved arrow) and stricture formation of the pelvis (arrow head).

Reflux nephropathy (chronic pyelonephritis)

Reflux nephropathy used to be called chronic pyelonephritis. It has been renamed because the condition is due to reflux of infected urine from the bladder into the kidneys, leading to destruction and scarring of the renal substance. Most damage occurs in the first year of life. The severity of reflux diminishes as the child gets older and may have ceased by the time the diagnosis of reflux nephropathy is made. The condition is often bilateral.

The signs of reflux nephropathy are (Fig. 7.34):

• *Local reduction in renal parenchymal width (scar formation)*. The distance between the calix and the adjacent renal outline is usually substantially reduced and may be as little as 1 or 2 mm. The upper and lower calices are the most susceptible to damage from reflux. It may, therefore, be easy to miss the fact that extensive scarring exists. DMSA radionuclide scans and ultrasound are both useful for demonstrating cortical scars.

• *Dilatation of the calices in the scarred areas*. The dilatation is the result of destruction of the pyramids.

• *Overall reduction in renal size* partly from loss of renal substance and partly because the scarred areas do not grow.

• *Dilatation of the affected collecting system* from reflux may be seen.

• *Vesicoureteric reflux* may be demonstrated at micturating (voiding) cystography.

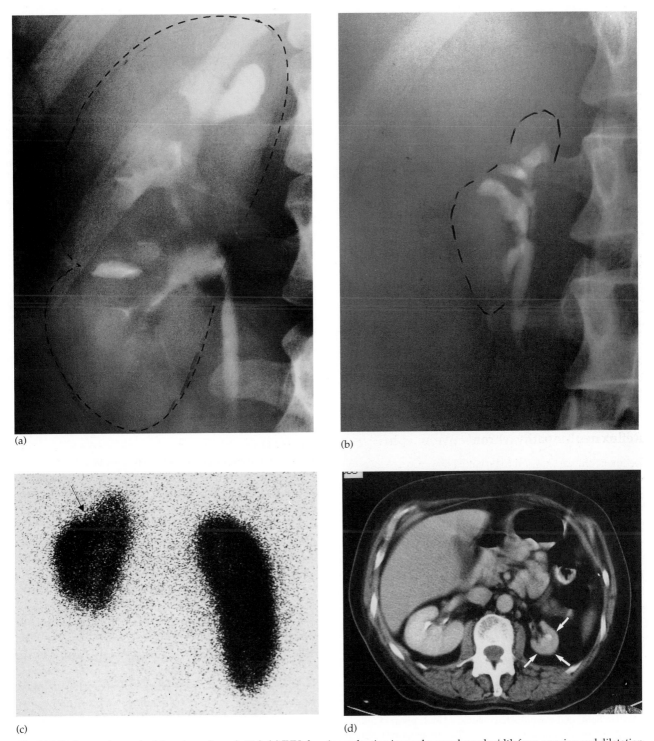

(a)

(b)

(c)

(d)

Fig. 7.34 Reflux nephropathy (chronic pyelonephritis). (a) IVU showing reduction in renal parenchymal width from scarring and dilatation (clubbing) of the adjacent calices. (b) IVU showing a severely shrunken kidney with multiple scars and clubbed calices. (c) DMSA scan (posterior view) showing shrunken left kidney with a focal scar in upper pole (arrow). (d) CT scan (after i.v. contrast enhancement) showing shrunken left pyelonephritic kidney (arrows).

Papillary necrosis (Fig. 7.35)

In papillary necrosis, part or all of the renal papilla sloughs and may fall into the pelvicaliceal system. These necrotic papillae may remain within the pelvicaliceal system, sometimes causing obstruction, or they may be voided. There are a number of conditions with strong associations with papillary necrosis. The most frequent are:

- high analgesic intake
- diabetes mellitus
- sickle cell disease
- infection, but usually only with very severe infections.

The pattern of destruction of the papilla takes many forms; the disease is usually patchy in distribution and severity. If the papilla is only partially separated, contrast can be seen tracking into it, but if the papilla is totally

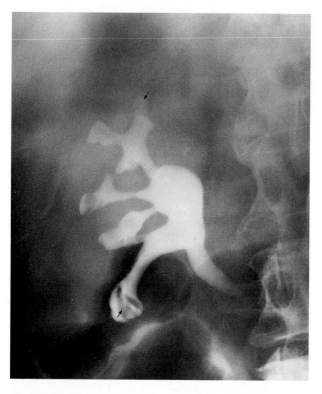

Fig. 7.35 Papillary necrosis showing dilated calices from loss of the papillae. Some of the papillae have sloughed and appear as filling defects within the calices (lower arrow). The upper arrow points to a contrast-filled cavity within a papilla.

sloughed the calix appears spherical, having lost its papillary indentation. When sloughed, the papilla may then be seen as a filling defect in a spherical calix or it may have passed down the ureter, often causing obstruction as it does so.

The necrotic papilla can calcify prior to sloughing. A sloughed, calcified papilla within the collecting system may closely resemble a urinary calculus.

Renal trauma

The kidney, along with the spleen, is the most frequent internal abdominal organ to be injured. Blunt trauma, particularly road traffic accidents and contact sports are the mechanisms of injury in well over three-quarters of patients, the remainder being caused by penetrating injury. Loin pain and haematuria are the major presenting features.

The indications for imaging tests depend on the clinical features and surgical approach. The IVU is usually the first test performed, followed by CT if necessary. Computed tomography has the advantage that it can also show or exclude damage to other abdominal structures. In general, these tests are used to:

- demonstrate the presence or absence of perfusion to the injured kidney;
- ensure that the opposite kidney is normal;
- show the extent of renal parenchymal damage;
- demonstrate injuries to other organs, a feature of great importance in penetrating injury, where other organs are frequently lacerated.

The appearances on IVU or CT depend on the extent of injury. Minor injury (contusion and small capsular haematomas) produces swelling of the parenchyma which compresses the calices. If the kidney substance is torn, the renal outline is irregular and the calices are separated. Large subcapsular and extracapsular blood collections may be present and extravasation of contrast may be seen (Fig. 7.36). Retroperitoneal haemorrhage may displace the kidney. Fragmentation of the kidney is a serious event, often, although by no means always, requiring nephrectomy or surgical repair. If thrombosis or rupture of the renal artery occurs, there will be no nephrogram. Renal infarction is a very serious condition demanding urgent restoration of blood flow or nephrectomy.

Hypertension in renal disease

Renal artery stenosis can be a cause of hypertension. It is, however, found fairly frequently at post mortem or angiographically in normotensive patients. The common cause is atheroma.

Radionuclide renography (Fig. 7.37) and colour-flow Doppler can be used to diagnose the condition. Renography shows delay in peak activity and a relative reduction of function on the affected side if renal artery stenosis is present. Angiography is the most definitive technique.

There are several other diseases, both renal and non-renal, that are associated with hypertension. The renal conditions include chronic glomerulonephritis, chronic pyelonephritis, renal artery stenosis, polycystic disease,

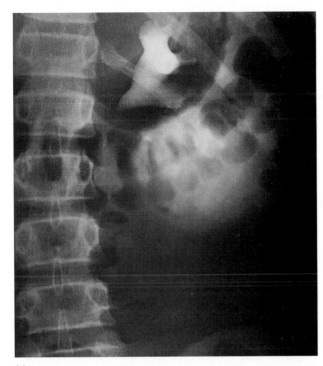

(a)

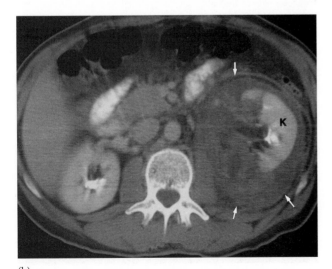

(b)

Fig. 7.36 Renal trauma. (a) The lower pole of the kidney has been ruptured and a pool of extravasated contrast can be seen. (b) CT scan showing extensive haematoma (arrows) surrounding a fragmented left kidney (K).

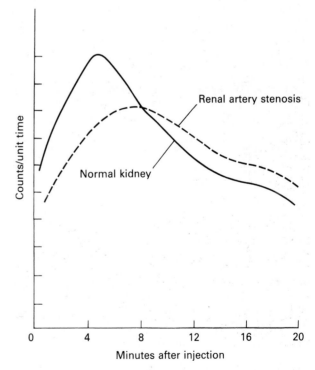

Fig. 7.37 Renal artery stenosis. Renogram curve. Accumulation and excretion of the radionuclide is delayed and reduced, so the peak of the curve is later and lower than normal.

polyarteritis nodosa, Kimmelstiel–Wilson kidney and, occasionally, renal masses. The common feature is a reduction in blood supply to all or part of the kidney.

In glomerulonephritis, polyarteritis nodosa and the Kimmelstiel–Wilson kidney, there is usually bilateral uniform reduction in renal size without other specific features. Essential hypertension may cause identical changes at IVU and the decision whether the small kidneys are the cause or the result of hypertension cannot be made radiologically.

Nowadays, because of improved drug therapy, the search for a renal cause is largely limited to children with severe hypertension and those patients whose hypertension is inadequately controlled.

Renal failure

The main roles of imaging in patients with impaired renal function are to detect obstruction to the urinary tract and to determine renal size. Bilateral small kidneys suggest chronic, often irreversible, renal failure.

Renal failure from obstructive uropathy

The cardinal sign of obstructive uropathy is dilatation of the pelvicaliceal system. Ultrasound has now replaced the IVU as the initial investigation to confirm or exclude obstruction (Fig. 7.38). Plain radiographs should be taken to exclude urinary calculi in any patient with renal failure and urinary tract obstruction demonstrated by ultrasound. The demonstration of a normal pelvicaliceal system rules out an obstructive cause for renal failure.

Renal failure from intrinsic renal disease ('end stage kidney')

Once obstruction and prerenal conditions have been excluded, intrinsic renal disease is assumed to be responsible for the renal failure.

Chronic pyelonephritis is the only specific diagnosis that can be made by imaging with any frequency. Most end-stage kidneys are small or normal in size with smooth outlines and normal calices. There are many causes for these appearances, notably chronic glomerulonephritis and diabetes (see Table 7.1, p. 224). An alteration of parenchymal

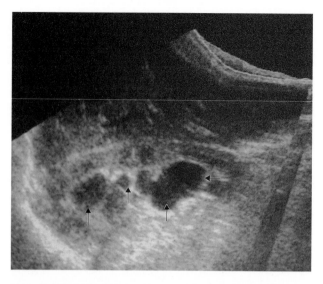

Fig. 7.38 Ultrasound of obstructive renal failure. The dilated collecting system is arrowed. The hydronephrosis was bilateral in this case of retroperitoneal fibrosis.

texture may be demonstrated by ultrasound (Fig. 7.39) but the appearances are rarely specific.

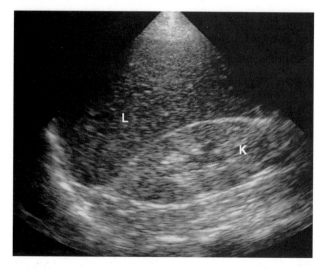

Fig. 7.39 Intrinsic renal disease. Ultrasound of right kidney (longitudinal scan). The kidney is small and the cortical echoes are increased and therefore the central echo is less obvious. Normally, the liver is more echo-reflective than the renal cortex. L, liver; K, kidney.

Acute tubular necrosis

In acute tubular necrosis, from whatever cause, the ultrasound scan shows kidneys that are normal or enlarged with normal pelvicaliceal systems. Early films during an IVU show a definite nephrogram – one which is often denser than normal (Fig. 7.40). The diagnostic feature is that the nephrogram persists for up to 24 hours without visible caliceal filling.

Congenital variations of the urinary tract

Congenital variations in the anatomy of the urinary tract are frequent. Only the more common anomalies are discussed here (congenital pelviureteric junction obstruction is discussed on p. 236).

Bifid collecting systems

Bifid collecting systems (Fig. 7.41) are the most frequent congenital variations. The condition may be unilateral or bilateral. Sometimes just the pelvis is bifid, an anomaly of no importance. At the other extreme, the two ureters may be separate throughout their length and have separate openings into the bladder. The ureter draining the upper moiety may drain outside the bladder, e.g. into the vagina or urethra, producing incontinence if the opening is beyond the urethral sphincter. Such ureters, known as *ectopic ureters*, are frequently obstructed (Fig. 7.42) and lead

to dilatation of the entire moiety; the dilated lower ureter in this condition is known as a *ureterocele*. The lower end of the dilated ureter often causes a smooth filling defect in the bladder.

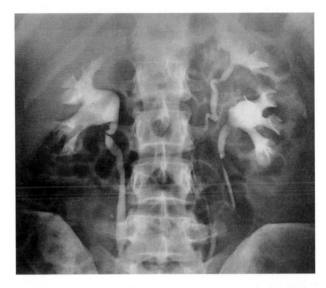

Fig. 7.41 Bifid collecting systems. There is a bifid collecting system on the left with the two ureters joining at the level of the transverse process of L5. Note how the left kidney is larger than the right.

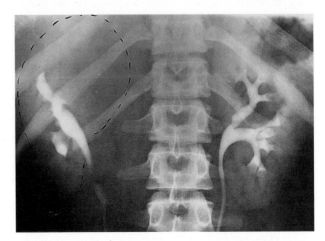

Fig. 7.42 Obstructed ectopic ureterocele. There is a bifid collecting system on the right. The upper moiety is obstructed and dilated causing deformity of the lower moiety. The obstructed moiety does not opacify.

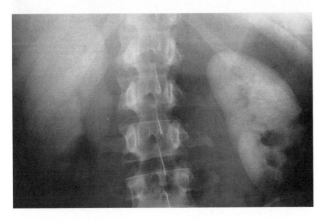

Fig. 7.40 Acute tubular necrosis. This film, taken 9 hours after injection of contrast, shows a dense persistent nephrogram with no opacification of the collecting systems.

Ectopic kidney

During fetal development the kidneys ascend within the abdomen. An ectopic kidney results if this ascent is halted. They are usually in the lower abdomen and rotated so that the pelvis of the kidney points forward. The ureter is short and travels directly to the bladder. Chronic pyelonephritis, hydronephrosis and calculi are all more common in ectopic kidneys, but ectopic kidneys are often incidental findings of no consequence to the patient, except as a cause of diagnostic confusion with other causes of lower abdominal masses.

Horseshoe kidney

The kidneys may fail to separate, giving rise to a horseshoe kidney. Almost invariably it is the lower poles that remain fused (Fig. 7.43).

The anomaly may be an incidental finding and of no significance, but obstruction to the collecting systems and calculi formation are both fairly common.

Congenital cystic disease of the kidneys

There are many varieties of cystic renal disease varying from simple cysts (see p. 239), which may be single or multiple, to complex renal dysplasias. The most frequent complex dysplasia encountered in clinical practice is polycystic disease, a familial disorder which, although congenital in origin, usually presents between the ages of 35 to 55 years with features of hypertension, renal failure or haematuria, or following the discovery of bilaterally enlarged kidneys. The reason for the late presentation is that the cysts are initially small and do not cause trouble for a long time.

At IVU, both kidneys are enlarged and the calices are stretched and distorted (Fig. 7.44a).

The diagnosis can be readily made at CT or ultrasound examination (Figs 7.44b and c) and is recognizable at an early age, even in childhood. The liver and pancreas may also contain cysts and these organs are routinely examined in such patients.

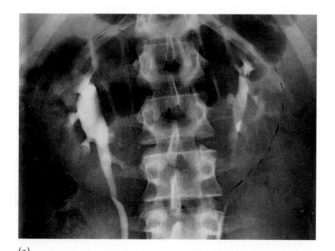

(a)

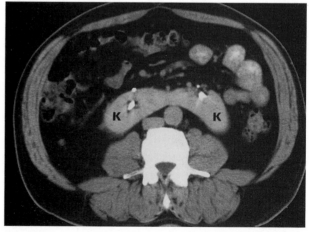

(b)

Fig. 7.43 Horseshoe kidneys. (a) The two kidneys are fused at their lower poles. The striking feature is the alteration in the axis of the kidneys: the lower calices are closer to the spine than the upper calices. The kidneys are rotated so that their pelves point forward and the lower calices point medially. The medial aspects of the lower poles cannot be identified. (b) CT scan of different patient, following i.v. contrast enhancement, showing fusion of the lower poles of the kidneys. K, kidney.

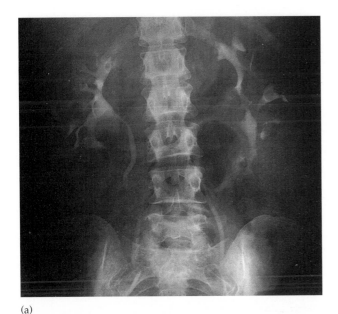

(a)

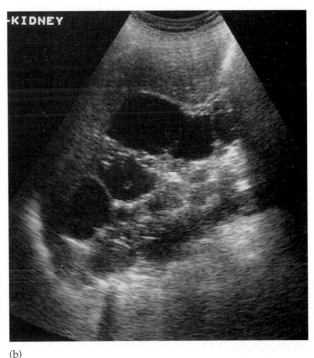

(b)

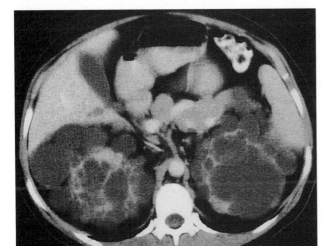

(c)

Fig. 7.44 Advanced polycystic disease in adults. (a) IVU. The kidneys are greatly enlarged and the renal outlines cannot be identified. The pelvicaliceal systems are stretched and deformed by innumerable cysts. (b) Ultrasound of a similar case showing the kidney consists almost entirely of large cysts. The other kidney looked the same. (c) CT scan, taken after intravenous contrast enhancement, of similar case showing that both kidneys are almost entirely replaced by cysts of variable size.

Renal agenesis

In renal agenesis, the opposite kidney, providing it is normal, will show compensatory hypertrophy. Complete absence of blood flow and function on the affected side will be shown on radionuclide studies, and no renal tissue can be identified with ultrasound or CT examination.

Bladder

The bladder is well demonstrated on all imaging modalities. At ultrasound, the simplest routine method of imaging, the bladder lumen should be free of echogenic structures and its wall should be uniformly thick. When the bladder is distended, the wall should be less than 3 mm thick.

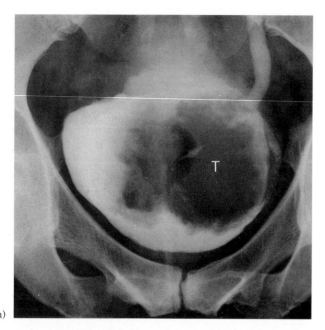

(a)

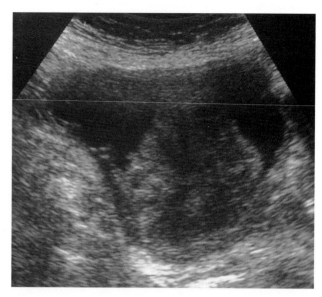

Fig. 7.45 Bladder neoplasm. (a) There is a large filling defect in the left side of the bladder from a transitional cell carcinoma. Note the obstructive dilatation of the left ureter. (b) Ultrasound scan from a different patient showing a large tumour (T) within the bladder.

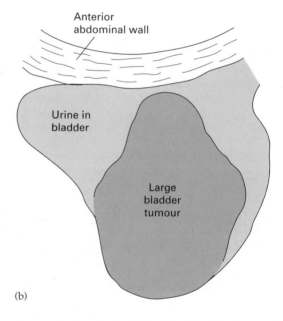

(b)

Bladder tumours

The bladder is the most frequent site for neoplasms in the urinary tract. Almost all are transitional cell carcinomas of varying degrees of malignancy. They vary in shape: some are delicate fronded papillary lesions, some are sessile irregular masses, and others form flat, plaque-like growths that infiltrate widely. At IVU they produce filling defects in the bladder (Fig. 7.45). Gas and faeces in the sigmoid colon or rectum, projected over the bladder outline on IVU, may closely resemble a bladder neoplasm. Usually, it is possible to show on oblique and postmicturition views that bowel contents lie at least partly outside the bladder, whereas the filling defect of a bladder tumour of necessity always lies wholly within the bladder shadow, regardless of projection. On rare occasions, there is visible calcification on the surface of the tumour.

The nature and extent of a tumour in the bladder is best observed at cystoscopy, so the main value of the IVU is to demonstrate ureteric obstruction. Small lesions readily identifiable at cystoscopy may be invisible on IVU.

On ultrasound examination (Fig. 7.45b) bladder tumours are seen as soft tissue masses protruding into the fluid-filled bladder or as localized bladder wall thickening, but the technique is poor for detecting extravesical spread.

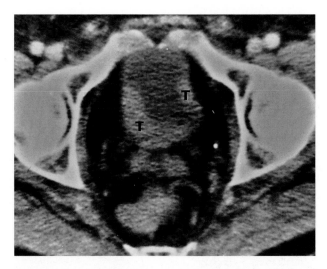

Fig. 7.46 CT scan of carcinoma of bladder, showing an extensive tumour (T) involving the bladder wall but still confined to the bladder.

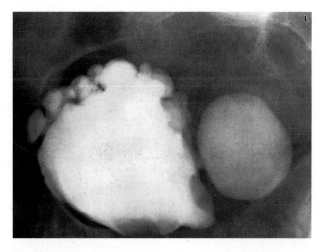

Fig. 7.47 Bladder diverticula. Cystogram showing numerous out-pouchings from the bladder with a very large diverticulum projecting to the left.

On CT and MRI, a tumour of the bladder is seen as a soft tissue mass projecting from the wall. Since the diagnosis is best established by cystoscopy and biopsy, the roles of CT and MRI are to determine the extent of spread of tumour beyond the bladder wall (Fig. 7.46). No imaging technique has adequate accuracy for assessing the depth of invasion within the muscle of the bladder.

Bladder diverticula (Fig. 7.47)

Bladder diverticula may be congenital in origin but are usually the consequence of chronic obstruction to bladder outflow. Because of urinary stasis, diverticula predispose to infection and stone formation and tumours may, on occasion, arise within them. Most diverticula fill at urography and cystography. They are readily demonstrated at ultrasound, CT and MRI. When large, diverticula may deform the adjacent bladder or ureter.

Bladder calcification

The most frequent cause of calcification in the bladder is calculi. Such calculi are frequently large and laminated. Calcification in the wall of the bladder is rare. When seen, it is usually due to schistosomiasis or bladder tumour.

Neurogenic bladder

There are two basic types of neurogenic bladder (attempts to correlate these types with specific neurological lesions have not been satisfactory):
• The large atonic smooth walled bladder with poor or absent contractions and a large residual volume.
• The hypertrophic type, which can be regarded as neurologically induced bladder outflow obstruction. In this condition, the bladder is of small volume, has a very thick, grossly trabeculated wall and shows marked sacculation (Fig. 7.48). The ureters and pelvicaliceal systems may be dilated.

Full assessment of neuropathic bladder dysfunction requires voiding cystourethrography combined with pressure measurements, so-called videourodynamics.

Trauma to the bladder and urethra

Rupture of the bladder may result from a direct blow to the distended bladder or may be part of extensive injury such as occurs with fractures of the pelvis. If the rupture is intraperitoneal, contrast introduced into the bladder will leak out into the peritoneal cavity.

A common site of rupture is at the bladder base, in which

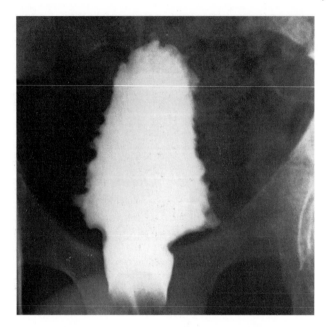

Fig. 7.48 Neurogenic bladder. The outline of the bladder is very irregular due to trabeculation of the bladder wall. The bladder has a small volume with an elongated shape. This appearance has been described as a 'Christmas tree bladder'. There is a balloon catheter in the dilated posterior urethra.

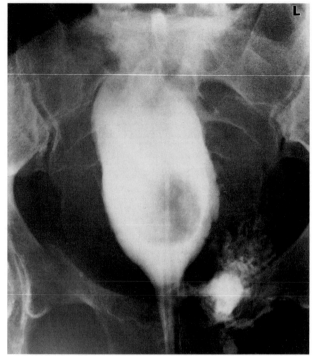

Fig. 7.49 Rupture of the base of the bladder. Cystogram showing extravasation of contrast into the extraperitoneal space on the left, and deformity of the bladder due to surrounding haematoma and urine. There is a fracture of the right pubic bone.

case the bladder shows elevation and compression from extravasated urine and haematoma.

Rupture of the bladder may be revealed sonographically by the presence of a perivesicular fluid collection but the actual site of a tear will not be seen.

Computed tomography may demonstrate fresh haematomas within the pelvis (which are of high density) or urine collections (which are of low density). It also demonstrates the associated fractures, some of which may not be apparent on plain radiographs. Cystography remains the best way of demonstrating the actual site of leakage from the bladder (Fig. 7.49).

Damage to the urethra is a serious complication of pelvic fractures. An ascending urethrogram with a water-soluble contrast medium may show rupture of the urethra with extravasation of contrast into the adjacent tissues.

Prostate and urethra

Prostatic enlargement

Prostatic enlargement is very common in elderly men. It is usually due to benign hypertrophy but may be due to carcinoma. The diagnosis of enlargement is made by digital rectal examination and needle biopsy is undertaken if carcinoma is suspected.

The IVU provides little information about the prostate itself, although an enlarged prostate may be visible as a filling defect in the bladder base (Fig. 7.50).

Prostatic ultrasound uses a transducer designed to be introduced into the rectum. Transrectal ultrasound can show the overall size of the prostate and can diagnose relatively small masses within its substance (Fig. 7.51).

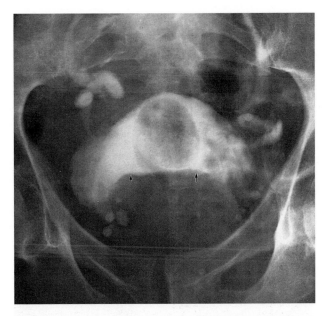

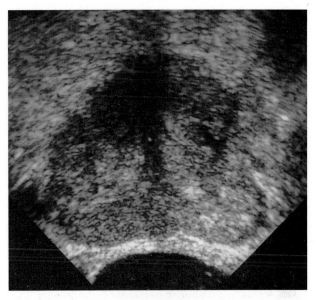

Fig. 7.50 Prostatic enlargement. The bladder base is lifted up and shows an impression from the enlarged prostate (arrows). The ureters are tortuous and enter the bladder horizontally. A balloon catheter is in the bladder.

Unfortunately, ultrasound cannot distinguish benign from malignant disease when confined to the prostate, except on the basis that masses in the peripheral zone are likely to be malignant and those in the central zone are more likely to be benign.

The prostate can be seen quite well at CT, but CT cannot distinguish benign from malignant disease, unless the disease has spread. However, in cases of known prostatic carcinoma, it is helpful in determining the extent of local spread as well as lymph node metastases (Fig. 7.52).

Magnetic resonance imaging is a promising method for imaging the prostate. Carcinoma produces a mass in the peripheral zone of the prostate of different intensity to the adjacent normal tissue. The major role for MRI is in staging the periprostatic extent of tumour and to show invasion of the seminal vesicles (Fig. 7.53). The best quality images are obtained with the use of a coil placed into the rectum adjacent to the prostate.

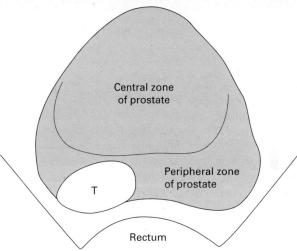

Fig. 7.51 Prostate carcinoma shown by transrectal ultrasound. T, tumour.

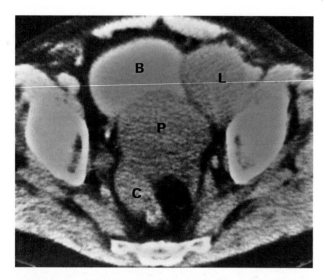

Fig. 7.52 Carcinoma of the prostate. CT scan showing massively enlarged prostate (P) indenting the bladder. The tumour has spread to involve pelvic lymph nodes. A huge lymph node mass is seen (L). B, bladder; C, colon.

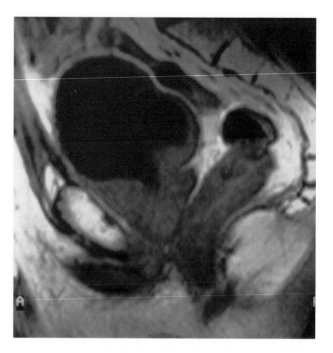

Prostatic calcification

Prostatic calcification is due to numerous prostatic calculi. It is so common that it can be regarded as a normal finding in older men. It shows no correlation with the symptoms of prostatic hypertrophy nor any relation to prostatic carcinoma. It always appears as numerous flecks of calcification of varying size, approximately symmetrical about the midline just beneath the bladder (Fig. 7.54).

Bladder outflow obstruction

The most frequent cause of bladder outflow obstruction is enlargement of the prostate. Other causes include bladder tumours, urethral strictures and, in little boys, posterior urethral valves. As discussed above, patients with neurological deficit may have neurogenic obstruction to bladder emptying. Regardless of the specific cause, the imaging signs of bladder outflow obstruction are:
• increased trabeculation and thickness of the bladder wall, often with diverticula formation;
• residual urine in the bladder after micturition;
• dilatation of the collecting systems.

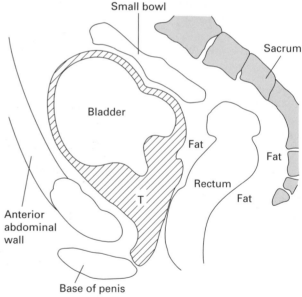

Fig. 7.53 Prostate carcinoma (T) invading lower part of bladder, shown on MRI scan (T1-weighted sagittal section).

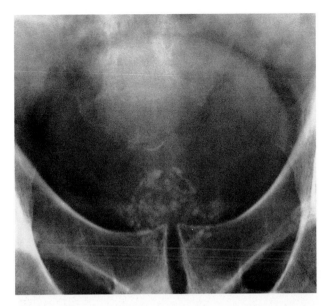

Fig. 7.54 Prostatic calcification. Numerous calculi just above the pubic symphysis are present in the prostate.

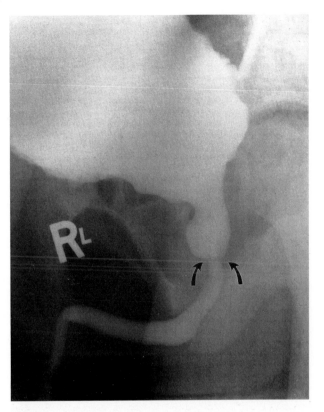

Fig. 7.56 Posterior urethral valves in a 6-year-old boy. On this micturating (voiding) cystogram the site of the valves is arrowed. The presence of the valves is recognized by dilatation of the posterior urethra. Note the irregular outline of the thick-walled bladder due to chronic obstruction.

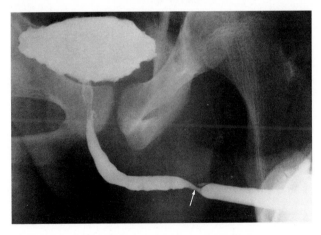

Fig. 7.55 Urethral stricture. An ascending urethrogram showing a stricture in the penile urethra (arrow). The patient had gonorrhoea.

the urethra to external trauma. Such strictures are usually smooth in outline and relatively short. Inflammatory strictures, which are usually gonococcal in origin, may be seen in any portion of the urethra, but are usually found in the anterior urethra. Urethral strictures are imaged by urethrography (see p. 230).

Posterior urethral valves (Fig. 7.56)

Congenital valves may occur in the posterior urethra. They cause significant obstruction and are almost invariably discovered in boys during infancy or childhood. The IVU in such children will show hydronephrosis, hydroureter and a

Urethral stricture (Fig. 7.55)

The majority of urethral strictures are due to previous trauma or infection. Post-traumatic strictures are usually in the proximal penile urethra – the most vulnerable portion of large, poorly emptying bladder. Urethral valves cannot be demonstrated by retrograde urethrography since there is no obstruction to retrograde flow. They are easily demonstrated at micturating cystourethrography where substantial dilatation of the posterior urethra is seen which terminates abruptly in a convex border formed by the valves. The valves are not visible at ultrasound, though the hydronephrosis and thickened bladder wall are readily demonstrated.

Scrotum and testes

The scrotal contents are usually imaged with ultrasound, but radionuclide examination and MRI are occasionally used.

Ultrasound is used to investigate scrotal swelling. The main indications are a suspected testicular tumour (Fig. 7.57a) or abscess. Benign epididymal cysts (Fig. 7.57b) are common and can be readily distinguished from testicular tumours on ultrasound examination.

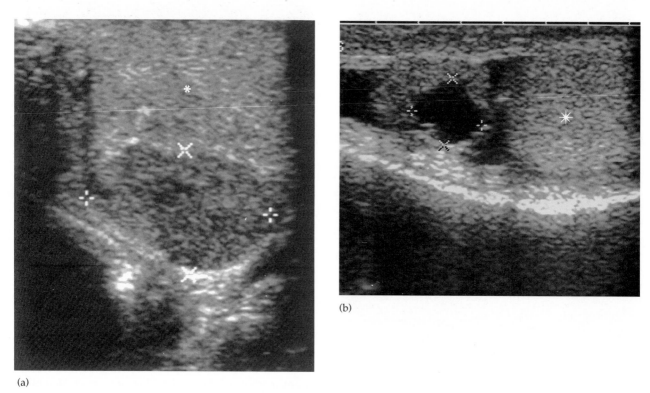

(a)

(b)

Fig. 7.57 Ultrasound of testis. (a) Seminoma (indicated by the crosses) arising within an otherwise normal testis*. (b) Epididymal cyst (indicated by the crosses) at the upper pole of an otherwise normal testis (*).

Doppler ultrasound, or radionuclide imaging, can be used for patients with acute testicular pain and swelling to distinguish between testicular torsion, in which testicular perfusion is dramatically decreased, and acute epididymitis/orchitis in which testicular perfusion is normal or increased.

MRI can produce highly detailed images of the scrotal contents (Fig. 7.58) and is used in those cases where ultrasound does not provide sufficient information.

Ectopic testis in the inguinal canal, the commonest site, can be diagnosed by ultrasound. In those few cases where the ectopic testis lies within the abdomen, MRI is the investigation of choice.

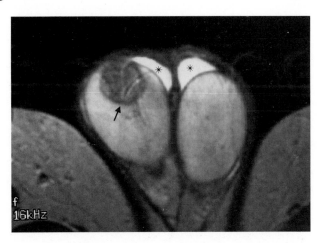

Fig. 7.58 MRI of seminoma (arrow) in right testis. The two testes are well demonstrated. The high signal adjacent to both testes is normal fluid between the layers of the tunica vaginalis(*).

8

Female Genital Tract

Ultrasound, computed tomography (CT) and magnetic resonance imaging (MRI) have important roles to play in gynaecological disease. Because of its ease and ready availability, ultrasound is usually the principal examination. Conventional radiology plays almost no part – the major exception being hysterosalpingography.

Normal appearances

Ultrasound

Ultrasound of the pelvis can be carried out two ways: either by scanning through the abdominal wall or transvaginally with a specialized ultrasound probe inserted directly into the vagina. With the transvaginal route the pelvic organs are nearer the ultrasound probe so image quality is much improved. Moreover it is not necessary for the patient to have a full bladder.

When abdominal scanning is undertaken it is essential for the patient to have a full bladder to act as a 'window' through which the pelvic structures can be seen. Scans are usually made in the longitudinal and transverse planes.

On a midline longitudinal scan the *vagina* can be recognized as a tubular structure, with a central linear echo arising from the opposing vaginal surfaces. The *uterus* lies immediately behind the bladder, and the body of the uterus can be seen to be in continuity with the cervix and vagina. The myometrium shows low level echoes, whereas the endometrial cavity gives a high amplitude linear echo (Fig. 8.1). The precise appearances of the uterus depend on the age and parity of the patient and also on the lie of the uterus. The normal *fallopian tubes* are too small to be visualized sonographically.

The *ovaries* are suspended from the broad ligament and usually lie lateral to the uterus near the side walls of the pelvis (Fig. 8.2). During the child bearing years, the ovaries measure 2.5–5 cm in greatest diameter, but after the menopause, they atrophy. The endocrine changes occurring during the menstrual cycle have a great effect on the appearance of the ovaries. During the early phase, several cystic structures are seen representing developing follicles. Around the eighth day of the cycle, one follicle becomes

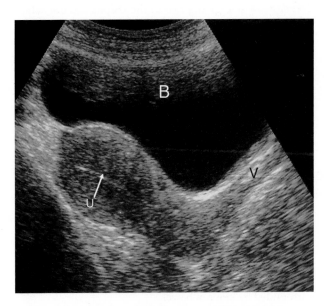

Fig. 8.1 Normal uterus and vagina. Longitudinal section. The central echo of uterus (U) corresponds to the endometrial cavity; the uterus itself has a homogeneous echo texture; V, vagina; B, bladder.

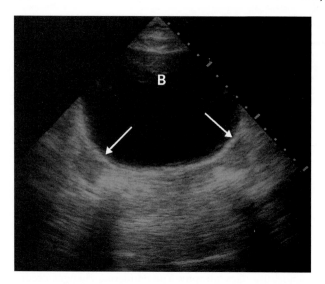

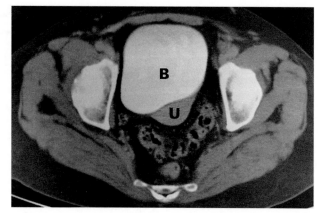

Fig. 8.3 Normal uterus, CT scan. B, bladder; U, uterus.

Fig. 8.2 Normal ovaries (arrows). Transverse section in 25-year-old woman. B, bladder.

dominant and may reach 2–2.5 cm in diameter prior to ovulation. At ovulation, the follicle ruptures and immediately decreases in size giving rise to the corpus luteum which degenerates if there is no intervening pregnancy. By observing these changes it is possible to determine whether an infertile woman is ovulating.

CT

In order to identify the *vagina*, a tampon is usually placed within it. Because of the air trapped in the tampon, it appears black on the CT images. Immediately above the tampon, the *cervix* is seen as a rounded soft tissue structure approximately 3 cm in diameter. The body of the *uterus* (Fig. 8.3) merges with the cervix, its precise appearance depending on the lie of the uterus. The fallopian tubes and broad ligaments are not visible and the ovaries cannot usually be identified. The parametrium is of fat density, the interface with the pelvic musculature being clearly visible. Since the peritoneal cavity extends into the pelvis, the uterus may be surrounded by loops of bowel.

MRI

The pelvic anatomy is very well demonstrated because of the excellent soft tissue contrast afforded by MRI. Images are usually taken in the transverse and sagittal planes but may be supplemented by coronal images, particularly for examining the ovaries. Images in the transverse plane give appearances similar to CT. The sagittal plane shows the vagina and cervix in continuity with the body of the uterus which can be readily recognized on a T2-weighted scan because the endometrium has a high signal (Fig. 8.4). The ovaries and broad ligaments can also be identified.

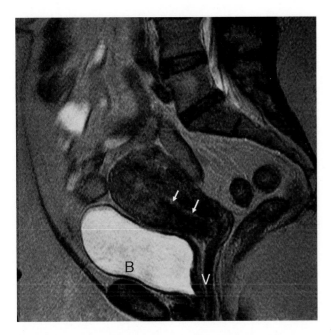

Fig. 8.4 Normal uterus, sagittal T2-weighted MRI scan. There is a high signal from the endometrium (arrows). B, bladder; V, vagina.

Pelvic masses

CT, ultrasound and MRI will be abnormal in virtually any patient in whom a mass can be felt on physical examination. With ultrasound, it is possible to tell whether the mass is cystic or solid. Unfortunately, there is no clear association of cystic with benign disease, or of solid characteristics with malignant disease. A limitation of imaging is that it is sometimes not possible to determine from which organ the mass arises; an ovarian mass which lies in contact with the uterus may appear similar to a mass arising within the uterus and vice versa.

Ovarian masses

Ovarian cysts

Sometimes a follicle or corpus luteum persists as a follicular or corpus luteum cyst, both of which are easily recognized by ultrasound, CT or MRI (Fig. 8.5). Follicular cysts are mostly asymptomatic and regress spontaneously. Corpus luteum cysts are most often seen in the first trimester of pregnancy; they usually resolve, but may rupture or twist. Haemorrhage into both types of cyst may occur and gives a characteristic appearance on MRI.

Ovarian tumours

The commonest ovarian tumours are the cystadenoma and the cystadenocarcinoma. Ovarian tumours can be cystic, solid or a mixture of the two (Fig. 8.6). Those that are cystic may be multilocular. Evidence of invasion of neighbouring structures or metastasis indicates a malignant tumour. Although ultrasound, CT and MRI are reliable at showing the size, consistency and location of an ovarian mass, it is often not possible to say whether the mass is benign or malignant unless there is evidence of local invasion or distant spread. A malignant nature is suggested if the septa are thick and there are coexisting solid nodules within or adjacent to the cyst. With disseminated malignancy, ascites may be visible, but frequently omental and peritoneal metastases are difficult to detect due to their small size. Computed tomography, MRI and ultrasound may show hydronephrosis from ureteric obstruction by the tumour and may also demonstrate enlarged lymph nodes and liver metastases.

Treatment of ovarian carcinoma is usually by hysterectomy, oophorectomy and surgical removal of all macroscopic tumour and staging is carried out during surgery. The main role of imaging is for follow-up to assess response to treatment and disease recurrence.

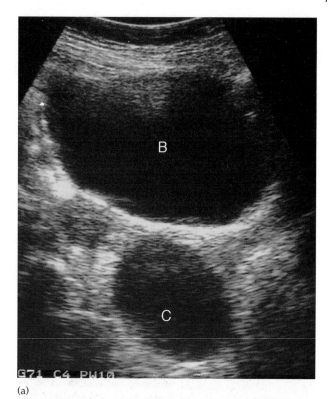

(a)

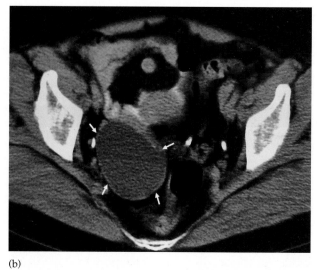

(b)

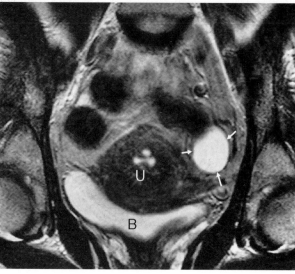

(c)

Fig. 8.5 Ovarian cyst. (a) Longitudinal ultrasound scan to right of midline showing a 5 cm cyst (C) in right ovary with no internal echoes. B, bladder. (b) CT scan of same patient showing the cyst in the right ovary (arrows). Note the uniform water density centre of the cyst. (c) Coronal T2-weighted MRI scan showing a left sided ovarian cyst (arrows) in a patient with an enlarged uterus due to adenomyosis. B, bladder; U, uterus.

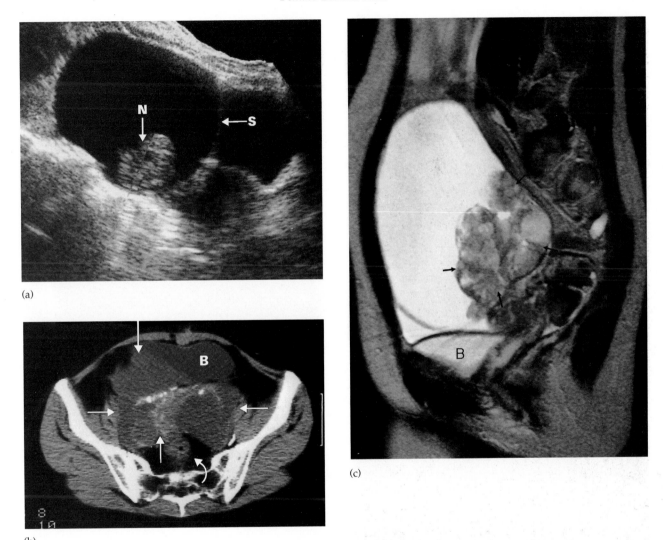

(a)

(b)

(c)

Fig. 8.6 Ovarian carcinoma. (a) Longitudinal ultrasound scan showing a very large multilocular cystic tumour containing septa (S) and solid nodules (N). The lesion was a cystadenocarcinoma. (b) CT scan showing large partly cystic, partly solid ovarian carcinoma (arrows). The tumour, which contains irregular areas of calcification, has invaded the right side of the bladder (B). The rectum is indicated by a curved arrow. (c) MRI scan showing a partly solid (arrows) and partly cystic tumour. The cystic component shows as a high signal on this T2-weighted scan. B, bladder.

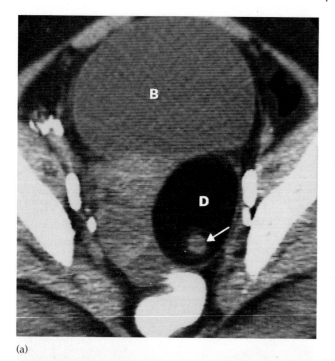

(a)

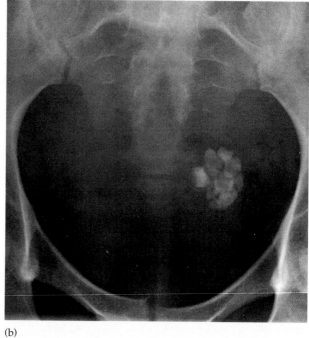

(b)

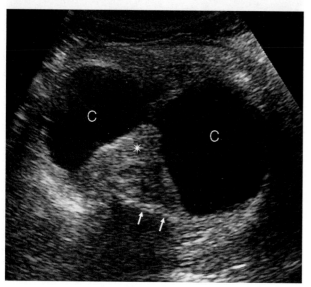

(c)

A dermoid cyst can sometimes be confidently diagnosed because of the fat within it, and it may contain various calcified components, of which teeth are the commonest. The findings can be recognized at ultrasound, CT or MRI and sometimes on plain radiographs (Fig. 8.7). Otherwise, only very large ovarian tumours are recognizable on plain abdominal radiographs as a soft tissue mass, occasionally containing calcium, arising from the pelvis.

Fig. 8.7 Dermoid cyst. (a) CT scan shows oval shaped fat density of a dermoid cyst (D) containing calcified material (arrow). B, bladder. (b) Plain film of another patient showing well-developed teeth within the cyst. (c) Transverse ultrasound scan showing a dermoid consisting of cystic (C) and solid components (∗) with calcification (arrows) owing to teeth within it.

Uterine tumours

Fibroid

Leiomyomas (fibroids) are common in women over 30 years of age. They are often asymptomatic but may cause menorrhagia or present as a palpable mass. When sufficiently large, a fibroid can be seen on a plain film as a mass in the pelvis and may show multiple irregular but well-defined calcifications (see Fig. 4.12, p. 142). Ultrasound and CT both show a spherical or lobular uterine mass. At ultrasound, the mass may be either sonolucent or echogenic, whereas at CT, fibroids are usually the same density as the adjacent myometrium (Fig. 8.8). Magnetic resonance imaging can readily identify fibroids as they have a different signal characteristic from the normal uterus. Degenerating and non-degenerating fibroids can also be distinguished.

Carcinoma of the cervix and body of the uterus (Fig. 8.9)

Neither CT, MRI nor ultrasound play much part in the initial diagnosis of these conditions, which is normally made by physical examination and biopsy or cytology.

Carcinoma of the cervix may be staged by CT or preferably by MRI because the stage determines whether the patient is managed with surgery, radiotherapy or a combination of treatments. In essence the observations to be made are whether the tumour is confined to the cervix or whether it extends into the parametrium, rectum or pelvic side walls. Computed tomography and MRI also enable detection of enlarged lymph nodes and dilatation of the ureters in cases where the tumour has caused ureteric obstruction.

Endometrial carcinoma is usually treated by surgical removal of the uterus, ovaries and pelvic lymph nodes. Therefore the use of imaging to stage the tumour at presentation is limited. Magnetic resonance imaging can predict the depth of myometrial invasion by tumour, and both CT and MRI can demonstrate lymph node involvement.

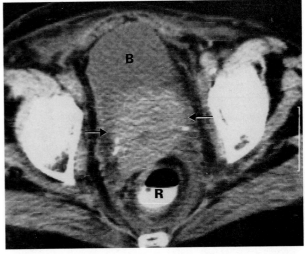

(a)

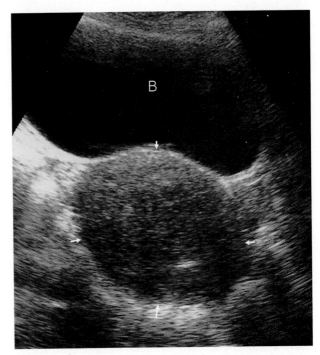

(b)

Fig. 8.8 Uterine tumour. (a) CT scan showing enlarged uterus (arrows) which was due to fibroids. It is not possible to distinguish this appearance from adenocarcinoma confined to the uterus. B, bladder; R, rectum. (b) Transverse ultrasound scan showing a large fibroid in the uterus. Its extent is indicated by the arrows. B, bladder.

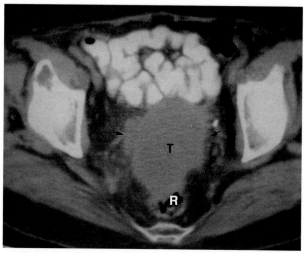

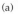

(a)

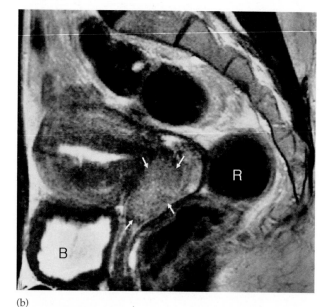

(b)

Fig. 8.9 Carcinoma of cervix. (a) CT scan showing a large tumour of the cervix (T) invading the parametrium (arrows) and extending into the rectum (R) posteriorly. (b) Sagittal MRI scan showing a tumour confined to the cervix (arrows). B, bladder; R, rectum.

Pelvic inflammatory disease

Pelvic inflammatory disease may be due to venereal infection, commonly gonorrhoea, which in the acute stages gives rise to a tubo-ovarian abscess. Pelvic inflammation and abscess formation may also occur following pelvic surgery, childbirth or abortion and may be seen in association with intrauterine contraceptive devices, appendicitis or diverticular disease. The usual imaging technique is ultrasound. Irrespective of the cause of the infection, ultrasound will show a hypoechoic or complex mass in the adnexal region or pouch of Douglas (cul-de-sac) (Fig. 8.10). Blockage of the fallopian tubes may cause a hydrosalpinx which can be recognized as a hypoechoic adnexal mass, which is often tubular in shape.

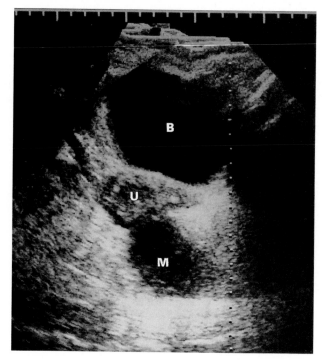

Fig. 8.10 Pelvic abscess. Transverse ultrasound scan showing a hypoechoic mass (M) behind the uterus (U). B, bladder.

The appearance of pelvic inflammatory disease may be indistinguishable from endometriosis and ectopic pregnancy (p. 283), conditions which both occur in women of reproductive years.

Endometriosis

In endometriosis, there is endometrial tissue outside the uterus, most commonly confined to the pelvis. At ultrasound, endometriosis is usually seen as a cystic or hypoechoic mass in the adnexal region and/or pouch of Douglas corresponding to the chocolate cysts found on pathological examination. Because of the recurrent haemorrhage in these endometriomas they often have a characteristic appearance on MRI (Fig. 8.11). If the endometriosis has bled into the peritoneal cavity, as it commonly does at the time of menstruation, fluid may be detectable in the pouch of Douglas.

Detection of intrauterine contraceptive devices

The lost intrauterine contraceptive device (IUCD) is a common problem and ultrasound should be the first investigation. Different devices have characteristic appearances. They are seen as highly reflective structures and their relationship to the uterine cavity can be determined (Fig. 8.12). If the IUCD cannot be located in the pelvis, then a plain film of the abdomen should be taken in case the device has migrated through the uterus. If there is a coexisting pregnancy, it becomes very difficult to locate the IUCD by ultrasound after the first trimester.

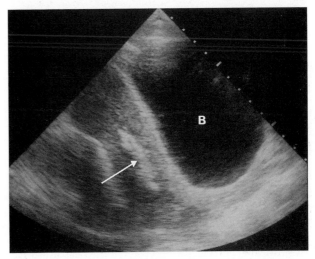

Fig. 8.12 Intrauterine contraceptive device (arrow) seen as reflective echoes within the uterine cavity, shown on a longitudinal ultrasound scan. B, bladder.

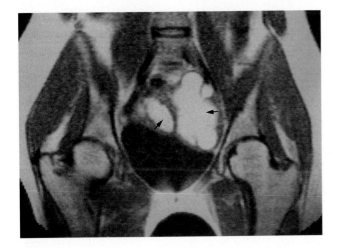

Fig. 8.11 Endometriosis. Coronal MRI showing haemorrhagic cysts in the pelvis (arrows) which give a high signal on this T1-weighted sequence.

Hysterosalpingography

Hysterosalpingography is performed in selected cases in the investigation of infertility in order to assess the patency of the fallopian tubes. A catheter with a seal to prevent leakage from the external cervical os is inserted into the uterus. Sufficient contrast is then injected under fluoroscopic control to fill the uterus and fallopian tubes (Fig. 8.13). If the fallopian tubes are patent, there is free spill into the peritoneum, recognized by the demonstration of contrast between loops of bowel. Congenital variations in uterine morphology which may prevent maintenance of pregnancy can also be assessed.

Ultrasound hysterosalpingography may be performed to detect tubal patency. This technique, which avoids the use of ionizing radiation, involves injecting an ultrasound contrast agent into the uterus through a catheter and following the passage of contrast through the fallopian tubes with ultrasound.

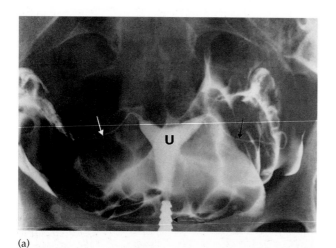
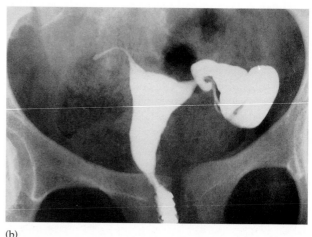

(a)   (b)

Fig. 8.13 Hysterosalpingogram. (a) Normal. Contrast has been injected to fill the uterus (U) and both fallopian tubes (vertical arrows). Free spill into the peritoneum has occurred to outline loops of bowel. Note the cannula in the cervical canal (horizontal arrow). (b) Hydrosalpinx. Both fallopian tubes are obstructed and dilated, the left one massively. There is no spill of contrast into the peritoneum.

9

Obstetrics

Ultrasound of the pregnant patient is simple to perform and has proved reliable in examining the fetus and in detecting the complications of pregnancy. Unlike x-ray examination (see p. 14 for discussion of radiation hazards) no biological damage has yet been attributed to ultrasound examination as currently used in obstetric practice. No fetal abnormalities have been attributable to ultrasound during pregnancy over more than three decades that the technique has been in use.

The developing fetus

Ultrasound in the first trimester

Ultrasound examination during early pregnancy may be undertaken using a probe placed on the abdomen. The patient should have a full bladder that will lift the small bowel out of the pelvis and act as a window to provide better visualization of the uterus. Alternatively, transvaginal scanning may be carried out, which produces superior images and does not need a full bladder.

The normal gestational sac is seen as a small cystic structure lying within the uterus. It first appears at the fifth week of amenorrhoea*. By the sixth week, internal echoes representing the developing fetus are seen within the gestational sac and by the seventh week movement of the fetal heart should be visible (Fig. 9.1). In the early stages, the volume of the gestational sac can be used to estimate gestational development. Later, as fetal echoes become visible, the pregnancy can be dated by measuring the crown rump length (Fig. 9.2),

*In this book the gestational age is always expressed as weeks from the last menstrual period.

i.e. the longest demonstrable length of the fetus within the gestational sac. This length is a highly reliable method of dating from the seventh to twelfth weeks of pregnancy. Multiple pregnancies can be recognized by the presence of two or more gestation sacs.

Ultrasound in the second and third trimesters

After the first trimester, fetal maturity can be assessed by measuring both the biparietal diameter and the femur length, both of which can be precisely defined. The apposi-

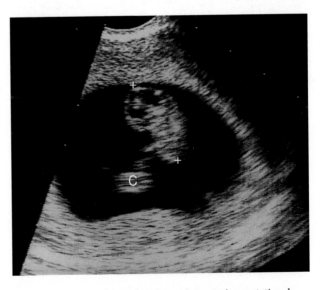

Fig. 9.1 Transvaginal scan showing an intrauterine gestational sac containing an 8-week-old fetus. Small crosses indicate the crown–rump length (15 mm). C, part of umbilical cord.

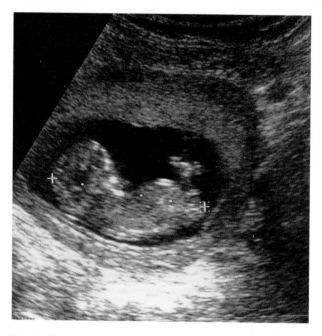

Fig. 9.2 Eleven-week-old fetus. Crown–rump length is indicated by the crosses. The fetus is seen in sagittal section and the head is clearly visible on the left and body to the right.

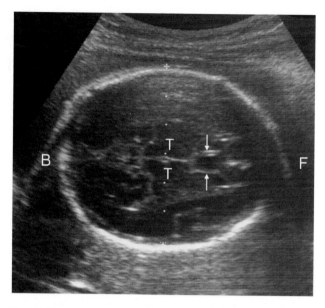

Fig. 9.3 Biparietal diameter in an 18-week-old fetus. The midline echo is interrupted by the box-like cavum septum pellucidum (arrows). The crosses indicate measurement points for the biparietal diameter. B, back; F, front; T, thalamus.

tion of the two cerebral hemispheres adjacent to the falx gives a well-defined midline echo. A small 'box like' structure, the cavum septum pellucidum, interrupts the midline echo one-third of the way between the sinciput and occiput (Fig. 9.3). This structure identifies the position, at the level of the thalami, where the biparietal diameter should be measured. By comparing the measurements with a standard growth chart an estimate of gestational age can be obtained. The chart for the biparietal diameter (Fig. 9.4) shows that there is a greater deviation from the mean in late pregnancy than in the early stages, which means that accurate dating based on the biparietal diameter must be carried out before 24–26 weeks. The ventricles can be measured at the same time as the biparietal diameter, to exclude hydrocephalus (Fig. 9.5). An estimate of fetal maturity can also be obtained by measuring the femur length; the ultrasound beam is directed down the long axis of the femur, this length then compared with a standard growth chart.

At 18–20 weeks gestation the fetus is well formed and this is an appropriate time to obtain an accurate biparietal dia-

meter to estimate fetal maturity. Also, 18–20 weeks is a suitable time to examine the fetus for fetal abnormalities, so enabling a therapeutic abortion to be performed if a lethal abnormality is seen. Accurate dating is very helpful if problems arise in late pregnancy, as the obstetrician then knows the maturity of the fetus should induction or caesarian section become necessary.

Obtaining serial biparietal diameters and comparing them with growth curves permits observation of fetal growth. However, growth retardation may be first manifested by lack of growth of the fetal body. To detect this, the abdominal circumference is measured at the level of the umbilical vein, as it passes through the liver (see Fig. 9.13, p. 278).

Identification of the sex of the fetus is frequently possible. Though parents often like to know the sex, its medical importance is confined to those situations where there is a risk of sex-linked inherited disease. Sexual differentiation is most reliable in the third trimester, when the penis and scrotum can usually be defined.

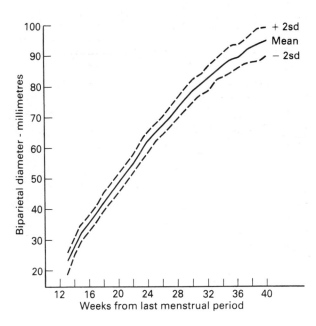

Fig. 9.4 Growth chart of biparietal diameter against gestational age, showing the mean and two standard deviations from the mean.

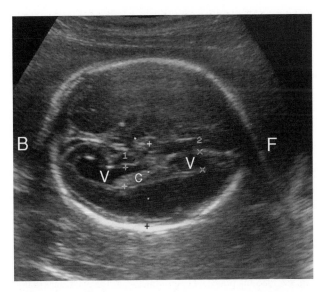

Fig. 9.5 Ventricular measurements. Transverse section through the fetal head in a 20-week-old fetus. The two sets of crosses labelled 1 and 2 measure the width of the lateral ventricle (V). The width should be less than one-third of the distance between the midline and the internal surface of the skull (crosses). The lateral ventricles normally measure less than 10 mm in width. B, back; C, choroid plexus; F, front.

The placenta

The placenta is easily evaluated sonographically. By the ninth week, it is seen as a well-defined intrauterine structure lining the inner wall of a portion of the uterine cavity. The surface of the placenta, the chorionic plate, may be recognized as a thin line of bright echoes (Fig. 9.6). As the placenta matures it undergoes successive changes in texture but these changes are not thought to be of clinical significance.

Haemorrhage from placenta praevia, the condition in which the placenta encroaches on the lower uterine segment, is a common cause of bleeding in the third trimester, occurring in about 0.5% of pregnancies. Sonography permits accurate delineation of the placental position and its relationship to the presenting part of the fetus (Fig. 9.7). Although the internal cervical os cannot always be identified as such, the position of the cervix can usually be inferred from the position of other structures.

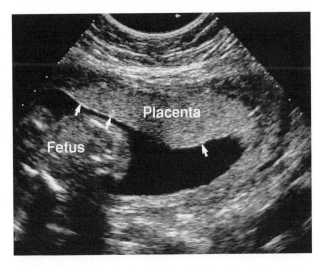

Fig. 9.6 Placenta seen on a longitudinal scan at 18 weeks gestation. The chorionic plate is seen as a thin line of bright echoes (arrows).

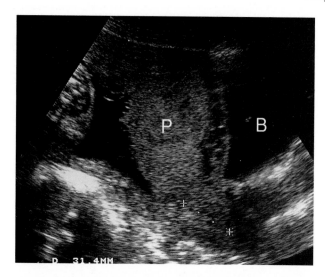

Fig. 9.7 Placenta praevia. Longitudinal scan. The placenta is in the lower uterine segment and covers the position of the internal cervical os. The crosses outline the position of the cervical canal. B, bladder; P, placenta.

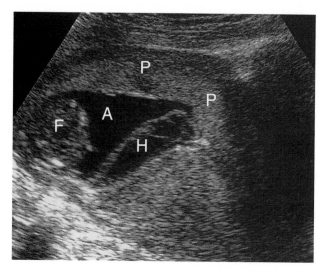

Fig. 9.8 Retromembranous haemorrhage. Longitudinal scan in a 14-week-old pregnancy. There is separation of the membranes by haemorrhage (H). A, amniotic fluid; F, fetus; P, placenta.

During the second trimester, a third to a half of all placentas are low lying, thus raising the question of placenta praevia. However, when followed through to term the vast majority of these do not turn out to be true placenta previa. This is because of the differential growth rate of the uterus during pregnancy; the lower uterine segment grows more than the rest of the uterus and, therefore, as pregnancy progresses, placental tissue is carried towards the fundus and away from the cervical os. Consequently, the diagnosis of a marginal placenta praevia before the 36th week should always be confirmed with a repeat scan before delivery.

Abruptio placentae (accidental haemorrhage) occurs in approximately 1–2% of pregnancies. The majority of cases present with vaginal bleeding, but some are concealed. Ultrasound can be of help in making this diagnosis, if a collection of blood is seen separating the amniotic membranes from the uterine surface. However, frequently there is no such collection, as the blood has drained into the amniotic cavity or out through the vagina. Retromembranous haemorrhage under the chorionic membrane may be seen particularly in early pregnancy (Fig. 9.8). The haemorrhage is usually resorbed within a few weeks.

'Large for dates' uterus

A common problem in obstetric care is the patient whose uterus is larger than expected. Often the cause is a false estimate of the gestational age, usually due to a mistake in calculating the date of conception. With the use of the methods outlined earlier in this chapter, it is possible to determine the fetal age with great accuracy.

The most common causes for a uterus larger than expected for true gestational age include:
• multiparity;
• trophoblastic disease;
• associated ovarian or uterine tumours, either of which may be mistaken for generalized enlargement of the uterus;
• polyhydramnios.

Multiparity is readily diagnosed by sonography (Fig. 9.9). More than one gestational sac is seen early on. Later, two or more fetal heads and bodies can be identified and the biparietal diameters can be measured. Ultrasound is helpful in detecting any fetal abnormalities, which are more frequent in multiple pregnancies. Because of the risks associated with multiple pregnancies, fetal growth is subsequently monitored throughout pregnancy.

Trophoblastic disease is a spectrum of pathology ranging

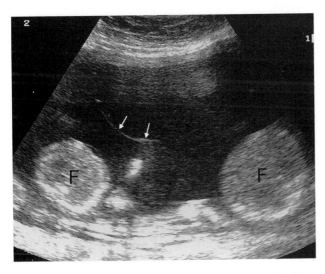

Fig. 9.9 Twin pregnancy. Two fetuses (F) are seen and in addition there is increased liquor volume. Part of the amniotic membrane separating the pregnancies is seen (arrows).

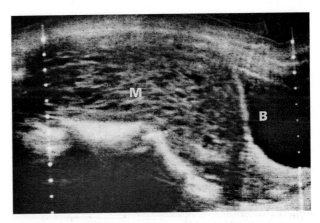

Fig. 9.10 Hydatidiform mole. Longitudinal scan showing multiple irregular vesicular structures within an enlarged uterus. M, mole; B, bladder.

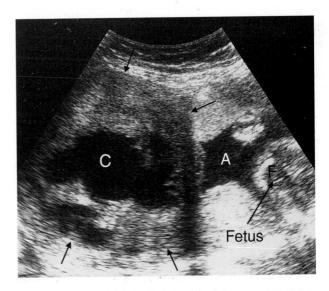

Fig. 9.11 Transverse section through a 16-week pregnancy showing cystic degeneration (C) within a large fibroid (arrows). A, amniotic fluid.

from the relatively benign hydatidiform mole to the malignant choriocarcinoma. The enlarged uterus is filled with multiple vesicular (cystic) structures within a background of echoes of varying densities (Fig. 9.10). In most cases no fetal parts will be identified, but very rarely trophoblastic disease may coexist with a living pregnancy. Although it is occasionally possible to identify invasion of the myometrium by malignant trophoblastic disease, benign and malignant forms are in general indistinguishable on ultrasound examination. In about a third of cases multilocular ovarian cysts, called theca lutein cysts, may be identified. They are caused by the high output of FSH by the disordered pregnancy.

Uterine tumours are present in about 1% of pregnant patients, the most common variety being leiomyoma (fibroid) which can increase in size under the hormonal influences of pregnancy. Usually they arise in the body or fundus but, when situated low in the uterus, they can obstruct labour. Occasionally, fibroids undergo cystic degeneration during pregnancy (Fig. 9.11).

Ovarian tumours may be confused clinically with uterine enlargement. Those associated with pregnancy are usually corpus luteum cysts. At ultrasound they are seen as simple cysts adjacent to, but separate from, the gravid uterus; they frequently involute as the pregnancy progresses.

Polyhydramnios is defined as twice the volume of amniotic fluid expected for the period of gestation. Although mathematical formulae exist, in practice a visual estimate is

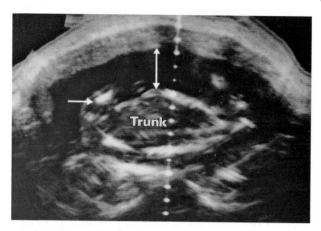

Fig. 9.12 Polyhydramnios. Transverse section showing a large echo-free space (arrowed) due to fluid anterior to the fetal trunk. This 22 week fetus was anencephalic. The horizontal arrow points to the skull base – no cranial vault was present.

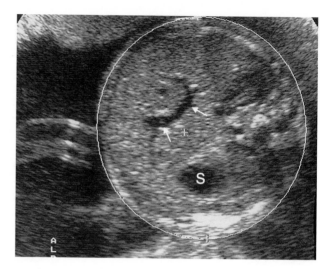

Fig. 9.13 Abdominal circumference. Transverse section through the fetal trunk at the level of the umbilical portion of the portal vein (arrows) and the fetal stomach (S). When two calipers are placed across the fetal abdomen, the ultrasound machine produces a circle around the fetal abdomen and gives a measurement of the abdominal circumference.

usually made (Fig. 9.12). Polyhydramnios is associated with maternal abnormalities such as diabetes and with a number of fetal conditions. The fetal abnormalities include neural tube defects, in which the hydramnios is probably due to excessive production of cerebrospinal fluid, and obstruction of the alimentary tract, e.g. oesophageal or duodenal atresia, where the hydramnios is due to an impaired circulation of swallowed amniotic fluid. Polyhydramnios also occurs with normal multiple pregnancies.

'Small for dates' uterus: intrauterine growth retardation

An important cause for a fetus that is small for dates is intrauterine growth retardation, which carries a greatly increased risk of perinatal death and will alter obstetrical management. However, it is important not to misdiagnose a fetus as being small for dates because of an error in calculating the age from the menstrual history: hence the need for accurate dating early in pregnancy.

Growth retardation can be divided into two groups. Symmetrical growth retardation affects the head and body equally and is associated with congenital abnormalities and intrauterine infections. Asymmetrical growth retardation affects growth of the fetal body (Fig. 9.13) before that of the fetal brain. Therefore, measurements of the biparietal diameter may not detect any abnormality early on. Asymmetri-

cal growth retardation occurs in the third trimester and is associated with placental insufficiency, either primary disease of the placenta, or is due to maternal causes such as hypertension or diabetes. Standards are available for biparietal diameter and abdominal circumference in order that fetal growth may be assessed. In some centres, scans are performed routinely around 32 weeks in order to diagnose intrauterine growth retardation.

Fetal monitoring

In those fetuses with intrauterine growth retardation or at risk from any cause, ultrasound can be used to assess fetal well-being and may influence the decision to effect early delivery of the baby.

Doppler ultrasound of the umbilical artery enables the blood flow in the placental circulation to be studied. In normal pregnancy, placental resistance is low and a large proportion of the fetal cardiac output flows through the placenta. There is, therefore, a high diastolic flow shown by the flow velocity waveform in the umbilical artery. In conditions such as intrauterine growth retardation and maternal hypertension, the placental resistance increases so the diastolic flow in the umbilical artery is reduced or in extreme cases may be absent (Fig. 9.14).

Fetal abnormalities

It is important to recognize fetal abnormalities as early as possible during the pregnancy so that the appropriate management can be instituted. The commonest abnormalities detected by ultrasound are neural tube defects, particularly spina bifida and anencephaly. Both should be identified by 18 weeks, at a time when therapeutic abortion is still an option. These conditions are associated with elevated serum and amniotic alpha fetoprotein levels.

Many of the anomalies which result in structural defor-mity of the fetus can be detected *in utero* during the second trimester. An indication of fetal abnormality is polyhydramnios, since polyhydramnios is due to fetal anomaly in 20% of cases.

Head

The two common cranial anomalies that can be identified are hydrocephalus and anencephaly.

The lateral ventricles are easily visualized from 16 weeks onwards. The walls of the ventricles are seen as white lines. Abnormal dilatation of the lateral ventricles precedes excessive enlargement of the calvarium in most cases. Hydrocephalus is diagnosed sonographically when the distance between the lateral walls of the lateral ventricles are greater than 50% of the biparietal diameter. Hydrocephalus frequently accompanies spina bifida.

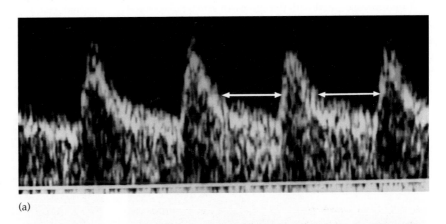

(a)

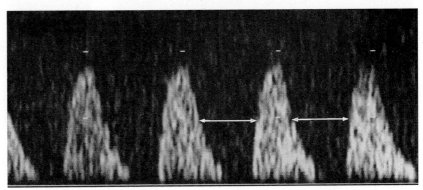

(b)

Fig. 9.14 Doppler flow velocity waveform of the umbilical artery. The peaks represent systolic flow. The arrows indicate the period of the diastolic flow. (a) Normal – note the flow during diastole. (b) Abnormal – there is an absence of flow during diastole in this fetus at risk because of maternal hypertension.

The echogenic choroid plexuses occupy the posterior parts of the lateral ventricles. Cysts within the choroid plexuses are a fairly common finding but these cysts are usually of no significance.

Anencephaly may be diagnosed after the 12th week by the absence of a visible skull vault. Echoes from the skull base and face may be seen, however. The fetal body is usually well formed and moves actively.

Spine

Spina bifida is due to incomplete closure of the neural tube. It is recognized at ultrasound as an absence or a widening of the paired echoes that represent the normal fetal spine (Fig. 9.15). Severe cases are associated with meningocele or meningomyelocele, which are recognized as a sac arising from the back at the level of the widened canal. Limb motion may be absent, but even if the limbs are moving, there may be significant neurological impairment.

Tumours associated with the spine can also be diagnosed *in utero*. The most common of these is the sacral teratoma (Fig. 9.16). They may be solid, cystic or complex and may contain calcifications.

Chest

The size and configuration of the chest may aid in the diagnosis of syndromes associated with pulmonary hypoplasia. Congenital diaphragmatic hernia is the commonest abnormality and in this condition the stomach and intestines herniate into the chest and compress the lungs.

The heart is readily seen and it is possible to diagnose some serious causes of congenital heart disease. Because the four-chamber view is the most reliable view in such situations, diagnosis of the hypoplastic left heart syndrome, single ventricle and Fallot's tetralogy may be made. More complex abnormalities may be inferred but cannot be diagnosed with confidence.

Gastrointestinal tract

The commonest congenital anomalies of the gastrointestinal tract to be diagnosed *in utero* are duodenal atresia, omphalocele and gastroschisis. Oesophageal atresia may be associated with polyhydramnios but cannot be directly demonstrated.

In duodenal atresia, two round cystic structures are seen

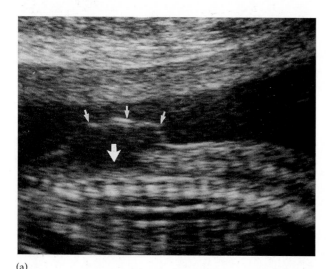

(a)

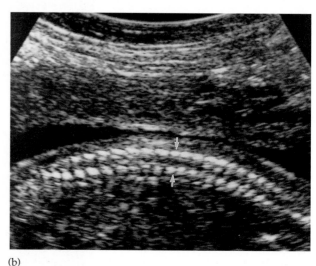

(b)

Fig. 9.15 Spina bifida. (a) There is a defect in the lumbar spine (large arrow) with a mass projecting from the baby's back representing a meningomyelocele (small arrows). (b) Normal for comparison showing the parallel paired echoes (arrows) of the normal thoracic and lumbar spine.

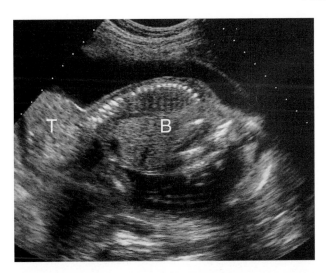

Fig. 9.16 Sacrococcygeal teratoma. A longitudinal scan through the fetus showing the body (B) and sacral tumour (T) arising from the sacrum. The head is out of the plane of the scan.

representing the distended stomach and duodenum (Fig. 9.17).

Omphalocele and gastroschisis are diagnosed by the presence of loops of bowel or liver outside the abdominal cavity (Fig. 9.18).

Urinary tract

The kidneys contribute significantly to the amniotic fluid volume. The presence of profound oligohydramnios, although most frequently due to premature rupture of the membranes, should raise the possibility of a renal abnormality. The normal kidneys are seen as circles of diminished echoreflectivity on either side of the fetal spine. The kidneys may fail to develop at all (agenesis) or be severely dysplastic. At times, even if normal, it may be difficult to visualize the kidneys. Therefore, an attempt is made to find the fetal bladder, since the presence of urine in the

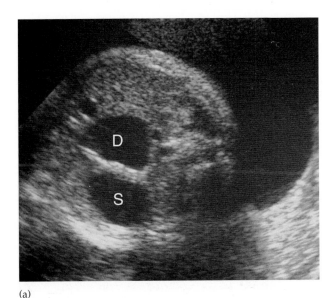

(a)

Fig. 9.17 Duodenal atresia. (a) Transverse section through the fetal abdomen showing a dilated fluid filled stomach (S) and duodenum (D) – 'the double bubble sign'. (b) Plain abdominal film after birth showing dilated air-filled stomach and duodenum with no gas in the rest of the bowel.

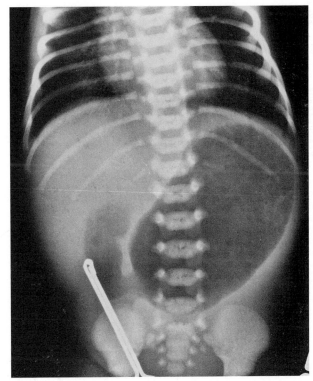

(b)

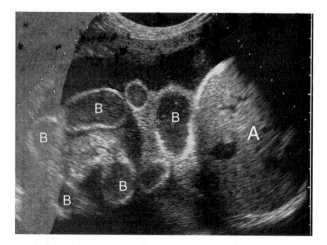

Fig. 9.18 Gastroschisis. Transverse section through the fetal trunk showing fluid-filled loops of bowel (B) outside the fetal abdomen (A) floating in the amniotic fluid.

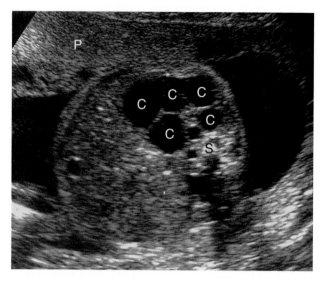

Fig. 9.19 Multicystic kidney. Transverse section through the fetal abdomen showing multiple cysts (C) in the right kidney. P, placenta; S, spine.

bladder indicates functioning renal tissue. However, note that the bladder may be empty at any given moment from fetal voiding.

The commonest identifiable abnormalities are hydronephrosis and the dysplastic condition, multicystic kidney (Fig. 9.19). They are difficult to distinguish from each other with ultrasound. Both are usually unilateral conditions showing multiple fluid-filled rounded spaces within the kidney. If the opposite kidney is normal, as is often the case, the liquor volume is normal.

Chronic bladder outlet obstruction, the usual cause of which is posterior urethral valves, can lead to bilateral hydronephrosis and hydroureters and a massively dilated thick-walled bladder (Fig. 9.20).

Skeleton

Skeletal anomalies giving rise to dwarfism can be recognized by the presence of short limbs. The lethal forms are usually associated with polyhydramnios.

Ultrasound for karyotyping

There are three main techniques for fetal karyotyping, which all require ultrasound to guide the needle to the required position:

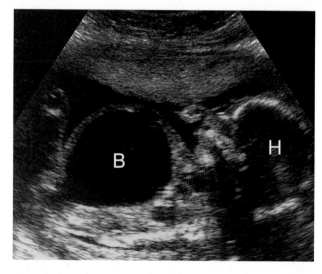

Fig. 9.20 Bladder outlet obstruction. Longitudinal scan through an 18-week-old fetus showing massive dilatation of the fetal bladder (B). H, head.

- Chorion villus sampling is usually carried but between 8 and 12 weeks gestation and involves taking a sample of placental tissue.
- Amniocentesis is usually carried out at 16 weeks gestation and involves passing a needle through the maternal abdominal wall in order to withdraw a sample of amniotic fluid. In addition to analysis for chromosome abnormalites, the alpha fetoprotein level in the amniotic fluid may be measured.
- Cordocentesis involves puncturing the umbilical vein to obtain a sample of fetal blood.

Amniocentesis is the simplest technique but it may take up to two weeks for karyotyping. With chorion villus sampling or cordocentesis the results may be available within two to three days.

Fetal death

With ultrasound it is possible to see the heart beating and observe fetal movement from the seventh week of pregnancy onward. Failure to observe these phenomena suggests fetal death, but in the early stages of pregnancy one must be careful that the gestational age has been calculated correctly. It is, therefore, important to repeat the scan after a

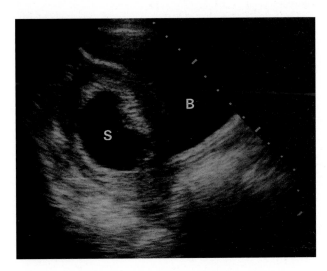

Fig. 9.21 Blighted ovum. Longitudinal scan. Nine weeks amenorrhoea, showing a gestational sac (S) with no fetal parts within it. B, bladder.

suitable interval, if there is any doubt. After the ninth week, fetal death can be readily diagnosed by the absence of a visible heart beat.

A blighted ovum is diagnosed if the size of the gestational sac is greater than 3 cm in diameter but no fetal structures are seen within it (Fig. 9.21). In a twin pregnancy there may be two gestational sacs, one of which contains a live fetus and the other one being anembryonic. So long as the patient is not bleeding at the time of examination, there is a good possibility that the empty sac will resolve and a normal baby will be delivered at term.

Ectopic pregnancy

Ectopic pregnancy generally presents with sudden pain due to rupture of the ectopically placed gestational sac. The ruptured ectopic pregnancy itself is not always visible. When seen sonographically, it is identified as an adnexal mass having both solid and cystic characteristics and occasionally a fetus can be seen within it (Fig. 9.22). There should be no intrauterine pregnancy. Free fluid may be seen in the pouch of Douglas (cul de sac) from haemorrhage. These signs, by themselves, are not enough to make the diagnosis of ectopic gestation, since pelvic inflammatory disease, rupture of adnexal cysts and various neoplasms can appear identical.

In clinical practice, if the pregnancy test is positive and no intrauterine gestation can be identified, the obstetrician may assume that there is an ectopic pregnancy.

Puerperium

Retained products of conception can readily be detected sonographically as echoes within the uterine cavity.

Abdominal problems in pregnancy

The safety of ultrasound enables certain maternal abnormalities, which may coexist with pregnancy, to be examined so avoiding the dangers of radiation to the fetus. Diseases of the biliary tract and urinary tract, in particular, may be readily diagnosed and Doppler ultrasound can be used for suspected venous thrombosis.

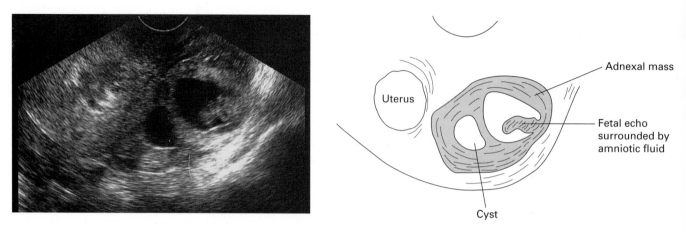

Fig. 9.22 Ectopic pregnancy. Transvaginal scan in the transverse plane in a patient whose pregnancy test was positive. The uterus is seen containing no gestational sac and there is a predominantly cystic adnexal mass containing a fetal echo surrounded by amniotic fluid.

Pelvimetry

Pelvimetry is a method used to determine the relative pelvic and fetal head dimensions. An erect lateral radiograph is taken from which anteroposterior measurements of the pelvic inlet and outlet can be made. In some centres, a supine AP film is added so that the transverse pelvic diameters can be calculated. These diameters are of limited use because the measurements are made from bone surface to bone surface. This does not take into account the thickness of soft tissues which may be very important in determining the effective diameter available to the fetus during delivery.

10

Peritoneal Cavity and Retroperitoneum

Peritoneal cavity

Ascites

Ultrasound, CT and MRI can demonstrate very small amounts of ascites, far less than the amount needed for clinical or plain film detection, but no imaging technique can reliably distinguish the nature of the fluid, e.g. pus or ascitic fluid.

Peritoneal fluid, when free to move, collects in a predictable manner. With the patient supine, the fluid tends to fall to the most dependent portions of the peritoneal cavity, namely in the pelvis anterior to the upper rectum (known as the pouch of Douglas in females), in the space anterior to the right kidney (known as Morrison's pouch), and in the paracolic gutters. If larger amounts of fluid are present, fluid will be seen throughout the peritoneal cavity and stomach, or loops of bowel may be seen floating in the ascites.

At CT (Fig. 10.1) ascites is of lower density than the liver, spleen and kidney and these organs stand out clearly compared to the adjacent fluid.

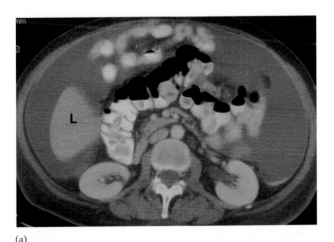

(a)

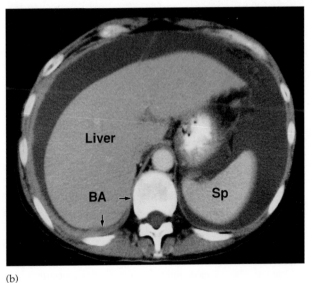

(b)

Fig. 10.1 CT scan of ascites. (a) At the level of the kidneys. The fluid is seen surrounding the lower portion of the liver (L) and the bowel loops. (b) At the level of the liver and spleen (Sp). Note that the ascites cannot collect posteromedial to the right lobe of the liver because of the peritoneal reflections of the bare area (BA).

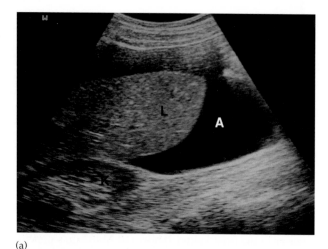

(a)

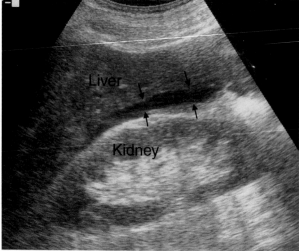

(b)

Fig. 10.2 Ultrasound of ascites. (a) The ascites (A) appears as a transonic area. The liver is clearly seen surrounded by the ascitic fluid. K, right kidney; L, liver. (b) Only a very small amount of ascites is present in this patient. The ascites (arrows) is lying between the liver and kidney in Morrison's pouch.

One of the easiest sites in which to recognize ascites is adjacent to the liver. A uniform band of low density is readily identified between the liver and the diaphragm or abdominal wall. It is worth noting that ascites

cannot collect posterior to the upper liver because of the peritoneal reflection forming the so-called bare area (Fig. 10.1b).

When loculated, ascites is seen as discrete collections of fluid partly surrounded by bands of adhesions and partly by the edges of normal abdominal structures, e.g. bowel wall or liver edge. Loculated collections of ascites may not be distinguishable from fluid in abscesses because the density of infected and uninfected fluid can be identical.

Ascites is readily detected by ultrasound (Fig. 10.2) as echo-free regions with excellent transmission of sound. Therefore, ascites is easy to demonstrate provided no bowel gas is in the path of the ultrasound beam. Bowel dilatation with excess gas frequently accompanies all types of ascites and often limits the information available. It is almost always possible, however, to demonstrate at least some of the ascites.

Plain film detection of ascites is discussed in Chapter 4.

Peritoneal tumours

By far the most frequent neoplastic disease of the peritoneum is metastases from an abdominal or pelvic tumour, particularly carcinoma of the ovary. Ultrasound and CT may show only ascites. Sometimes peritoneal nodules are demonstrated. In ovarian carcinoma, particularly, numerous nodules may coalesce to form what is known as an 'omental cake' (Fig. 10.3).

Intraperitoneal abscesses

Intraperitoneal abscesses may follow a perforation of the bowel or biliary tract, either spontaneous or post-traumatic, particularly following surgery. The common locations are subphrenic, subhepatic, paracolic and pelvic. The expected site of the abscess depends on the site of perforation, e.g. duodenal leakage usually results in subhepatic or subphrenic abscess, whereas a leak from the left colon often results in paracolic or pelvic abscess. Multiple abscesses are not uncommon. Ascites frequently accompanies abdominal and pelvic abscesses.

Computed tomography finds most abscesses and rarely gives false positive results. Ultrasound can be just as informative, provided it is positive, and may be preferred

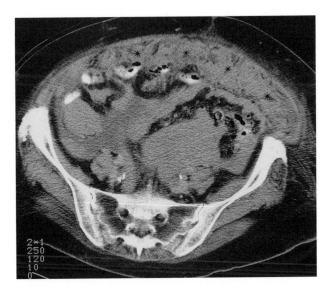

Fig. 10.3 Extensive intraperitoneal spread of ovarian carcinoma. Note the ascites separating the bowel loops and the massive 'omental cake' of tumour deposits (∗).

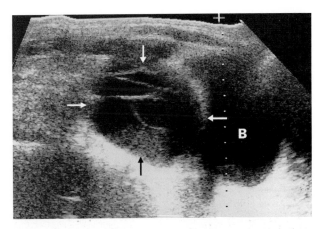

Fig. 10.4 Pelvic abscess. Ultrasound scan showing a large complex mass (arrows) just above the bladder (B). This young man had Crohn's disease.

because it is quick and simple to perform. The disadvantage of ultrasound is that gas in dilated loops of bowel can interfere with the images. Also, surgical wounds and dressings may make it impossible to place the transducer in direct contact with the skin; without such contact it is impossible to obtain images.

Ultrasound appearances

The areas best suited for ultrasound examination are the right upper quadrant and the true pelvis.

The ultrasonographer searches for any localized fluid collections lying outside the bowel (Fig. 10.4). Fluid within the bowel is recognized by observing peristaltic activity. Abscesses assume many different configurations depending on the adjacent organs. They often have slightly irregular walls and may contain internal echoes due to septations or debris. These internal echoes are not, however, specific for infection. Gas in an abscess appears echogenic and produces acoustic shadowing but it can be difficult to distinguish from gas within the bowel.

The major differential diagnosis is from loops of bowel

and uninfected loculations of ascites, blood or lymph, all of which can occur postoperatively. The distinction may require needle aspiration of the fluid.

Computed tomography appearances

The basic principles are similar to those described for ultrasound. The fluid centre of the abscess is identified as a homogeneous density surrounded by a definite wall of soft tissue lying within the peritoneal cavity but outside the bowel (Fig. 10.5a). Gas within the abscess is seen in approximately half the patients and is a very useful sign because it helps distinguish infected from uninfected fluid loculations. The gas may take the form of multiple small streaks or bubbles or it may collect as one large bubble. Air–fluid levels may be present within the larger collections. The wall of the abscess often shows enhancement following intravenous contrast administration. Subphrenic abscesses (Fig. 10.5b) may be difficult to distinguish from pleural empyemas at CT; the peritoneal and pleural cavities are, after all, separated only by the diaphragm, a structure that can be difficult to identify at CT. In such cases, ultrasound will usually be very helpful because it can demonstrate the abscess and also directly demonstrate the position of the diaphragm.

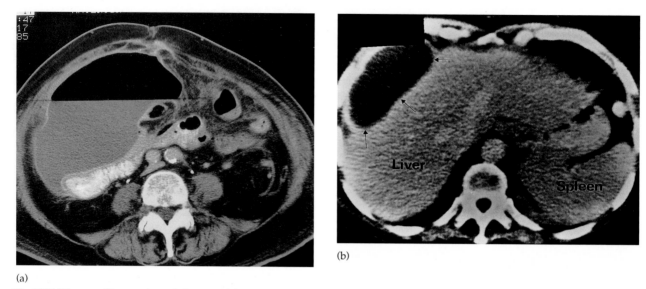

(a)

(b)

Fig. 10.5 CT scans of intraperitoneal abscesses. (a) Large abscess in the right side of the abdomen at the level of the umbilicus. Note the large air – fluid collection with a thin enhancing wall. The abscess displaces adjacent bowel loops (containing air and oral contrast). (b) Subphrenic abscess (arrows) lying anterior to liver.

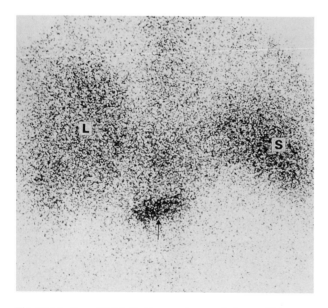

Fig. 10.6 Indium-111 labelled leucocyte scan of abscess. This abscess (arrow) followed small bowel surgery with subsequent anastomotic leak. Normal uptake is seen in the liver (L) and spleen (S).

The major differential diagnosis of intraperitoneal abscesses is:

• Fluid within distended or matted loops of bowel. The distinction at CT can usually be made by opacifying the bowel. Oral contrast agent is routinely given for this purpose before the examination in most centres. With ultrasound, peristalsis of bowel loops can be observed.

• Loculated uninfected fluid. It may not be possible to make the distinction between infected and uninfected fluid loculations and needle aspiration may have to be performed.

Radionuclide examinations

If CT and ultrasound have been unsuccessful in locating an abscess, then some of the patient's own white blood cells can be labelled with ^{99m}Tc or with indium-111 which will accumulate in an abscess (Fig. 10.6).

Retroperitoneum

Computed tomography, MRI and ultrasound all provide information about retroperitoneal structures. Plain films are limited to showing: very large masses or calcification within a mass; the occasional case where gas is seen in an abscess, and the curvilinear calcification of an aortic aneurysm. The discussion in this chapter will be confined to: the adrenal glands; lymphadenopathy; aortic aneurysms; retroperitoneal tumours; haematomas and abscesses. The urinary tract and pancreas are covered elsewhere. When considering the retroperitoneum it is useful to appreciate the anatomy of the anterior and posterior renal fascia which divides the retroperitoneum into three compartments: the anterior pararenal, the perinephric and the posterior pararenal spaces (Fig. 10.7). Infection in one of these compartments tends to be limited to that compartment.

Imaging techniques

Computed tomography

Retroperitoneal CT is particularly informative in obese subjects because fat surrounds the important structures.

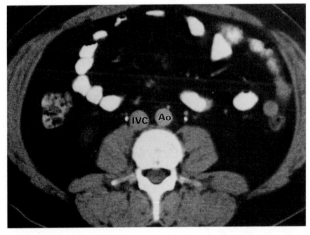

(a)

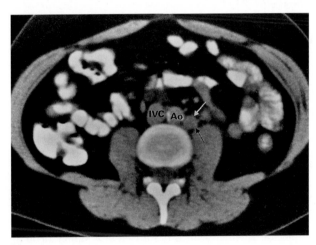

(b)

Fig. 10.8 (a) CT scan of normal retroperitoneum. Note that the aorta (Ao) and IVC are clearly outlined by fat and that there is a fat-containing space to the left of the aorta. The small white dots in the retroperitoneum are the opacified ureters. (b) An enlarged lymph node is shown to the left of the aorta (arrow).

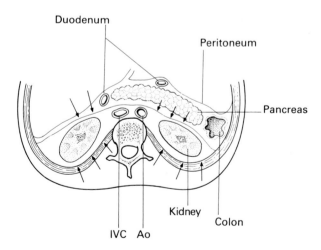

Fig. 10.7 Diagram of anterior (downward pointing arrows) and posterior (upward pointing arrows) renal fascia. Ao, aorta; IVC, inferior vena cava; K, kidney.

Indeed, retroperitoneal CT can be difficult to interpret in subjects with little or no fat – children are a particular problem in this regard.

When CT scans of the retroperitoneum are reviewed, the following normal features should be looked for (Figs 10.8 and 10.11):

- The complete outline of the aorta and inferior vena cava should be clearly visible throughout their lengths, except where the inferior vena cava (IVC) passes through the liver. The aorta is round in cross-section and normally measures 2.0–2.5 cm in diameter. The IVC varies in shape from round to oval.
- There is usually a fat-containing space to the left of the aorta, which is a good area in which to look for lymphadenopathy (Fig. 10.8b). The only structures other than lymph nodes to be seen in this space are the left renal vein and, on rare occasions, a loop of small bowel.
- The psoas muscles are seen as symmetrical, rounded structures outlined anteriorly by fat.
- Both adrenals are well seen in most subjects.

Ultrasound

Retroperitoneal fat, which is very echo reflective, surrounds the various retroperitoneal structures, which are seen as relatively sonolucent areas. The aorta and inferior vena cava, as expected, are easily identified. Normal adrenal glands are rarely visible. Enlarged lymph nodes can be identified.

Magnetic resonance imaging

Magnetic resonance imaging plays a small part in diagnosing retroperitoneal disorders as it provides few advantages over CT or ultrasound. The ability to display the body in any plane can be an advantage. MRI can, for example, help to decide whether a mass has arisen in a kidney or in an adrenal gland. Also the ability to display intravascular spread of tumour can be of value in showing the spread of renal carcinoma into the renal vein, IVC and heart (Fig. 10.9).

Retroperitoneal lymphadenopathy

The normal para-aortic lymph nodes vary in size from invisible to a short-axis diameter of 1 cm. In the retrocrural area, a diameter of 6 mm is the upper limit of normal. Size is the only criterion of abnormality since normal, inflammatory and neoplastic nodes usually have the same features and texture at CT, ultrasound, and even MRI. Metastatic neoplasm and primary lymphoma appear identical.

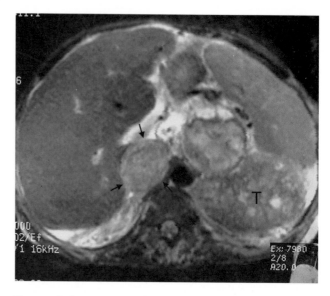

Fig. 10.9 Inferior vena caval spread of renal carcinoma. The tumour in the left kidney (T) has spread into the inferior vena cava (arrows) where it is clearly visible on this MRI scan.

Mild enlargement is seen with inflammatory as well as with neoplastic disease, whereas enlargement of over 2 cm almost always indicates neoplasm. Individually enlarged nodes may be seen (Fig. 10.8b), but not infrequently several nodes are matted together to form a lobular mass engulfing the aorta or inferior vena cava (Fig. 10.10).

Adrenal glands

The normal adrenal glands are thin, bilobed structures surrounded by fat (Fig. 10.11). The right adrenal gland is situated above the upper pole of the right kidney. The left adrenal gland is usually situated just anterior to the upper pole of the left kidney.

Calcification of the adrenal glands (Fig. 10.12) may follow old intra-adrenal haemorrhage or old healed tuberculosis. Severe destruction and calcification of the adrenal glands may lead to Addison's disease.

Enlargement of the adrenal glands can be recognized at CT, ultrasound and MRI. Enlargement may be due to neoplasm, hyperplasia, cyst, abscess or haemorrhage. CT is the best routine technique for diagnosing adrenal enlargement because it consistently shows the size and shape of the glands. Both ultrasound and MRI have one advantage over CT: they can display the retroperitoneum in any plane and can, therefore, show the relationship of masses to adjacent organs. This can be of real benefit when there is doubt about the origin of a mass, e.g. kidney or adrenal gland.

Functioning adrenal tumours

Patients with tumours producing an excess of hormones will have had their endocrine disorder diagnosed clinically and biochemically prior to the imaging examination. CT, or occasionally MRI, is used in this group primarily to localize the tumour. Such tumours, which are usually benign adenomas but which may be carcinomas, cause spherical enlargement of the adrenal gland. The distinction between pituitary tumour, adrenal adenoma and adrenal hyperplasia as a cause of Cushing's syndrome is usually based on biochemical findings but, on occasions, the precise diagnosis can be in doubt. Adrenal adenomas giving rise to Cushing's disease are nearly always larger than 2 cm and can virtually always be localized with CT (Fig. 10.13). Most hyperplastic glands in pituitary-dependent Cushing's disease appear normal or only slightly enlarged at CT.

Aldosteronomas (Conn's tumour) are usually less than 1 cm in size and may, on occasion, be difficult to identify.

Phaeochromocytomas are frequently very large at presentation and virtually all are demonstrable at CT or MRI (Fig. 10.14). Ten per cent of phaeochromocytomas are bilateral and, therefore, the opposite adrenal gland must be looked at carefully if a phaeochromocytoma is diagnosed. It

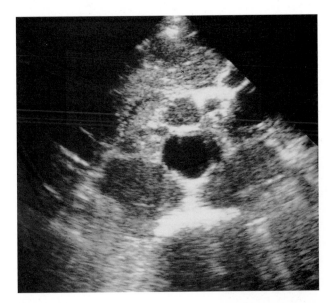

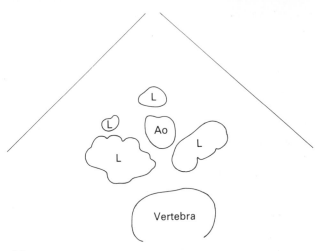

(a)

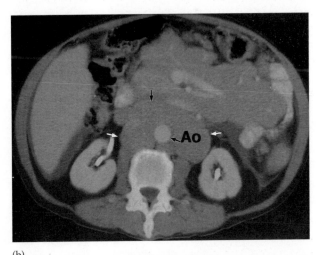

(b)

Fig. 10.10 Massive retroperitoneal lymphadenopathy (L). (a) Ultrasound showing multiple greatly enlarged lymph nodes surrounding the aorta. (b) CT scan of same patient. The arrows point to the enlarged nodes. Enlarged mesenteric nodes are also present. Ao, aorta.

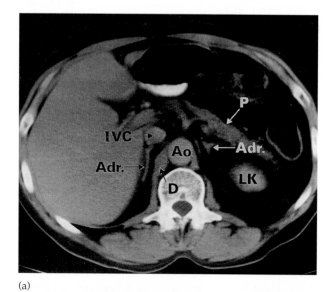

(a)

Fig. 10.11 Normal adrenal glands. (a) CT scan. Both adrenal glands (Adr.) are visible in this section. Note the different shape of the two glands. Ao, aorta; D, diaphragmatic crus; IVC, inferior vena cava; LK, left kidney; P, pancreas. (b) and (c) MRI scans (T1-weighted images) showing the right and left adrenal glands (arrows).

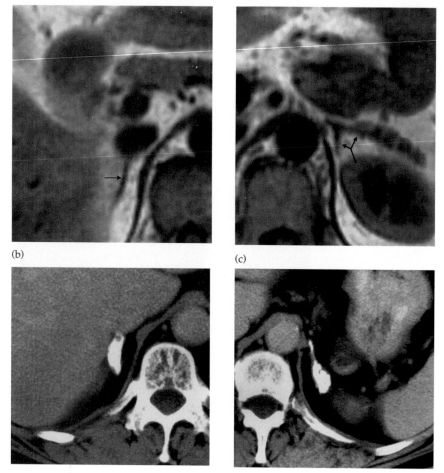

(b)

(c)

(a)

(b)

Fig. 10.12 Adrenal calcification shown by CT. (a) Heavily calcified right adrenal gland. (b) Heavily calcified left adrenal gland.

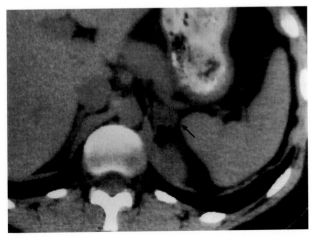

(a)

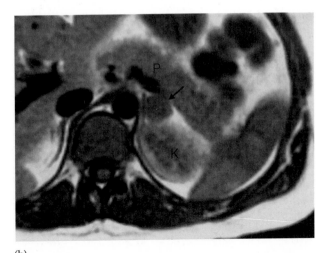

(b)

Fig. 10.13 Functioning adrenal adenoma causing Cushing's syndrome. (a) CT scan showing 2 cm mass in left adrenal (arrow). (b) MRI scan (T1-weighted) also showing the lesion (arrow). K, kidney; P, pancreas.

should also be remembered that 10% of phaeochromocytomas arise outside the adrenal gland, usually in another retroperitoneal site.

Radionuclide scans can be used to localize functioning adrenal tumours. The only radionuclide in widespread use, now that CT has become the prime method of localizing cortisol and aldosterone-producing tumours, is iodine-123 labelled MIBG (meta-iodo-benzyl guanidine), an agent which is concentrated by phaeochromocytomas (Fig. 10.14c). As already mentioned, the great majority of phaeochromocytomas are single, but a few are multiple, either in both adrenal glands or extra-adrenal in location, and a radioiodine-labelled MIBG scan is an excellent survey technique for finding all sites of phaeochromocytoma.

Non-functioning adrenal masses

A small non-functioning adenoma is indistinguishable by CT or ultrasound from a small metastasis. This can pose a major dilemma for patients undergoing staging for a cancer in whom a small adrenal mass (up to 3 cm in diameter) is discovered. Special MRI sequences can, on occasion, be very helpful when deciding between non-functioning adenoma and metastasis. In some patients, percutaneous biopsy will be needed, but as with all needle biopsy techniques it is only possible to prove, not exclude, the diagnosis of metastatic cancer.

Non-functioning adenomas larger than 3 cm are very rare and therefore larger adrenal masses are likely to be metastases or, rarely, primary adrenal carcinoma. The common malignant adrenal tumour of early childhood is *neuroblastoma*.

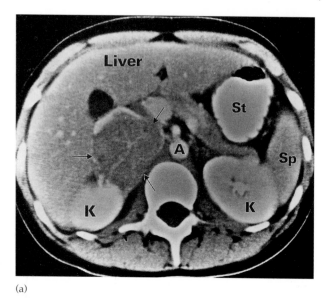

(a)

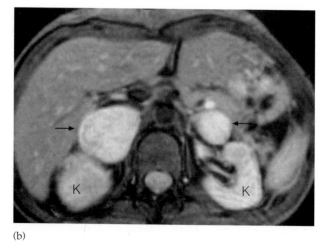

(b)

Fig. 10.14 Phaeochromocytoma. (a) CT scan showing large phaeochromocytoma (arrows) between right kidney, liver and spine. The inferior vena cava is compressed. A, aorta; K, kidney; Sp, spleen; St, stomach. (b) MRI scan showing bilateral phaeochromocytomas (arrows). K, kidney. (c) Radio-iodine labelled MIBG scan of a phaeochromocytoma (arrows) in the left adrenal gland.

(c)

Metastases to the adrenal gland are common; they are frequently bilateral (Fig. 10.15). Many different tumours metastasize to the adrenal glands. It is a particular feature of lung carcinoma; it is for this reason that the adrenals are frequently added to CT scans of the chest in patients being staged for bronchial carcinoma.

Adrenal abscesses and haemorrhage are usually bilateral and are indistinguishable from one another at CT and ultrasound. The clinical features usually suggest the correct diagnosis.

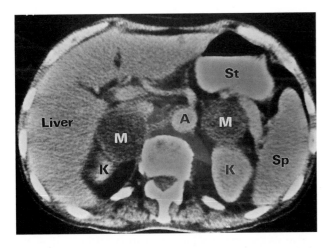

Fig. 10.15 CT scan showing large bilateral adrenal metastases (M). These masses are separate from the kidneys (K). Only the extreme top of the right kidney is visible on this particular section. A, aorta; Sp, spleen; St, stomach.

Retroperitoneal tumours

The term retroperitoneal tumour covers tumours arising primarily in retroperitoneal muscles, fat or connective tissue, the commonest being liposarcoma and fibrosarcoma. All these tumours appear as masses on CT, ultrasound or MRI. Sometimes, the edge of the mass is well defined, but sometimes there is invasion of the adjacent tissue. A liposarcoma (Fig. 10.16a) almost always contains significant amounts of recognizable fat interspersed between strands or masses of soft-tissue density; a combination that permits a specific diagnosis to be made at CT. Otherwise, it is usually impossible to determine histologically the nature of the tumour (Fig. 10.16b).

Aortic aneurysm

Abdominal aortic aneurysms are readily diagnosed at ultrasound, CT and MRI, although MRI is rarely used for this purpose (Fig. 10.17). Ultrasound is being used in some centres as a screening examination to find asymptomatic aortic aneurysms in older men.

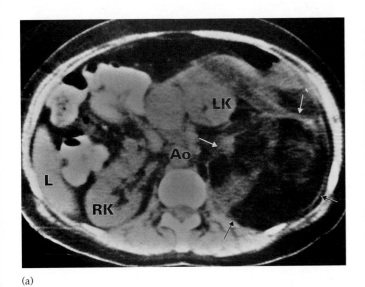

(a)

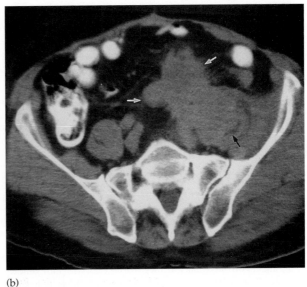

(b)

Fig. 10.16 Retroperitoneal tumours. (a) Liposarcoma. CT scan showing large partially fatty tumour (arrows) displacing the left kidney forward. The right kidney is in normal position. Ao, aorta; L, liver, LK, left kidney; RK, right kidney. (b) Malignant tumour (recurrent colon carcinoma) in left retroperitoneum (arrows). Note the asymmetry of the retroperitoneal tissues.

Both CT and ultrasound allow the true maximum diameter of the aneurysm to be measured and to identify separately the wall and any lining thrombus. It is also relatively easy to see any retroperitoneal bleeding from an aneurysm at CT. It is generally held that aneurysms of greater than 6 cm in diameter are in serious danger of rupture, whether or not the patient has had any demonstrable retroperitoneal bleeding.

It is the thrombus, not the wall, that forms the outline of the aortic lumen at angiography. Aortography is, therefore, of limited use in assessing the true diameter of an aneurysm, although it is a good technique for showing the aorta above the aneurysm as well as for showing stenoses of branches of the aorta.

Aortic aneurysms may also be recognizable on plain films of the abdomen (p. 143), but only if substantial calcification is present in the wall.

Retroperitoneal haematoma

Retroperitoneal bleeding is usually due to trauma or to bleeding from an aortic aneurysm. It is occasionally spontaneous in patients with bleeding disorders or in those on anticoagulant therapy.

The diagnosis is readily made by CT, MRI or ultrasound. Haematomas may have similar CT and ultrasound features to the non-fatty retroperitoneal tumours, but frequently CT numbers are higher or lower than muscle, depending on how recently the bleeding occurred (Fig. 10.18). Recent haemorrhage may show areas of high density, an appearance that can be pathognomonic, whereas older haematomas have often undergone liquefaction, the liquefied areas then being of low attenuation. MRI may show the characteristic features of haematoma.

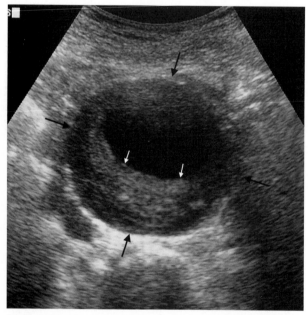

(a)

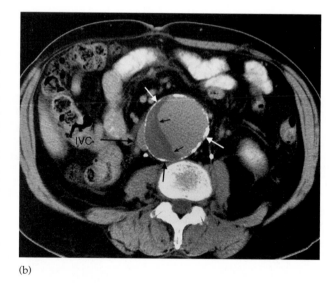

(b)

Fig. 10.17 Abdominal aortic aneurysm. (a) Ultrasound. Transverse scan showing a blood clot lining the wall (small white arrows) within the aneurysm (large black arrows). (b) CT scan with intravenous contrast enhancement. A 7 cm aneurysm (arrows) with a lower density blood clot (small black arrows) lining the wall. The wall shows patches of calcification. The inferior vena cava (IVC) is displaced by the aneurysm.

Retroperitoneal and psoas abscesses

Retroperitoneal and psoas abscesses are usually due to spread of infection from the appendix, colon, kidney, pancreas or spine. They are often found close to the organ of origin.

Retroperitoneal abscesses have many similar features to tumours and haematomas at both CT and ultrasound (Fig. 10.19). Usually, however, there is evidence of a fluid centre and then there may also be gas present within the abscess, best seen at CT. Abscesses can be confused with normal colon unless the colon is carefully identified on each image at CT. This is much easier to do if bowel opacification has been used. The wall of the abscess may enhance with contrast medium, a feature that is also seen with neoplasms. The radionuclide findings of retroperitoneal abscesses are the same as with intraperitoneal abscesses (see p. 289).

Psoas abscesses may occasionally be seen as an isolated entity. A psoas abscess will show enlargement of the psoas muscle. In order to make this diagnosis, it is helpful to compare the two psoas muscles, as they are normally symmetrical.

Retroperitoneal fibrosis

See p. 237.

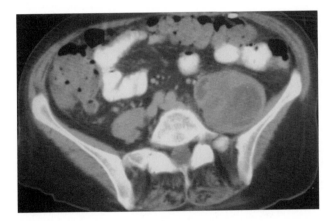

Fig. 10.18 CT scan of a large haematoma in the left iliopsoas muscle. Note the variable density, much of which is of lower density than the normal muscles.

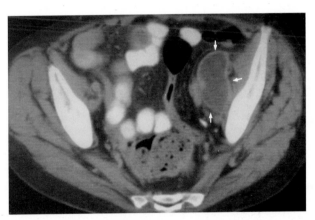

Fig. 10.19 Psoas abscess. CT scan showing left psoas abscess (arrows). Note the uniformly thick wall and the uniform low density of the contents.

11

Bone Disease

Imaging techniques

Plain bone radiographs

It is helpful to understand the anatomical terms used to describe a normal long bone. These are shown in Fig. 11.1.

The radiological responses of bone to pathological process are limited; thus similar x-ray signs occur in widely different conditions. It should be noted that it takes time for the various signs to develop; for example, in adults, it takes several weeks for a periosteal reaction to be visible after trauma and, in a child with osteomyelitis, the clinical

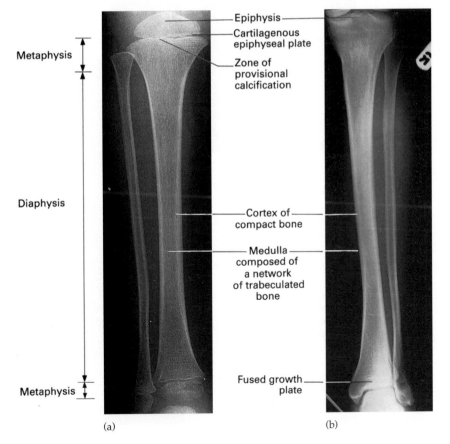

Fig. 11.1 Normal long bones in (a) child and (b) adult. Increase in length takes place at the cartilagenous epiphyseal plate. In the growing child, calcification of cartilage occurs at the interface between the radiolucent growing cartilage and the bone to give the zone of provisional calcification, which is seen as a dense white line forming the ends of the shaft and surrounding the bony epiphyses. This calcified cartilage becomes converted to bone. (If there is temporary cessation of growth then the zone of provisional calcification may persist as a thin white line, known as a 'growth line', extending across the shaft of the bone.) As the child grows older the epiphyseal plate becomes thinner until, eventually, there is bony fusion of the epiphysis with the shaft.

Metaphysis

Diaphysis

Metaphysis

Epiphysis
Cartilagenous epiphyseal plate
Zone of provisional calcification

Cortex of compact bone
Medulla composed of a network of trabeculated bone

Fused growth plate

(a)

(b)

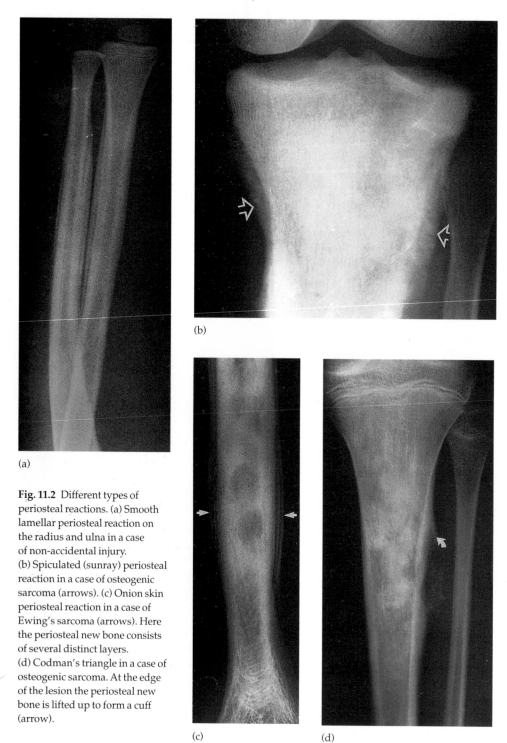

(a)

(b)

(c)

(d)

Fig. 11.2 Different types of periosteal reactions. (a) Smooth lamellar periosteal reaction on the radius and ulna in a case of non-accidental injury.
(b) Spiculated (sunray) periosteal reaction in a case of osteogenic sarcoma (arrows). (c) Onion skin periosteal reaction in a case of Ewing's sarcoma (arrows). Here the periosteal new bone consists of several distinct layers.
(d) Codman's triangle in a case of osteogenic sarcoma. At the edge of the lesion the periosteal new bone is lifted up to form a cuff (arrow).

features are present from seven to ten days before the first sign is visible on the radiograph. In general, the signs take longer to develop in adults than they do in children.

The signs of bone disease are:
• *Decrease in bone density* which may be focal or generalized. Focal reduction in density is usually referred to as a 'lytic area' or an area of 'bone destruction'. When generalized, decrease in bone density is best referred to as 'osteopenia' until a specific diagnosis such as osteomalacia or osteoporosis can be made.
• *Increase in bone density (sclerosis)* which may also be focal or generalized.
• *Periosteal reaction.* The periosteum is not normally visible on a radiograph. The term 'periosteal reaction' refers to excess bone produced by the periosteum, which occurs in response to such conditions as neoplasm, inflammation or trauma. Several patterns of periosteal reaction are seen (Fig. 11.2) but they do not correlate with specific diagnoses. At the edge of a very active periosteal reaction there may be a cuff of new bone known as a Codman's triangle (Fig. 11.2d). Although often seen in highly malignant primary bone tumours, e.g. osteosarcoma, a Codman's triangle is also found in other aggressive conditions.
• *Cortical thickening* also involves the laying down of new bone by the periosteum (Fig. 11.3), but here the process is very slow. The result is that the new bone, although it may be thick and irregular, shows the same homogeneous density as does the normal cortex. There are no separate lines or spicules of calcification as seen in a periosteal reaction. The causes are many, including chronic osteomyelitis, healed trauma, response to chronic stress or benign neoplasm. The feature common to all these conditions is that the process is either very slowly progressive or has healed.
• *Alteration in trabecular pattern* is a complex response usually involving a reduction in the number of trabeculae with an alteration in the remaining trabeculae, e.g. in osteoporosis and Paget's disease. In osteoporosis the cortex is thin and the trabeculae that remain are more prominent than usual, whereas in Paget's disease the trabeculae are thickened and trabeculation is seen in the normal compact bone of the cortex (Fig. 11.4).
• *Alteration in the shape of a bone* is another complex response with many causes. Many cases are congenital in origin; some are acquired, e.g. acromegaly and expanding bone tumours.

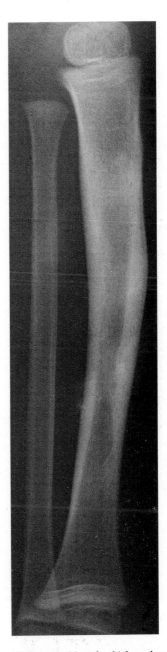

Fig. 11.3 Cortical thickening. Note the thickened cortex in the midshaft of the tibia from old, healed osteomyelitis. Same case as in Fig. 11.17, taken one year later.

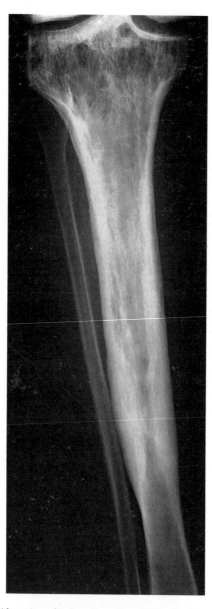

Fig. 11.4 Alteration of trabecular pattern in Paget's disease involving the upper part of the tibia leaving the lowest part of the tibia and the fibula unaffected. Note the coarse trabeculae. The other features of Paget's disease – thickened cortex and bone expansion – are also present.

• *Alteration in bone age.* The time of appearance of the various epiphyseal centres and their time of fusion depends on the age of the child. Sets of standard films have been published which provide an indication of skeletal maturation. For the measurement of 'bone age' it is usually most convenient to take a film of the hand and wrist but, in the neonatal period, films of the knee provide the most accurate assessment.

Radionuclide bone scanning

Technetium-99m (^{99m}Tc)-labelled phosphate complexes given as an intravenous injection are the agents used for bone scanning. They are taken up selectively by the bones (Fig. 11.5) and also excreted in the urine. These agents may be concentrated by certain soft tissue tumours, by soft tissue calcifications and by sites of tissue damage.

Increased uptake on the radionuclide bone scan is seen in conditions where there is an increased blood supply and high bone turnover. Many bone abnormalities including fractures, benign or malignant tumours, infection, infarction and Paget's disease give positive scans, so correlation with plain radiographs is usually essential.

Indications for radionuclide bone scanning are:
• detection of metastases;
• detection of osteomyelitis;
• determination of whether a lesion is solitary or multifocal;
• investigation of a clinically suspected bone lesion despite a normal radiograph (this may occur with metastases, trauma (particularly stress injury), osteoid osteoma or early osteomyelitis (Figs 11.6 and 11.15));
• determination, in equivocal cases, of whether an abnormality seen on the radiograph is significant or not (a positive bone scan makes it likely that a true lesion exists and a negative one reduces the probability of disease considerably);
• investigation of painful hip prostheses.

Computed tomography in bone disease

Plain radiographs are usually very informative and CT is only needed in selected cases. Routine window settings on brain, chest and abdomen CT scans, although clearly not

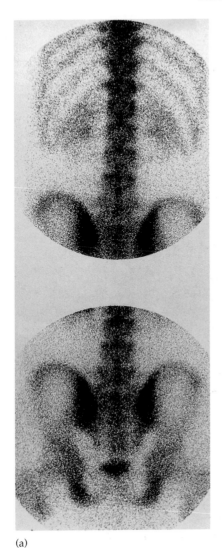

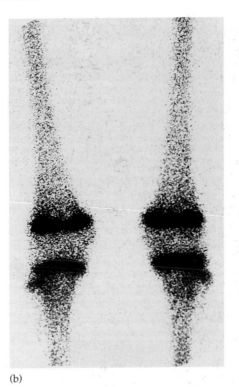

Fig. 11.5 Normal radionuclide bone scan.
(a) Adult. Posterior scans of thorax, abdomen
and pelvis. Note the radionuclide in the bladder.
(b) Child. Scan of lower thighs and knees. Note
the bands of increased uptake in the epiphyseal
plates where bone growth is occurring.

(a)

(b)

optimal, should nevertheless be carefully scrutinized for skeletal abnormalities. For specific bone details, special 'bone windows' are needed.

The indications for bone CT are:
• Evaluation of complex shaped bones, such as the spine and pelvis (Fig. 11.7), where plain films are frequently very difficult, or even impossible, to interpret. The transaxial display is particularly useful for diagnosing the presence and extent of tumours or fractures of these bones (see Fig. 14.13, p. 383).

• With more advanced scanners, three-dimensional reconstructions can be made. These are particularly useful for planning corrective surgery of bone fractures and deformity.

• Demonstrating the extent of bone tumours both within the bone and in adjacent soft tissues, where this information

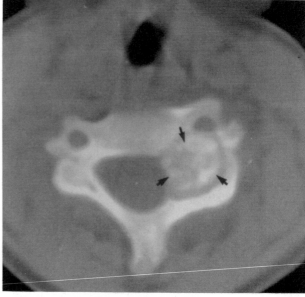

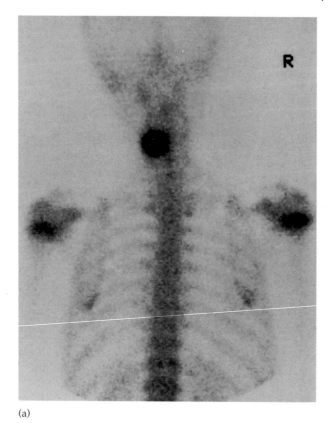

(a)

(b)

Fig. 11.6 Giant osteoid osteoma (osteoblastoma) which was difficult to appreciate on plain films. (a) Bone scan (posterior view) showing a focal area of intense increased uptake in the cervical spine. (b) CT of the cervical spine demonstrates the tumour arising from the pedicle (arrows).

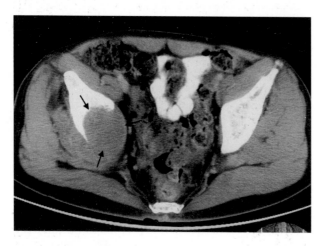

Fig. 11.7 CT scan of pelvis showing a large mass (arrows) due to a metastasis destroying the medial half of the right iliac bone with extension into the adjacent soft tissues.

will materially affect management, e.g. most pelvic and spinal tumours and those peripheral tumours where conservative surgery is a possibility (Fig. 11.6b).
• Diagnosis of disc herniation and spinal stenosis.

Magnetic resonance imaging in bone disease

Calcified tissues such as bone produce no signal with MRI, but MRI can demonstrate the bone marrow directly, making it possible to see the full extent of disease such as metastases, other tumours and infections, even in areas where bone destruction is not yet evident on plain films or CT. (Fig. 11.8). MRI is also particularly good for showing soft tissue abnormalities.

The major indications for musculoskeletal MRI are:
• to demonstrate disc herniation and spinal cord compression;

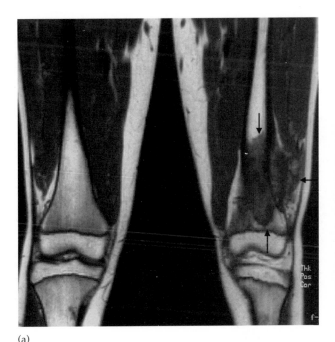

(a)

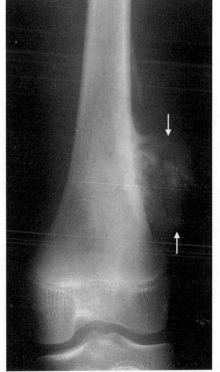

(b)

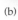

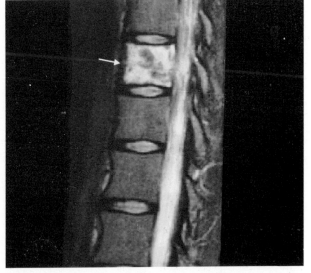

Fig. 11.8 Magnetic resonance imaging of bone tumours. (a) T1-weighted scan of osteosarcoma in the lower shaft and metaphysis of the left femur. The extent of tumour (arrows) within the bone and the soft tissue extension are both very well shown. This information is not available from the plain film (b), although the plain film provides a more specific diagnosis, because the bone formation within the soft tissue extension (arrows) is obvious. (c) T2-weighted scan of lymphoma in the T10 vertebral body (arrow). The very high signal of the neoplastic tissue is very evident even though there is no deformity of shape of the vertebral body.

(c)

- to show the extent of primary bone tumours and to demonstrate bone metastases, myeloma and lymphoma (Fig. 11.8);
- to image soft tissue masses (Fig. 11.9);

- to diagnose avascular necrosis and other joint pathologies and to image injury to joint cartilages, ligaments and other intra-articular soft tissues. These topics are discussed in the next chapter on joint diseases.

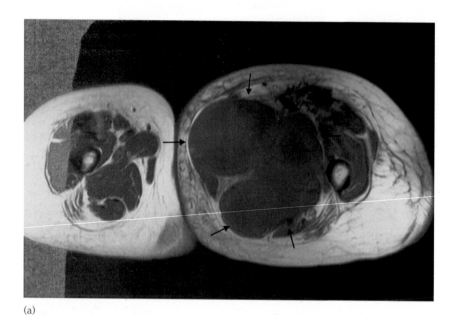

(a)

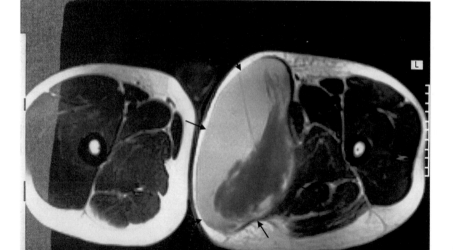

(b)

Fig. 11.9 Magnetic resonance imaging of soft tissue masses. (a) Soft tissue sarcoma producing an obvious soft tissue mass (arrows) in the medial compartment of the left thigh. (b) Large haematoma (arrows) in the medial compartment of the left thigh showing mixed signal including the characteristic high signal of recent haemorrhage on T1-weighted sequence. (Both scans are T1-weighted.)

BONE DISEASES

When considering the diagnosis and differential diagnosis of bone diseases, it is convenient to divide disorders into those that:

• cause solitary lytic or sclerotic lesions;
• produce multiple focal lesions, i.e. several discrete lytic or sclerotic lesions in one or more bones;
• cause generalized lesions where all the bones show diffuse increase or decrease in bone density;
• alter the trabecular pattern;
• change the shape of the bone.

Solitary lesions (fractures are dealt with separately in Chapter 14)

Solitary areas of lysis, sclerosis or a combination of the two, are usually one of the following:

• bone tumours
  (a) malignant (primary or secondary)
  (b) benign
• osteomyelitis
• bone cysts, fibrous dysplasia or other non-neoplastic defects of bone
• conditions of uncertain nature such as Langerhans histiocytosis and osteoid osteoma.

Primary malignant bone tumours and osteomyelitis are usually accompanied by periosteal reaction. Pathological fractures may be seen through benign and malignant bone tumours and through bone cysts.

The radiological diagnosis of a localized bone lesion can be a problem. Some conditions are readily diagnosed but, in others, even establishing which broad category of disease is present can be difficult. The initial radiological decision is usually to try and decide whether the lesion is benign, i.e. stable or very slow growing, or whether it is aggressive, i.e. a malignant tumour or an infection. It is also important to know the age of the patient, since certain lesions tend to occur in a specific age range.

The features to look for on plain radiographs and CT when trying to decide the nature of a localized bone lesion are:

1 *The edge.* The edge of any lytic or sclerotic lesion should be examined carefully to see whether it is well demarcated or whether there is a wide zone of transition between the normal and the abnormal bone. There are two extremes: a lesion with a well-defined sclerotic edge is almost certainly benign, e.g. a fibrous cortical defect (Fig. 11.10a) or a bone island (Fig. 11.10b), whereas a lytic or sclerotic area with an ill-defined edge is likely to be aggressive (Fig. 11.10c). In the middle of this spectrum lies the lytic area with no sclerotic rim, which may be a benign or malignant lesion. Metastases and myeloma (Fig. 11.10d) are a frequent cause of this pattern.

2 *The adjacent cortex.* Any destruction of the adjacent cortex indicates an aggressive lesion such as a malignant tumour or osteomyelitis (Fig. 11.10e).

3 *Expansion.* Bone expansion with an intact well-formed

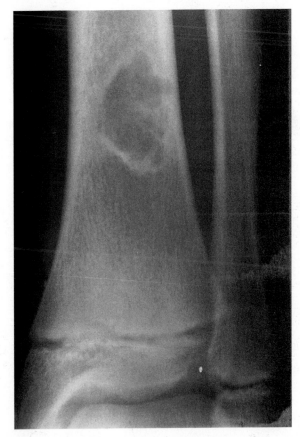

(a)

Fig. 11.10 The localized lesion. (a) A well-defined sclerotic edge indicating a benign lesion – a fibrous cortical defect. *Continued on pp. 308–9.*

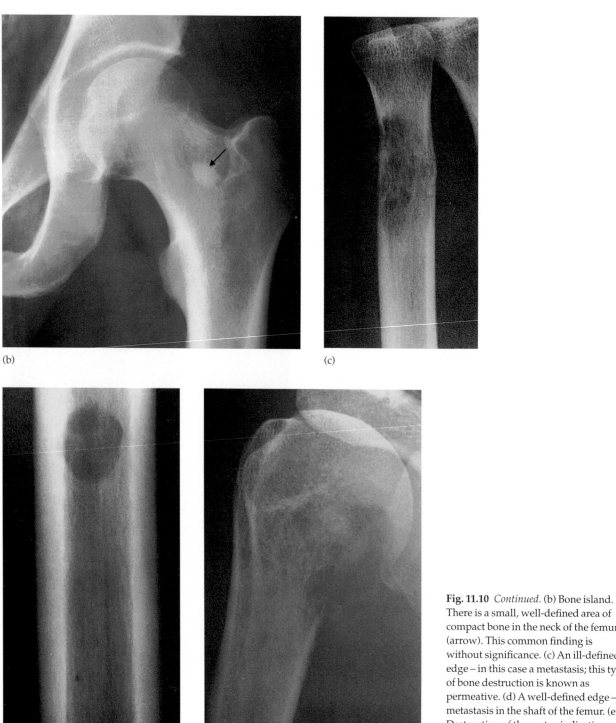

(b)

(c)

(d)

(e)

Fig. 11.10 *Continued.* (b) Bone island. There is a small, well-defined area of compact bone in the neck of the femur (arrow). This common finding is without significance. (c) An ill-defined edge – in this case a metastasis; this type of bone destruction is known as permeative. (d) A well-defined edge – a metastasis in the shaft of the femur. (e) Destruction of the cortex indicating an aggressive lesion – another metastasis.

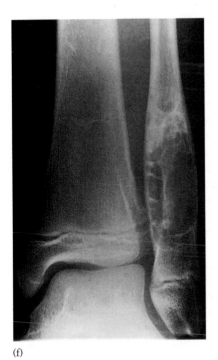

(f)

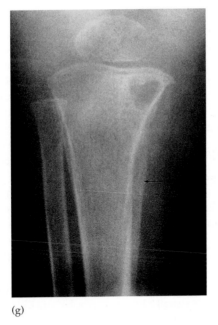

(g)

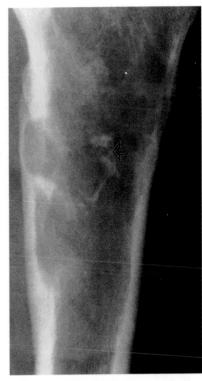

(h)

Fig. 11.10 *Continued.* (f) Expansion of the cortex – fibrous dysplasia. (g) Periosteal reaction (arrow) – osteomyelitis. (h) Containing calcium (arrow) – a cartilage tumour, in this case a chondrosarcoma.

cortex usually indicates a slow-growing lesion such as an enchondroma or fibrous dysplasia (Fig. 11.10f).

4 *Periosteal reaction.* The presence of an active periosteal reaction in the absence of trauma usually indicates an aggressive lesion (Fig. 11.10g). The causes of localized periosteal reactions adjacent to a lytic or sclerotic lesion are:

- osteomyelitis;
- malignant bone tumour, particularly Ewing's sarcoma and osteosarcoma;
- occasionally metastasis, particularly neuroblastoma;
- Langerhans histiocytosis.

A periosteal reaction is also a feature of trauma to a bone, but trauma while it causes fracture does not cause focal bone destruction.

5 *Calcific densities within the lesion.* Calcification within an area of bone destruction occurs in specific conditions; for example, patchy calcification of a popcorn type usually indicates a cartilage tumour (Fig. 11.10h), whereas diffuse ill-defined calcification suggests osteoid formation and indicates an osteosarcoma.

6 *Soft tissue swelling.* The presence of a soft tissue mass suggests an aggressive lesion; the better defined it is, the more likely it is that the lesion is a neoplasm. Ill-defined soft tissue swelling adjacent to a focal destructive lesion suggests infection. Sometimes a tumour arising primarily in the soft tissues may destroy bone by pressure erosion or direct invasion.

7 *Site.* The site of a lesion is important since certain lesions tend to occur at certain sites; for example, osteomyelitis characteristically occurs in the metaphyseal areas, particularly of the knee and lower tibia, whereas giant cell tumours are subarticular in position.

Bone tumours

The precise diagnosis of a bone tumour can be notoriously difficult both for the radiologist and the pathologist. Accurate histological diagnosis is essential for all malignant lesions and it is important to realize that separate portions of a tumour may show different histological appearances. In general, plain film radiography is the best imaging technique for making a diagnosis, whereas CT and/or MRI often show the full extent of a tumour to advantage. The main role for radionuclide bone scanning is to diagnose metastatic bone disease. Metastatic malignant tumours are by far the commonest bone neoplasm, outnumbering many times primary malignant tumours. They are discussed on p. 316.

Primary malignant tumours

On plain films, primary malignant tumours usually have poorly defined margins, often with a wide zone of transition between the normal and abnormal bone. The lesion may destroy the cortex of the bone. A periosteal reaction is often present and a soft tissue mass may be seen.

Radionuclide bone scans show substantially increased activity in the lesion.

Although CT is no better than plain radiographs at making a diagnosis, CT scans can be used to show the extent of a tumour. Extension within the marrow cavity can be recognized by increased density of what should normally be a density close to that of fat. Extension into the soft tissues can be accurately defined, as can the relationship to important nerves and arteries.

Similar information can be obtained using MRI with the advantage that images may be produced in the sagittal or coronal planes and bone marrow and soft tissue involvement is more acurately demonstrated. Magnetic resonance imaging is therefore the best imaging tool for determining the local extent of the primary tumour.

Osteosarcoma (osteogenic sarcoma) (Fig. 11.8) occurs mainly in the 5–20-year-old age group, but is also seen in the elderly following malignant change in Paget's disease. The tumour often arises in a metaphysis, most commonly around the knee. There is usually bone destruction with new bone formation and typically a florid spiculated periosteal reaction is present, the so-called 'sunray appear-

ance' (Fig. 11.2b). The tumour may elevate the periosteum to form a Codman's triangle (Fig. 11.2d).

Chondrosarcoma occurs mainly in the 30–50-year-old age group, most commonly in the pelvic bones, scapulae, humeri and femora. A chondrosarcoma produces a lytic expanding lesion containing flecks of calcium, a sign that indicates its origin from cartilage cells. It can be difficult to distinguish from its benign counterpart, the enchondroma, but a chondrosarcoma is usually less well defined in at least one portion of its outline and it may show a periosteal reaction. Pelvic chondrosarcomas often have large extraosseus components best seen with CT or MRI (Fig. 11.11). A chondrosarcoma may arise from malignant degeneration of a benign cartilagenous tumour.

Fibrosarcoma and malignant fibrous histiocytoma are rare bone tumours with similar histological and radiological features. They most often present in young and middle-aged adults, usually around the knee. The feature on plain radiographs is an ill-defined area of lysis with periosteal reaction. Frequently the cortex is breached. There are no imaging features that distinguish these tumours from metastases or lymphoma.

Ewing's sarcoma is a highly malignant tumour, commonest in children, arising in the shaft of long bones. It produces ill-defined bone destruction with periosteal reaction that is typically 'onion skin' in type (Fig. 11.2c, p. 300).

Giant cell tumour has features of both malignant and benign tumours. It is locally invasive but rarely metastasizes. It occurs most commonly around the knee and at the wrist after the epiphyses have fused. It is an expanding destructive lesion which is subarticular in position (Fig. 11.12). The margin is fairly well defined but the cortex is thin and may in places be completely destroyed.

Primary lymphoma of bone is rare; most osseous malignant lymphoma is associated with generalized lymph node disease. When solitary primary lymphomas are encountered they may produce sclerotic bone lesions or they may cause destruction of bone, indistinguishable on imaging grounds from fibrosarcoma/malignant fibrous histiocytoma.

Benign tumours and tumour-like conditions

Included under this heading are benign tumours such as enchondroma, certain benign conditions similar to

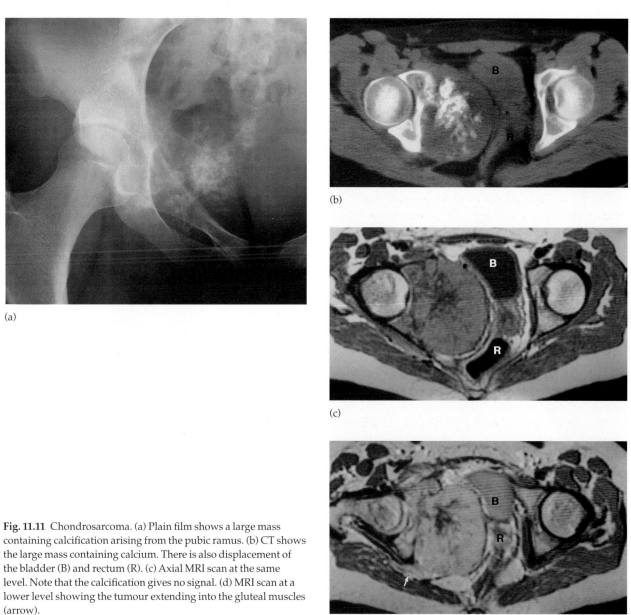

(a)

(b)

(c)

(d)

Fig. 11.11 Chondrosarcoma. (a) Plain film shows a large mass containing calcification arising from the pubic ramus. (b) CT shows the large mass containing calcium. There is also displacement of the bladder (B) and rectum (R). (c) Axial MRI scan at the same level. Note that the calcification gives no signal. (d) MRI scan at a lower level showing the tumour extending into the gluteal muscles (arrow).

tumours, such as fibrous dysplasia and some abnormalities which are difficult to classify, such as osteoid osteoma and Langerhans histiocytosis. Some of these lesions are discussed below. In general, benign lesions have an edge which is well demarcated from the normal bone by a sclerotic rim. They cause expansion but rarely breach the cortex. There is no soft tissue mass and a periosteal reaction is unusual unless there has been a fracture through the lesion.

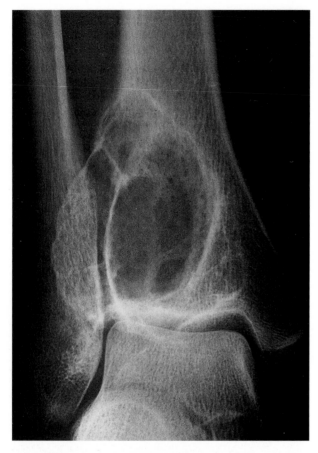

Fig. 11.12 Giant cell tumour. Eccentric expanding lytic lesion which has thinned the cortex crossed by strands of bone. The subarticular position is characteristic of this tumour.

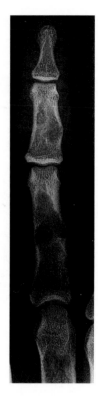

Fig. 11.13 Enchondromas in the metacarpal, proximal and middle phalanges showing lytic areas that expand but do not breach the cortex.

Radionuclide scans in benign tumours usually show little or no increase in activity, provided no fracture has occurred. CT and MRI scanning are rarely needed in the evaluation of benign tumours.

Enchondromas are seen as lytic expanding lesions most commonly in the bones of the hand (Fig. 11.13). They often contain a few flecks of calcium.

Fibrous cortical defects (non-ossifying fibromas) are common chance findings in children and young adults. They produce well-defined lucent areas in the cortex of long bones (Fig. 11.10a, p. 307).

Fibrous dysplasia may affect one or several bones. It occurs most commonly in the long bones and ribs as a lucent area with a well-defined edge and may expand the bone (Fig. 11.10f, p. 309). There may be a sclerotic rim around the lesion.

A *simple bone cyst* has a wall of fibrous tissue and is filled with fluid. It occurs in children and young adults, most commonly in the humerus and femur. Bone cysts form a lucency across the width of the shaft of the bone, with a well-defined edge. The cortex may be thin and the bone expanded (Fig. 11.14). Often, the first clinical feature is a pathological fracture.

Aneurysmal bone cysts are not true neoplasms, but they probably form secondarily to an underlying primary tumour. Mostly they are seen in children and

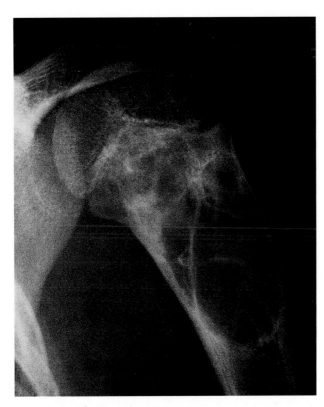

Fig. 11.14 Bone cyst. There is an expanding lesion crossed by strands of bone in the upper end of the humerus in a child. The lesion extends to but does not cross the epiphyseal plate.

young adults in the spine, long bones or pelvis. These lesions are purely lytic and cause massive expansion of the cortex, hence the name 'aneurysmal'. They may grow quickly and appear very aggressive but are nevertheless benign lesions. CT and MRI may show the blood pools within the cyst. The major differential diagnosis is from giant-cell tumour.

An *osteoid osteoma* is a painful condition found most commonly in the femur and tibia in young adults. It has a characteristic radiological appearance: a small lucency, sometimes with central specks of calcification, known as a nidus, surrounded by dense sclerotic rim. A periosteal reaction may also be present (Fig. 11.15). CT shows these features to advantage and osteoid osteomas can also be shown

by MRI. An important imaging investigation is radio-nuclide bone scanning which shows marked focal increased activity. Radionuclide bone scanning is particularly useful when the osteoid osteoma is difficult to see on plain film (Fig. 11.15b and c).

Eosinophil granuloma is the mildest and most frequent form of Langerhans histiocytosis (previously referred to as histiocytosis X). It occurs in children and young adults and produces lytic lesions which may be single or multiple, most frequently in the skull, pelvis, femur and ribs. Extensive lesions may be seen giving rise to the so-called 'geographic skull' (see Fig. 15.9, p. 395). Long bone lesions show bone destruction which may be well defined or ill defined and may have a sclerotic rim. A periosteal reaction is sometimes seen.

Osteomyelitis

Osteomyelitis is most often caused by *Staphylococcus aureus* and usually affects infants and children. The initial radiographs are normal as bone changes are not visible until 10–14 days after the onset of the infection but the ^{99m}Tc radionuclide bone scan shows increased uptake after two to three days. Radionuclide-labelled white cells can be used for confirmation. Increased activity on the early (blood pool) images of a radionuclide bone scan occurs in cellulitis as well as in osteomyelitis, reflecting the hyperaemia common to both conditions. However, the delayed images are normal with cellulitis but show persistent increased activity if osteomyelitis is present (Fig. 11.16).

Typically, acute osteomyelitis affects the metaphysis of a long bone, usually the femur or tibia. The earliest signs on plain radiographs are soft tissue swelling and bone destruction in the metaphysis with a periosteal reaction that eventually may become very extensive and surround the bone to form an involucrum (Fig. 11.17b). A part of the original bone may die and form a separate dense fragment known as a sequestrum (Fig. 11.17c). A recent development is the use of ultrasound which can demonstrate subperiosteal collections of pus well before bone changes are evident on plain film. Magnetic resonance imaging also shows the changes early in the course of disease showing evidence of bone oedema and pus accumulation.

In chronic osteomyelitis, the bone becomes thickened and

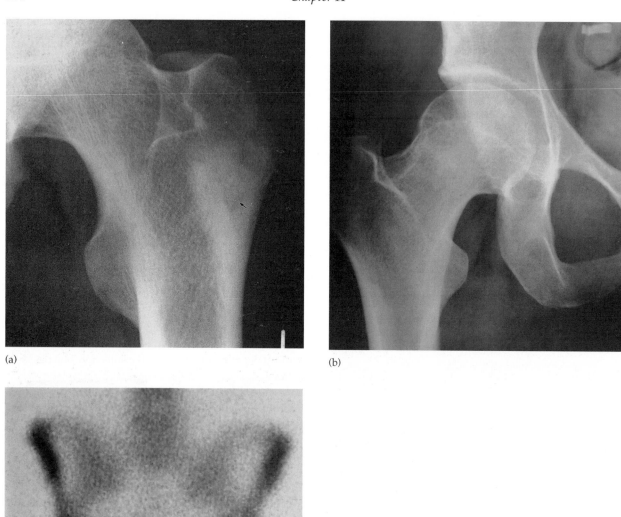

(a)

(b)

(c)

Fig. 11.15 Osteoid osteoma. (a) Typical plain film showing an area of sclerosis in the upper end of the femur containing a central lucency (arrow) known as a nidus. (b) and (c) Osteoid osteoma in neck of femur which is very difficult to see on plain film but is clearly shown as an area of focal high activity (arrow) on radionuclide bone scan.

Fig. 11.17 (*Opposite.*) Osteomyelitis. (a) Initial films reveal no abnormality. (b) Films taken 3 weeks later show some destruction of the upper end of the tibia and an extensive periosteal reaction along the tibia, particularly the medial side (arrow). (c) Late acute osteomyelitis in another young child. The upper part of the humerus has separated to form a sequestrum. It is surrounded by an extensive periosteal reaction to form an involucrum. (d) Chronic osteomyelitis (Brodie's abscess) in a teenager showing a lucency surrounded by substantial sclerosis. A faint periosteal reaction is present (arrow).

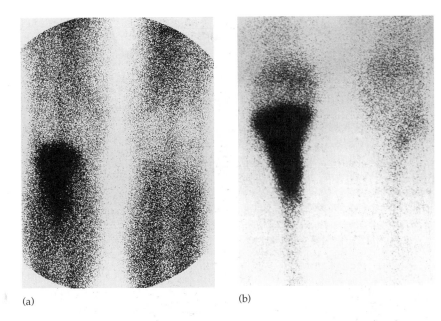

Fig. 11.16 Osteomyelitis. Radionuclide scans of knees. (a) The blood pool scan taken 1 min after injection of radionuclide shows increased uptake in the upper part of the leg due to hyperaemia. (b) The delayed scan taken 3 hours later shows substantially increased uptake in the bone itself.

(a)

(b)

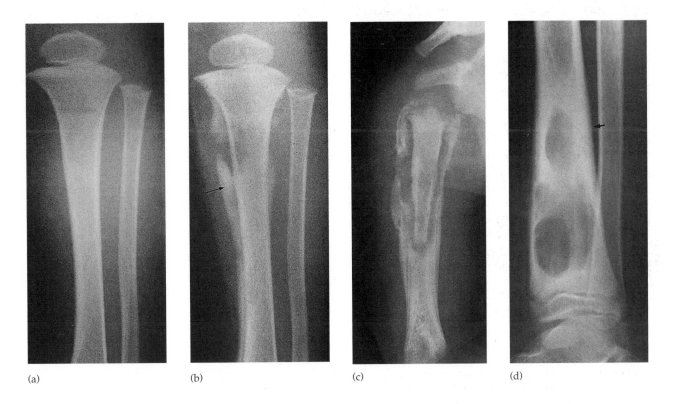

(a)

(b)

(c)

(d)

sclerotic with loss of differentiation between the cortex and the medulla. Within the bone there may be sequestra and areas of bone destruction. This type of lesion is known as a Brodie's abscess (Fig. 11.17d). Computed tomography can be used in selected cases to show sequestra and sinus tracks. Magnetic resonance imaging shows the extent of infection better than plain films or CT, but is rarely necessary.

Tuberculous osteomyelitis is a particular problem in African and Asian populations and is being seen with increased frequency in patients with AIDS. The spine is the most frequent site of infection, followed by the large joints, but any bone may be affected. The disease is relatively indolent and produces large areas of bone destruction which, unlike pyogenic osteomyelitis, may be relatively asymptomatic in the early stages.

Distinction of neoplasm from osteomyelitis

It is not always possible using imaging tests to distinguish osteomyelitis from a bone tumour and biopsy is then needed. The clinical history is clearly important. With malignant bone tumours, the radiographs are usually abnormal when the patient first presents, whereas with osteomyelitis the initial films are often normal. But if early films are not available, difficulties may arise in distinguishing acute osteomyelitis from a highly malignant tumour such as Ewing's tumour or osteosarcoma. Chronic osteomyelitis may simulate a benign bone tumour on imaging examinations, but the presence of fever, and sometimes of discharging sinuses, usually helps to diagnose an infective lesion. Computed tomography and magnetic resonance imaging, are more informative because they show the lesion better, but even with these imaging modalities there can be considerable difficulty deciding between infection and neoplasm.

The ^{99m}Tc bone scan is positive in both osteomyelitis and malignant tumours and cannot be used in differentiation.

Bone infarction

Bone infarction occurs most often in the intra-articular portions of the bones and is therefore described in the chapter on joint disease (p. 342). However, infarcts can occur in the shaft of a bone in several diseases including caisson disease, sickle cell disease or following radiation therapy. Some-

times, they are found incidentally in older people with no known cause. In the acute phase no abnormality is visible, other than a very occasional periosteal reaction. Once healed, they appear as irregular calcification in the medulla of a long bone (Fig. 11.18).

Multiple focal lesions

Metastases

Metastases are by far the commonest malignant bone tumour, outnumbering many times primary tumours. Metastases may be sclerotic, lytic or a mixture of lysis and sclerosis. Those bones containing red marrow are the ones most frequently affected, namely the spine, skull, ribs, pelvis, humeri and femora.

Many tumours metastasize to bone but lytic metastases in adults most commonly arise from a carcinoma of the prostate, breast and bronchus, and in children from neuroblastoma or leukaemia. Lytic metastases give rise to well-defined or ill-defined areas of bone destruction without a sclerotic rim. The lesions vary from small holes to large areas of bone destruction (Fig. 11.19). In the long bones metastases usually arise in the medulla and as they grow they enlarge and destroy the cortex. Metastases and myeloma are virtually the only causes of multiple obvious lytic lesions in bone.

Sclerotic metastases appear as ill-defined areas of increased density of varying size with ill-defined margins. In men, they are most commonly due to metastases from carcinoma of the prostate (Fig. 11.20), and in women from carcinoma of the breast.

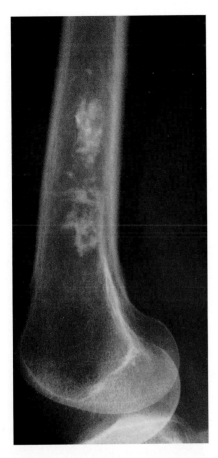

Fig. 11.18 Bone infarct. There is calcification in the medulla of the lower end of the femur.

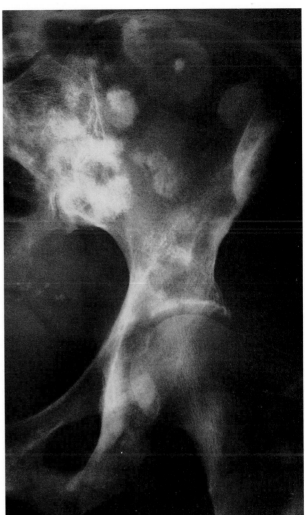

Fig. 11.20 Sclerotic metastases showing scattered areas of increased density.

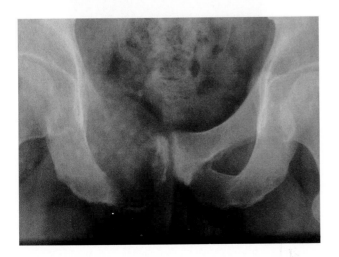

Fig. 11.19 Metastasis from a carcinoma of the kidney causing a large area of bone destruction with an ill-defined edge in the right superior and inferior pubic rami.

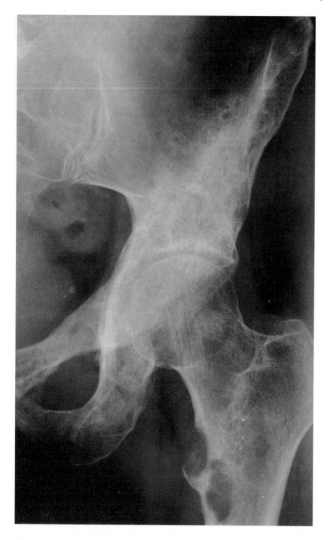

Fig. 11.21 Multiple metastases from carcinoma of the breast showing both lytic and sclerotic areas.

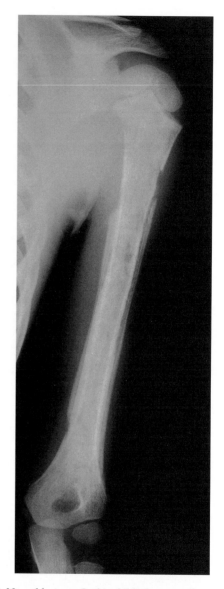

Fig. 11.22 Neuroblastoma. In this child's humerus there are several lytic areas and a florid periosteal reaction.

Mixed lytic and sclerotic metastases are not uncommon. They are often seen with carcinoma of the breast (Fig. 11.21).

A periosteal reaction is uncommon with metastases, except in neuroblastoma (Fig. 11.22).

A radionuclide bone scan is much more sensitive for detecting metastases than plain films. Not only are more lesions detected, it is also an easier examination for the patient than a radiographic skeletal survey, which involves taking numerous films. Approximately 30% of metastases seen on a bone scan will not be visible on plain films. Increased radionuclide uptake in a patient with a known primary tumour but normal bone radiographs suggests metastases. If numerous areas of increased activity are seen

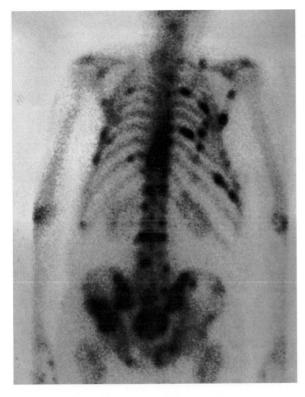

Fig. 11.23 Metastases. Radionuclide bone scan showing numerous discrete areas of increased uptake in bones.

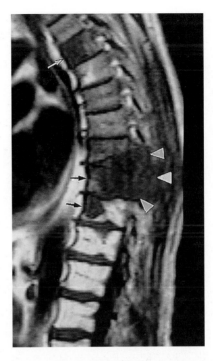

Fig. 11.24 Metastases from carcinoma of the prostate. Sagittal MRI scan showing low signal intensity in several vertebral bodies (arrows). Note the metastases also involve the posterior elements of two adjacent vertebrae (arrow heads).

in a patient with a known primary carcinoma, then the diagnosis of metastases is virtually certain (Fig. 11.23). If only one or a few areas of increased activity are present, radiographs will be needed to exclude the possibility of a benign condition such as degenerative change or fracture being responsible for the increased uptake of the radionuclide. If the bone scan is normal, it is most unlikely that radiographs will show metastases.

Radionuclide bone scanning can be used to examine the whole skeleton with one procedure whereas a skeletal survey using MRI is more time-consuming and very expensive. This means that MRI is only used in selected cases, even though MRI is better than radionuclide scanning for the detection of metastases (Fig. 11.24). Computed tomography has little to offer for detecting metastases as it is less sensitive than MRI and is unsuitable for surveying large portions of the skeleton.

Multiple myeloma

Although myeloma deposits may be found in any bone, they are most frequently seen in bones with active haemopoiesis. The bone lesions may resemble lytic metastases in every way (Fig. 11.25) but are often better defined and may cause expansion of the bone. Diffuse marrow involvement may give rise to generalized loss of bone density, producing a picture similar to that of osteoporosis.

Most myeloma deposits show increased activity on radionuclide bone scans. In some instances, however, even large areas of bone destruction, which are clearly visible on plain radiographs, show no abnormality on the scan. Nevertheless, it is rare for all the lesions in a particular

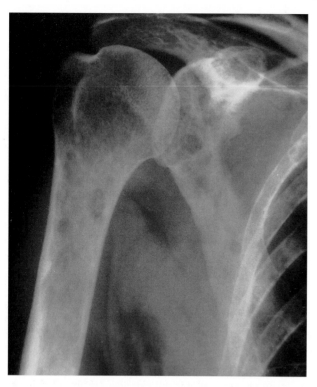

Fig. 11.25 Myeloma deposits causing multiple well-defined lytic lesions.

patient to be invisible, so bone scanning is still used for survey purposes, with radiographic skeletal surveys held in reserve. The limited role of CT and MRI for detecting metastases applies also to multiple myeloma.

Malignant lymphoma and leukaemia

Malignant lymphoma involving bone may give rise to lesions closely resembling metastases on all imaging modalities (Fig. 11.8c, p. 305).

Bone involvement in acute leukaemia in children is not uncommon. Leukaemic deposits produce ill-defined permeative bone destruction, mostly in the metaphyseal regions. Bone lesions are very rare in adult leukaemias.

Multiple periosteal reactions

Multiple periosteal reactions are seen in conjunction with other signs in:
- non-accidental injury;
- widespread bone infection, e.g. congenital syphilis, neonates with infected intravenous catheters;
- venous stasis and ulceration of the legs, where low-grade periosteal reaction and cortical thickening of the tibia and fibula may be encountered;
- hypertrophic pulmonary osteoarthropathy. In this condition, there is widespread periosteal reaction around the bones of the forearms and lower legs which, when severe, extends to involve the hands and feet (Fig. 11.26). Finger clubbing is invariably present. Hypertrophic pulmonary osteoarthropathy is seen in a number of conditions, mostly intrathoracic, of which carcinoma of the bronchus is by far the commonest;
- scurvy.

Generalized decrease in bone density (osteopenia)

The radiographic density of bone is dependent on the amount of calcium present in the bones. Calcium content may be reduced due to a disorder of calcium metabolism, as in osteomalacia or hyperparathyroidism, or to a reduction in protein matrix, as in osteoporosis. The radiological diagnosis of decreased bone density is often difficult, especially as the appearances of the bones are markedly affected by radiographic exposure factors.

The main causes of generalized decrease in bone density are:
- osteoporosis;
- osteomalacia;
- hyperparathyroidism;
- multiple myeloma, which may cause generalized loss of bone density, with or without focal bone destruction.

Each of these conditions may have other radiological features that enable the diagnosis to be made, but when they are lacking, as they frequently are in osteoporosis and osteomalacia, it becomes very difficult to distinguish between them radiologically.

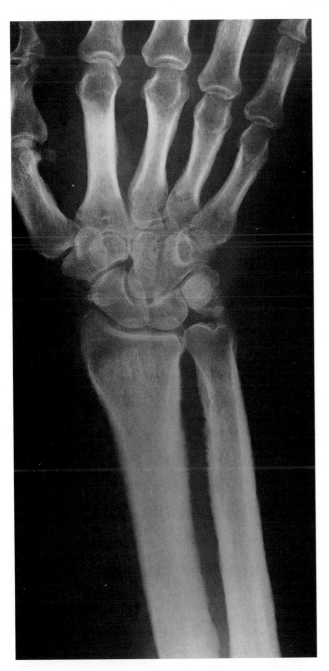

Fig. 11.26 Hypertrophic pulmonary osteoarthropathy. There is a periosteal reaction which was present bilaterally along the shafts of the radius and ulna and the metacarpals. In this case it was associated with a bronchial carcinoma.

Osteoporosis

Osteoporosis is the consequence of a deficiency of protein matrix (osteoid). The remaining bone is normally mineralized and appears normal histologically, but because the matrix is reduced in quantity there is necessarily a reduction in calcium content. Osteoporosis predisposes to fractures, particularly of the vertebral bodies and hips.

The more frequent causes of osteoporosis are:
• idiopathic, often subdivided according to age of onset, e.g. juvenile, postmenopausal, senile; postmenopausal and senile osteoporosis are the commonest forms: up to 50% of women over 60 years of age have osteoporosis;
• Cushing's syndrome and steroid therapy;
• disuse.

A radiological diagnosis of osteoporosis is only made after other diseases have been excluded. Bone destruction, which could indicate metastatic carcinoma or myeloma, and evidence of hyperparathyroidism and osteomalacia should be sought, because these conditions can closely resemble osteoporosis.

The changes of osteoporosis are best seen in the spine (Fig. 11.27). Although there is an overall decrease in bone density the cortex stands out clearly, as if pencilled in. An important feature is collapse of the vertebral bodies, representing compression fractures, which result in the vertebral bodies appearing wedged or biconcave. Several vertebrae may be involved and the disc spaces often appear widened.

The long bones have thin cortices. Many of the trabeculae are resorbed but those that remain stand out clearly.

Disuse osteoporosis can be caused by localized pain or immobilization of a fracture (Fig. 11.28). Besides a reduction in density and thinning of the cortex, the bone may sometimes have a spotty appearance.

Sudeck's atrophy (reflex sympathetic dystrophy syndrome) is a disorder of the sympathetic nervous system comprising severe osteoporosis and oedema of the soft tissues following a fracture. The degree of osteoporosis is disproportionate to the trauma or the degree of disuse.

Screening for osteoporosis

Because osteoporosis is such a prevalent problem and, once established, is difficult to treat, attempts have been made to develop screening tests for the at-risk population in order

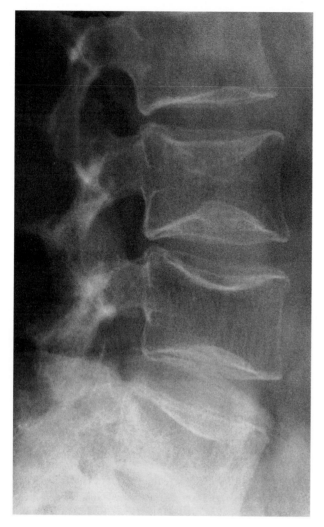

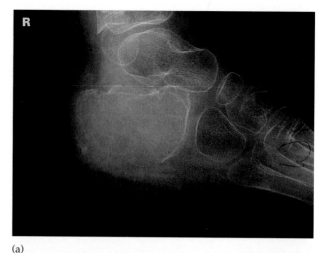

(a)

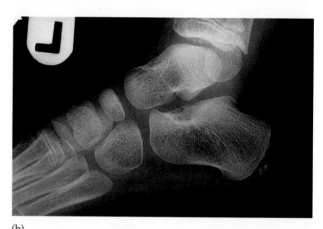

(b)

Fig. 11.27 Senile osteoporosis. There is decreased bone density but the edge of the vertebral bodies are well demarcated. Note the partial collapse of several of the vertebral bodies and the widening of the disc spaces.

Fig. 11.28 (a) Disuse osteoporosis due to osteomyelitis of the right calcaneum. The calcaneum is partly destroyed by infection. The remaining bones of the right foot show a marked reduction in bone density with well-defined cortex. Compare these bones with those in the normal left foot (b).

to institute preventive treatment, e.g. hormone replacement therapy. Bone mass may be measured by dual energy x-ray absorption, often abbreviated to DEXA, or quantitative computed tomography (QCT). Although bone density can be accurately and reproducibly measured, it is not yet clear how useful bone densitometry will prove to be in selecting patients for preventive therapy on a population-wide basis.

Rickets and osteomalacia

In these conditions there is poor mineralization of osteoid. If this occurs before epiphyseal closure, the condition is known as rickets – in adults the condition is known as osteomalacia.

The main causes of rickets and osteomalacia are:
1 Dietary deficiency of vitamin D, or lack of exposure to

sunlight, resulting in decreased production of endogeneous vitamin D.

2 Malabsorption, resulting in impaired absorption of calcium or vitamin D.

3 Renal disease, where rickets develops despite normal amounts of vitamin D in the diet, hence the term 'vitamin D-resistant rickets':

- tubular defects: hypophosphataemia, Fanconi syndrome and renal tubular acidosis
- chronic renal failure: impaired ability to activate vitamin D.

Regardless of the cause of the osteomalacia or rickets, the bone changes are similar. When it is due to chronic renal failure, the changes of hyperparathyroidism may also be present.

In *rickets* the changes are maximal where bone growth is occurring, so they are best seen at the knees, wrists and ankles. The zone of provisional calcification is deficient and the metaphyses are irregularly mineralized, widened and cupped (Fig. 11.29). This results in an increased distance between the visible epiphysis and the calcified portion of the metaphysis. The generalized decrease in bone density, however, may not be very obvious. Deformities of the bones occur because the undermineralized bone is soft. Greenstick fractures are common.

In *osteomalacia* the characteristic features are loss of bone density, thinning of the trabeculae and the cortex, and Looser's zones (pseudofractures) (Fig. 11.30a). Looser's zones are short lucent bands running through the cortex at right-angles, usually going only part way across the bone. They may have a sclerotic margin making them more obvious. They are commonest in the scapulae, medial aspects of the femoral necks and in the pubic rami.

Bone deformity, consequent upon bone softening, is an important feature. In the spine, the vertebral bodies are biconcave (Fig. 11.30b), the femora may be bowed and in severe cases the side walls of the pelvis may bend inwards, giving the so-called 'triradiate pelvis'.

Hyperparathyroidism

Excess parathyroid hormone secretion mobilizes calcium from the bones, resulting in a decrease in bone density.

Hyperparathyroidism may be primary, from hyperplasia or a tumour of the parathyroid glands, or secondary to

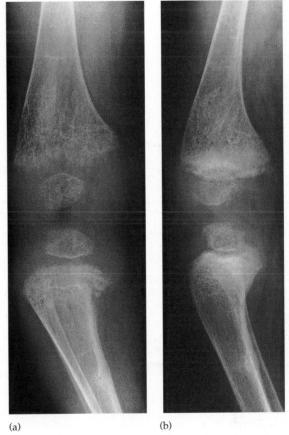

(a)   (b)

Fig. 11.29 (a) Rickets. Dietary rickets showing widening and irregular mineralization of the metaphyses which have a frayed appearance. There is reduced bone density and bowing of the limbs. (b) After commencement of vitamin D treatment mineralization of the metaphyses has occurred.

chronic renal failure (see next section on renal osteodystrophy).

Many patients with primary hyperparathyroidism present with renal stones and only a small minority have bone changes radiologically.

The signs of hyperparathyroidism in the bones are:

- A generalized loss of bone density, with loss of the differentiation between cortex and medulla. The trabecular pattern may have a fine lacework appearance. With advanced disease there may be marked deformity of the skeleton.

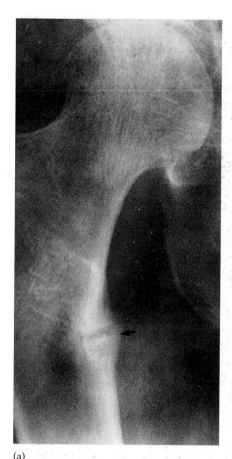

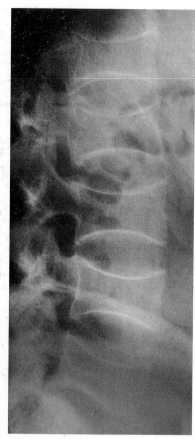

(a)   (b)

Fig. 11.30 Osteomalacia. (a) Looser's zone showing the horizontal lucent band with sclerotic margins running through the cortex of the medial side of the upper femur (arrow). (b) There is decreased bone density and partial collapse of all the vertebral bodies to approximately the same extent.

• The hallmark of hyperparathyroidism is subperiosteal bone resorption (Fig. 11.31a), which occurs particularly in the hands on the radial side of the middle phalanges and at the tips of the terminal phalanges. There may be also be resorption of the outer ends of the clavicles.
• Soft tissue calcification, vascular calcification and chondrocalcinosis sometimes occur.
• Brown tumours are occasionally present. These are lytic lesions, which may be single or multiple. They are of varying size and may expand the bone. They occur most commonly in the mandible and pelvis but any bone may be involved (Fig. 11.31b).

The bone changes in primary and secondary hyperparathyroidism are similar except that 'brown tumours' are much rarer and vascular calcification is commoner in secondary hyperparathyroidism.

Renal osteodystrophy

Three distinct bone lesions can occur, often together, in patients with chronic renal failure:
1 osteomalacia in adults; rickets in children;
2 hyperparathyroidism;
3 sclerosis, an infrequent feature. It may be seen in the spine as bands across the upper and lower ends of the vertebral bodies, giving the so-called 'rugger jersey' spine (Fig. 11.32) or at the metaphyses of the long bones.

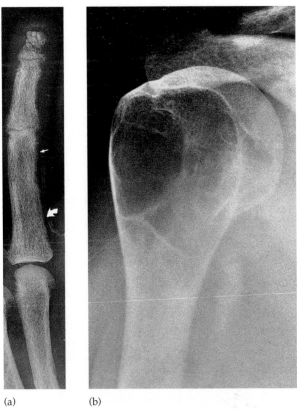

(a)   (b)

Fig. 11.31 Hyperparathyroidism. (a) Note the characteristic features of subperiosteal bone resorption (straight arrow), resorption of the tip of the terminal phalanx and the altered bone architecture. Arterial calcification is also present (curved arrow). (b) Brown tumour. There is a lytic area in the upper end of the humerus with a well-defined edge.

Generalized increase in bone density

Several conditions can cause a generalized increase in bone density, including:

• *Sclerotic metastases*, particularly from prostatic or breast carcinoma. These may affect the skeleton diffusely (Fig. 11.33).

• *Osteopetrosis (marble bone disease)*. In this congenital disorder of bone formation the bones are densely sclerotic (Fig. 11.34). The bones are brittle and may fracture readily but if fractured they heal easily.

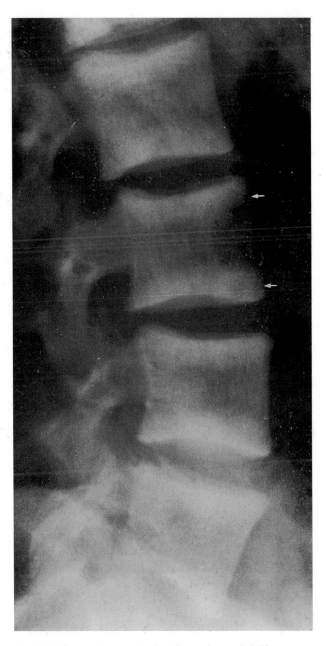

Fig. 11.32 Rugger jersey spine (renal osteodystrophy). There are sclerotic bands running across the upper and lower ends of the vertebral bodies of the lumbar spine (arrows).

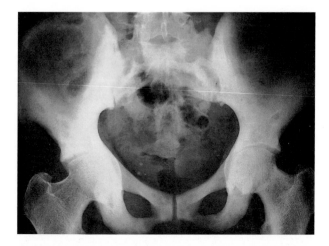

Fig. 11.33 Metastases from carcinoma of the breast causing a widespread increase in bone density.

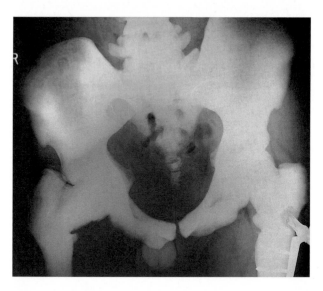

Fig. 11.34 Osteopetrosis. There is a marked generalized increased bone density affecting all bones. There are multiple healed fractures, with a pin and plate in the left femur.

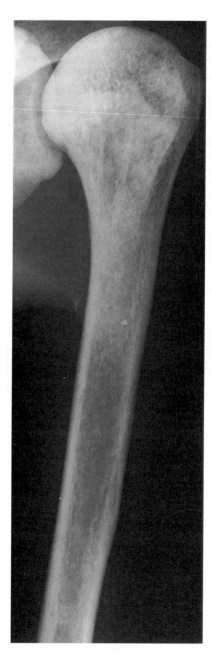

Fig. 11.35 Myelosclerosis. Patchy increase in bone density in the humerus is seen. In this condition the bone marrow becomes replaced with bone.

• *Myelosclerosis* is a form of myelofibrosis in which, in addition to the replacement of bone marrow by fibrous tissue, the process extends to lay down extratrabecular bone, usually in a rather patchy fashion (Fig. 11.35). The spleen is invariably enlarged because it becomes the site of haemopoiesis. It may reach a very large size and forms an important sign on abdominal radiographs.

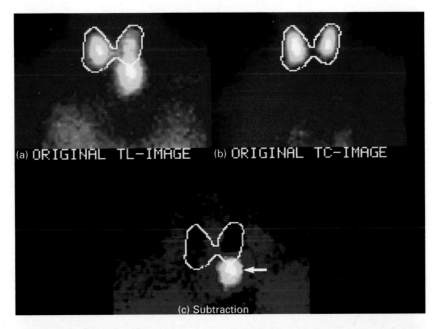

Plate 6 Parathyroid adenoma. (a) Thallium scan. Uptake occurs in the parathyroid adenoma and in the thyroid gland. (b) Pertechnetate scan. The pertechnetate is taken up by the thyroid gland and its outline has been drawn in. (c) Subtraction of the pertechnetate from the thallium scan reveals uptake in the parathyroid adenoma (arrow).

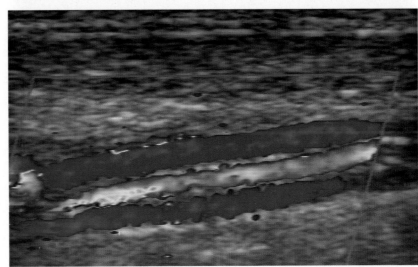

Plate 7 Doppler ultrasound of normal calf veins. The veins, shown in blue, lie on either side of the posterior tibial artery, shown in red.

Alteration of trabecular pattern

Paget's disease

The incidence of Paget's disease varies greatly from country to country, being common in the UK but rare in the USA. It is usually a chance finding in an elderly patient. One or more bones may be affected, the usual sites being the pelvis, spine, skull and long bones. Bone softening causes bowing and deformity of the bones and basilar invagination in the skull. Pathological fractures may also occur (Fig. 14.19, p. 386).

Although there is a rare lytic form of Paget's disease, e.g. osteoporosis circumscripta of the skull, the cardinal features are thickening of the trabeculae and of the cortex, leading to loss of corticomedullary differentiation and increased bone density, together with enlargement of the affected bone (Fig. 11.36).

In the skull there are many circumscribed areas of sclerosis scattered in the skull vault giving a mottled appearance which has been likened to cotton wool. An increased thickness of the calvarium is a particularly obvious feature (Fig. 15.12, p. 396).

These changes of sclerosis, cortical thickening, coarse trabeculae and most particularly, increase in the size of the bone, distinguish Paget's disease from metastases due to prostatic or breast carcinoma, which are also common in the elderly.

Malignant degeneration, with development of an osteosarcoma in abnormal bone, is an occasional occurrence (Fig. 11.37).

There is greatly increased uptake of radionuclide at bone scanning in bones involved by Paget's disease (Fig. 11.38), which can be useful to define the extent of disease and response to treatment. Perhaps more importantly, it should be realized that Paget's disease may mimic tumours on radionuclide bone scans as well as on plain radiographs.

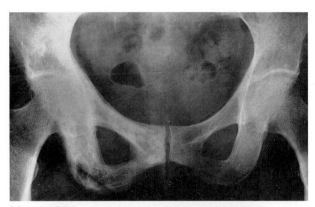

(a)

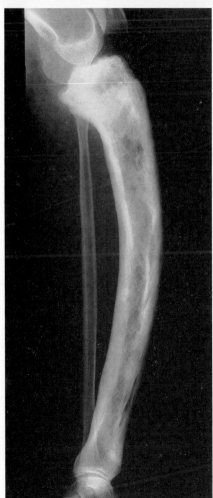

(b)

Fig. 11.36 (a) Paget's disease showing typical sclerosis with coarse trabeculae in the right pubic and ischial rami. Note that the width of the affected bones is increased. (b) Similar signs in the tibia of another patient. Note the bowing of the bone from softening.

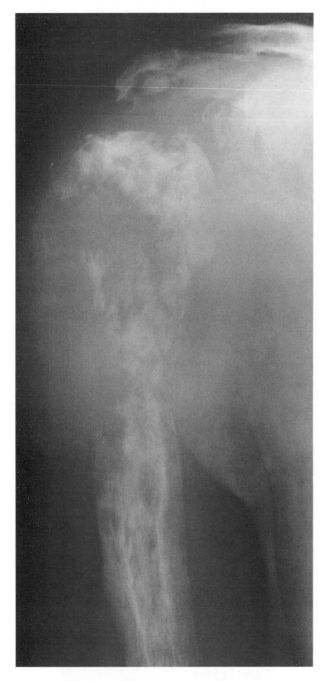

Fig. 11.37 Sarcoma in Paget's disease. There is extensive bone destruction in the humeral head and shaft. Evidence of the underlying Paget's disease can be seen.

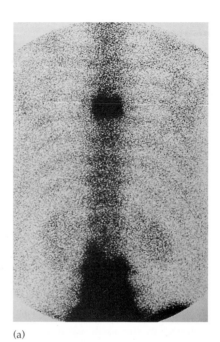

(a)

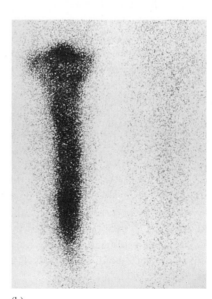

(b)

Fig. 11.38 Paget's disease. Radionuclide bone scan showing increased uptake in (a) a midthoracic vertebra, several lower lumbar vertebrae, the iliac bones and (b) the right tibia. Note the resemblance to metastases. Also note that individual lesions, e.g. in the spine, are indistinguishable from malignant neoplasm.

Haemolytic anaemia

There are several types of haemolytic anaemia but radiological changes are seen in two main types: thalassaemia and sickle-cell disease. Both show changes of marrow hyperplasia, but sickle-cell anaemia may also show evidence of bone infarction and infection.

Marrow hyperplasia

Overactivity and expansion of the bone marrow causes thinning of the cortex and resorption of some of the trabeculae so that those that remain are thickened and stand out more clearly. In the skull, there is widening of the diploë and there may be perpendicular striations giving an appearance known as 'hair-on-end' (Fig. 11.39a). The ribs may enlarge and the phalanges may become rectangular (Fig. 11.39b).

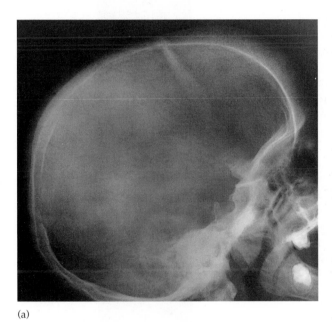

(a)

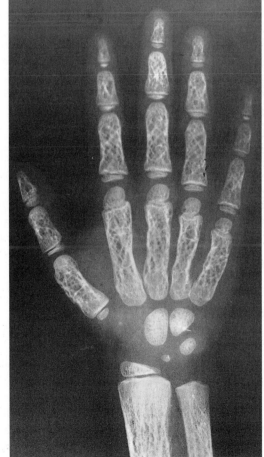

(b)

Fig. 11.39 Haemolytic anaemia – thalassaemia. (a) Skull showing thickened diploë. (b) Hand. Due to marrow expansion the bones are expanded and those trabeculae that remain are very thickened.

Infarction and infection

Infarction at bone ends causes flattening and sclerosis of the humeral and femoral heads.

Areas of bone destruction with periosteal new bone formation, or just a periosteal reaction, may be seen in the shafts of the bones. These signs are due to bone infarction. It is not possible to determine from the radiographs whether or not these infarcts are infected.

Sarcoidosis

Sarcoidosis occasionally involves the bones. The phalanges of the hands and feet are virtually the only bones affected. The signs are either small cysts with a well-defined edge or areas of bone destruction showing a lace-like pattern (Fig. 11.40). If the bones are involved, there is invariably evidence of sarcoidosis in the chest and sarcoid skin lesions are usually present.

Radiation-induced disease of bone

Radiotherapy may damage bones in the radiation field or may induce a bone neoplasm. Early change may be limited to osteoporosis. In severe cases, the bone thins and shows patchy increased density with small lytic areas. Pathological fracture is a serious complication. The commonest sites are in the ribs following radiotherapy for breast cancer and in the pelvis or femora following treatment for cervical carcinoma.

Changes in bone shape

Bone dysplasias

Bone dysplasias are congenital disorders resulting in abnormalities in the size and shape of the bones. There are a large number of different dysplasias; many of them are hereditary and all of them are rare. Only two examples will be mentioned here: achondroplasia and diaphyseal aclasia. Osteopetrosis has been described on p. 325.

In *achondroplasia* there is defective ossification of the bones formed in cartilage. The condition results in dwarfism characterized by shortening of the shafts of the long bones (Fig. 11.41) and the pelvis is contracted.

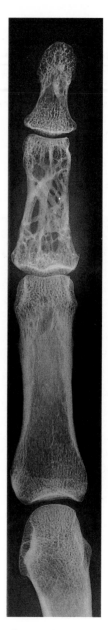

Fig. 11.40 Sarcoidosis, showing the characteristic lace-like trabecular pattern in the middle phalanx.

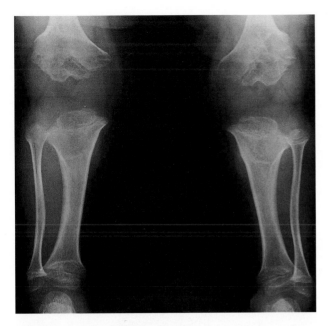

Fig. 11.41 Achondroplasia. This child shows shortening of the bones with expansion of the metaphyses.

In *diaphyseal aclasia (multiple exostoses)* there are multiple bony projections known as osteochondromas or exostoses. They have a cartilagenous cap which may contain calcification. When osteochondromas occur on the long bones they are near the metaphyses and are directed away from the joint (Fig. 11.42).

Occasionally, a chondrosarcoma may develop in the cartilage cap. This should be suspected if there is either rapid growth, an ill-defined edge to the bone, or extensive calcification extending into the soft tissues.

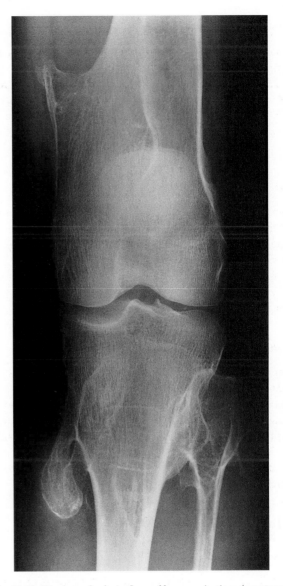

Fig. 11.42 Diaphyseal aclasia. Several bony projections (exostoses) are seen arising around the knee, directed away from the joint. The opposite knee was similarly affected.

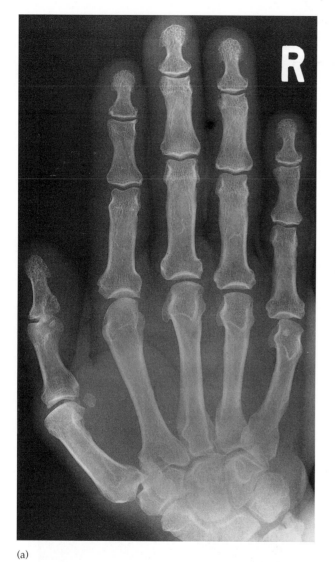

(a)

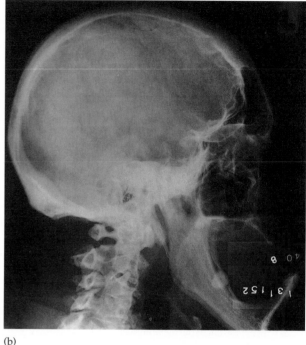

(b)

Fig. 11.43 Acromegaly. (a) The hand is large with prominent tufts to the terminal phalanges. There is widening of metacarpophalangeal joint spaces from overgrowth of articular cartilage. (b) Note the enlarged pituitary fossa, thickened skull vault, large frontal sinuses and prognathous jaw.

Acromegaly

In acromegaly, the bone and soft tissue overgrowth is maximal in the hands, feet and face. The tufts of the terminal phalanges enlarge and overgrowth of the articular cartilage in the hands and feet results in widened joint spaces. The outline of the bones becomes irregular (Fig. 11.43a). The changes, however, may be difficult to differentiate from a normal hand in a manual worker.

In the skull, the pituitary fossa is frequently enlarged by the growth hormone-secreting adenoma responsible for the excess growth hormone. The skull vault may be thickened and the sinuses and mastoid air cells enlarged (Fig. 11.43b). A typical feature is the prognathous jaw with an increase in the angle between the body and ramus of the mandible.

12

Joints

Imaging techniques

The *plain film* examination remains important for imaging joint disease (Fig. 12.1), but MRI is being used with increasing frequency to show meniscal and ligamentous tears in the knee, rotator cuff tears of the shoulder and avascular necrosis of the hip.

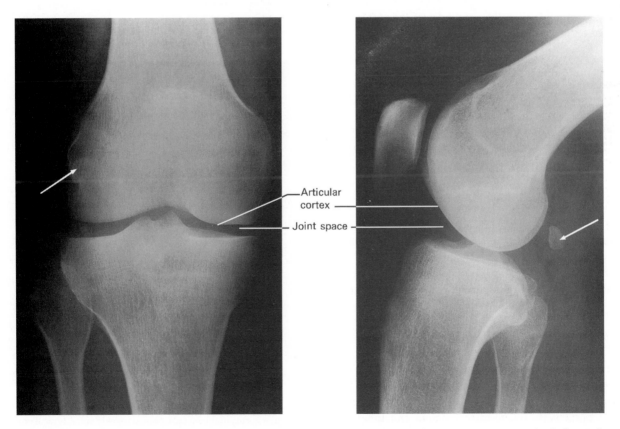

Fig. 12.1 Normal knee joint. Note the fabella (arrow), a sesamoid bone in the gastrocnemius. The 'joint space' consists of articular cartilage and synovial fluid.

Arthrography involves injecting contrast medium into the joint space directly and taking plain films or CT scans. The main use of arthrography is to demonstrate meniscal tears of the knee and occasionally rotator cuff tears of the shoulder, but it has been largely replaced by MRI.

Plain film signs of joint disease

Synovial joints have articular surfaces covered by hyaline cartilage. Both articular and intra-articular cartilage (such as the menisci in the knee) are of the same radiodensity on plain films as the soft tissues and therefore are not visualized as such; only the space between the adjacent articular cortices can be appreciated (Fig. 12.1). The synovium, synovial fluid and capsule also have the same radiodensity as the surrounding soft tissues and, unless outlined by a plane of fat, cannot be identified as discrete structures. The articular cortex forms a thin, well-defined line which merges smoothly with the remainder of the cortex of the bone.

Signs indicating the presence of an arthritis

Joint space narrowing

Joint space narrowing is due to destruction of articular cartilage. It occurs in practically all forms of joint disease, except avascular necrosis.

Soft tissue swelling

Swelling of the soft tissues around a joint may be seen in any arthritis accompanied by a joint effusion and whenever periarticular inflammation is present. It is, therefore, a feature of inflammatory, and particularly infective, arthritis. Discrete soft tissue swelling around the joints can be seen in gout due to gouty tophi.

Osteoporosis

Osteoporosis of the bones adjacent to joints occurs in many painful conditions. Underuse of the bones seems to be an important mechanism, but is not the only factor. Osteoporosis is particularly severe in rheumatoid and tuberculous arthritis.

Signs that point to the cause of an arthritis

Articular erosions

An erosion is an area of destruction of the articular cortex and the adjacent trabecular bone (Fig. 12.2), usually accompanied by destruction of the articular cartilage. Erosions are easily recognized when seen in profile, but when viewed *en face* the appearances can be confused with a cyst. Oblique views designed to show erosions in profile are often taken.

There are several causes of erosions:

1 Inflammatory overgrowth of the synovium (pannus) which occurs in:
   • rheumatoid arthritis, which is by far the commonest cause of an erosive arthropathy
   • juvenile rheumatoid arthritis (Still's disease)
   • psoriasis
   • Reiter's disease
   • ankylosing spondylitis
   • tuberculosis.

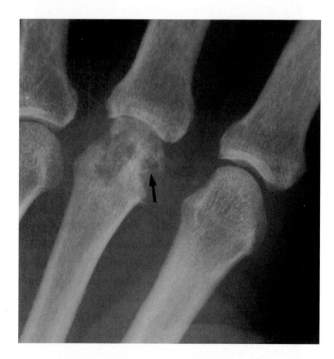

Fig. 12.2 Erosions. Areas of bone destruction are seen affecting the articular cortex of the metacarpophalangeal joint. A typical erosion is arrowed. The joint space is also narrowed.

2 Response to the deposition of urate crystals in gout.
3 Destruction caused by infection:
- pyogenic arthritis.
- tuberculosis.

4 Synovial overgrowth caused by repeated haemorrhage in haemophilia and related bleeding disorders.
5 Neoplastic overgrowth of synovium, e.g. synovial sarcoma.

Osteophytes, subchondral sclerosis and cysts

Osteophytes, subchondral sclerosis and cysts are all features of osteoarthritis. A characteristic increase in the density of subchondral bone is seen in avascular necrosis (see p. 342).

Alteration in the shape of the joint

Several conditions lead to characteristic alterations in the shape or relationship of the bone ends, e.g. slipped epiphysis, congenital dislocation of the hip, osteochondritis dissecans and avascular necrosis in its later stages.

Diagnosis of arthritis

When dealing with an arthritis it is important to have the following information:
1 *Is more than one joint involved?* Certain diseases typically involve several joints, e.g. rheumatoid arthritis, while others rarely do, e.g. infections and synovial tumours.
2 *Which joints are involved?* Many arthropathies have a predilection for certain joints and spare others:
- Rheumatoid arthritis virtually always involves the hands and feet, principally the metacarpo- and metatarsophalangeal joints, the proximal interphalangeal joints and the wrist joints. Psoriatic arthritis usually affects the terminal interphalangeal joints.
- Gout, characteristically involves the metatarsophalangeal joint of the big toe.
- When osteoarthritis is seen in the hands it almost always involves the terminal interphalangeal joints and often affects the carpometacarpal joint of the thumb. In the feet, it is almost always the first metatarsophalangeal joint that is affected. In the large joints, osteoarthritis is common in the hips and knees but relatively rare in the ankle, shoulders and elbows unless there is some underlying deformity or disease.
- The distribution of neuropathic arthritis depends on the neurological deficit; for example, diabetes affects the ankles and feet, whereas syringomyelia affects the shoulders, elbows and hands.

3 *Is a known disease present?* Sometimes an arthritis is part of a known disease, e.g. haemophilia or diabetes.

Rheumatoid arthritis

Rheumatoid arthritis is a polyarthritis caused by inflammatory overgrowth of synovium known as pannus.

The earliest change is periarticular soft tissue swelling and osteoporosis. This osteoporosis is believed to be due to a combination of disuse and synovial hyperaemia. Destruction of the articular cartilage by pannus leads to joint space narrowing. Further destruction leads to small bony erosions which occur, initially, at the joint margins (Fig. 12.3). These erosions are often seen first around the metatarso- or metacarpophalangeal joints, proximal interphalangeal joints and on the styloid process of the ulna. Later, extensive erosions may disrupt the joint surfaces. Ulnar deviation is usually present at this stage. With very severe destruction the condition is referred to as arthritis mutilans (Fig. 12.4).

Similar changes are seen in the large joints (Fig. 12.5). In such cases osteoarthritis may be superimposed on the rheumatoid arthritis and may dominate the picture.

With severe disease, there may be subluxation at the atlantoaxial joint (Fig. 12.6) due to laxity of the transverse ligament which holds the odontoid peg against the anterior arch of the atlas. Atlantoaxial subluxation may only be demonstrable in a film taken with the neck flexed. Even though it is frequently asymptomatic, there is always the possibility of neurological symptoms from compression of the spinal cord by the odontoid process. Atlantoaxial instability can be well demonstrated with MRI.

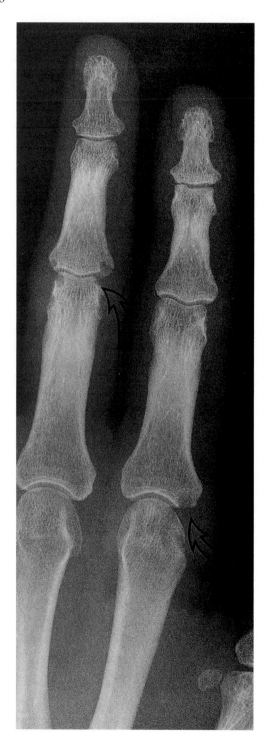

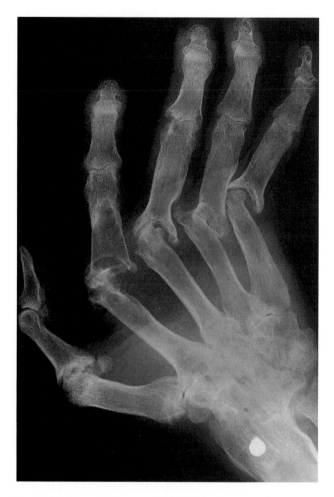

Fig. 12.4 Advanced rheumatoid arthritis (arthritis mutilans). There is extensive destruction of the articular cortex of the metacarpophalangeal joints with ulnar deviation of the fingers. Fusion of the carpal bones and wrist joint has occurred.

Fig. 12.3 (*Left.*) Early rheumatoid arthritis. Small erosions are present in the articular cortex (arrows) and there is soft tissue swelling around the proximal interphalangeal joints.

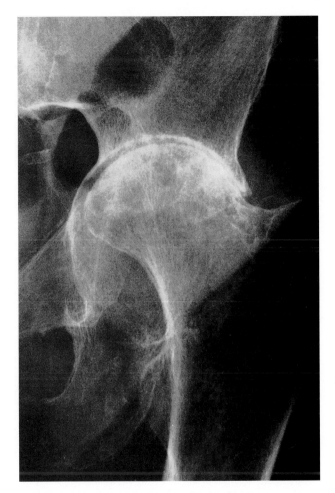

Fig. 12.5 Rheumatoid arthritis. Uniform loss of joint space is seen in this hip joint. Sclerosis is also present due to associated osteoarthritis.

Role of radiology in rheumatoid arthritis

Radiographs assist in the diagnosis of doubtful cases. To this end, the detection of erosions is extremely helpful. A widespread erosive arthropathy is almost diagnostic of rheumatoid arthritis. X-ray films are also useful in assessing the extent of the disease and in observing the response to treatment.

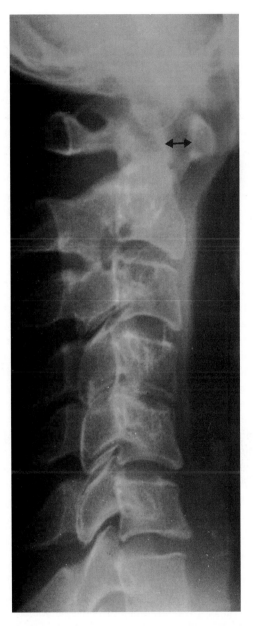

Fig. 12.6 Rheumatoid arthritis – atlantoaxial subluxation. C1 is displaced anteriorly upon C2. The distance between the arch of the atlas and the odontoid peg (arrow) is increased from the normal value (2 mm) to 8 mm. (This is the same patient whose hand is illustrated in Fig. 12.4.)

Other erosive arthropathies

A number of other arthropathies, such as juvenile rheumatoid arthritis, psoriasis and Reiter's disease produce articular erosions.

Juvenile rheumatoid arthritis (Still's disease; juvenile chronic polyarthritis) shows many features similar to rheumatoid arthritis but erosions are less prominent. The knee, ankle and wrist are the joints most commonly affected. Hyperaemia from joint inflammation causes epiphyseal enlargement and premature fusion.

In *psoriasis*, there is an erosive arthropathy with predominant involvement of the terminal interphalangeal joints (Fig. 12.7).

Gout

In gout, the deposition of urate crystals in the joint and in the adjacent bone gives rise to an arthritis which most commonly affects the metatarsophalangeal joint of the big toe.

The earliest change is soft tissue swelling. At a later stage, erosions occur that, unlike rheumatoid arthritis, may be at a distance from the articular cortex. These erosions have a well-defined, often sclerotic, edge and frequently have overhanging edges (Fig. 12.8a). They are due to urate deposits in the bone. These deposits may be very large, causing extensive bony destruction. There is usually no osteoporosis.

Localized soft tissue lumps caused by collections of sodium urate, known as tophi, may occur in the periarticular tissues (Fig. 12.8b). These swellings can be large and occasionally show calcification.

Joint infection

Joint infection is most often due to pyogenic bacterial infection or tuberculosis. Usually only one joint is affected.

Synovial biopsy or examination of the joint fluid is necessary in order to identify the infecting organism.

Pyogenic arthritis

In pyogenic arthritis, which is usually due to *Staphylococcus aureus*, there is rapid destruction of the articular cartilage followed by destruction of the subchondral bone. A pyo-

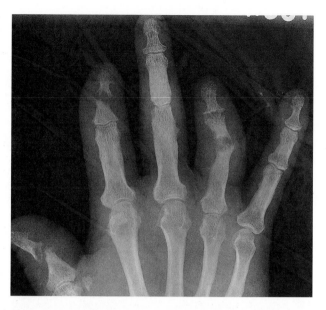

Fig. 12.7 Psoriatic arthropathy. There are extensive erosive changes affecting the interphalangeal joints but sparing the metacarpophalangeal joints.

genic arthritis may occasionally be due to spread of osteomyelitis from the metaphysis into the adjacent joint. Soft tissue swelling around the joint may be visible (Fig. 12.9).

Tuberculous arthritis

An early pathological change is the formation of pannus, which explains why tuberculous arthritis may be radiologically indistinguishable from rheumatoid arthritis. The hip and knee are the most commonly affected peripheral joints. The features to look for are joint space narrowing and erosions, which may lead to extensive destruction of the articular cortex. A very important sign is a striking osteoporosis, which may be seen before any destructive changes are visible (Fig. 12.10).

At a late stage there may be gross disorganization of the joint with calcified debris near the joint.

Haemophilia and bleeding disorders

In haemophilia and Christmas disease repeated haemor-

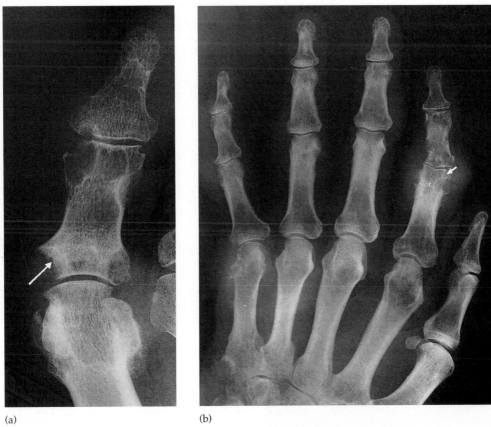

(a) (b)

Fig. 12.8 Gout. (a) Erosion: there is a typical well-defined erosion with an overhanging edge (arrow) at the metatarsophalangeal joint of the big toe. (b) Tophi: these are the large soft tissue swellings. A good example is seen around the proximal interphalangeal joint of the index finger. Several erosions are present (one of these is arrowed).

rhages into the joints result in soft tissue swelling, erosions and cysts in the subchondral bone. The epiphyses may enlarge and fuse prematurely (Fig. 12.11).

Osteoarthritis

Osteoarthritis is the commonest form of arthritis. It is due to degenerative changes resulting from wear and tear of the articular cartilage. The hip and the knee are frequently involved but, despite being a weight-bearing joint, the ankle is infrequently affected. The wrist, joints of the hand and the metatarsophalangeal joint of the big toe are also frequently involved.

In osteoarthritis, a number of features can usually be seen (Fig. 12.12):
• *Joint space narrowing.* The loss of joint space is maximal in the weight-bearing portion of the joint; for example, in the hip it is often maximal in the superior part of the joint, whereas in the knee it is the medial compartment that usually narrows the most. Even when the joint space is very narrow it is usually possible to trace out the articular cortex.
• *Osteophytes* are bony spurs, often quite large, which occur at the articular margins.
• *Subchondral sclerosis* usually occurs on both sides of the joint; it is often worse on one side.

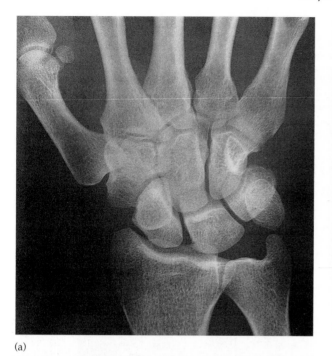

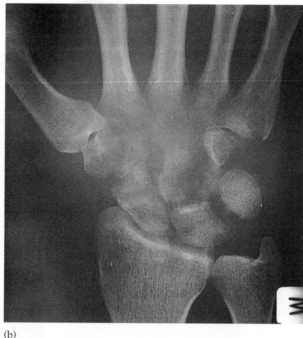

(a)   (b)

Fig. 12.9 Pyogenic arthritis. (a) Initial film of the wrist was normal. (b) Film taken three weeks later shows destruction of the carpal bones and bases of the metacarpals.

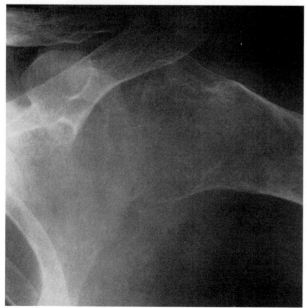

Fig. 12.10 Tuberculous arthritis of the shoulder. Note the striking osteoporosis and erosion of the humeral head.

• *Subchondral cysts* may be seen beneath the articular cortex often in association with subchondral sclerosis. Normally, the cysts are easily distinguished from an erosion as they are beneath the intact cortex and have a sclerotic rim but occasionally, if there is crumbling of the joint surfaces, the differentiation becomes difficult.

• *Loose bodies* are discrete pieces of calcified cartilage or bone lying free within the joint, most frequently seen in the knee. It is important not to call the fabella, a sesamoid bone in the gastrocnemius, a loose body in the knee joint (see Fig. 12.1, p. 333).

Osteoarthritis and rheumatoid arthritis are the two types of arthritis most commonly encountered. They show many distinguishing features which are listed in Table 12.1.

Neuropathic (Charcot) joint

An extreme form of degenerative change develops in neuropathic joints. Typical examples are the shoulder and elbow in syringomyelia and the knee in tabes dorsalis. Complete disorganization with much sclerosis of the surrounding bone may be seen. The joint is often subluxed with bone fragments or calcified debris around it (Fig. 12.13).

A different appearance is seen in the feet of diabetics with peripheral neuropathy and in leprosy. In these conditions, the predominant feature is resorption of the bone ends. Calcification of the arteries in the feet is often present in diabetes. There may also be bone destruction due to infection (Fig. 12.14). Diagnosing osteomyelitis in the bones of the

Table 12.1 Comparison of osteoarthritis and rheumatoid arthritis.

Osteoarthritis	Rheumatoid arthritis
Joint space narrowing maximal at weight-bearing site	Joint space narrowing uniform
Erosions do not occur but crumbling of the joint surfaces may mimic erosions	Erosions a characteristic feature
Subchondral sclerosis and cysts may be seen	Not a feature but erosions *en face* may mimic cysts
Sclerosis is a prominent feature	Sclerosis not a feature unless there is secondary osteoarthritis
No osteoporosis	Osteoporosis often present

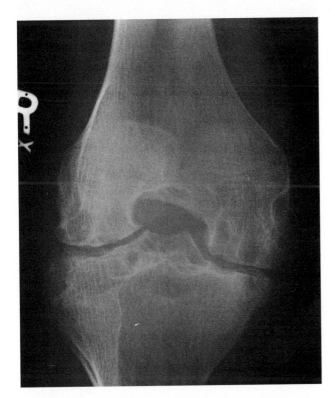

Fig. 12.11 Haemophilia. Subchondral cysts have formed caused by repeated haemorrhages into the joint. Note the soft tissue swelling around the joint and the deep intercondylar notch – a characteristic feature of haemophilia.

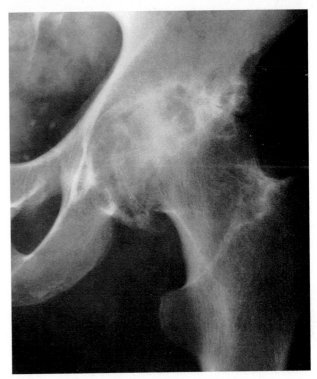

Fig. 12.12 Severe osteoarthritis of the hip. Note the narrowed superior part of the joint space, subchondral sclerosis and cyst formation and osteophytes.

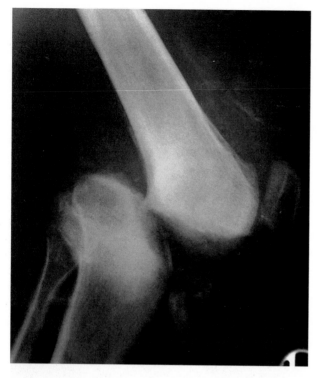

Fig. 12.13 Neuropataic joint. This knee in a patient with tabes dorsalis is grossly disorganized with sclerosis, calcified debris and bone fragments around the joint.

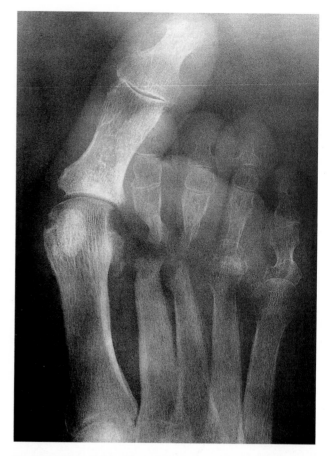

Fig. 12.14 Diabetic foot. There is resorption of the heads of the second and third metatarsals and bases of the proximal phalanges causing disorganization of the metatarsophalangeal joints. The patient had a peripheral neuropathy with an anaesthetic foot.

feet in diabetic patients can be difficult because bone destruction can be due to neuropathy or infection, or to a combination of the two.

Chondrocalcinosis

Chondrocalcinosis is a descriptive term for calcification occurring in articular cartilage. In the knee, which is the most frequently affected joint, calcification may occur in the fibrocartilage of the menisci (Fig. 12.15) as well as the articular cartilage. Chondrocalcinosis is usually due to calcium pyrophosphate deposition disease, which may give rise to an arthritis clinically simulating gout, hence the alternative name 'pseudogout'. A severe arthritis resembling degenerative disease may follow. Chondrocalcinosis may, however, be an incidental asymptomatic finding.

Synovial sarcoma (synovioma)

This tumour appears as a soft tissue mass adjacent to a joint. Bone destruction on one or both sides of the joint occurs at a later stage. The soft tissue mass may contain visible calcification. The diagnosis is most readily made by MRI, which can demonstrate the full extent of the soft tissue mass.

Avascular (aseptic) necrosis

Avascular necrosis occurs most commonly in the intra-articular portions of bones. It is associated with numerous underlying conditions including:

- steroid therapy
- collagen vascular diseases
- radiation therapy
- sickle-cell anaemia
- exposure to high pressure environments, e.g. tunnel workers and deep-sea divers (caisson disease)
- fractures.

The plain radiographic features of avascular necrosis are increased density of the subchondral bone with irregularity of the articular contour or even fragmentation of the bone (Fig. 12.16). A characteristic crescentic lucent line may be seen just beneath the articular cortex. The cartilage space is preserved until secondary degenerative changes supervene. The diagnosis of avascular necrosis may be made with a radionuclide bone scan, but MRI has now become the imaging modality of choice for demonstrating avascular necrosis. The appearances at MRI depend on the stage of disease, but the typical vascular distribution and signal pattern allows a specific diagnosis to be made (Fig. 12.17).

After a *fracture* the blood supply may become interrupted and avascular necrosis may then supervene, particularly in subcapital fractures of the femoral neck (Fig. 12.18) and fractures through the waist of the scaphoid. The femoral head and proximal pole of the scaphoid become fragmented and dense due to the ischaemia.

Osteochondritis

There is also a group of conditions, some of which are called osteochondritis, in which no associated cause for avascular necrosis can be found. The osteochondrites are now regarded as being due to impaired blood supply associated with repeated trauma.

Perthe's disease, an avascular necrosis of the femoral head

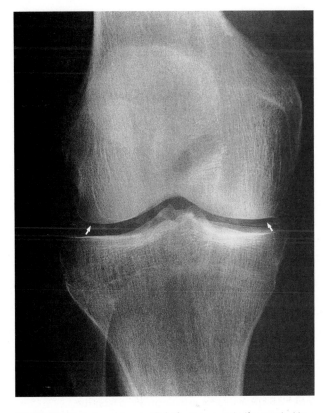

Fig. 12.15 Chondrocalcinosis. Calcification seen in the menisci in the knee (arrows).

in children, is the most important example. The earliest plain radiographic change is increase in density and flattening of the femoral epiphysis which later may progress to collapse and fragmentation (Fig. 12.19). The epiphysis may

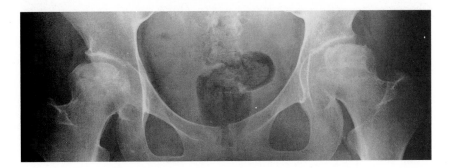

Fig. 12.16 Avascular necrosis. There is fragmentation with some sclerosis of both femoral heads.

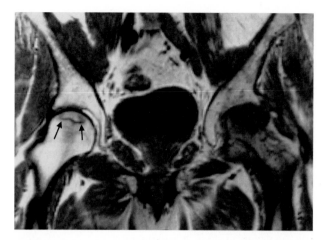

Fig. 12.17 Bilateral avascular necrosis of both femoral heads. Coronal MRI scan. The changes on the left are very severe and advanced. The changes in the right hip are relatively early and show a rim of low signal demarcating the ischaemic area (arrow).

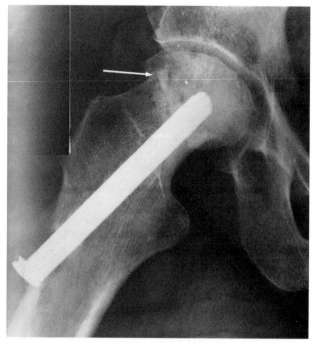

widen and, in consequence, the femoral neck enlarges and may contain small cysts. The joint space is widened but the acetabulum is not affected. With healing, the femoral head reforms but may remain permanently flattened and, therefore, be responsible for osteoarthritis in later life.

Other forms of avascular necrosis are: *Freiberg's disease*,

Fig. 12.18 Post-traumatic avascular necrosis. A pin has been inserted because of a subcapital fracture of the femoral neck (arrow) which occurred 10 months before this film was taken. Avascular necrosis has occurred in the head of the femur which has become sclerotic.

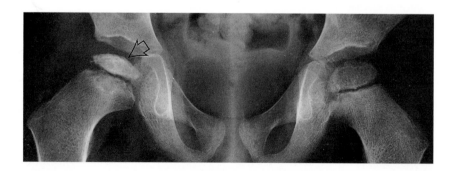

Fig. 12.19 Perthe's disease. The right femoral epiphysis (arrow) in this child is sclerotic and flattened. Compare it with the normal left side.

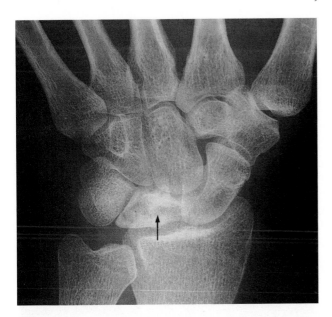

Fig. 12.20 Kienböck's disease. The lunate is flattened and sclerotic (arrow).

which affects the metatarsal heads; *Kohler's disease*, which affects the navicular bone of the foot; *Osgood–Schlatter's disease* of the tibial tuberosity and *Kienböck's disease* of lunate bone in the wrist (Fig. 12.20).

Osteochondritis dissecans is thought to be a localized form of avascular necrosis. A small fragment of bone becomes separated from the articular surface of a joint leaving a defect and the bony fragment can often be detected lying free within the joint. It occurs most frequently in the knee and ankle. The diagnosis can be established with plain film radiography (Fig. 12.21). Computed tomography and MRI are excellent imaging methods to diagnose small lesions or osteochondritis dissecans in portions of the articular bone that are difficult to see in standard plain film projections.

Slipped femoral epiphysis

Slipped femoral epiphysis occurs between the ages of 9 and 17 years and may present with pain in the hip or pain referred to the knee. The epiphysis slips posteriorly from its normal position: this is best appreciated on a lateral film of the hip (Fig. 12.22). With a greater degree of slip the condition can be recognized on the frontal view as a downward displacement of the epiphysis.

The films of the hip must be very carefully evaluated if the diagnosis is suspected clinically, because the diagnosis is easy to miss in the early stage at a time when further slip can be prevented surgically.

Congenital dislocation of the hip

Ultrasound has now replaced x-rays for detecting dislocation or subluxation of the hip in the infant in whom clinical examination is suspicious but not diagnostic. Ultrasound allows visualization of cartilagenous structures which are not seen on x-ray films, so the relationship of the cartilagenous femoral head and acetabulum can be determined.

Later in life, the condition is easier to diagnose on plain radiographs, but fortunately such cases are now rare, since the condition is usually treated in the neonatal period, the diagnosis having been made clinically. The features to look for are lateral and upper displacement of the head of the femur (Fig. 12.23). Increased slope to the acetabular roof is sometimes present.

Osteitis condensans ilii

Osteitis condensans ilii occurs almost exclusively in women who have borne children. The condition is thought to be a stress phenomenon associated with childbearing and is usually asymptomatic. There is a zone of sclerosis on the iliac side of the sacroiliac joints, but the sacroiliac joints themselves are normal (Fig. 12.24).

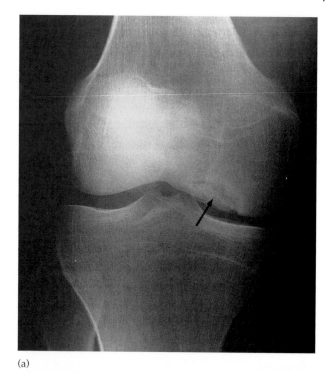

(a)

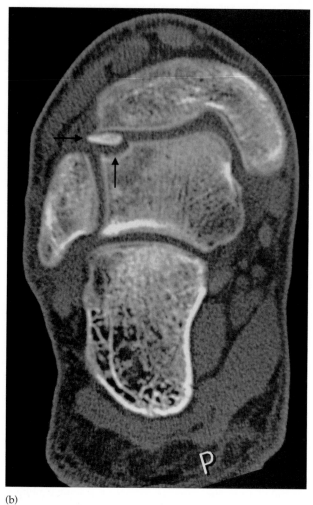

(b)

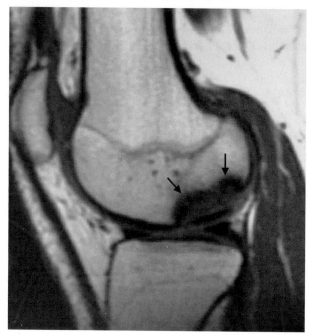

(c)

Fig. 12.21 Osteochondritis dissecans. (a) A fragment (arrow) has become separated from the articular cortex of the medial femoral condyle. (b) Coronal CT scan through an ankle showing small osteochondritis dissecans fragment (horizontal arrow) separated from the rest of the talus with a well-corticated defect in the underlying bone (vertical arrow). (c) MRI scan of the knee showing an osteochondritis defect (arrows) of the medial femoral condyle.

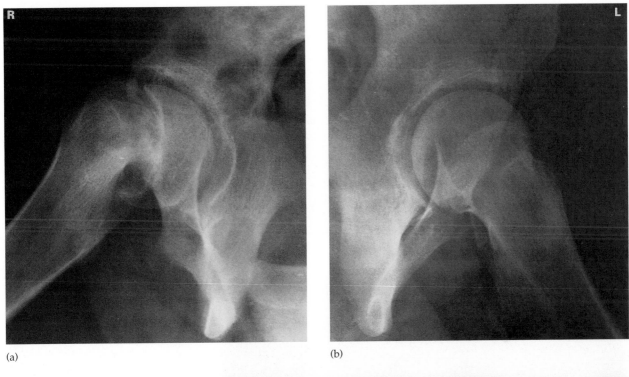

(a)

(b)

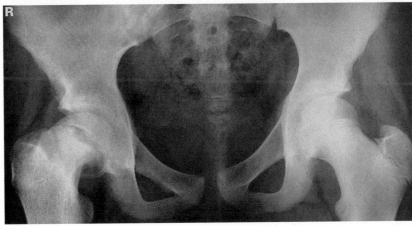

Fig. 12.22 Slipped femoral epiphysis.
(a) and (b) Lateral view of the hips
showing the right femoral epiphysis
displaced posteriorly (compare with the
normal left side). (c) Frontal view of same
patient showing the right femoral
epiphysis displaced downwards.

(c)

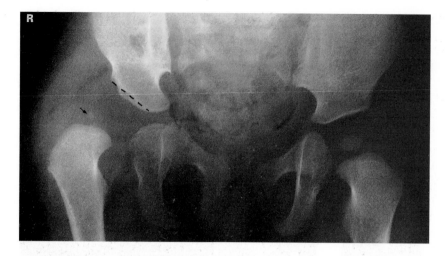

Fig. 12.23 Congenital dislocation of right hip. The right femoral epiphysis (arrow) is smaller than on the normal left side and it does not lie within the acetabulum. Note the sloping roof of the right acetabulum (dotted lines).

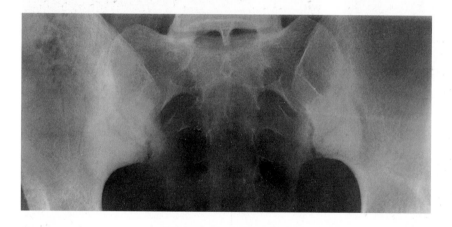

Fig. 12.24 Osteitis condensans ilii. AP view. Sclerosis is seen in both iliac bones just adjacent to the sacroiliac joints. The joints themselves, however, are normal. The patient was a young woman who had borne children.

Scleroderma

Scleroderma may cause calcification and atrophy of soft tissues of the hands with loss of the tips of the terminal phalanges (Fig. 12.25).

Internal derangements of the knee

Most knee injuries produce soft tissue damage, notably meniscal or ligamentous tears, either alone or in conjunction with bony fracture. Plain film examination can only demonstrate the state of the bones. Magnetic resonance imaging is the best imaging modality for detecting internal derangement. The key question for clinicians nowadays is which patients should be referred for MRI and which should have arthroscopy without prior MRI.

Magnetic resonance imaging

The menisci, which are composed of fibrocartilage, are well demonstrated on MRI as they have a different signal intensity from the hyaline cartilage covering the adjacent femoral condyles and tibial plateau. The normal menisci are of uniform low signal on all sequences. A meniscal tear (Fig. 12.26) can be recognized as a break in the meniscus allowing

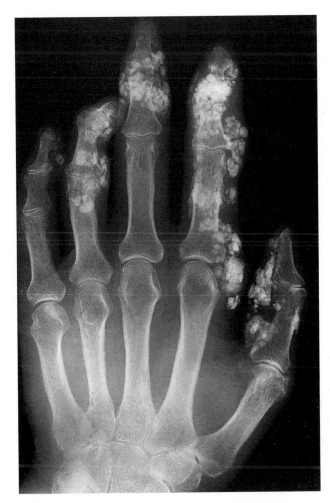

Fig. 12.25 Scleroderma. Extensive soft tissue calcification is present as well as atrophy of soft tissues at the ends of the fingers.

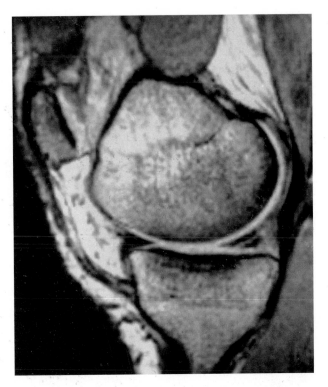

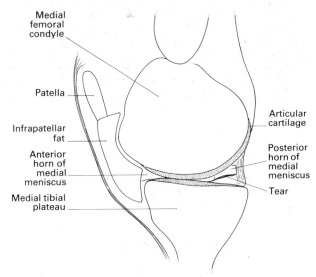

Fig. 12.26 Tear of medial meniscus. Sagittal MRI through the medial part of the knee joint showing a tear in the posterior horn of the medial meniscus. The anterior horn appears normal.

synovial fluid, which has a higher signal intensity, to enter the substance of the meniscus. Tears of the cruciate and collateral ligaments are also readily identified.

Some surgeons proceed directly to arthroscopy in patients with clear-cut clinical features of internal derangement, reserving MRI for those patients with suspicious but not definite clinical signs or symptoms. Magnetic resonance imaging can show bone bruises and other pathology adjacent to, but not within, the joint, entities that cannot

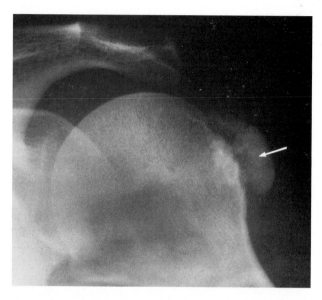

Fig. 12.27 Supraspinatus tendinitis. Calcification is present in the supraspinatus tendon (arrow).

be diagnosed at arthroscopy. Magnetic resonance imaging can also, on occasion, show meniscal tears not seen at arthroscopy and is, therefore, used in selected patients with persistent symptoms following an apparently normal arthroscopy.

Shoulder rotator cuff degeneration/tear

The rotator cuff of the shoulder consists of the supraspinatus, infraspinatus, teres minor and subcapularis muscles together with their tendons. Tears of the supraspinatus tendon are common and can lead to acute or chronic symptoms. On plain radiographs there may be amorphous calcification adjacent to the greater tuberosity of the humerus (Fig. 12.27). Magnetic resonance imaging and/or ultrasound can be useful in selected patients when corrective surgery is being considered. On MRI the normal black signal of the supraspinatous tendon is interrupted by the higher signal of fluid, and in complete tears it may be possible to see the retracted ends of the torn tendon–muscle junction. Arthrography, which involves needling the joint and demonstrating extravasation of contrast medium from the joint through the ruptured tendon is performed in some centres.

Spine

Plain films still have an important role in the diagnosis of disorders of the spine, especially in spinal trauma, but spinal imaging has been revolutionized over the past decade following the introduction of MRI. The spinal cord and spinal nerves are invisible on plain films but MRI is able to visualize not only the vertebrae and the intervertebral discs but the spinal canal and contents as well. Magnetic resonance imaging is the preferred examination for degenerative, inflammatory and malignant conditions of the spine.

The detailed structure of the vertebrae differs in the cervical, thoracic and lumbar regions, but the general structure is similar. The appearances of a normal vertebra is illustrated in Fig. 13.1. In the lateral projection, the vertebral bodies are approximately rectangular in shape. There may be shallow indentations on the upper and lower surfaces due to protrusion of disc material into the vertebral end plates. These indentations are known as Schmorl's nodes and are of no clinical significance (Fig. 13.2).

The appearances of normal vertebrae at MRI are illustrated in Fig. 13.3. On a T1-weighted MRI scan, fat appears as high signal while cerebrospinal fluid (CSF) and the intervertebral discs are of low signal. On a T2-weighted scan normal discs and CSF are of high signal. It should be appreciated that bone produces no signal at MRI; the signal responsible for showing the spine on an MR image comes from the bone marrow, thecal contents and discs. Normal bone marrow has a different MRI signal to most soft tissues and, in particular, has a different signal to tumour and infection.

Other imaging methods for examining the spine are *radionuclide bone scans* which are particularly useful for the detection of bony metastases and *CT* which has an important role in spinal trauma. *Myelography*, which entails injecting contrast into the subarachnoid space by lumbar puncture to detect suspected disc protrusion and spinal cord compression, has now been almost exclusively replaced by MRI.

Signs of abnormality

Disc space narrowing (Fig. 13.4)

The intervertebral discs are radiolucent on plain radiographs as they are composed of fibrous tissue and cartilage. Normally, the disc spaces are the same height at all levels in the cervical and thoracic spine. In the lumbar spine the disc spaces increase slightly in height going down the spine, except for the disc space at the lumbosacral junction, which is usually narrower than the one above it. MRI shows the internal structure of the disc, and any loss of disc height together with alteration of the normal signal characteristics can be readily appreciated. Disc space narrowing occurs with degenerative disease and with disc space infection.

Collapse of vertebral bodies

A collapsed vertebral body is one which has lost height. Loss of height is most easily appreciated on plain lateral radiographs of the spine, though it is, of course, well demonstrated on sagittal sections with MRI. If any collapse is present, it is essential to look at the adjacent disc to see if it is narrowed and to check if part of any pedicle is destroyed. The commoner causes of vertebral collapse are listed below together with a synopsis of the signs of importance in differential diagnosis:

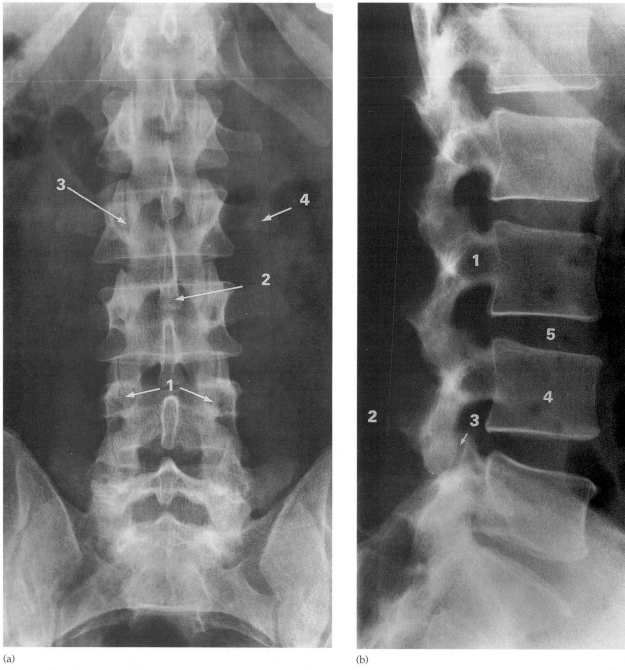

(a)   (b)

Fig. 13.1 Plain film of normal lumbar spine. (a) Frontal. **1**, pedicles; **2**, spinous process; **3**, facet joint; **4**, transverse process. (b) Lateral. **1**, pedicles; **2**, spinous process; **3**, facet joint; **4**, vertebral body; **5**, disc space. Note how the height of the disc spaces increases from L1–L5 with the exception of the L5–S1 disc space which is normally narrower than the one above.

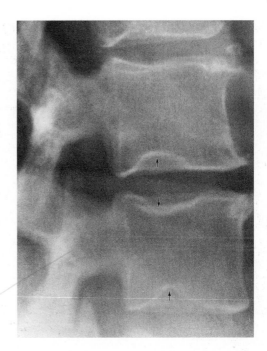

Fig. 13.2 (*Right.*) Schmorl's nodes. These are indentations into the end plates of the vertebral bodies (arrows) and are without significance.

Fig. 13.3 (*below*) MRI of normal lumbar spine. (a) T1-weighted scan. The discs and spinal cord (arrow) are of intermediate signal. (b) T2-weighted scan. The discs and CSF appear as high signal. The spinal cord is arrowed. (c) Axial T$_1$-weighted scan through the L5/S1 disc space. Note the high signal fat surrounding the S1 nerve roots (arrows). F, facet joints; LF, ligamentum flavum; SP, spinous process; TS, thecal sac.

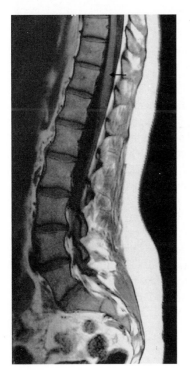

(a)

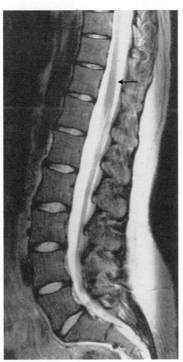

(b)

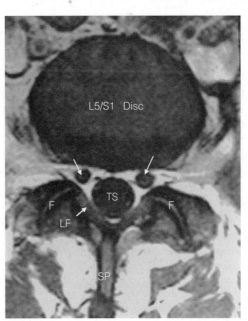

(c)

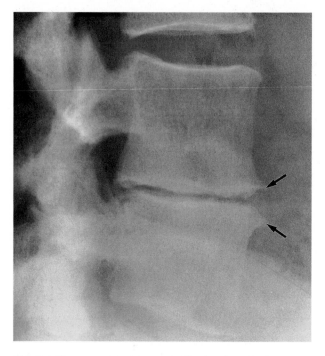

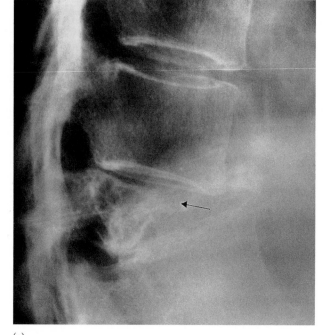

(a)

Fig. 13.4 Disc space narrowing caused by disc degenerative changes between L3 and L4. Note the osteophytes (arrows) and sclerosis of the adjoining surfaces of the vertebral bodies.

Fig. 13.5 Collapsed vertebra. (a) Metastasis (arrow) causing complete collapse of the vertebral body. The adjacent vertebral discs are unaffected. (*b–e, opposite.*)

• *Metastases and myeloma.* Bone destruction, or replacement of normal marrow signal by tumour in the case of MRI, may be visible. The pedicles are a good place to look for evidence of bone destruction on plain film examination. The disc spaces are usually normal (Fig. 13.5a).

• *Infection.* The adjacent disc space is nearly always narrow or obliterated. There may be bone destruction next to the affected disc but the pedicles are usually intact (Fig. 13.5b). MRI will show altered signal within the affected vertebral body and disc.

• *Osteoporosis and osteomalacia.* There is generalized reduction in bone density. The disc spaces are normal or even slightly increased in height and the pedicles are intact. Marrow signal at MRI is normal.

• *Trauma.* A compression fracture is commonly due to forward flexion of the spine, causing the vertebral body to become wedge shaped. The superior surface is usually concave (Fig. 13.5c,d). The discs are normal but may be impacted into the fractured bone – a feature well shown on sagittal MRI. Associated fractures may be seen in the pedicles or neural arch, but otherwise the bone and discs are normal.

• *Eosinophil granuloma.* Complete collapse of one or more vertebral bodies may occur in children or young adults with Langerhans histiocytosis (eosinophil granuloma). The vertebral body is flattened and sometimes referred to as a 'vertebra plana' (Fig. 13.5e). The adjacent discs are normal and the pedicles are usually preserved.

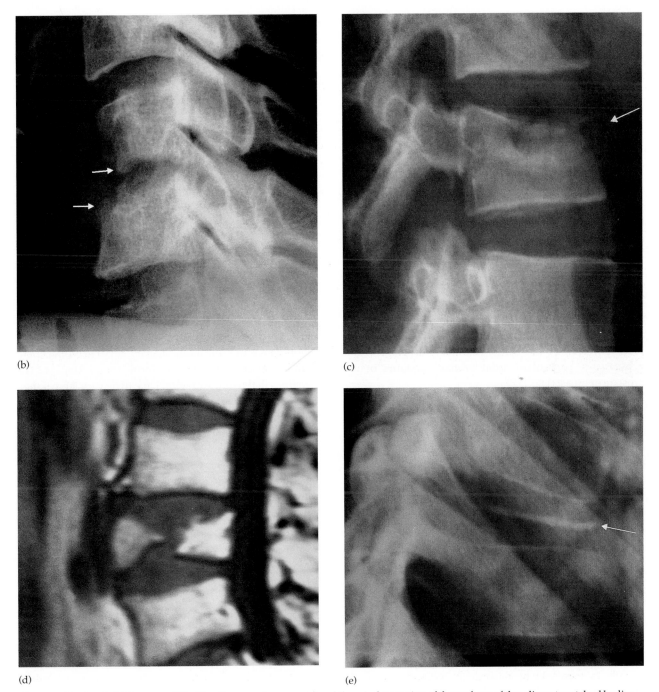

(b)

(c)

(d)

(e)

Fig. 13.5 *Continued.* (b) Osteomyelitis. The disc space is narrowed and there is destruction of the surfaces of the adjacent vertebral bodies (arrows). (c) Traumatic collapse. Note the concave superior surface of the collapsed vertebral body. Some fragments have been extruded anteriorly (arrow). (d) MRI of traumatic collapse. Note how well the fractured vertebral body is shown and that there is no abnormality of the bone marrow of the collapsed vertebra. (e) Collapse due to eosinophil granuloma. In this child the vertebral body is so collapsed that it resembles a thin disc (arrow).

Pedicles

On plain films the pedicles are best assessed in the frontal view, except in the cervical spine where oblique views are necessary. They are very well demonstrated on CT scans. Destruction of one or more of the pedicles (Fig. 13.6) is a fairly reliable sign of spinal metastases.

Flattening and widening of the distance between the pedicles occurs with tumours arising within the spinal canal, e.g. neurofibroma or meningioma. Although neurofibromas may be completely intradural, some have a dumbbell shape with a portion lying outside the spinal canal. In these instances the intervertebral foramen is enlarged (Fig. 13.7).

Dense vertebrae

Sclerosis, which is demonstrated on plain films or CT, may affect just one vertebra or may be part of a generalized process involving many bones. Common causes are:
• *metastases*, particularly from primary tumours of the prostate or breast (Fig. 13.8);
• *malignant lymphoma*;
• *Paget's disease*, which may be difficult to distinguish from neoplastic disease. (An important diagnostic feature is increase in the size of the vertebra. A coarse trabecular pattern typical of Paget's disease is usually but not invariably present (Fig. 13.9).);
• *haemangioma*, which gives rise to characteristic vertical striations in a vertebra that is normal in size (Fig. 13.10).

Lysis within a vertebra

As with sclerosis, lysis, which is demonstrated on plain films or CT, may be part of a widespread process or may be confined to one vertebra. The common causes are:
• metastases, particularly from primary tumours of the lungs or kidneys (Fig. 13.6);
• multiple myeloma/plasmacytoma;
• malignant lymphoma occasionally gives rise to a lytic lesion;
• infection. Here the lysis usually involves one body or two adjacent bodies and the adjacent disc space is almost invariably narrowed (see below).

Paravertebral shadow

A paravertebral soft tissue shadow may first draw attention to an abnormality in the spine. The easiest place to recognize such swelling on plain radiographs is in the thoracic region where the soft tissue density adjacent to the spine assumes a characteristic fusiform shape (Fig. 13.11). Swellings in the lumbar region have to be very large if they are to displace the psoas outline and be recognizable on plain films. Anterior swelling in the cervical region can be recognized by the forward displacement of the pharyngeal air shadow. Paravertebral soft tissue swelling is readily recognized at all levels with CT and MRI scanning.

Paravertebral soft tissue swelling occurs with infection, with malignant neoplasms and with haematomas following trauma. Specific diagnostic signs are often present in such cases in the adjacent bones.

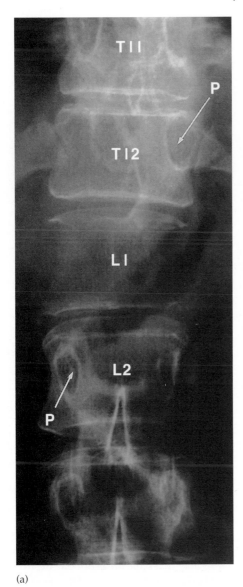

(a)

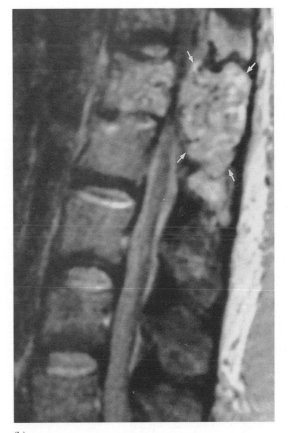

(b)

Fig. 13.6 Destruction of the pedicles due to metastatic renal cell carcinoma. (a) The pedicles of L1 have both been destroyed, as has the right pedicle of T12. Arrows point to representative normal pedicles (P). (b) MRI scan in the same patient showing extensive tumour in the vertebral body and a posterior mass of tumour (arrows) which is compressing the dural sac. (c) CT scan in another patient showing destruction of the left pedicle of a lower thoracic vertebra and the adjacent body, transverse process and medial end of rib.

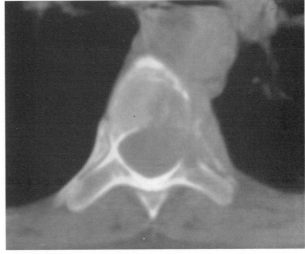

(c)

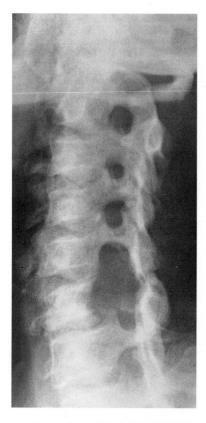

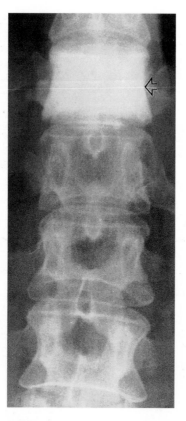

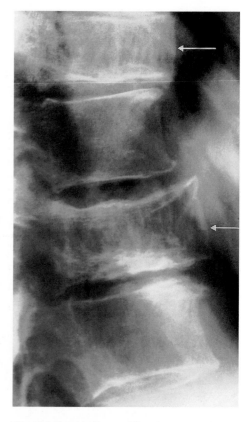

Fig. 13.7 A dumb-bell neurofibroma has enlarged the intervertebral foramina in the cervical spine to cause a large bony defect.

Fig. 13.8 Dense vertebra (arrow) due to metastases from carcinoma of the breast.

Fig. 13.9 Paget's disease. Note the increased density and coarse trabeculae in the vertebral bodies (arrows). They are also wider than the normal ones.

Metastases/myeloma/lymphoma

As with the remainder of the skeleton, the important signs of metastases and lymphoma on plain films or CT are areas of lysis or sclerosis, or a mixture of the two (Fig. 13.12). Multiple myeloma, which almost always gives rise to lytic lesions in the vertebral bodies, is frequently indistinguishable from lytic metastases. A point of difference is that metastases often involve the pedicles as well as the bodies.

Collapse of one or more vertebral bodies may occur with metastases and is a particular feature of myeloma. The collapse may mask the areas of bone destruction in the vertebral body. True destruction of the disc space does not occur with metastases or myeloma.

Radionuclide bone imaging may reveal increased activity around neoplastic tumour deposits, because of increased bone turnover, but myeloma lesions may or may not give rise to focal areas of increased activity.

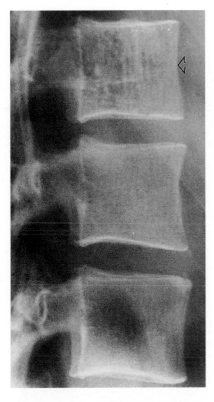

Fig. 13.10 Haemangioma. Vertical striations are present in this normal-sized vertebra (arrow).

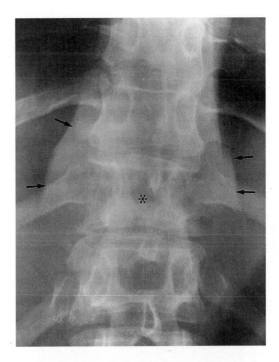

Fig. 13.11 Fusiform paravertebral shadow (arrows) around a thoracic vertebra partially destroyed by Hodgkin's disease (asterisk).

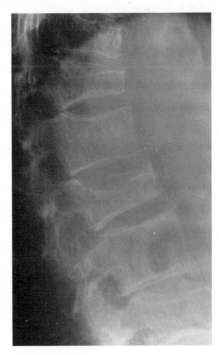

Magnetic resonance imaging is the most accurate test for demonstrating metastases, lymphoma and myeloma. Tumour tissue has significantly different signal characteristics (low signal on T1-weighted images, high signal on T2-weighted images) than normal bone marrow (Fig. 13.13), and thus the tumour deposits stand out clearly from the adjacent marrow. The normal bone does not generate any signal and therefore does not impair the visibility of the tumour. Magnetic resonance imaging has the advantage that it can additionally detect any spinal cord or nerve root compression (Figs 13.6 and 13.26).

Fig. 13.12 (*Right.*) Metastases. Lateral view of the upper lumbar spine. Note the abnormal bony architecture and varying degrees of collapse of several of the vertebral bodies.

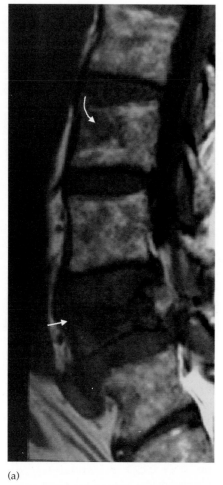

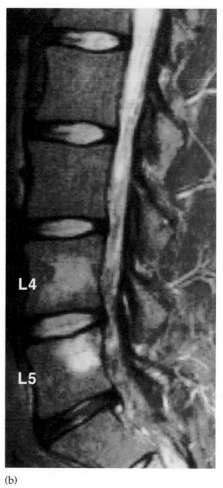

(a)   (b)

Fig. 13.13 (a) Metastases. T1-weighted MRI scan showing widespread metastases that have replaced the normal marrow signal and appear as low signal areas: a particularly large metastases seen in L2 (curved arrow). L4 is collapsed (straight arrow). (b) Lymphoma. T2-weighted scan showing high signal areas in L4 and L5.

Infection

The hallmark of infection is destruction of the intervertebral disc and adjacent vertebral bodies. Early in the course of the disease, there is narrowing of the disc space with erosion of the adjoining surface of the vertebral body. Later, bone destruction may lead to collapse of the vertebral body, resulting in a sharp angulation known as a gibbus (Fig. 13.14). A paravertebral abscess is usually present.

Computed tomography shows the bone destruction and paravertebral soft tissue swelling to advantage but is a poor technique for demonstrating disc space narrowing. MRI has the advantage that it can, with one examination, demonstrate disc space narrowing, altered signal in the adjacent vertebral body and adjacent soft tissue swelling. Needle biopsy/aspiration of the infected disc or adjacent vertebral body under plain film or CT control is a very useful technique to confirm the diagnosis and identify the

Bony fusion of the vertebral bodies across the obliterated disc spaces occurs with healing. Eventually, tuberculous paravertebral abscesses may calcify.

Spinal trauma

Plain films are the initial investigation for trauma to the spine and the following should be looked for:
• fractures of the vertebral bodies, pedicles, laminae, spinous processes;
• alignment of fractures and interarticular facets;
• alignment of the vertebral bodies.

Computed tomography can be very helpful in major trauma, as it will show the extent of any fractures. It is particularly useful for showing fractures of the neural arch and any associated dislocation, because these injuries may result in an unstable spine. CT will also show any bone fragments displaced into the spinal canal – the so-called burst fracture. These fragments may need surgical removal (Fig. 13.15). Because of the excellent demonstration of bony structures with CT and the difficulties of monitoring severely ill patients in the MR scanner, CT is used preferentially in patients with major trauma. However, MRI is useful for demonstrating haemorrhage and contusion of the spinal cord in these patients.

In trauma it can be helpful to divide the spine into the anterior, middle and posterior columns (Fig. 13.16), since spinal stability depends on the integrity of the middle and posterior columns. Fractures confined to the anterior column are stable and these include the commonly seen wedge fractures such as those which occur in osteoporosis.

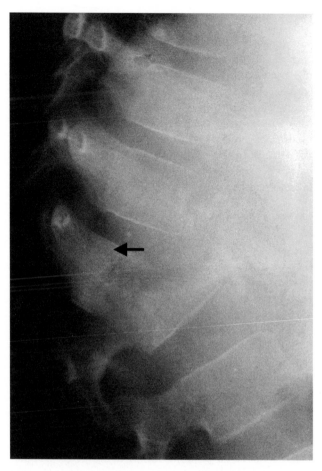

Fig. 13.14 Tuberculosis of the spine. Destruction of the vertebral bodies and the intervening discs has occurred with the formation of a sharp angulation (gibbus). One vertebral body is almost completely destroyed (arrow) and there is destruction of the upper part of the one below it.

responsible organism. It should be remembered, however, that positive cultures are rare once antibiotics have been commenced.

The common infecting organisms are *Mycobacteruim tuberculosis* and *Staphylococcus aureus*. Though there are some differences in the signs produced by these two infections, there is considerable overlap. The lesion in tuberculosis is usually purely lytic, whereas some sclerosis is often seen in pyogenic infection. Paravertebral abscesses tend to be larger in tuberculosis.

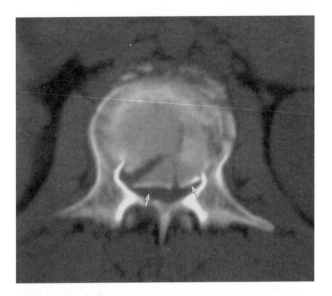

Fig. 13.15 CT scan of fractured vertebral body showing fragments (arrows) displaced backwards into the spinal canal.

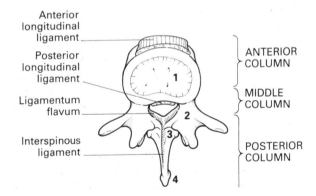

Fig. 13.16 Diagram to show the three columns of the spine. The anterior column includes the anterior longitudinal ligament and anterior two-thirds of the vertebral body. The middle column includes the posterior third of the vertebral body and the posterior longitudinal ligament. The posterior column includes the pedicles, laminae and spinous processes. **1**, vertebral body; **2**, pedicle; **3**, lamina; **4**, spinous process. Redrawn from Dr T. Jaspan, with permission.

Degenerative disc disease

Spondylosis results from degeneration of the intervertebral disc. The degenerate disc may herniate into the surrounding tissues and if the herniated disc presses on the spinal cord or spinal nerves, pain and/or neurological deficit may result. Degenerate discs often stimulate the formation of osteophytes, which together with thickening of the soft tissues, may press upon the spinal cord or nerve roots. Osteoarthritic changes in the apophyseal joints may exacerbate this problem. Spondylosis occurs maximally in the lower cervical and lower lumbar regions.

Plain radiographs in spondylosis

In most cases in which spondylosis is seen, the patient is asymptomatic. When neurological symptoms or signs are present, radiographs of the spine have limited clinical value, as there is little correlation between the symptoms, the signs and the radiological changes. Even when there is disc protrusion producing neurological signs, plain films of the spine may be normal. Usually, the major purpose of requesting radiographs of the spine is to exclude other diseases that may be present.

The signs of spondylosis on plain films (Fig. 13.17) are:
• disc space narrowing;
• osteophyte formation and sclerosis, which frequently occur on the adjoining surfaces of the vertebral bodies. Osteophytes on the posterior surface of the vertebral bodies narrow the spinal canal and may encroach on the exit foramina through which the spinal nerves travel. In the cervical spine osteophytic encroachment of the exit foramina is best shown on oblique views.

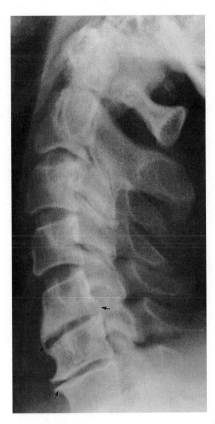

Fig. 13.17 Cervical spondylosis. The C5–C6 and C6–C7 disc spaces are narrowed and there are osteophytes on the anterior and posterior aspects of these vertebral bodies (arrows).

MRI in spondylosis and disc herniation (prolapse)

With advancing age the intervertebral discs lose their normal hydration and become degenerate, recognized by signal reduced on the T2-weighted images. The discs lose height and may bulge. Small tears which can cause back pain may occur in the discs. Changes in the adjoining end plates may be associated with the disc degeneration.

Another feature of degenerative spinal disease is facet joint arthropathy. These joints may become inflamed giving rise to pain. Inflammation causing facet joint hypertrophy and osteophyte formation may cause compression of the nerve root sheath in the exit canal. In the cervical region osteophytes may impinge on and compress the spinal cord eventually leading to ischaemic damage.

Disc protrusion. Disc protrusions vary in size from small central bulges of little significance to larger, posterolateral or far lateral herniation of disc material. The herniated disc can migrate a considerable distance and may become detached from the parent disc when it is known as a sequestrated disc. The common sites for disc herniation are the lower cervical and lower lumbar regions. Sagittal and axial MRI scans of the spine are taken together with axial views limited to those levels likely to show disc herniation of clinical importance.

Lumbar disc herniation. The majority of disc herniations occur posterolaterally at the L4/5 and L5/S1 levels (Fig. 13.18). They are directly visualized on both the axial and sagittal views as small focal projections that point towards the neural exit foramen and therefore compress the adjacent nerve root or root sheath. Loss of visualization of the fat which normally surrounds the nerve roots and root sheaths is a helpful indication of nerve root compression by a herniated disc. It should be appreciated that more than a third of demonstrably herniated discs are asymptomatic, so the criteria for surgery must be clear-cut evidence of compression of the clinically affected nerve root.

Magnetic resonance imaging is also useful in patients who continue to have symptoms following surgery for back pain. Postoperative scarring can be distinguished from disc herniation with a high degree of accuracy if contrast-enhanced images are obtained. Scarring enhances and is of high signal in contradistinction to disc herniation which does not enhance (Fig. 13.19).

Cervical disc herniation. Herniation of a cervical disc may press on a nerve root sheath as in the lumbar region or may compress the spinal cord at multiple levels. These changes may be aggravated by hypertrophy of the adjacent spinal ligaments. The majority of protrusions occur at the lower three disc levels. MRI can assess the discs, identify protrusions indenting the thecal sac and spinal cord, and detect nerve root compression (Fig. 13.20). Plain films are sometimes employed to detect osteophytes, which may compress exiting nerves, since small bony abnormalities may be difficult to assess with MRI.

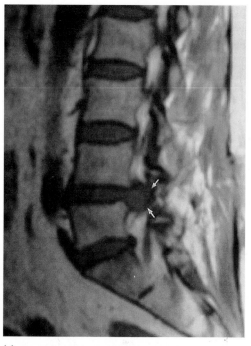

(a)

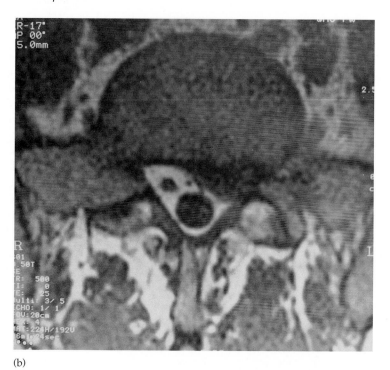

(b)

Fig. 13.18 Disc herniation. MRI scans. (a) Sagittal T1-weighted scan showing a large posterior herniation of the L4/5 disc (arrows). (b) Axial T1-weighted scan of an L5/S1 disc showing a disc herniation compressing the adjacent nerve root. The opposite equivalent nerve root can be clearly seen.

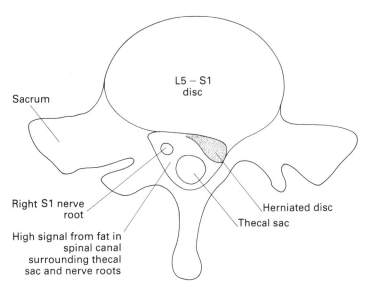

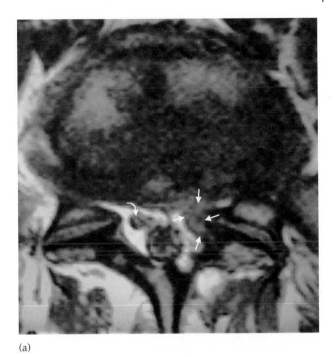

(a)

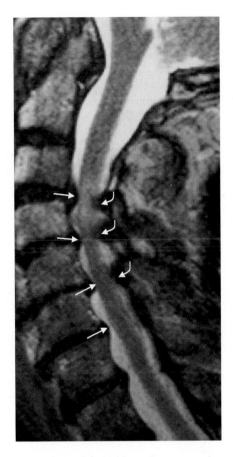

Fig. 13.20 Cervical spondylosis. Magnetic resonance image scan showing the thecal sac is indented anteriorly (arrows) by a combination of disc protrusion and osteophyte formation. Posteriorly the thecal sac is indented by hypertrophied ligamenta flava (curved arrows). This encroachment upon the thecal sac has produced stenosis of the spinal canal and subsequent spinal cord compression.

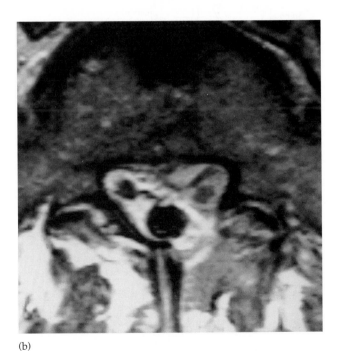

(b)

Fig. 13.19 (*Opposite.*) Postoperative fibrosis. Magnetic resonance imaging T1-weighted scans at L5/S1 level in a patient with sciatica following L5/S1 laminectomy six months previously. (a) The scan shows a normal right S1 nerve root (curved arrow) but around the left S1 nerve root there is a mass (arrows) which could be either fibrosis or recurrent disc herniation. (b) After gadolinium the mass enhances indicating it is fibrosis. A disc herniation would not enhance.

CT in disc herniation

Computed tomography for disc herniation has been largely replaced by MRI. At CT the disc is of lower density than bone and of uniform opacity. The contents of the dural sac without contrast are all of the same density; therefore, swelling of the intrathecal nerves and of the spinal cord are not recognizable. The nerve root sheaths are seen as circular dots adjacent to the dural sac surrounded by fat within the spinal cord. The posterior margin of the disc is outlined by fat and it is displacement of this fat that allows one to recognize disc herniation seen as focal projections from the disc (Fig. 13.21).

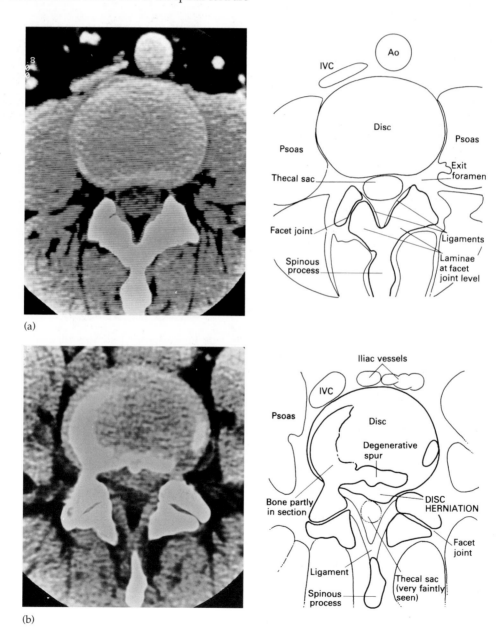

(a)

(b)

Spinal stenosis

A narrow spinal canal may give rise to cord or nerve root compression especially when spondylotic changes supervene. Symptomatic spinal stenosis is encountered in the cervical and lumbar regions.

MRI is the ideal method of demonstrating the size and shape of the spinal canal and thus diagnosing spinal stenosis. It also shows disc protrusions and any bony or soft tissue encroachment upon the narrowed spinal canal.

Ankylosing spondylitis

Ankylosing spondylitis affects principally the sacroiliac joints and the spine, although occasionally other joints may be involved as well. Both sacroiliac joints are invariably affected by the time spinal involvement has occurred. The earliest radiological change is fuzziness of the joint margins, followed by frank erosions (Fig. 13.22a). Eventually, the process leads to obliteration of the joint space.

In the spine the spinal ligaments ossify, forming vertically oriented bony bridges between the vertebral bodies. The posterior apophyseal and the costotransverse joints become fused. In advanced cases the whole spine is rigidly fused and becomes a solid block of bone. From its plain radiographic appearance this is known as a 'bamboo spine' (Fig. 13.22b).

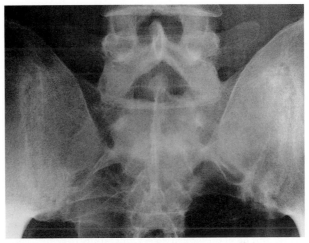

(a)

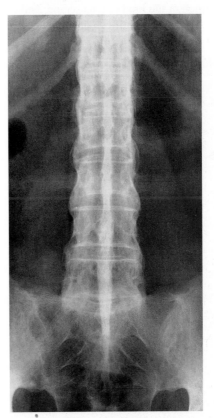

(b)

Fig. 13.22 (*Right.*) Ankylosing spondylitis. (a) The sacroiliac joints have an irregular fuzzy outline. (b) With advanced disease the whole spine becomes fused (bamboo spine). Note that the sacroiliac joints are also fused.

Fig. 13.21 (*Left.*) Computed tomography scan of disc herniation. (a) Normal lumbar disc. Note the normal shape of the disc with no protrusions into the spinal canal or exit foramina. Ao, aorta; IVC, inferior vena cava. (b) Disc herniation. There is a large posterior herniation, maximal on the left and centrally. The thecal sac (very difficult to see at these settings) is pushed backward. IVC, inferior vena cava.

Spina bifida

Spina bifida is a result of incomplete closure of the vertebral canal, usually in the lumbosacral region, and may be associated with an abnormality affecting the spinal cord. In severe cases presenting at birth there may be protrusion of the spinal cord (meningomyelocele) or its membranes (meningocele) from the spinal canal. In these cases the laminae of several vertebrae will be absent and the distance between the pedicles will be increased. Complex malformations of the vertebral bodies and the contents of the spinal canal (spinal dysraphism) may also be present. In such cases, CT/MRI can provide useful information. Nowadays, the diagnosis is made antenatally by ultrasound.

Frequently, the patient has no externally visible abnormality and no neurological defect, but failure of bony fusion of the two laminae is seen radiologically. This may occur at any level but is common in the lumbosacral region, and in these cases it is without significance (Fig. 13.23).

Spondylolisthesis

The term spondylolisthesis refers to forward slip of one vertebral body on the one below it, a condition which occurs most frequently at the lumbosacral junction and between L4 and L5 vertebral bodies. It is usually the result of a defect between the superior and inferior articular facets (the pars interarticularis). The defect in the pars interarticularis is thought to be a stress fracture. It can usually be identified on the lateral projection but may sometimes be better seen on oblique films (Fig. 13.24). Minor degrees of slip can also occur without a break in the pars interarticularis, if there is degenerative disc disease with osteoarthritis in the apophyseal joints.

Spondylolysis is the term given to a defect in the pars interarticularis without a forward slip of one vertebral body on the other.

Defects in the pars interarticularis are readily identified with CT or MRI but the plain film examination usually suffices. Radionuclide scanning may show increased uptake before the defect is visible on plain films.

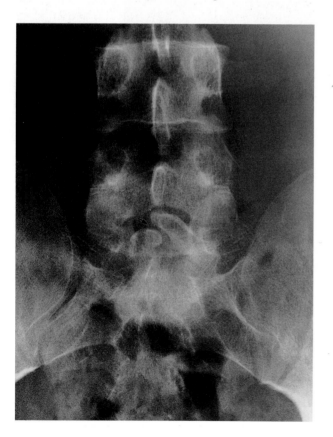

Fig. 13.23 Failure of bony fusion of the two laminae of the first part of the sacrum (arrow) is a common finding without significance.

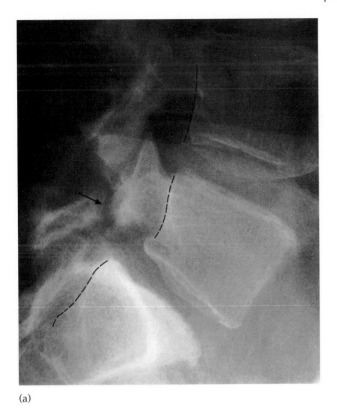

(a)

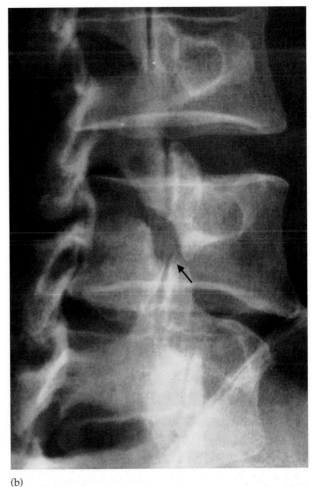

(b)

Fig. 13.24 Spondylolisthesis. (a) Lateral view. There is forward slip of L5 upon S1. The dotted lines which mark the posterior aspects of the vertebral bodies should form a smooth curve. The defect in the pars interarticularis is arrowed. (b) Oblique view showing the defect in the pars interarticularis (arrow). On the oblique view a shape resembling the front end of a 'scottie dog' can be recognized. (c) The 'scottie dog'. A defect in the pars interarticularis is seen as a break in the dog's neck.

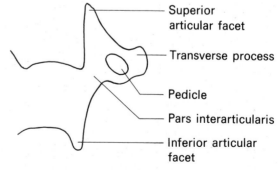

Superior articular facet

Transverse process

Pedicle

Pars interarticularis

Inferior articular facet

(c)

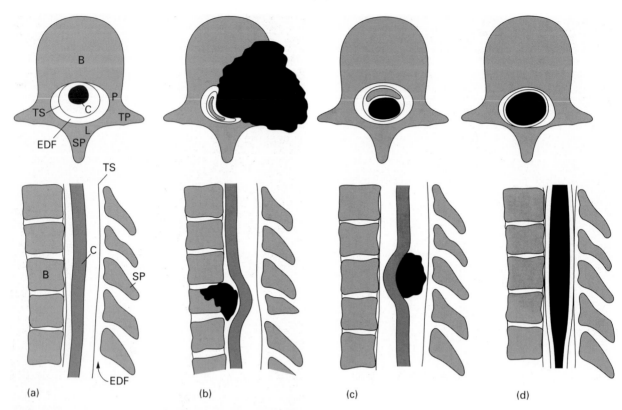

Fig. 13.25 Spinal cord compression. Schematic axial and sagittal sections. (a) Normal view. B, vertebral body; C, spinal cord; EDF, extradural fat; L, lamina; P, pedicle; SP, spinous process; TP, transverse process; TS, thecal sac. (b) Extradural metastatic tumour. Extrinsic compression of the thecal sac and spinal cord which are compressed and displaced away from the tumour. (c) Intradural extramedullary tumour. The tumour is contained within the undisplaced thecal sac but compresses and displaces the spinal cord. (d) Intradural intramedullary spinal cord tumour. The spinal cord is expanded but undisplaced with little or no visualization of the cerebrospinal fluid in the thecal sac around the spinal cord. Illustration redrawn from Dr T. Jaspan with permission.

Spinal cord compression

Although the level of cord compression can be correctly predicted by clinical examination, MRI of the spine can demonstrate the site and often the nature and extent of the abnormality and any other sites involved, information that is important should surgery be necessary. Magnetic resonance imaging is particularly suitable for demonstrating cord compression because it shows the spine, extradural tissues, subarachnoid space and intrathecal contents with just one examination.

The causes of compression of the spinal cord are usually divided according to the site of origin of the responsible space-occupying lesion (Fig. 13.25).
• Extradural lesions, e.g. metastases (Fig. 13.26), spinal tuberculosis, cervical disc herniation and the bone and soft tissue reactions that accompany cervical spondylosis. It is worth remembering here that lumbar disc herniations are too low to compress the spinal cord, which does not extend below L1.
• Intradural but extramedullary lesions, i.e. within the

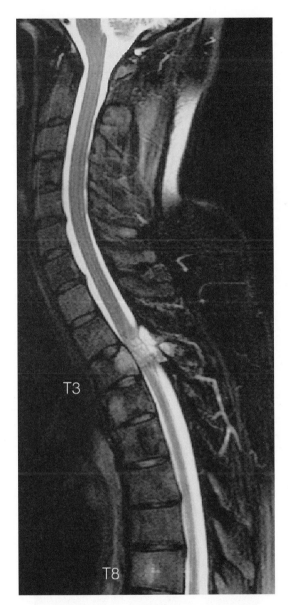

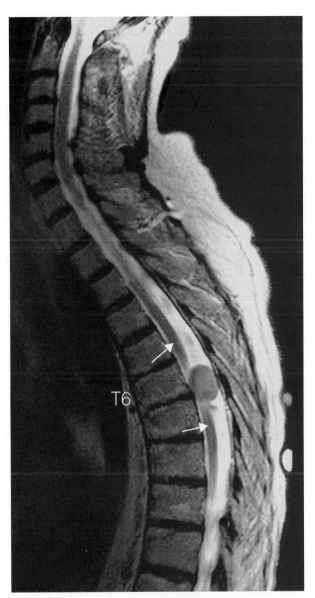

Fig. 13.26 Spinal cord compression. Magnetic resonance imaging T2-weighted scan showing metastases from a breast carcinoma in the body and pedicle of T3 causing compression of the spinal cord. Further metastases can be seen in the bodies of T4 and T8.

Fig. 13.27 Intradural neurofibroma. Magnetic resonance imaging T2-weighted scan showing the tumour at the T6/7 level compressing and displacing the spinal cord anteriorly (arrows).

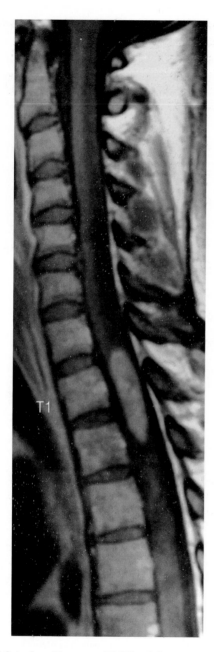

dura but not within the spinal cord, e.g. neurofibroma (Fig. 13.27) and meningioma.

• Intramedullary lesions, i.e. within the spinal cord, e.g. spinal cord tumour or haemorrhage into the spinal cord (Fig. 13.28).

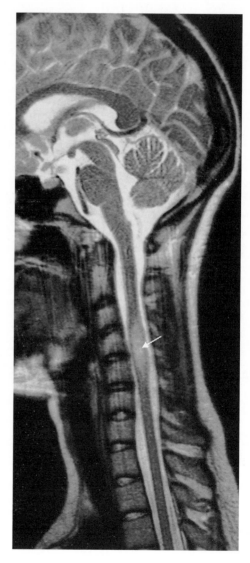

Fig. 13.28 Spinal cord tumour at T1/2 level shown on a gadolinium-enhanced T1-weighted MRI scan.

Fig. 13.29 Magnetic resonance imaging T2-weighted scan showing plaque of demyelination (arrow) in this patient with multiple sclerosis.

Intrinsic disorders of the spinal cord

Magnetic resonance imaging is able to give an excellent demonstration of the whole of the spinal cord. Conditions which expand the cord, such as tumours, syringomyelia and hydromyelia, and some haematomas, are readily diagnosed by a combination of altered signal within the cord and expansion of its outline. It is also possible to diagnose some conditions which do not give rise to space-occupying lesions, such as plaques of demyelination in multiple sclerosis (Fig. 13.29) and small areas of haemorrhage, because the signal from these pathological processes is very different to that of the adjacent normal nerve tissue.

14

Bone Trauma

Imaging techniques

Plain radiographs

Plain radiography in bone trauma is invaluable in order to:
- diagnose the presence of a fracture or dislocation;
- determine whether the underlying bone is normal or whether the fracture has occurred through abnormal bone (pathological fracture);
- show the position of bone ends before and after treatment of a fracture;
- assess healing and complications of fractures.

The latter two subjects and details of individual fractures will not be discussed as they are best dealt with in textbooks of orthopaedics. Head injury is discussed on p. 415.

In any case of trauma it is essential to take at least two views, preferably at right angles to one another. Sometimes a fracture or dislocation will be seen on only one view and so may be missed unless two views are taken. Similarly, the position of a fracture should never be assessed from a single film (Fig. 14.1).

Some injuries are likely to produce fractures in more than one site. With tibial fractures, for example, the fibula is frequently also broken but the fractures may be a considerable distance apart. Certain bones, e.g. the pelvis and mandible, often fracture in two sites, only one producing severe symptoms. In these situations all likely fracture sites should be included on the films.

Fracture

Frequently, a fracture is very obvious but in some cases the changes are more subtle. Fractures may be recognized or suspected by the following signs:
- *Fracture line*. The fracture usually appears as a lucent line.

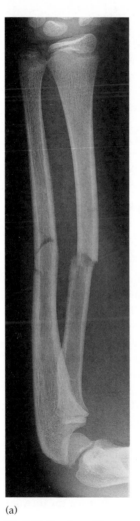 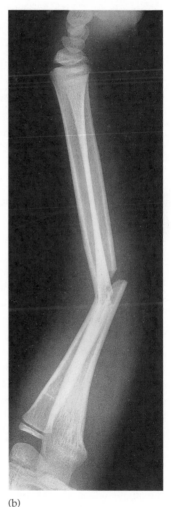

(a)   (b)

Fig. 14.1 Fracture of forearm showing the value of two views. (a) The fractures of the radius and ulna show little displacement on the frontal projection. (b) The lateral view, however, shows a marked angulation.

375

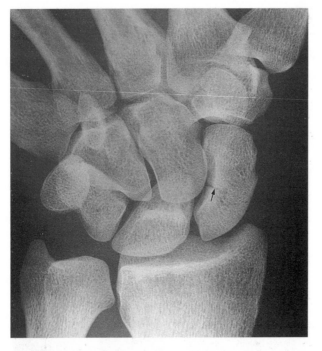

Fig. 14.2 Fracture of the scaphoid appearing as a lucent line (arrow).

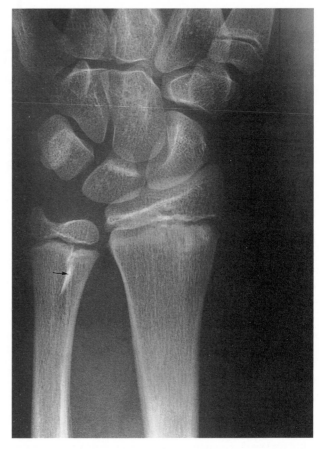

Fig. 14.3 Fracture of the ulna appearing as a sclerotic line (arrow).

This may be very thin and easily overlooked (Fig. 14.2). Occasionally, the fracture appears as a dense line from overlap of the fragments (Fig. 14.3).

• *A step in the cortex* may be the only evidence of a fracture (Fig. 14.4).

• *Interruption of bony trabeculae* is of use in impacted fractures where there is no visible lucent line. This is, however, a difficult sign to evaluate (Fig. 14.5).

• *Bulging or buckling of the cortex* is a particularly important sign in children, where fractures are frequently of the greenstick type (Fig. 14.6).

• *Soft tissue swelling* may be a valuable guide to the presence of an underlying fracture.

• *A joint effusion* may become visible following trauma. In the elbow, where an effusion often indicates a fracture, fat pads lie adjacent to the joint capsule and, if there is an effusion, they will be displaced away from the shaft of the humerus on the lateral view (Fig. 14.7).

Dislocation

The joint surfaces no longer maintain their normal relationship to each other. An associated fracture should be carefully looked for.

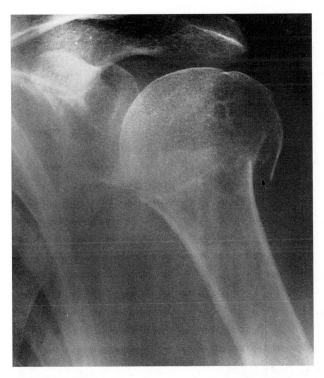

Fig. 14.4 Fracture of neck of humerus appearing as a step in the cortex (arrow).

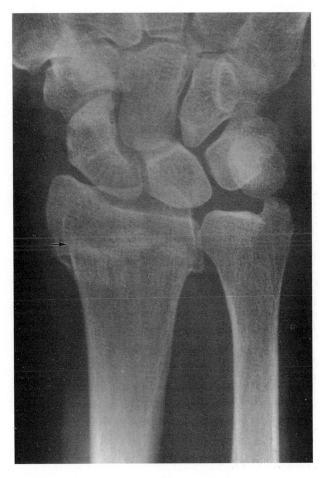

Fig. 14.5 Colles' fracture showing the bony trabeculae are interrupted across the fracture site (arrow). There is also a step in the cortex.

Further plain film views

Injuries may sometimes be invisible even with two views taken at right angles to each other. If the radiographic findings are equivocal, or if there is clinical suspicion of bony injury with normal radiographs, then further films should be taken as follows:

• *Different projections*, e.g. oblique views (Fig. 14.8).

• *Stress films*. A film taken with a joint under stress may show that it is unstable, due to ligamentous damage. Stress films are helpful in ankle injuries when forced inversion and eversion may show movement of the talus.

• *Flexion and extension views*. In the cervical spine, injury may cause alteration in the alignment of the posterior borders of the vertebral bodies. This is usually much more

obvious on a film taken with the neck flexed (Fig. 14.9). In the conscious patient pain will prevent damage to the spinal cord from instability of the cervical spine, providing the movement is carried out by the patient himself. Flexion and extension views should not be carried out on the unconscious patient.

• *X-ray of the other side.* Comparison with the normal side can be useful in the problem case, particularly if expert help is not available. This applies largely in children where epi-

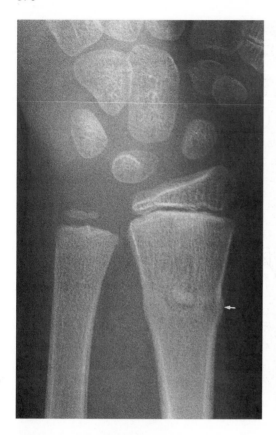

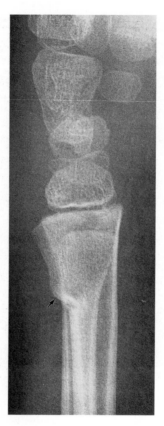

Fig. 14.6 Greenstick fracture of lower end of radius in a child. There is buckling of the cortex (arrows).

physeal lines and unusual patterns of ossification may simulate a fracture.

• *Delayed films*. If films are taken about two weeks after injury, resorption of the bone at the fracture site may then reveal the fracture line. This is particularly useful in detecting scaphoid fractures which may be invisible immediately after the injury (Fig. 14.10).

Although plain films suffice in almost all patients who have undergone trauma, in certain instances other imaging modalities are employed.

Radionuclide bone scanning in bone trauma (Fig. 14.11)

Fractures may not be visible on plain films and in these instances radionuclide bone scanning is particularly helpful. The bone scans show increased activity at injured sites within two to three days. Increased activity persists for as long as the fractures are healing, often lasting several months. Multiple fractures occasionally give a picture, resembling metastases, but usually the distribution suggests injury.

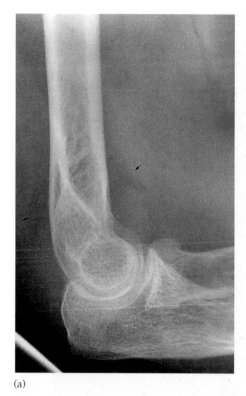

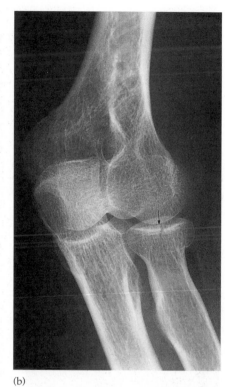

Fig. 14.7 Elbow effusion with fracture of radial head. (a) The anterior and posterior fat pads (arrows) are displaced away from the humerus which almost invariably means a fracture is present. (b) Oblique view in this patient shows the fracture of the radial head (arrow) which was only demonstrated on the oblique view.

(a)   (b)

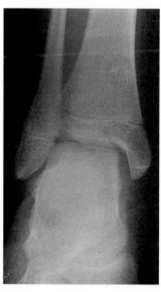

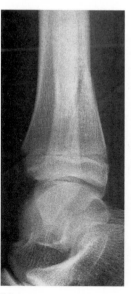

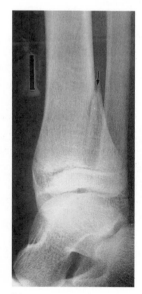

Fig. 14.8 Oblique view to demonstrate a fracture. (a) and (b) AP and lateral views in this child's ankle do not show an obvious fracture. (c) Oblique view clearly demonstrates the fracture (arrow).

(a)   (b)   (c)

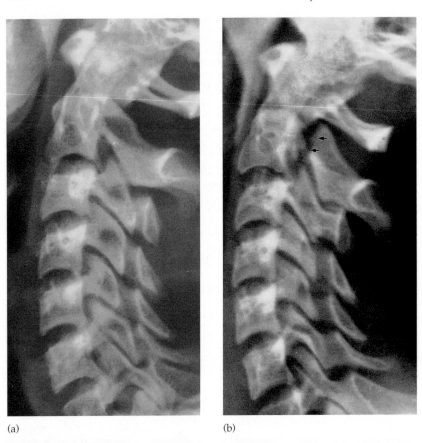

(a)

(b)

Fig. 14.9 Flexion and extension views to demonstrate a fracture. (a) Extension view of cervical spine does not reveal a fracture. (b) Flexion view clearly shows the fracture of the arch of C2 (arrows).

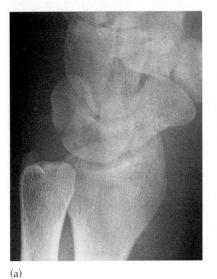

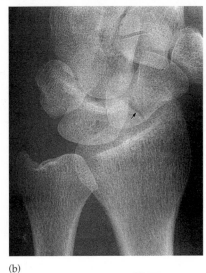

(a)

(b)

Fig. 14.10 Delayed films to demonstrate a fracture. (a) Films taken immediately after injury do not show a fracture. (b) Films taken two weeks after injury show a fracture through the scaphoid (arrow).

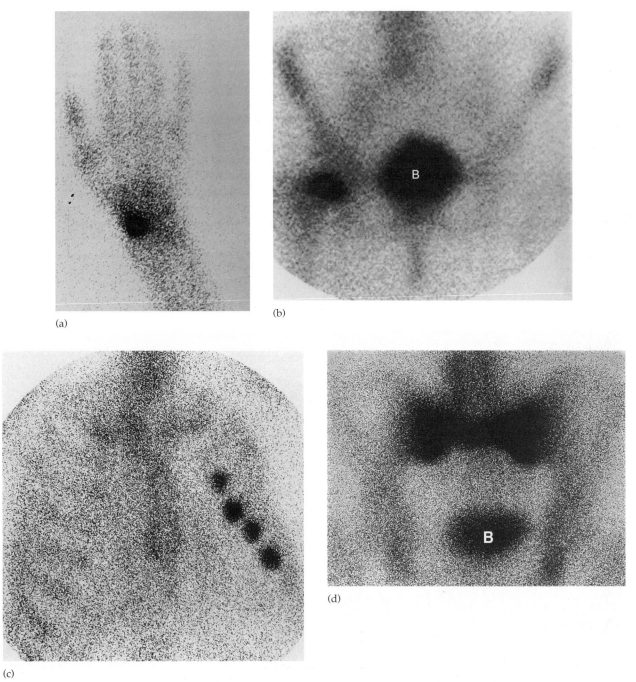

(a)

(b)

(c)

(d)

Fig. 14.11 Radionuclide bone scans in trauma. (a) Fracture of scaphoid. There is increased activity in the scaphoid in this patient who suffered continuing pain after trauma to the wrist. In spite of normal x-rays the bone scan indicates there is a fracture which was not visible on the radiographs. (b) Increased uptake in a fracture of the right femoral neck that was visible on MRI (Fig. 14.14a) but not on x-rays of the hip. B, bladder. (c) Fractures in the anterior ends of four adjacent ribs. The distribution of increased activity is diagnostic of injury; metastases would be more randomly distributed. (d) Insufficiency fracture. There is increased uptake in the sacrum in this elderly lady who had a normal pelvic x-ray. B, isotope in the bladder.

Computed tomography in bone trauma

The major advantages of computed tomography (CT) over plain films are:

• Better assessment of fractures in bones of complex shape, such as the spine and pelvis. The plan view and the multiplicity of sections are major advantages here. In the spine, fractures of the pedicles, laminae and articular facets as well as fragments displaced into the spinal canal are particularly well seen (Fig. 14.12). In fractures of the pelvis, especially those around the hip joints, CT shows the relationship of the fractures to the joint as well as loose fragments within the joint (Fig. 14.13). Fractures and their displacement, as well as bone fragments in pelvic fractures may be better appreciated by three-dimensional reconstruction of the CT image.

• Better assessment of the extent of soft tissue damage and haematomas and of internal visceral injuries.

• In general, less manipulation of the patient is required, so that the examination of the severely injured individual is more comfortable and often safer. With modern equipment the examination is quick, an important factor in patients with serious internal injuries.

Magnetic resonance imaging in bone trauma

Even though cortical bone does not produce an MR signal, a fracture can be seen as a dark line across the bright signal of the fat in the marrow on a T1-weighted scan (Fig. 14.14a). Altered signal is seen within the bone representing haemorrhage oedema. Sometimes a bone bruise may be visible at MRI even though there is no discernible fracture (Fig. 14.14b) on a conventional radiograph. Magnetic resonance imaging is also very useful for demonstrating injury to soft tissues such as muscle, tendons and ligaments.

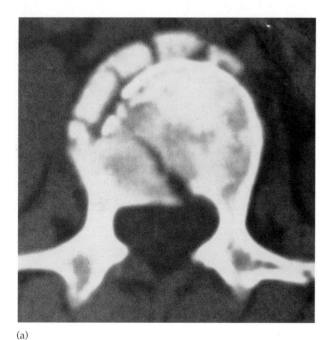

(a)

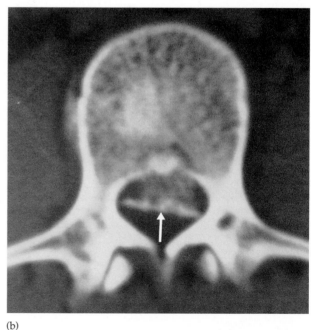

(b)

Fig. 14.12 CT scanning in fractures of the lumbar spine. (a) A comminuted fracture of a vertebral body with slight backward displacement of one half. (b) A large bone fragment (arrow) displaced into the spinal canal.

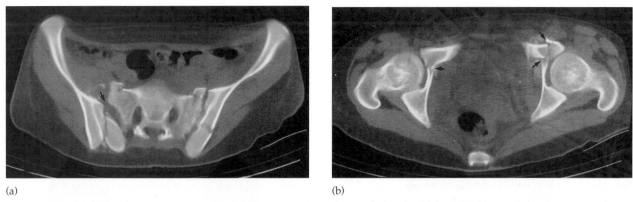

(a)   (b)

Fig. 14.13 Fracture of the pelvis. (a) A section through the sacrum shows fractures of the sacrum and iliac bones. There is separation of the right sacroiliac joint (arrow). (b) A lower section shows fractures through the acetabula (arrows). The fractures and their displacement were much better demonstrated with CT than with radiographs of the pelvis.

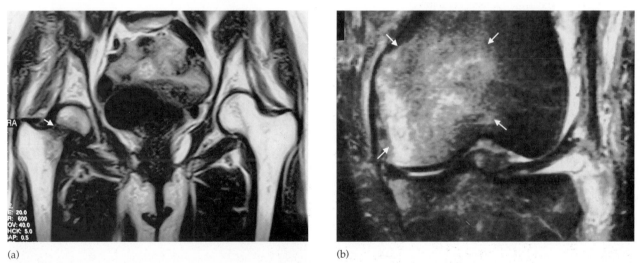

(a)   (b)

Fig. 14.14 (a) Coronal MRI showing a fracture of the right femoral neck (arrow) which was not visible on x-rays of the hip. The bone scan of this patient is illustrated in Fig. 14.11(b). (b) Bone bruise. Magnetic resonance imaging scan in a patient who suffered severe soft tissue damage to the lateral side of his knee. The high signal in the medial femoral condyle (arrows) is due to a bone bruise. The plain films of the knee showed no bony injury.

Specific injuries

Stress fracture

Stress fractures are due to repeated, often minor, trauma. They occur in athletes, particularly in the tibia and fibula.

Another example is the so-called march fracture occurring in the shafts of the metatarsals. Initially, despite the presence of pain, a radiograph will show no evidence of a fracture but if a further film is taken after 10–14 days a periosteal

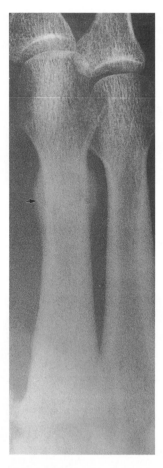

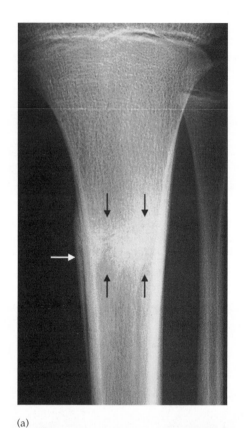

(a)

Fig. 14.15 Stress fracture. This film was taken two weeks after the onset of pain. It shows a periosteal reaction (arrow) around the metatarsal shaft although a fracture cannot be seen.

reaction may draw attention to the fracture site, where a thin crack may be visible (Fig. 14.15). A stress fracture may appear as a sclerotic band across the bone and a fracture line may not necessarily be visible (Fig. 14.16).

Fig. 14.16 (*Opposite.*) Stress fracture. (a) Fracture appearing as a sclerotic band (vertical arrows) across the tibia accompanied by a periosteal reaction (horizontal arrow). (b) In this calcaneum there is a sclerosis adjacent to the fracture (arrow).

(b)

Radionuclide bone scanning can be helpful in distinguishing stress fractures from other causes of pain, because a stress fracture will appear as an area of increased uptake before any changes are visible on the radiographs (Fig. 14.17).

Insufficiency fracture

An insufficiency fracture results from normal activity or minimal trauma in weakened bone commonly from osteoporosis or osteomalacia. Compression fractures of the verte- bral bodies are the commonest insufficiency fractures but they also characteristically occur in the sacrum, pubic rami and femoral necks though other bones may be involved.

Pathological fracture

A pathological fracture is one that occurs through abnormal bone. Pathological fractures may be the presenting feature of both primary and secondary bone tumours (Fig. 14.18). Often, the causative lesion is obvious. Sometimes, particu- larly in ribs, metastases responsible for fractures are ill

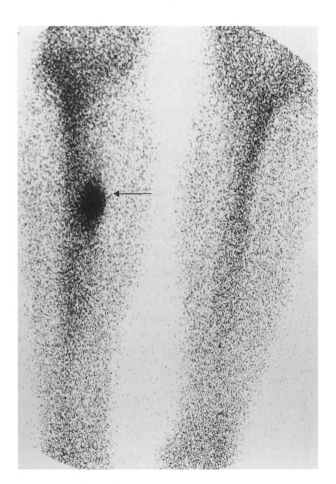

Fig. 14.17 Stress fracture. Radionuclide bone scan showing increased uptake in the tibia (arrow) of this athlete with pain in the leg. The radiographs at the time of the scan were normal.

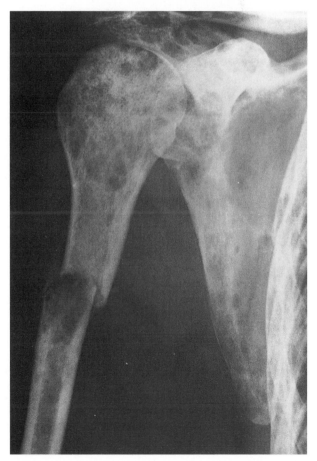

Fig. 14.18 Pathological fracture of the humerus. There are widespread lytic metastases from a carcinoma of the breast.

defined and difficult to see. In such cases the diagnosis rests on recognizing the irregularity of the margins of the fracture. If there is doubt about the diagnosis it is helpful to look elsewhere in the skeleton for other metastases.

Transverse fractures occur through abnormal bone, particularly in Paget's disease. In these instances the Paget's disease is always obvious (Fig. 14.19).

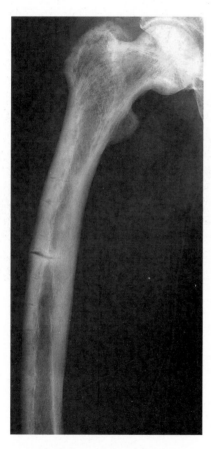

Fig. 14.19 Paget's disease showing incomplete fractures, known as infractions, of the lateral aspect of the femur. Note the marked thickening of the cortex and bowing of the femur.

Non-accidental injury (battered baby syndrome)

It is essential that everyone looking at radiographs should be fully aware of this condition, as the radiological findings may suggest the diagnosis in otherwise unsuspected cases. If child abuse is suspected the whole skeleton including the skull should be x-rayed, as clinically unsuspected injuries may be detected.

Certain patterns suggest that the injury is not accidental (Fig. 14.20):

- *Multiplicity of fractures* is an important sign, particularly if the fractures are of different ages, because the injuries often take place on separate occasions. Some fractures appear recent, while others show periosteal reaction indicating healing (see also Fig. 11.2a, p. 300).
- *Metaphyseal fractures* frequently appear as small chips from the metaphyses of the long bones. They most probably result from twisting and pulling the limbs of a struggling baby.
- *Metaphyseal sclerosis* is probably due to repeated injury and repair.
- *Epiphyseal separation* is frequently associated with a metaphyseal fracture.
- *Periosteal reactions.* Haemorrhage under the periosteum occurs easily in children. The elevated periosteum lays down new bone which may be so extensive that it envelops the shaft.

Radionuclide bone scanning is sometimes used to show multiple bone and joint injuries in the non-accidental injury. Such injuries appear as areas of increased uptake and detailed radiographs of these sites can be taken at presentation and again during the follow-up period if the initial radiographs show no abnormality.

A CT scan or ultrasound of head may be necessary to detect brain damage or subdural haemorrhage.

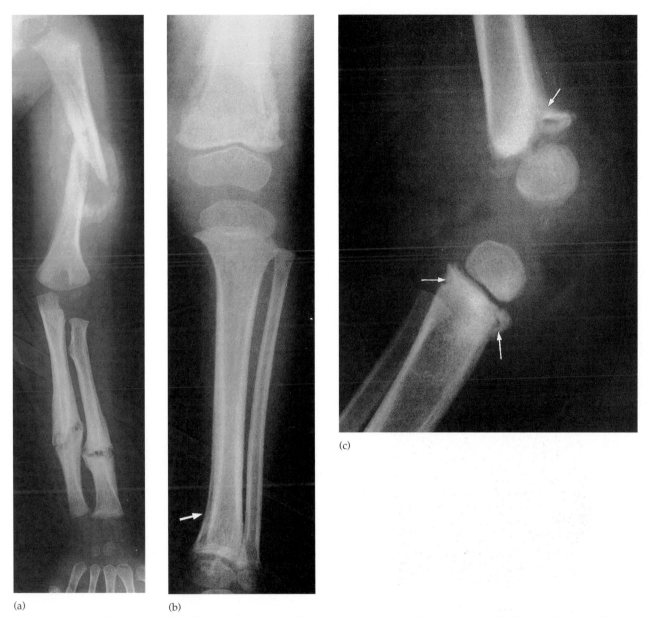

(a)

(b)

(c)

Fig. 14.20 Non-accidental injury. (a) Multiplicity of fractures. There is a recent fracture of the humerus with florid callus formation. The fractures of the radius and ulna are of longer duration and show healing with organized callus. (b) Periosteal reaction along the shaft of the tibia (arrow) from previous trauma with haemorrhage under the periosteum. There has been recent trauma to the lower end of the femur with marked periosteal reaction. (c) Metaphyseal fractures (arrows) and sclerosis around the knee.

15

Skull and Brain

The newer imaging modalities have had a greater impact on the diagnosis of diseases of the central nervous system than on any other body system. Computed tomography (CT) and magnetic resonance imaging (MRI) have become the standard investigations for most disorders of the brain. Plain films are still the initial investigation for disorders of the bones of the skull – particularly fractures, but otherwise have limited uses. Radionuclide imaging has been almost entirely replaced by CT and MRI. Arteriography is now limited to demonstrating arterial stenoses, aneurysms and some arteriovenous malformations.

Plain skull films

Normal

The standard views of the normal skull and pituitary fossa are shown in Figure 15.1a–e.

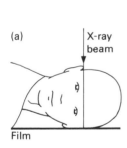

(a)

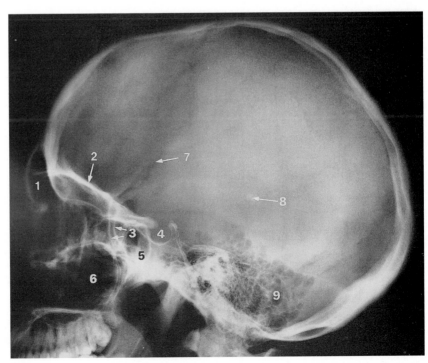

(a)

Fig. 15.1 Standard view of the skull (diagrams show the position in which the films are taken). (a) Lateral view: **1**, frontal sinus; **2**, roof of right and left orbits superimposed; **3**, anterior border of middle cranial fossa; **4**, pituitary fossa; **5**, sphenoid sinus; **6**, maxillary antrum; **7**, vascular groove; **8**, pineal; **9**, mastoid air cells. *Continued on pp. 392–3.*

389

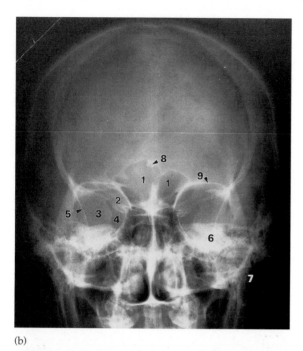

(b)

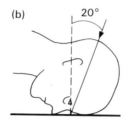

(b)

Fig. 15.1 *Continued.* (b) Posteroanterior view: **1**, frontal sinuses; **2**, lesser wing of sphenoid; **3**, greater wing of sphenoid; **4**, superior orbital fissure; **5**, wall of middle cranial fossa, **6**, petrous bone; **7**, mastoid air cells; **8**, pineal; **9**, superior orbital margin.

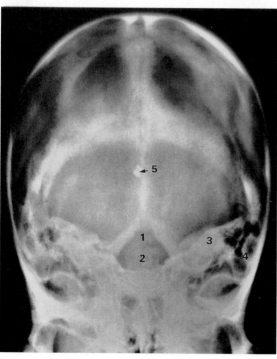

(c)

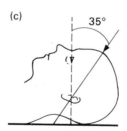

(c)

Fig. 15.1 *Continued.* (c) Towne's view: **1**, foramen magnum; **2**, dorsum sellae of pituitary fossa; **3**, petrous bone; **4**, mastoid air cells; **5**, pineal.

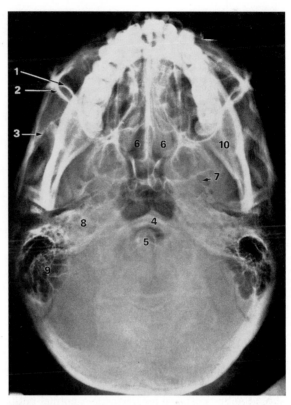

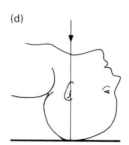

(d)

(d)

Fig. 15.1 *Continued.* (d) Base or submentovertical view: **1**, lateral border of maxillary sinus; **2**, lateral border of orbit; **3**, anterior border of middle cranial fossa; **4**, anterior arch of atlas; **5**, odontoid peg; **6**, sphenoid sinus; **7**, foramen ovale; **8**, petrous bone; **9**, mastoid air cells; **10**, mandible.

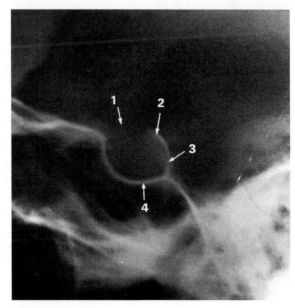

Fig. 15.1 *Continued.* (e) Normal pituitary fossa: **1**, anterior clinoid process; **2**, posterior clinoid process; **3**, dorsum sellae; **4**, floor. The white line forming the floor and the dorsum sellae is known as the lamina dura.

(e)

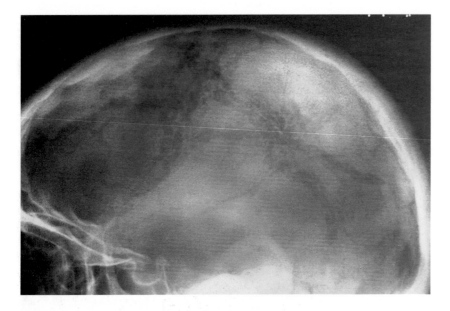

Fig. 15.2 Vascular markings. In this normal skull the vascular markings are very prominent. Note how they form a star-shaped translucency in the parietal region.

The bones of the normal vault have an inner and outer table of compact bone with spongy bone (diploë) between them; the sutures remain visible even when fused and should not be mistaken for fractures. A normal but inconstant suture – the metopic suture – is sometimes seen dividing the frontal bone. Blood vessels cause impressions on the bones of the vault, resulting in linear or star-shaped translucencies (Fig. 15.2) and small lucencies are often seen in the inner table near the vertex caused by normal arachnoid granulations; they may be difficult to distinguish from small lytic lesions.

The position of a *calcified pineal gland* is the only method of identifying the midline of the brain on plain films.

Abnormal plain films

A good method of reviewing plain skull films is to look first for intracranial calcification, then to examine the pituitary fossa and, lastly, to review the bones for areas of lysis or sclerosis and for fractures.

The important plain film signs of intracranial disease are calcification and signs of raised intracranial pressure. Pituitary tumours can be recognized by enlargement of the pituitary fossa (Fig. 15.3).

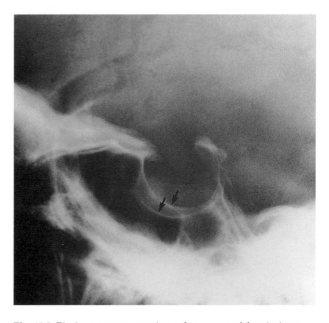

Fig. 15.3 Pituitary tumour causing enlargement of the pituitary fossa with a sloping floor. The floor appears as a double line on the lateral view (arrows).

Intracranial calcifications on plain films

Most intracranial calcification is normal and of no significance to the patient. These calcifications can usually be readily identified from their site (Fig. 15.4). It is, however, very important to recognize those few occasions where the calcification is pathological. The major causes of focal areas of calcification are primary tumours (Fig. 15.5), notably meningioma and glioma, craniopharyngioma, arteriovenous malformation, large aneurysms and old abscesses. CT

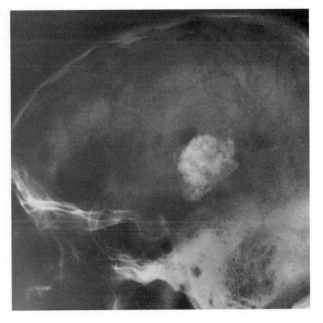

Fig. 15.5 Calcification in a glioma.

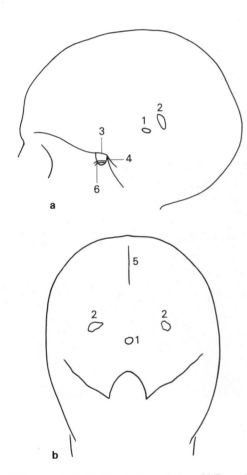

Fig. 15.4 Innocent calcification. (a) Lateral view. (b) Towne's view: **1**, pineal; **2**, choroid plexus, the calcification may be asymmetrical and only one side may calcify; **3**, interclinoid ligament; **4**, petroclinoid ligament; **5**, falx, best seen on frontal projection; **6**, atheromatous calcification in carotid artery.

or MRI is almost invariably required, either to make the diagnosis or to show the shape and extent of the underlying abnormality.

Raised intracranial pressure

Plain film abnormalities are only seen in prolonged cases of raised intracranial pressure. In children under eight the sutures are widened (Fig. 15.6), whereas in older children and adults there is erosion of the lamina dura of the dorsum sellae, i.e. it becomes ill defined (Fig. 15.7). This form of erosion may be very hard to evaluate, particularly in older people.

Bone lysis

Focal areas of bone lysis usually indicate metastasis or myeloma (Fig. 15.8). Large areas of bone destruction are seen in Langerhans histiocytosis (histiocytosis X), giving the appearance known as 'geographical skull' (Fig. 15.9), and in a form of Paget's disease known as osteoporosis circumscripta.

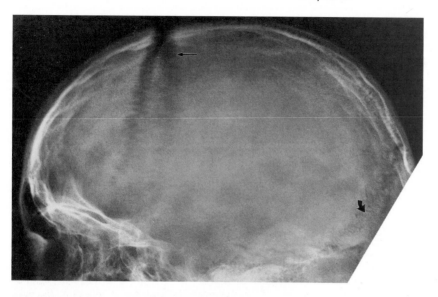

Fig. 15.6 Raised intracranial pressure in a child. The sutures become widened affecting the coronal suture first (straight arrow). Compare this widened suture with the normal lambdoid suture (curved arrow).

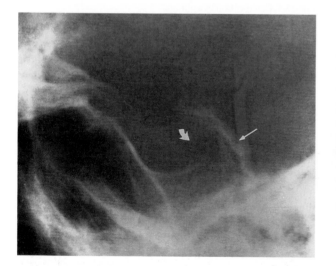

Fig. 15.7 Raised intracranial pressure in an adult. The dorsum sellae of the pituitary fossa (curved arrow) has lost its sharp outline and appears indistinct. The petroclinoid ligament is calcified (arrow).

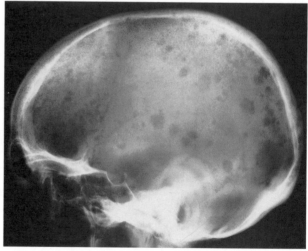

Fig. 15.8 Myeloma. Many well-defined lytic lesions of various sizes are seen in all areas of the skull vault.

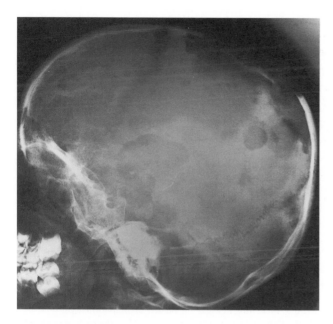

Fig. 15.9 Langerhans histiocytosis. In this child's skull vault there are large irregularly shaped lytic areas. This appearance is known as a geographical skull.

Bone sclerosis

The commonest cause of bone sclerosis is hyperostosis frontalis interna, a condition of no clinical significance, in which there is irregular thickening of the inner table of the skull in the frontal regions sparing the midline (Fig. 15.10).

Localized sclerosis, sometimes mixed with lytic areas, may be caused by a meningioma (Fig. 15.11), metastasis or fibrous dysplasia.

Paget's disease (Fig. 15.12) is the commonest cause of widespread sclerosis in the United Kingdom, but is much less common in the United States. It may take the form of multiple patchy areas of increased density. A striking feature is thickening of the skull vault. Recognition of this thickening is important in distinguishing Paget's disease from sclerotic metastases. Basilar invagination may also be seen due to softening of the bone. In basilar invagination the odontoid peg encroaches on the foramen magnum and may press on the brain stem, giving rise to clinical symptoms and signs.

Skull fractures

Skull fractures are discussed on p. 415 together with the other plain film signs of head injury.

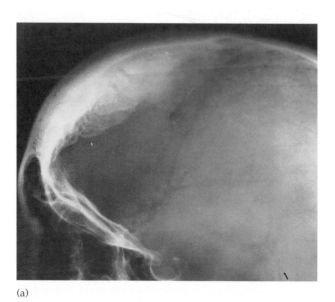

(a)

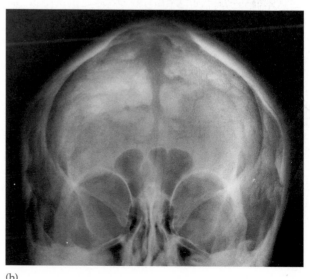

(b)

Fig. 15.10 Hyperostosis frontalis interna. (a) Lateral view showing sclerosis in the frontal region near the vertex. (b) The frontal view shows the characteristic sparing of the midline.

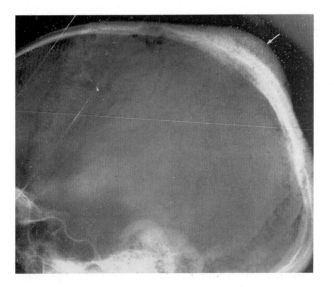

Fig. 15.11 Meningioma. A localized hyperostosis (arrow) is seen on the parietal bone.

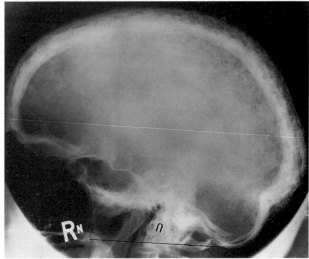

Fig. 15.12 Paget's disease. There is generalized sclerosis with marked thickening of the bone. Basilar invagination is present which can be detected by drawing a line from the back of the hard palate to the lowermost part of the occiput. The tip of the odontoid peg should not be more than 6 mm above this line. In this case it is 18 mm.

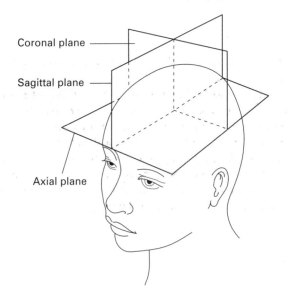

Fig. 15.13 Illustration of the axial, coronal and sagittal planes.

CT and MRI

In most neurological disorders, plain films are either normal or the abnormalities are too non-specific for the diagnosis to be made. CT and MRI give vastly more information and one or other investigation is indicated in practically all patients with intracranial disease.

Computed tomography of the brain

A routine CT examination of the brain involves making nine or ten axial sections. The axial plane is the routine projection but it is sometimes possible to obtain direct coronal scans. Alternatively computer reconstructions can, in selected circumstances, be made from the axial sections which then provide images in the coronal or sagittal planes (Fig. 15.13). The window settings are selected for the brain, but may be altered to show the bones.

Contrast enhancement for CT

An intravenous injection of contrast medium is often given because an abnormality not seen on precontrast scans may be rendered visible following contrast enhancement. Contrast enhancement is predominantly a consequence of breakdown of the blood–brain barrier allowing contrast to enter the lesion. Such breakdown occurs mainly with neoplasm, ischaemia and inflammation.

The use of contrast enhancement varies in different centres. It tends not to be used in patients who are known to have a very recent cerebral haemorrhage or infarct.

Normal head CT

A normal CT scan of the head is illustrated in Fig. 15.14. The cerebrospinal fluid (CSF) is seen as water density within the ventricular system and subarachnoid space, and is clearly different in density to the normal brain substance. With modern scanners and the use of intravenous contrast enhancement, it is possible to distinguish the white and grey matter of the brain. The larger arteries at the base of the brain as well as the venous sinuses can be recognized when opacified by contrast medium. The falx appears denser than the brain. The supratentorial regions are usually well shown, but details of the posterior fossa may be obscured by artefacts from the overlying temporal and occipital bones.

Abnormal head CT

the cardinal signs of an abnormality on a CT scan are:
- abnormal tissue density
- mass effect
- enlargement of the ventricles.

Abnormal tissue density

Abnormal tissue may be of higher or lower density than the normal surrounding brain. High density is seen with recent haemorrhage (see Fig. 15.27, p. 410), calcified lesions (see Fig. 15.22a, p. 405) and areas of contrast enhancement (see Fig. 15.21, p. 404). Low density is usually due to neoplasms or infarcts, or to oedema, which commonly surrounds neoplasms, infarcts, haemorrhages and areas of inflammation. Oedema characteristically shows finger-like projections and does not enhance with intravenous contrast medium (see Fig. 15.19a, p. 403). As a rule it is not possible to diagnose the nature of a mass based on attenuation values alone; an exception being lipoma which, because it contains fat, has a value of approximately – 100 Hounsfield units.

Mass effect

The lateral ventricles should be examined to see if they are displaced or compressed. Shift of midline structures, such as the septum pellucidum (the thin membrane separating the lateral ventricles), the third ventricle, or the pineal, is a common finding with intracranial masses. Ventricular dilatation will occur if the mass obstructs the flow of CSF. Specific diagnoses are suggested by combining the clinical features with information about multiplicity, size, shape, position and density of the lesion, all of which are known with great accuracy from CT.

Enlargement of ventricles

There are two basic mechanisms which cause the cerebral ventricles to enlarge:
- obstruction to the CSF pathway, either within the ventricular system (non-communicating hydrocephalus) or over the surface of the brain (communicating hydrocephalus);
- secondary to atrophy of brain tissue (Fig. 15.15).

Computed tomography or MRI can provide an accurate picture of the size of the various ventricles, cerebral sulci and subarachnoid cisterns. With this information it may be possible to predict the nature of hydrocephalus.

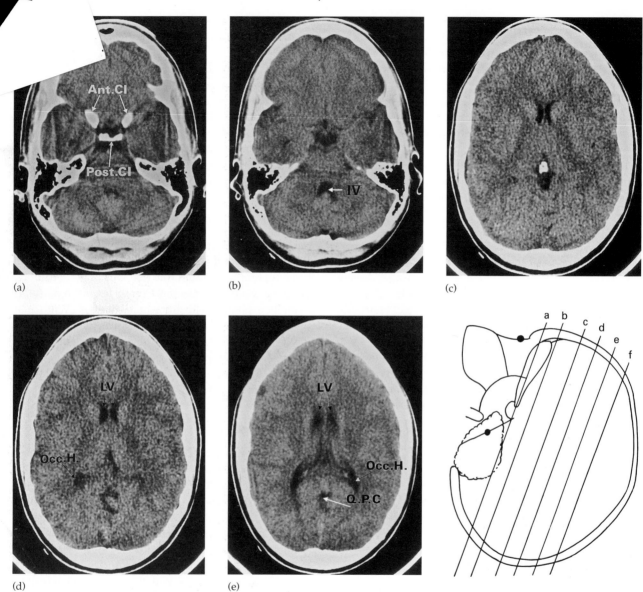

Fig. 15.14 Normal head CT. The images on the page opposite are representative sections from a postcontrast series. Those on this page are the precontrast images from the same patient. The levels at which the sections were taken are indicated in the diagram.

a.c.a.	anterior cerebral artery	m.c.a.	middle cerebral artery	Post. Cl	posterior clinoid process
Ant. Cl	anterior clinoid process	Occ. H	occipital horns	PS	pituitary stalk
CP	choroid plexus	P	pineal gland	Q.P.C.	quadrigeminal plate cistern
Fa	falx cerebri	p.c.a.	posterior cerebral artery	III	third ventricle
LV	lateral ventricle	Pe	petrous bone	IV	fourth ventricle

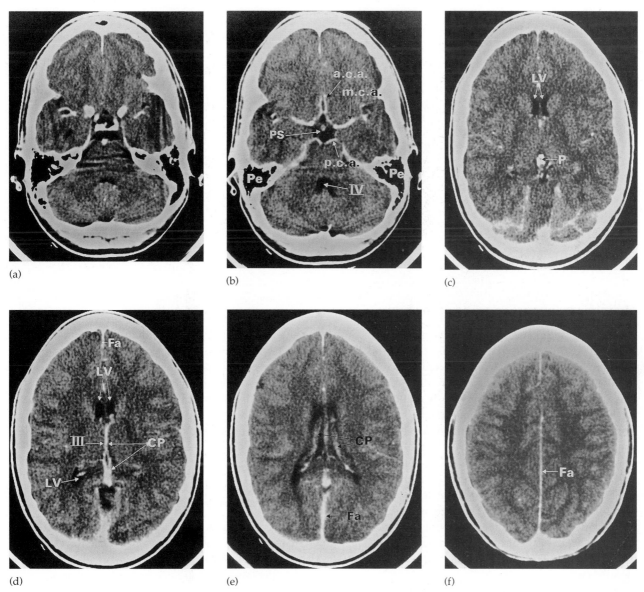

(a)

(b)

(c)

(d)

(e)

(f)

Fig. 15.14 (*Continued*).

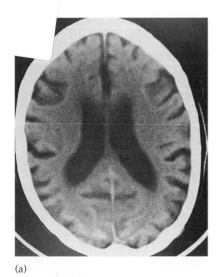

(a)

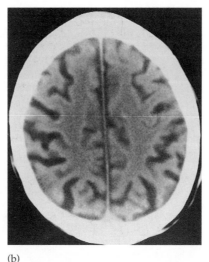

(b)

Fig. 15.15 Cerebral atrophy. CT scan. The ventricles are dilated from atrophy of the brain substance and the cortical sulci are widened. (a) Section through bodies of lateral ventricles. (b) Section above level of lateral ventricles (the midline linear density is the falx).

Magnetic resonance imaging of the brain

The routine techniques used for magnetic resonance imaging vary from centre to centre. Axial, coronal and sagittal projections are all considered standard (Fig. 15.16) and two of these are usually chosen for a routine examination. This multiplanar capability is particularly useful for assessing the extent of pituitary tumours and for visualizing structures in the posterior fossa and craniovertebral junction. A variety of signal sequences are used to create the images: particularly T1-weighted and T2-weighted images.

It is possible to recognize flowing blood and, therefore, the larger arteries and veins stand out clearly without the need for contrast medium. The characteristics of grey and white matter are different, and both are clearly different from the CSF in the ventricular system and subarachnoid space. Therefore, the anatomy of the brain can be exquisitely displayed.

The disadvantages of MRI compared to CT are the inability to show calcification, lack of bone detail, the relative expense of the technique, and the difficulty of monitoring seriously ill patients whilst lying within the scanner.

Contrast enhancement for MRI

The natural differences in MRI signal intensity are sufficiently great that the need for artificial contrast agents is less with MRI than it is with CT. Like the intravenous iodinated agents used for CT, the gadolinium compound used for MRI enhancement is excluded from the normal brain substance by the blood–brain barrier (it does, however, accumulate in the pituitary gland). Breakdown of the blood–brain barrier by tumours, abscess and infarcts means that gadolinium will accumulate within these pathological processes. The tissues containing the gadolinium show very high signal intensity (i.e. they appear white) on T1-weighted images.

Magnetic resonance angiography

Magnetic resonance angiography (MRA) of the vascular system (Fig. 15.17) has now developed to such an extent that it can be used to show arterial and venous anatomy as well as disorders such as severe stenoses and aneurysms.

Abnormal MRI of the brain

The range of abnormalities that can be shown by MRI is very great. Fat, subacute and chronic haemorrhage, oedema, CSF and flowing blood all have characteristic signal intensities. Thus it is more often possible to make a specific diagnosis of an intracranial disorder with MRI than with CT. Nevertheless, many mass lesions, such as the

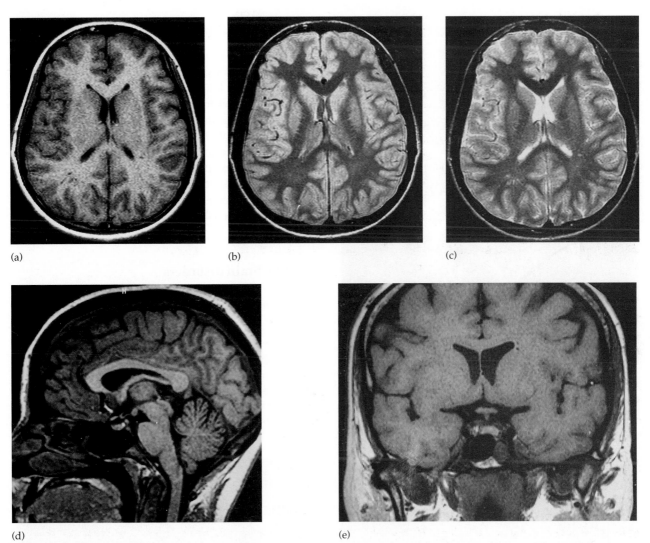

(a)   (b)   (c)

(d)   (e)

Fig. 15.16 Normal brain MRI. The top row of images are axial sections at the level of the lateral ventricles. (a) T1-weighted image. (b) Balanced image. (c) T2-weighted image. The bottom two images are (d) a midline sagittal section (T1-weighted) and (e) a coronal section through the level of the frontal horns (T1-weighted).

various cerebral neoplasms and infections, can appear similar to one another in all respects. A note-worthy feature of MRI is its ability to demonstrate plaques of demyelina-tion in multiple sclerosis (see Fig. 15.37, p. 415) and abnormal blood vessels such as arteriovenous malformations (see Fig. 15.33, p. 413).

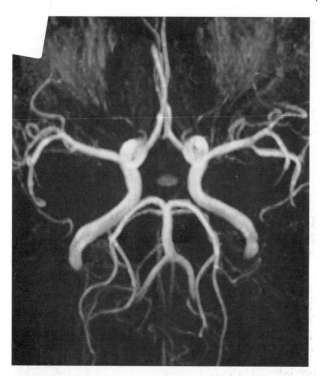

Fig. 15.17 Magnetic resonance angiography (MRA). The arteries at the base of the brain, the circle of Willis, are very well shown by MRA without the use of any contrast agent.

Neurosonography (Fig. 15.18)

With ultrasound it is simple to scan the heads of neonates and young babies to obtain images of the ventricular system and the adjacent brain. Scanning is best done through an open fontanelle where there is no bone to impede the transmission of ultrasound. Little discomfort is caused to the baby and the procedure is readily carried out even on ill babies in intensive care units. Neurosonography has proved particularly useful in detecting intracerebral haemorrhage and the ventricular dilatation that may follow. It has also been used to demonstrate the presence and cause of other forms of hydrocephalus and congenital abnormalities of the brain.

Specific brain disorders

Brain tumours

Glioma

At CT (Fig. 15.19), a glioma typically appears as a solitary, irregular mass surrounded by oedema. Compression or dis-

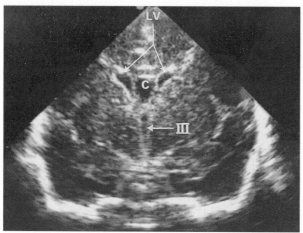

(a)

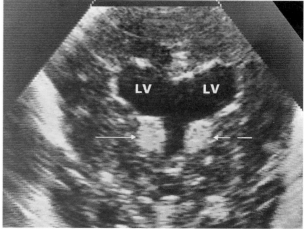

(b)

Fig. 15.18 Neurosonography. (a) Normal coronal section taken through the anterior fontanelle in a neonate. C, cavum septum pellucidum; LV, lateral ventricle; III, third ventricle. (b) Coronal section showing bilateral subependymal haemorrhages (arrows). The lateral ventricles are dilated.

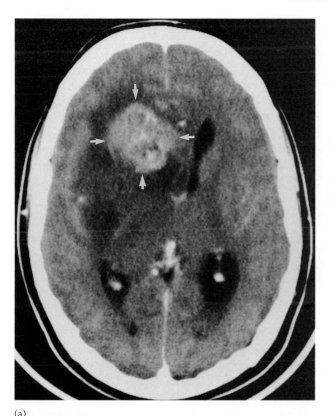

(a)

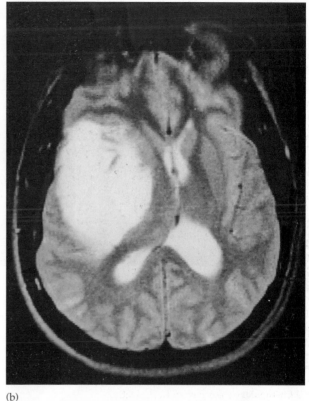

(b)

Fig. 15.19 Glioma. (a) CT scan, post i.v. contrast, showing round mass (arrows) with contrast enhancement and surrounding oedema. Note the compression and displacement of the adjacent lateral ventricles. (b) MRI scan (T2-weighted) in another patient, showing a large, high-intensity rounded lesion with displacement of the adjacent ventricular system.

placement of the ventricles can usually be demonstrated. The CT attenuation values of the tumour itself are usually low, but may be high or mixed. Gliomas may calcify; some, particularly the low grade tumours may be very densely calcified and even visible on plain film (see Fig. 15.5, p. 393). Most gliomas show partial enhancement with intravenous contrast medium (Fig. 15.19a); sometimes only the outer portion enhances, giving a so-called 'ring enhancement' pattern.

AT MRI, the signs are basically the same as for CT. The essential features are a mass, often with adjacent oedema. The mass may show a variety of signal intensities. In general, the tumour is lower in signal intensity than the normal brain on the T1-weighted images and higher in signal intensity on the T2-weighted images (Fig. 15.19b). Calcification, though sometimes recognizable as absence of

signal, is less evident than it is with CT. The enhancement pattern with gadolinium is similar to the pattern of contrast enhancement at CT (Fig. 15.20).

Brain metastases (Fig. 15.21)

Metastases in the brain may be of high or low density at CT. They usually show contrast enhancement and are often surrounded by substantial oedema. The MRI features are essentially similar. Metastases are typically multiple. A solitary metastasis is indistinguishable from a primary intra-cerebral brain tumour with either technique.

Meningioma

Meningiomas arise from the meninges of the vault, falx or

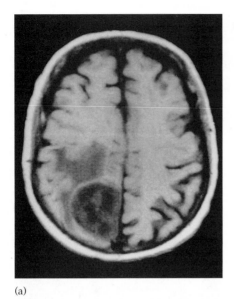 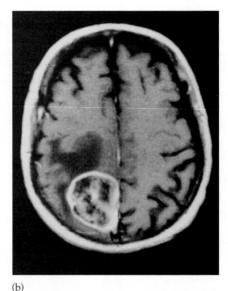

(a)   (b)

Fig. 15.20 (a) Pre- and (b) postcontrast enhancement (with intravenous gadolinium) shows the obvious partial enhancement of the tumour. Note the adjacent low intensity white matter oedema.

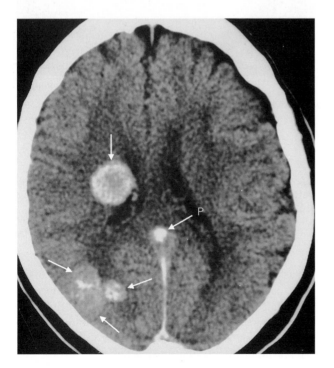

Fig. 15.21 Metastases. Enhanced CT scan showing several rounded areas of increased density (arrows). The round density in the midline is due to the pineal (P).

tentorium in characteristic sites, the commonest being the parasagittal region over the cerebral convexities and the sphenoid ridges. On an unenhanced CT scan, a meningioma is slightly denser than the brain because of fine calcium in the lesion (Fig. 15.22a). Following intravenous contrast injection the tumour shows marked enhancement (Fig. 15.22b). Sclerosis and thickening of the adjacent bone may also be seen (Fig. 15.11, p. 396).

The multiplanar imaging capability of MRI makes it possible to predict the site of origin of the tumour with greater confidence than is usually possible with CT (Fig. 15.23). Once it can be ascertained that the tumour is compressing the brain from outside the diagnosis of meningioma becomes highly likely.

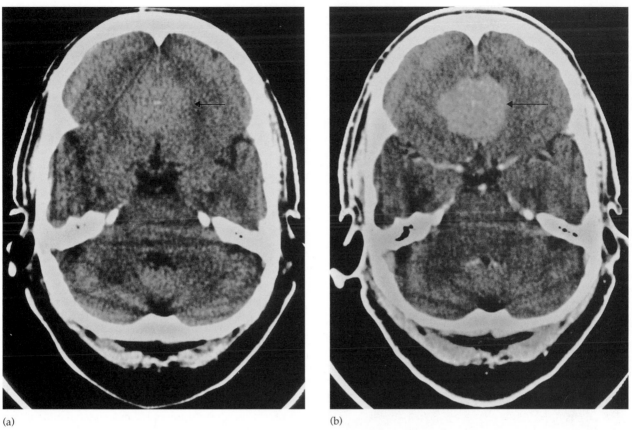

(a)   (b)

Fig. 15.22 Meningioma. (a) Precontrast image showing that the density of the meningioma (arrow) is slightly greater than the brain substance owing to fine calcification in the tumour. (b) Enhanced CT scan showing a large midline tumour (arrow) beneath the frontal lobes. Note the marked contrast enhancement.

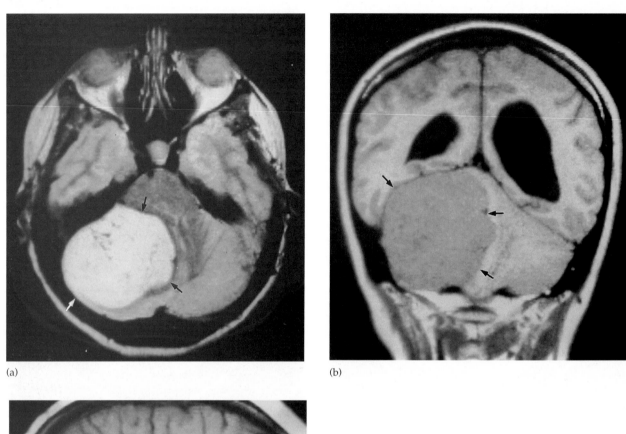

(a)

(b)

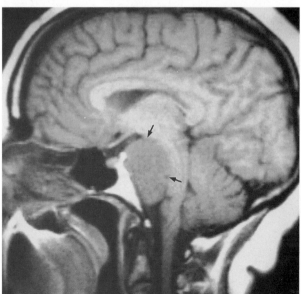

(c)

Fig. 15.23 Meningioma, illustrating the advantages of the multiplanar imaging capability of MRI in a patient with a large meningioma in the posterior fossa (arrows). (a) T2-weighted axial section. (b) T1-weighted coronal section. (c) Meningioma (arrows) of the clivus, in a different patient, pressing on the pons (T1-weighted midline sagittal section).

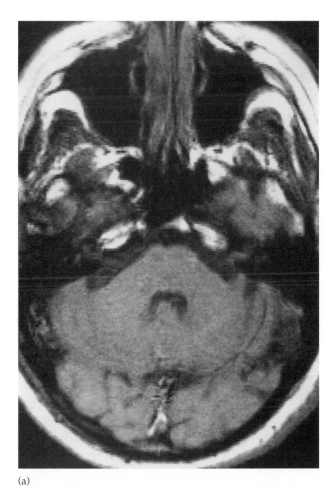

(a)

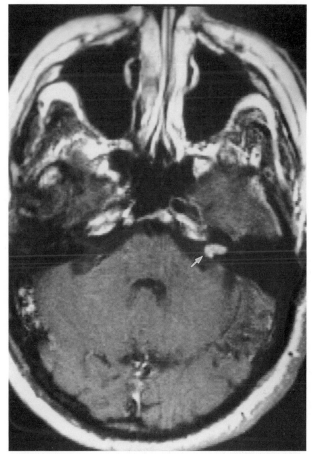

(b)

Acoustic neuroma

Neurofibromas of the acoustic nerve arise in the internal auditory canal or immediately adjacent to the internal auditory meatus in the cerebellopontine angle. When large, they can be recognized at CT or MRI (Fig. 15.24). When small, they may only be identifiable with MRI. Contrast enhancement improves their visibility with either technique (Fig. 15.24).

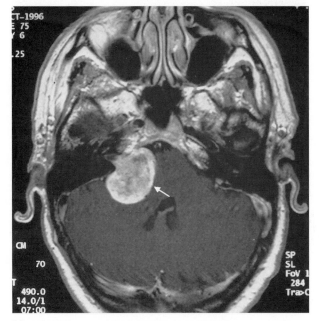

Fig. 15.24 Acoustic neuroma. (a) Precontrast MRI scan; the acoustic neuroma is virtually invisible. (b) Postgadolinium enhancement; the small acoustic neuroma (arrow) in the left internal auditory canal is clearly demonstrated. (c) A different patient with a larger right-sided acoustic neuroma (arrow) in the cerebellopontine angle (enhanced T1-weighted scan).

(c)

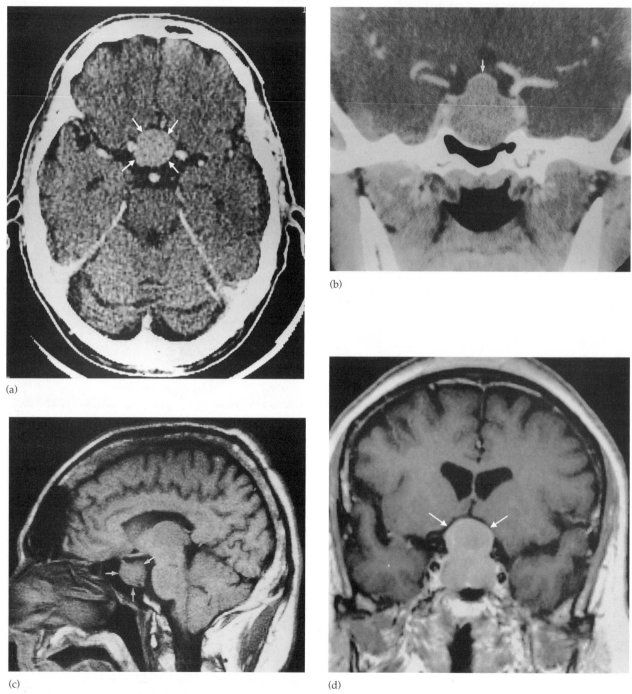

Fig. 15.25 Pituitary tumour. (a) Computed tomography scan after contrast shows a mass in the pituitary fossa which enhances vividly (arrows). (b) Direct coronal postcontrast CT scan in another patient, showing a large tumour expanding the pituitary fossa and projecting superiorly (arrow). (c) Sagittal MRI scan of a pituitary tumour (arrows) in another patient. (d) Coronal MRI scan, postcontrast, in a similar patient (the arrows point to the tumour).

Pituitary tumours

Computed tomography of the pituitary region requires thin sections through the pituitary fossa and suprasellar region in the axial and/or coronal plane (Fig. 15.25). Computed tomography can demonstrate the pituitary tumour directly, together with any suprasellar extension which may be pressing on the optic chiasm. A large pituitary adenoma may enhance vividly following intravenous contrast administration. Similar appearances, however, may be seen with a large aneurysm, a meningioma and a craniopharyngioma.

Magnetic resonance imaging is particularly suitable for demonstrating the presence and extent of a pituitary tumour (Figs 15.25 and 15.26). The combined sagittal and coronal imaging planes are ideal, showing very small tumours, smaller than can be seen with CT. Gadolinium enhancement is particularly useful for finding tumours less than 1 cm in diameter, so-called microadenomas of the pituitary. The upward extent of a pituitary tumour, particularly

its relationship to the optic chiasm and optic nerves, can be readily demonstrated with MRI.

Cerebral infarction and haemorrhage

Acute cerebral infarction and haemorrhage

Acute cerebral infarction and haemorrhage are often clinically similar. Computed tomography can help distinguish between these two entities, because acute intracerebral haemorrhage gives rise to a specific appearance, namely high density from the haematoma itself (Fig. 15.27). The high density area may be surrounded by a lower density region due to oedema. Depending on the site and amount of bleeding, blood may also be identified in the subarachnoid space and within the ventricles. The initial high density of the haemorrhage itself lessens over a week or two, eventually leaving a low density area indistinguishable from an infarct.

An acute infarct, on the other hand, does not produce any

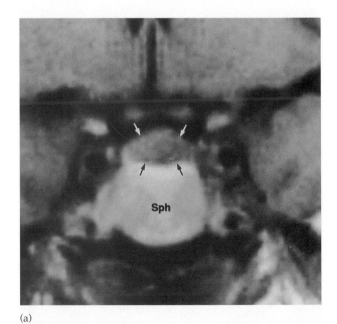

(a)

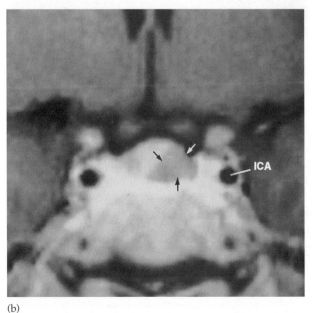

(b)

Fig. 15.26 Very small pituitary adenoma (microadenoma) demonstrated by MRI using gadolinium enhancement. (a) T1-weighted precontrast image, which shows slight enlargement of the pituitary. The arrows point to the pituitary. (b) Postcontrast image on which the normal portion of the gland enhances whereas the adenoma (arrows) does not enhance. ICA, internal carotid artery; Sph, sphenoid sinus.

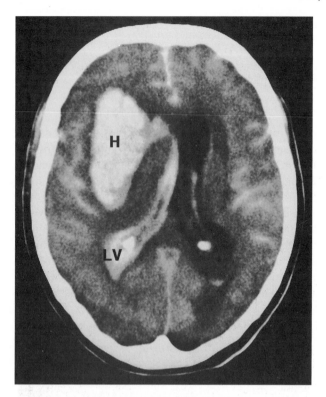

Fig. 15.27 Intracerebral haemorrhage. CT scan showing the
haematoma as a high density area (H). Blood is also seen in the
displaced lateral ventricle (LV) and in the subarachnoid spaces
over the cerebral hemispheres. The patient had suffered head
trauma.

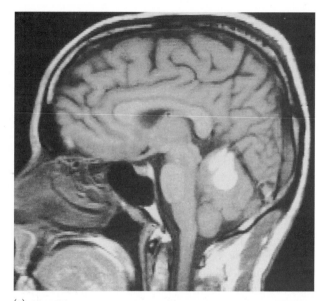

(a)

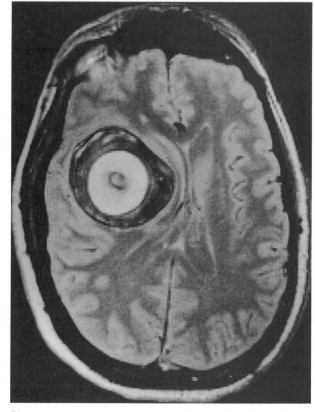

(b)

recognizable CT abnormality for the first 24 hours. Interestingly, MRI is not as useful as CT in the first 24 hours following an acute stroke. Even though MRI can demonstrate
altered signal from both infarction and haemorrhage, the
appearances in the two conditions are indistinguishable
from one another using MRI at this early stage.

In the ensuing few days after the onset of stroke, the
changes of intracerebral haemorrhage at MRI become more

Fig. 15.28 Cerebral haemorrhage on MRI. (a) A 7-day-old
haemorrhage into the superior portion of the cerebellum is clearly
shown as a high signal intensity collection on a T1-weighted
image. (b) A chronic haemorrhage in the right cerebral hemisphere
shows the complex mixture of high and low signals typical of old
haemorrhage.

specific. A subacute or chronic haemorrhage develops a specific signal pattern owing to breakdown products of haemoglobin, which have a paramagnetic effect that profoundly alters the MR signal in a highly characteristic way (Fig. 15.28).

Subacute and chronic infarction

Subacute and chronic infarction are recognizable at both CT and MRI. The changes are essentially those of oedematous brain conforming in shape to a known arterial distribution (Fig. 15.29), gradually resolving and sometimes leaving a recognizably atrophic area and/or persistent scar.

Subarachnoid haemorrhage

Subarachnoid haemorrhage is usually due to a ruptured intracranial aneurysm. Only the largest aneurysms are directly visualized at CT, even with intravenous contrast enhancement (Fig. 15.30). CT is nevertheless the best initial investigation as it may localize the site of bleeding. If multiple aneurysms are found at arteriography, the information from CT may indicate which aneurysm has bled. MRI can also demonstrate the presence of aneurysms. It will show smaller aneurysms than can be demonstrated with CT, but MRI is not as sensitive as arteriography in this regard. Like CT, MRI may show haematoma adjacent to a ruptured aneurysm (Fig. 15.31).

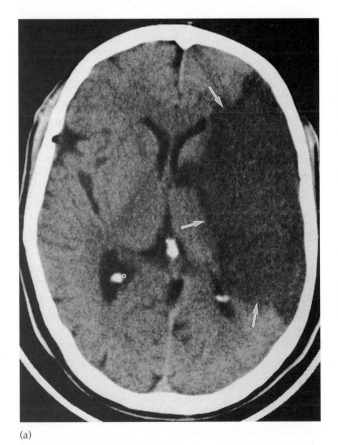

(a)

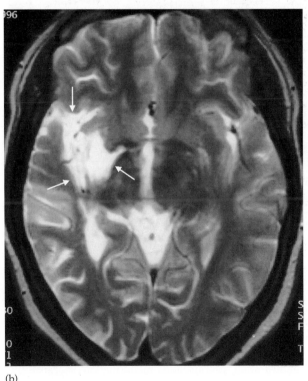

(b)

Fig. 15.29 Cerebral infarction. (a) Unenhanced CT scan showing a low density region of the left cerebral hemisphere conforming to the distribution of the middle cerebral artery (arrows). (b) MRI scan of another patient with a right middle cerebral artery territory infarct. The infarcted area (arrows) shows patchy high signal intensity on this T2-weighted image. The arrows point to the anterior and posterior extent of the infarcted brain tissue.

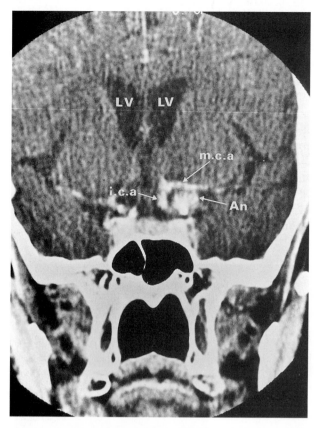

Fig. 15.30 Aneurysm (An) of the left internal carotid artery. This image, unlike most of the other CT scans in this chapter, is a direct coronal scan. LV, lateral ventricle; i.c.a., internal carotid artery; m.c.a., middle cerebral artery.

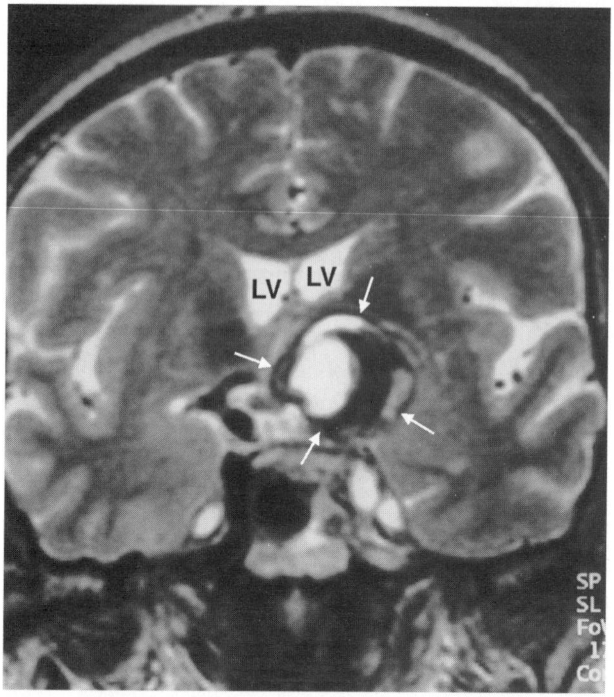

Fig. 15.31 MRI scan (T2-weighted) showing haemorrhage surrounding a ruptured middle cerebral artery aneurysm. The haemorrhage (arrows) shows the typical mixture of very high and very low signal intensity. LV, lateral ventricles.

Arteriovenous malformation

Arteriovenous malformations may present with haemorrhage. CT can demonstrate the abnormal vessels in the region of the haemorrhage, particularly with contrast enhancement (Fig. 15.32). MRI is particularly suitable for demonstrating arteriovenous malformations, because the signal from fast-flowing blood even without intravenous contrast agent is so very different to that of stationary tissues (Fig. 15.33). It has become the best method of investigation to confirm or exclude this particular diagnosis. As with aneurysms, angiography is then needed to define the vascular anatomy for those cases where surgery or percutaneous transvascular embolism is contemplated (Fig. 15.34).

Fig. 15.34 (*Opposite.*) Arteriovenous malformation. (a) Carotid angiogram showing a collection of large abnormal vessels (large open arrow) supplied by the middle cerebral artery (horizontal arrow.) On this injection the posterior cerebral artery (vertical arrow) but not the anterior cerebral artery has filled. (b) Subtraction. With this technique the shadowing due to the bones has almost been eliminated so that the contrast-filled vessels stand out more clearly.

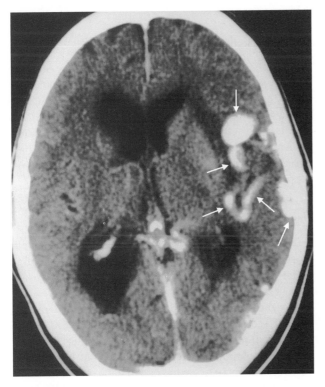

Fig. 15.32 Arteriovenous malformation. Enhanced CT scan showing the enlarged abnormal vessels (arrows).

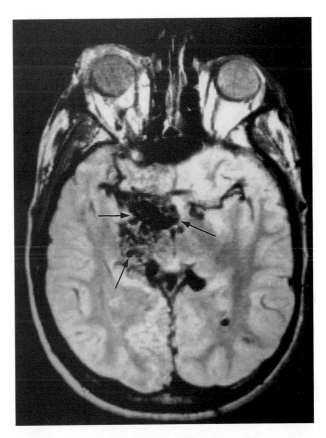

Fig. 15.33 Arteriovenous malformation. MRI scan (T1-weighted) showing signal void from fast-flowing blood in the vascular malformation (arrows).

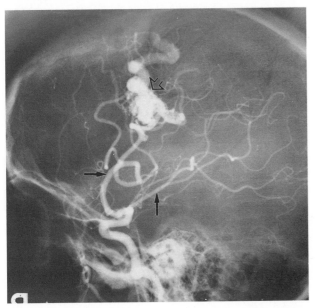

(a)

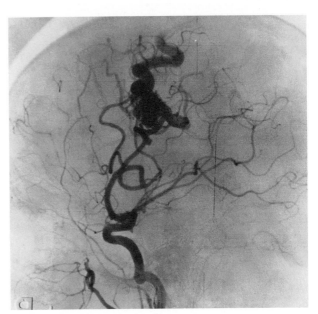

(b)

Infection

Inflamed tissue within the brain can be identified as increased contrast enhancement on CT. If abscess formation has occurred, the pus in the centre is of low density. Abscesses, therefore, typically show a 'ring enhancement' pattern (Fig. 15.35). The features at MRI are essentially similar.

Patients with AIDS have a high incidence of opportunistic brain infection. Herpes encephalitis may give a near diagnostic appearance of enhancing areas at CT, or altered signal intensity on MR scanning, in the temporal lobes. Multiple ring enhancing round lesions on CT or MRI are typical of toxoplasmosis or other cerebral abscesses (Fig. 15.36). Progressive multifocal leucoencephalopathy (PML) is due to the JC virus, which causes regions of demyelination. These are seen as oedematous areas of brain with no surrounding abnormal enhancement.

Multiple sclerosis (Fig. 15.37)

Prior to the introduction of MRI, there was no clinically useful imaging examination for diagnosing multiple sclerosis (MS). It is possible to see severe long-standing MS plaques on contrast-enhanced CT, but CT is too insensitive a test to be of clinical use. Magnetic resonance imaging, however, can demonstrate plaques at a time when the diagnosis of MS is not yet certain and can also be used to follow the progress of the disease.

Dementia

Only selected cases of dementia need imaging, for example, those under the age of 65 years and those in whom an underlying treatable lesion such as hydrocephalus or tumour is suspected on clinical examination.

In Alzheimer's disease, the commonest form of dementia, both CT and MRI shows dilated ventricles, widened cortical sulci and ill-defined white matter abnormalities. In multi-infarct dementia there are multiple areas of infarction of varying size. These two types of dementia can also be diagnosed with a radionuclide scan using ^{99m}Tc-HMPAO, an agent which crosses the blood–brain barrier.

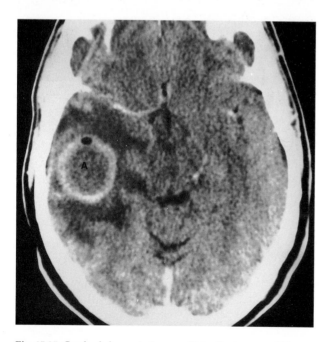

Fig. 15.35 Cerebral abscess in temporal lobe. Postcontrast CT scan showing a spherical mass with central low density and marked ring enhancement from the edge of the abscess (A). A small bubble of gas is seen at the top of the abscess.

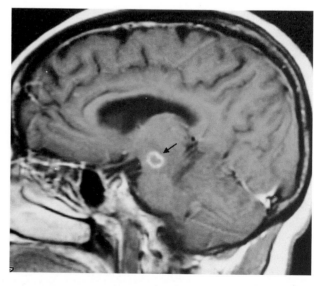

Fig. 15.36 Small cerebral abscess in a patient with AIDS. MRI scan (T1-weighted, postcontrast) shows ring enhancing lesion in the upper brain stem (arow).

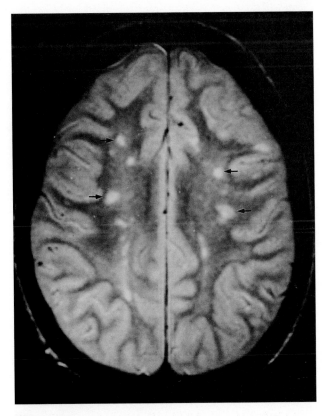

Fig. 15.37 Multiple sclerosis shown by MRI. The high signal intensity plaques of demyelination are well shown on this mildly T2-weighted image. (The arrows point to representative plaques.)

Head injury

Fractures

Most fractures of the skull are diagnosed on plain films. Fractures appear as linear translucencies, which can be difficult to distinguish from normal vascular markings and sutures. The following analysis may be helpful (Fig. 15.38):

• Fractures sometimes appear more translucent than vascular markings because they traverse the full thickness of the bone.

• Fractures may branch abruptly.

• Fractures have straight or jagged edges, and it is usually possible to see how these edges fit together. Conversely, venous channels have undulating irregular edges which cannot be fitted together.

• Arterial grooves have parallel sides and are therefore more easily mistaken for fractures, but they occur in known anatomical sites.

• Sutures also occur in recognized anatomical positions and show definite regular interdigitations. Widening of one suture has the same significance as a fracture.

A depressed fracture often has a different appearance. It appears dense rather than lucent because the fragments overlap. A tangential view is required to show the inward depression (Fig. 15.39).

An extradural haematoma should be carefully considered if a fracture crosses the groove for the middle meningeal artery.

Value of plain films following head injury

Although a fracture is a valuable sign of a head injury, the appearance of a fracture often bears little correlation to the underlying brain damage. Also, and very importantly, severe brain damage and subdural haematomas can occur in patients with normal skull films.

Plain film signs which indicate significant head injuries are:

• Shift of the pineal from the midline. This is an important sign as it often indicates an extradural or subdural haematoma. Swelling of one hemisphere owing to contusion of the brain can also cause pineal displacement.

• Fluid levels in the sinuses, or air in the subarachnoid space or ventricles, may indicate a fracture with a tear of the dura. Antibiotic treatment is often advocated with this type of injury to prevent meningitis. As with the detection of all fluid levels, it is necessary to take the lateral film with a horizontal ray.

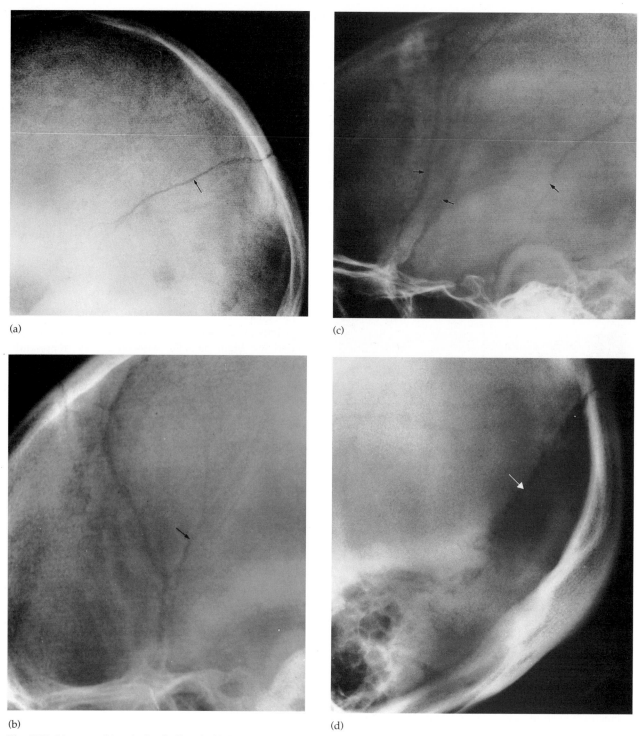

(a)

(c)

(b)

(d)

Fig. 15.38 Linear markings in the skull vault. (a) Fracture line with straight edges (arrow). (b) Arterial groove for middle meningeal artery (arrow) – line with straight edges occupying a recognized site. (c) Venous channels: wider, more undulating grooves (arrows) – the more posterior groove ends in a venous star. (d) Suture. These show regular interdigitations (arrow).

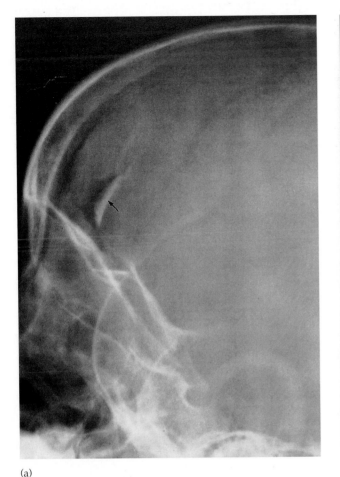
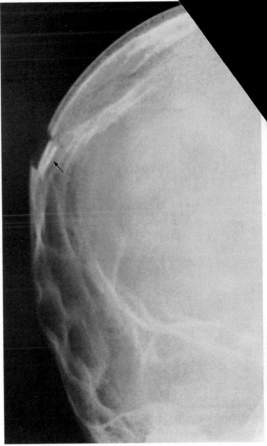

(a)   (b)

Fig. 15.39 Depressed fracture. (a) The fracture is seen as a curvilinear density (arrow) due to the overlapping fragments. (b) In a tangential view (another patient) the fragment can be seen to be depressed inwards (arrow).

Computed tomography in head injuries

Computed tomography of the brain should be carried out in all patients who have had a significant head injury, particularly if there is deterioration in the patient's conscious level or worsening of neurological deficit. (MRI can be used instead, but is rarely necessary). Computed tomography is initially performed without intravenous contrast administration. Selected cases are then given contrast. Computed tomography scans can distinguish between extracerebral and intracerebral lesions and can separate those patients with compressing haematomas who require immediate surgery from those in whom craniotomy might be of no benefit or might even be harmful.

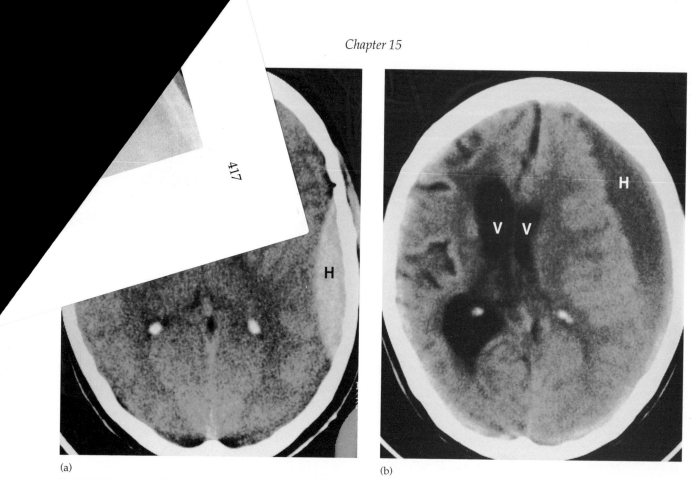

(a)   (b)

Fig. 15.40 Extracerebral haematoma. (a) CT scan showing a high density lentiform area typical of an acute extradural haematoma (H). (b) CT scan in another patient taken a month after injury showing a subdural haematoma (H) as a low density area. Note the substantial ventricular displacement. V, ventricles.

Extracerebral lesions

Extracerebral haematomas show a high density for about two weeks following the injury (Fig. 15.40a) but after three to four weeks the density decreases to become lower than that of the brain (Fig. 15.40b). In the intervening period, haematomas pass through a phase of being isodense with the brain and are therefore invisible on CT scans taken without contrast. Nevertheless, they should be suspected if there is midline or ventricular displacement. The displacement may not be obvious if the haematomas are bilateral.

Extradural haematoma is seen as a lens-shaped, smoothly demarcated high density area situated over the surface of the hemisphere associated with a skull fracture (Fig. 15.40a).

Subdural haematoma is similarly shaped and also situated over the surface of the cerebral hemisphere. A fracture somewhere in the skull may or may not be present.

Fractures of the skull base or vault. Fractures of the skull base and through the paranasal sinuses may be difficult or impossible to identify with plain films and should be carefully looked for on CT. Special settings, known as bone windows, may be needed to see subtle fractures.

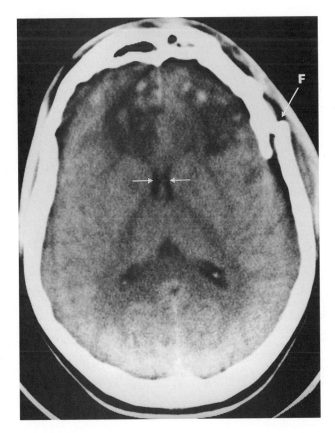

Fig. 15.41 Computed tomography scan showing several bilateral frontal lobe contusions. The widespread ill-defined low density is due to oedema: the small high density areas are focal haemorrhages. The lateral ventricles are compressed and therefore small (horizontal arrows). A depressed fracture (F) is also demonstrated.

Intracerebral lesions

Oedema. Post-trauma oedema may cause the whole brain to swell with homogeneous low density and compression of the ventricles (Fig. 15.41).

Contusions show as patchy areas of low density associated with swelling of the brain, causing displacement of the ventricles.

Intracerebral haematomas are seen as areas of high density which may be multifocal. There may be mass effect causing displacement of the ventricles and accompanying brain oedema.

 Occasionally a severe head injury can exist with no abnormal CT scan features.

16

Sinuses, Orbits and Neck

Sinuses

On plain radiographs the normal sinuses are transradiant because they contain air. Plain films have a role in showing mucosal thickening, fluid levels, bone destruction and fractures. However, in sinus disease CT is often the preferred technique as it gives much better images of the sinuses. Magnetic resonance imaging also demonstrates the sinuses well but is rarely needed as the primary investigation.

Thickened mucosa can be recognized providing there is some air in the sinus (Figs 16.1, 16.2 and 16.3), by noting the soft tissue density between the air in the sinus and the bony wall. The mucosal thickening may be smooth in outline or it may be polypoid. Polyps may be sufficiently large to extend into the nasopharynx.

Allergy and infection both cause mucosal thickening and

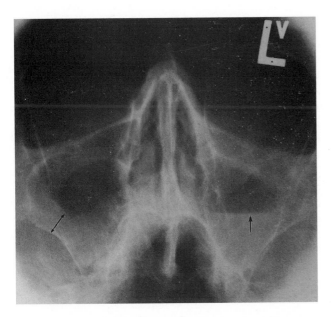

Fig. 16.1 Mucosal thickening and a fluid level. In the right antrum, thickening of the mucosa (arrows) results in the sinus no longer having a thin outline. The horizontal line in the left antrum on this erect film (arrow) indicates a fluid level which remains horizontal even when the patient's head is tilted.

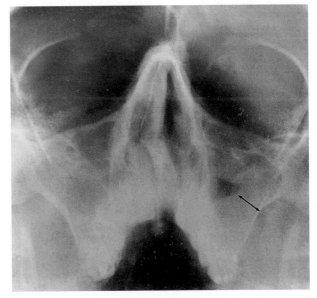

Fig. 16.2 Opaque antrum and mucosal thickening. The right antrum is completely opaque and it appears denser than the orbit. There is gross mucosal thickening in the left antrum (arrow) with only a small amount of air left in the antrum.

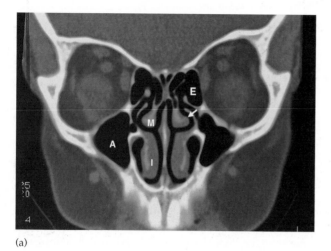

(a)

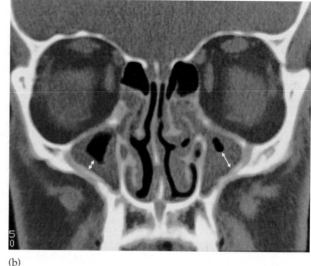

(b)

Fig. 16.3 Coronal CT scan. (a) Normal sinuses. Note the excellent demonstration of the bony margins. The arrow points to the middle meatus into which the maxillary antrum, frontal, anterior and middle ethmoid sinuses drain. A, maxillary antrum; E, ethmoid sinus; I, inferior turbinate; M, middle turbinate. (b) Sinusitis. Mucosal thickening prevents drainage of the sinuses. Both antra are almost opaque. The arrows indicate mucosal thickening in the antra.

it is impossible to say radiologically which condition is responsible.

Fluid in the sinuses is recognized by the presence of a fluid level. With the patient erect, a fluid level appears as a horizontal line across the sinus which remains horizontal even when the patient's head is tilted (Fig. 16.1). Fluid levels are seen with infection in the sinus and also with trauma, when a fracture allows blood or CSF to collect in the sinus.

Both CT and MRI can elegantly demonstrate mucosal thickening and fluid levels as well as displaying the bony walls of the sinuses. Sinus anatomy is ideally demonstrated with coronal CT sections. This information shows the drainage sites of the frontal, ethmoid and maxillary sinuses into the middle meatus and is a great aid for the surgeon planning endoscopic sinus surgery (Fig. 16.3).

The opaque sinus

The sinus becomes opaque when all the air is replaced and it then appears as dense or denser than the adjacent orbit on a plain film (Fig. 16.2).

The causes of an opaque sinus are:
• *Infection or allergy.* The air in the sinus is replaced by fluid, or a grossly thickened mucosa, or a combination of the two.

• *Mucocele.* Mucoceles are obstructed sinuses. Secretions accumulate and the sinus becomes expanded. A frontal sinus mucocele may erode the roof of the orbit and cause exophthalmos. Computed tomography clearly shows the size and extent of a mucocele.
• *Carcinoma of the sinus or nasal cavity.* In all opaque sinuses, particularly the antra, special attention should be paid on both plain films and CT to the bony margins, because if these are destroyed, the diagnosis of carcinoma becomes almost certain (Fig. 16.4). Computed tomography is superb at visualizing bone destruction, but its greatest value is in demonstrating tumour invasion, by showing the extent of any soft tissue mass which may extend beyond the sinus cavity. The same features can also be seen with MRI. Computed tomography and MRI have an important role in treatment planning and in assessing the response to radiotherapy.

Nasopharynx

The adenoids are normally seen on the lateral film in children as a bulge projecting into the nasopharyngeal air passage (Fig. 16.5). Computed tomography and MRI give excellent visualization of the nasopharynx and can demon-

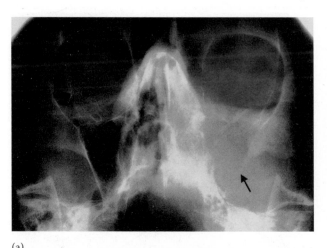

(a)

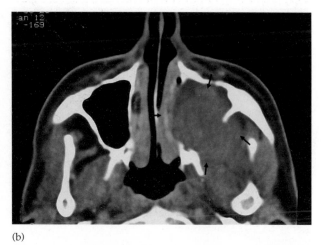

(b)

Fig. 16.4 (a) Carcinoma of the antrum. The left antrum is opaque and there is extensive destruction of its walls (arrow). Compare with the normal right antrum. (b) CT scan in another patient showing a large mass arising from the left antrum destroying its bony walls and extending into the adjacent soft tissues. The arrows point to the extent of the tumour. The opposite antrum is normal.

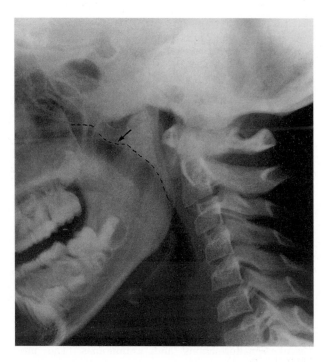

Fig. 16.5 Normal lateral view of postnasal space in a child. The posterior boundary of nasopharyngeal air passage has been marked with dotted lines and there is an impression into it (arrow) caused by the adenoids.

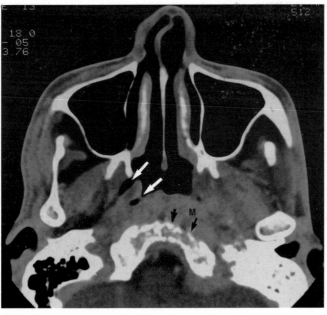

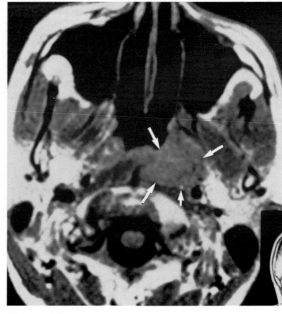

(a)   (b)

Fig. 16.6 Nasopharyngeal carcinoma. (a) CT scan showing a mass (M) in the nasopharynx on the left extending into the soft tissues of the postnasal space and eroding the skull base (black arrows). Note how the tumour obliterates the fossa of Rosenmuller and eustacian recess which are shown on the normal right side (white arrows). (b) MRI scan in another patient clearly showing the extent of the tumour (arrows).

strate the presence of tumour together with any spread into the skull base (Fig. 16.6).

Orbits

Computed tomography and MRI clearly demonstrate the anatomy of the orbits. Imaging is indicated in all patients with exophthalmos because it is possible to distinguish between masses arising within the orbit, masses arising outside the orbit and thyroid eye disease. With an intra-orbital mass its relationship to the optic nerve can be determined.

The main causes of intraorbital masses include various tumours, including tumours of the optic nerve (Fig. 16.7), vascular malformations and granulomas. The most common orbital masses originating outside the orbit are tumours or mucoceles of the frontal or ethmoid sinuses (Fig. 16.8), and a meningioma arising from the sphenoid ridge.

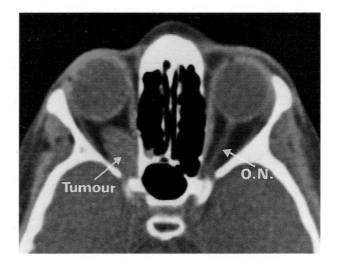

Fig. 16.7 Optic nerve glioma. CT scan showing a soft tissue mass arising from the optic nerve. The opposite orbit demonstrates the normal anatomy. O.N., optic nerve.

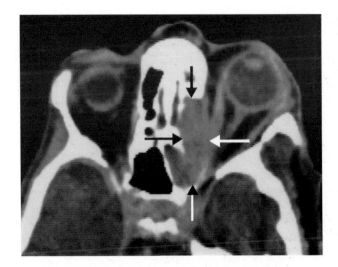

Fig. 16.8 Carcinoma of the ethmoid sinus invading the orbit and causing proptosis. The tumour is arrowed.

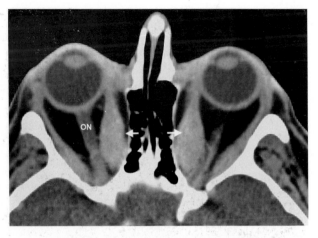

Fig. 16.9 Thyroid eye disease. CT scan through the orbits showing enlargement of the occulomotor muscles particularly the medial rectus (arrows). ON; optic nerve.

In thyroid eye disease, there is enlargement of the extraocular muscles (Fig. 16.9) which is frequently bilateral and may affect one, several, or all the eye muscles. There is also infiltration of the fat behind the eye which adds to the exophthalmos. When severe, these changes can lead to compression of the optic nerve in the apex of the orbit.

Salivary glands

Calculi, which occur most commonly in the submandibular duct or gland, normally contain calcium and can therefore be seen on plain films. In order to demonstrate the duct system sialography is necessary.

MRI is the preferred investigation for the investigation of masses thought to be in the salivary glands because the signal intensity of masses is often very different to the normal salivary tissue. Magnetic resonance imaging is excellent for demonstrating the presence of a mass (Fig. 16.10) and its relationship to the facial nerve, important information if surgery is contemplated, but MRI is often not able to predict the nature of the mass.

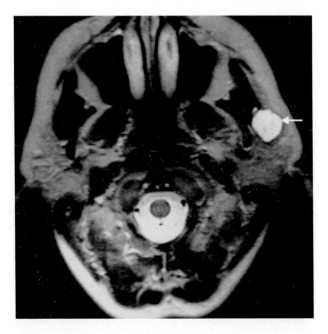

Fig. 16.10 MRI scan showing a high signal mass in the left parotid (arrow) which proved to be an adenoma.

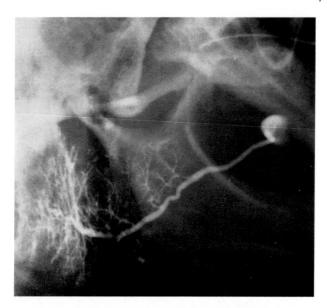

Fig. 16.11 Normal parotid sialogram. Note the long duct of even calibre and the fine branching of the ducts within the gland.

Sialography

A sialogram is performed by injecting contrast into the ducts of the salivary glands. Only the submandibular and parotid glands have ducts that can be cannulated (Fig. 16.11). Stones and strictures in the ducts can be identified. Dilatation of small ducts, which is known as *sialectasis*, may occur with obstruction to the main duct (Fig. 16.12) but may also be seen without obvious obstruction.

Neck

Computed tomography and MRI can be carried out to investigate a mass in the neck, to stage a primary tumour arising in the neck and to determine the presence and extent of enlarged cervical lymph nodes.

For CT, intravenous contrast enhancement is usually necessary as this opacifies the many vessels that might otherwise be mistaken for small lymph nodes. The thyroid gland,

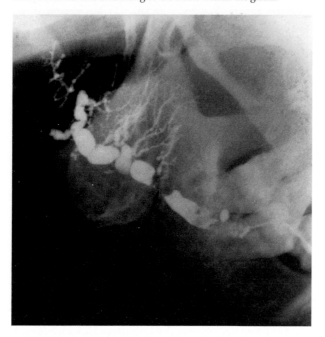

Fig. 16.12 Sialectasis. There is dilatation of the ducts due to a stone (arrow) in the main parotid duct.

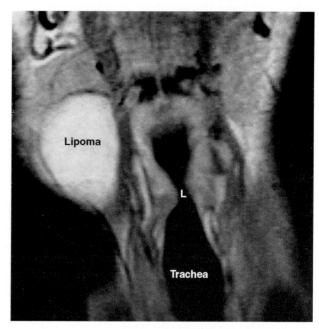

Fig. 16.13 Lipoma in the neck. Coronal MRI scan of a patient presenting with a lump in the neck. The signal characteristics of the mass indicate that it contained fat. Note how the larynx (L) has also been demonstrated.

which is situated on either side of the trachea, normally enhances quite markedly after intravenous contrast administration. Unless the mass is cystic, e.g. a branchial cleft cyst or cystic hygroma, or contains fat, (Fig. 16.13) it may be difficult to determine its nature using CT or MRI, although the size, shape and position may help in this regard.

Computed tomography can demonstrate enlarged lymph nodes in the neck that are too small to palpate or in sites not amenable to clinical examination. Enlarged nodes may be due to lymphoma, metastases (Fig. 16.14) or infection but their appearance on CT and MRI is similar irrespective of the cause.

Larynx

The larynx is best examined with MRI because of the excellent demonstration of soft tissues and the ability to produce images in the coronal plane. Alternatively, CT can be employed. Direct inspection by laryngoscopy reveals a great deal of information about the larynx, particularly in regard to the vocal cords. However, imaging can provide additional information regarding the spread of tumours outside the larynx, particularly into the subglottic space which cannot be inspected directly.

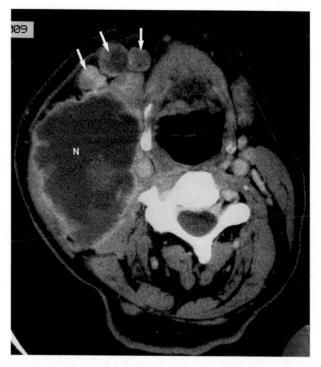

Fig. 16.14 Lymphadenopathy. There is a large lymph node (N) and several additional enlarged nodes (arrows) caused by metastases from a carcinoma of the floor of the mouth.

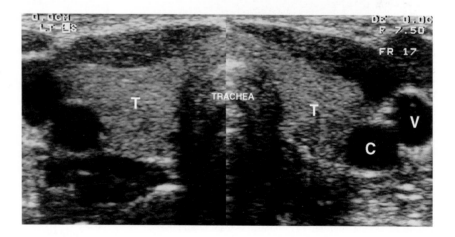

Fig. 16.15 Normal ultrasound of thyroid. The two lobes of the thyroid (T) lie on either side of the trachea. The carotid artery (C) and jugular vein (V) lie lateral to the thyroid gland.

Thyroid imaging

The thyroid is usually imaged by ultrasound (Fig. 16.15) or alternatively with nuclear medicine techniques by giving an intravenous injection of ^{99m}Tc pertechnetate or ^{123}I (Fig. 16.16). It is rarely necessary to use CT to examine the thyroid except in the case of a retrosternal goitre.

The commonest reason for imaging the thyroid is to determine the nature of a thyroid nodule, in particular to try and exclude malignancy. Ultrasound determines whether a nodule is cystic or solid or a mixture of both. Cysts are invariably benign and complex solid/cystic lesions are usually benign. A solid mass could be a carcinoma or an adenoma (Fig. 16.17). Ultrasound may show that the nodule is part of a multinodular goitre by demonstrating an enlarged gland with several nodules of varying size. The risk of malignancy in a multinodular goitre is little higher than in the general population.

Most solitary nodules do not take up radionuclide and are referred to as cold nodules and may be a cyst, adenoma or carcinoma (Fig. 16.18). Occasionally a nodule is functioning and takes up the radionuclide and sometimes referred to as a hot nodule. Such nodules are invariably benign adenomas. The remainder of the gland may show substantially reduced activity because of suppression of TSH production. As these nodules function independently of pituitary control they are known as autonomous nodules (Fig. 16.19).

The use of fine needle aspiration with cytological examination of the aspirate has increased considerably because of the limitations of both ultrasound and radionuclide

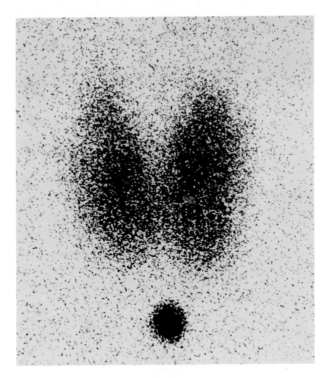

Fig. 16.16 Normal thyroid. ^{123}I radionuclide scan. The intense activity below the thyroid is a marker indicating the position of the suprasternal notch.

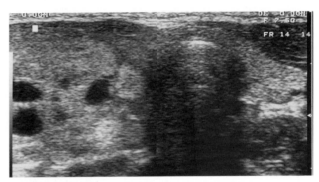

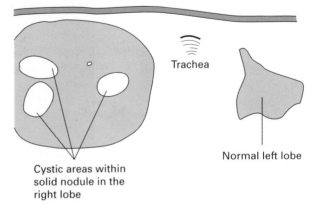

Fig. 16.17 Thyroid nodule. Ultrasound showing a colloid nodule in the right lobe of the thyroid showing solid and cystic areas. The left lobe of the thyroid is normal.

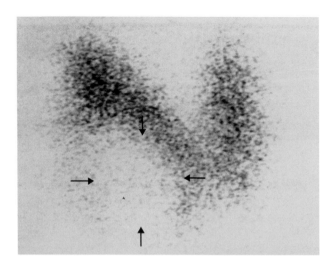

Fig. 16.18 Solitary non-functioning thyroid nodule. [123]I radionuclide scan showing a large 'cold' area in the lower pole of the right lobe of the thyroid (arrows). At surgery the nodule proved to be a carcinoma.

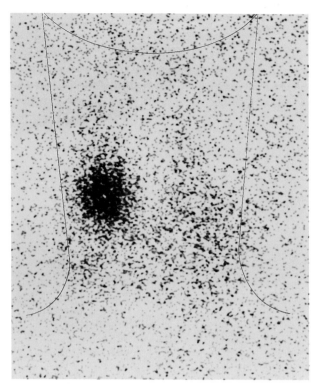

Fig. 16.19 Solitary functioning thyroid nodule. [123]I radionuclide scan showing intense uptake in the functioning adenoma. The remainder of the gland shows substantially reduced activity, because of suppression of TSH production. The outlines of the neck and jaw have been drawn in.

scanning. Many centres advocate aspiration as the initial investigation of a thyroid nodule because both solid and cystic lesions require confirmation of the diagnosis.

Thyroid masses may extend retrosternally into the mediastinum and thyroid imaging with ^{123}I or CT can be used to determine whether such a mass is due to thyroid tissue.

Iodine-131 has limited use because of high radiation dose to the thyroid. It has, however, an important role in the management of thyroid cancer. Most thyroid cancers present as 'cold' nodules. Imaging for metastatic spread at this stage is of no avail as the metastases do not take up sufficient radionuclide. However, after the normal thyroid tissue has been ablated by surgery or by a therapeutic dose of ^{131}I, thyroid stimulating hormone (TSH) levels rise and stimulate any functioning metastatic or recurrent tumour, which may be identified by radionuclide imaging and subsequently treated with a therapeutic dose of [131]I.

Parathyroid imaging

The usual cause of primary hyperparathyroidism is a parathyroid adenoma, which may be detected on ultra-

sound as a mass lying behind the thyroid. A parathyroid adenoma will take up thallium 201 when injected intravenously. The thyroid, which overlies the parathyroids, also accumulates thallium but if the thyroid is imaged using ^{99m}Tc, the thallium and technetium images can be subtracted electronically from one another so that the uptake of thallium in the thyroid is removed and the resulting image is that of the parathyroids. The normal parathyroid glands are too small to be visualized, but even a small adenoma can be detected (Plate 6, opposite p. 326). Localization of a parathyroid adenoma prior to surgery for hyperparathyroidism is important because about 10% of adenomas occur in an ectopic position, often in the mediastinum.

17

Vascular and Interventional Radiology

ANGIOGRAPHY

An angiogram is an x-ray examination in which the blood vessels are opacified by an iodine-containing contrast medium. The low-osmolar agents are used in order to avoid the pain and complications encountered with high-osmolar materials. Angiograms are broadly divided into arteriograms and venograms, depending on the vessels injected.

Arteriography

Although it is possible to inject the contrast medium directly through a needle, almost all arteriograms are done via a catheter. The most widely used method of catheterizing a blood vessel is the 'Seldinger technique' illustrated in Fig. 17.1. At the end of the procedure, the catheter is pulled out. A few minutes compressing the puncture site with the fingers is enough to stop the bleeding in most patients. The advantages of the Seldinger technique are that it is easy and quick to perform, that the hole in the artery is no bigger than the catheter and that catheters of any length may be used.

The punctured artery may occasionally become blocked, or alternatively it may be difficult to stop the bleeding once the catheter has been withdrawn. Either complication may require surgical intervention.

The major indications for arteriography are to demonstrate:
• disorders of the blood vessels, particularly occlusions, stenoses, thrombi, aneurysm formation and vascular malformations (Fig. 17.2);
• arterial anatomy before surgery, only necessary where such information will influence a subsequent surgical procedure;
• investigation of bleeding from the gastrointestinal tract;
• some tumours, by showing abnormal areas of vascularity, although this indication has now been largely replaced by other imaging modalities.

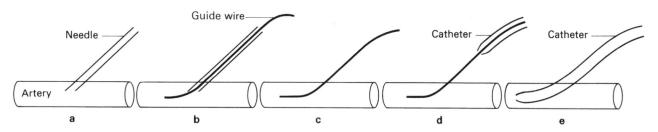

Fig. 17.1 Seldinger technique for catheterizing blood vessels. The femoral artery or vein are the usual vessels used. (a) A needle is inserted through the skin into the blood vessel. (b) A guidewire is passed through the needle into the lumen of the vessel. (c) The needle is withdrawn, leaving the guidewire in the lumen of the vessel. (d) A catheter is threaded over the guidewire and passed into the lumen of the vessel. (e) The guidewire is withdrawn, leaving the catheter in position in the lumen of the vessel.

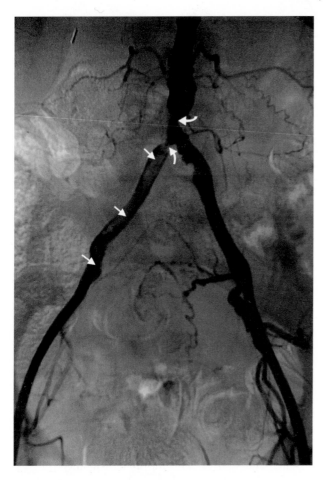

Fig. 17.2 Digital subtraction angiogram showing stenoses in the lower aorta and right common iliac artery (curved arrows). There is a long thrombus in the right common iliac artery (arrows) occluding the right internal iliac artery.

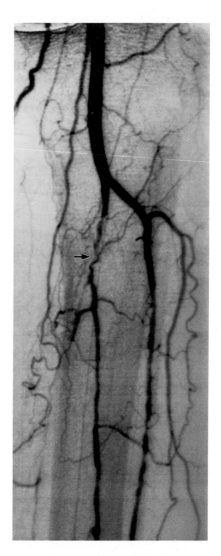

Fig. 17.3 Digital subtraction angiogram (DSA) following an intra-arterial injection of contrast medium. Note that the bones and soft tissues are barely visible. The angiogram shows the left popliteal artery and its branches with severe atheromatous stenosis of the proximal posterior tibial artery (arrow).

Subtraction angiography

It is possible to subtract the shadows that are present on the plain films from the films taken after the contrast has been injected for the angiogram. The result is an image containing details of the opacified structures only (Fig. 17.3). This principle is employed in digital subtraction angiography (DSA), also known as digital vascular imaging (DVI), in which the images are digitized and manipulated by a computer. Digital subtraction angiography is performed in the same way as conventional angiography but with the advantage that much smaller catheters can be used and much less contrast medium given.

Venography (phlebography)

Thrombi in the deep veins of the legs or in the iliac veins can be demonstrated by leg and pelvic phlebography. A large volume of contrast medium is injected into a small vein close to the toes. The contrast is forced into the deep venous system of the calf by means of tourniquets or by performing the examination with the patient semi-erect. Provided enough contrast is used, it is possible to demonstrate the pelvic veins and the inferior vena cava as well as the leg veins. Thrombi may cause a complete blockage or they may be seen as filling defects in the opacified veins (Fig. 17.4).

Ultrasound techniques in arterial and venous disorders

Ultrasound allows non-invasive examination of arteries and veins.

Ultrasound of the venous system has in many centres replaced venography for the detection of venous thrombosis. With a venous thrombosis, intraluminal echogenic material is visible and the veins lose their normal compressibility; thrombus-free veins should be compressible by direct pressure using the ultrasound transducer. Colour Doppler scanning shows that there is a lack of spontaneous flow in the affected veins.

Ultrasound can readily visualize the iliac, common femoral and popliteal veins although it can be sometimes difficult to visualize the calf veins (Plate 7, opposite p. 326). A disadvantage with ultrasound is that it is unreliable for examining the femoral vein within the adductor canal.

Ultrasound of the arterial system has been used extensively for examining the carotid arteries in patients with suspected cerebral ischaemia. Ultrasound techniques may also be used to visualize the aorta, iliac, femoral, popliteal and renal arteries.

The common, internal and external carotid arteries can be readily visualized in the neck. The location or size of any atheromatous plaques and the severity of any luminal narrowing can be determined. With colour Doppler imaging a stenosis in the artery can be visualized and an occlusion will show as an absence of flow (see Plate 2c, opposite p. 110). Because a stenosis disrupts the normal flow pattern, analysis of the flow velocity waveform can give further information regarding the degree of stenosis.

Magnetic resonance angiography

Angiography using magnetic resonance imaging is potentially a very useful non-invasive technique which is used principally for the arterial system although veins can also be

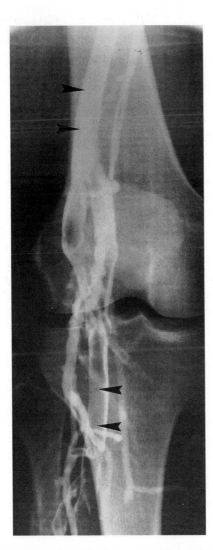

Fig. 17.4 Leg venogram showing deep vein thrombosis. The lower arrows point to the filling defect of the thrombus in the popliteal vein. Compare with the uniform opacity of the normal vein higher up (upper arrows).

imaged (Fig. 17.5). Several different imaging sequences are in use. Most depend on the signal obtained from flowing blood and do not require the injection of a contrast agent. Magnetic resonance angiography is particularly useful for showing the larger vessels, notably aortic aneurysms including dissecting aneurysms and for confirming the diagnosis of carotid artery disease and renal artery stenosis. Aneurysms and vascular malformations can also be detected in the intracranial circulation.

INTERVENTIONAL RADIOLOGY

The radiologist is now involved in carrying out various percutaneous techniques under imaging control. These include dilating stenoses, occluding vessels, draining abscesses and

other fluid collections, and obtaining biopsy samples. These procedures greatly assist and may modify surgery, or even replace it altogether. They are carried out with the help of a variety of imaging modalities, notably fluoroscopy, angiography, ultrasound, CT and, more recently, MRI. Interventional radiology is usually performed under local anaesthesia, causing only relatively minor discomfort to the patient. Only the basic principles of the interventional techniques in widespread use will be described here.

Angioplasty

Arterial stenoses and even occlusions may be traversed with a guidewire. A balloon catheter can be passed through the abnormal site, which has been previously determined by arteriography (Fig. 17.6). The stenosis is then dilated by inflating the balloon (Fig. 17.7). This percutaneous technique, which usually uses the femoral artery as an access route, has been widely employed in peripheral vascular disease and gives results as good as bypass surgery, particularly for iliac and superficial femoral artery disease. However, it can only be used in selected patients. Short stenoses are the ideal lesions to treat with angioplasty. Occlusions are less successfully treated and if the occlusion is very long, angioplasty may not be an appropriate treatment. Angioplasty has also been effective in renal artery stenosis in patients with renal vascular hypertension and in patients with coronary artery stenosis.

Therapeutic embolization

Arteries can be occluded by introducing a variety of materials through a catheter selectively placed in the vessel. Metal coils covered with thrombogenic filaments, gelatin foam, or even special cyanoacrylate glues that solidify on contact with blood, have all been used for therapeutic embolization. These techniques have been used primarily to control bleeding. Once arteriography has demonstrated the bleeding site, the offending vessel can then be embolized. Arterial embolization is also of use in patients with tumours, e.g. renal cell carcinoma, to reduce tumour vascularity prior to surgery, or inoperable tumours, or to treat intractable pain and bleeding (Fig. 17.8). Vascular occlusion has also been

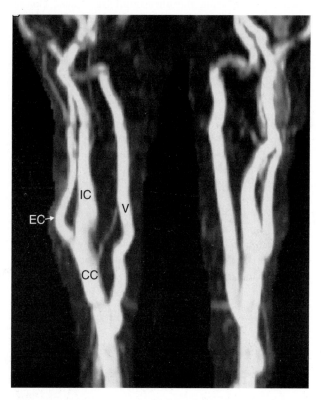

Fig. 17.5 MR angiography showing normal arteries in the neck. CC, common carotid; EC, external carotid; IC, internal carotid; V, vertebral artery.

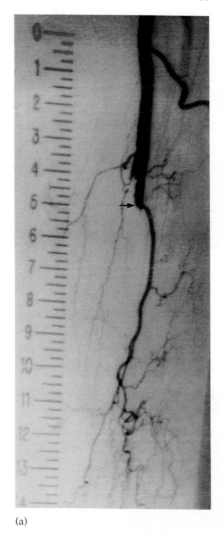

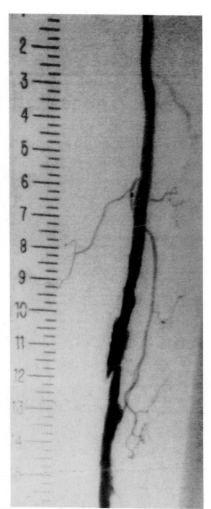

Fig. 17.6 Percutaneous transluminal angioplasty. (a) Preliminary arteriogram shows an occlusion in the left superficial femoral artery (arrow). (b) Following the angioplasty, the lumen has been restored. The residual irregularities usually improve within a few months. The distal run-off arteries are shown in Fig. 17.3.

(a)   (b)

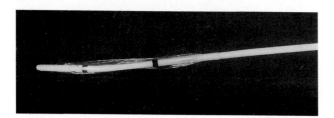

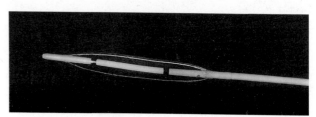

Fig. 17.7 Percutaneous angioplasty balloon catheters. The left image shows the catheter prior to inflating the balloon. The right image shows the catheter with the balloon distended as it would be if it were inside the artery.

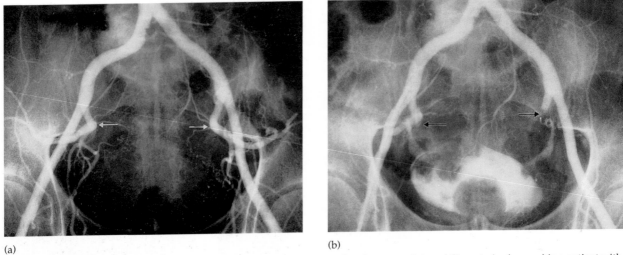

(a)

(b)

Fig. 17.8 Therapeutic embolization. (a) Arteriogram prior to embolization showing patent internal iliac arteries (arrows) in a patient with uncontrollable bleeding from a large bladder tumour. (b) Following embolization, both iliac arteries are occluded. The arrows point to the level of occlusion.

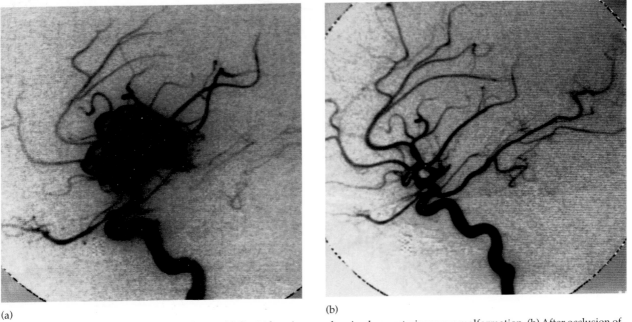

(a)

(b)

Fig. 17.9 Arteriovenous malformation occlusion. (a) Carotid angiogram showing large arteriovenous malformation. (b) After occlusion of the feeding vessels with cyanoacrylate glue the malformation is obliterated.

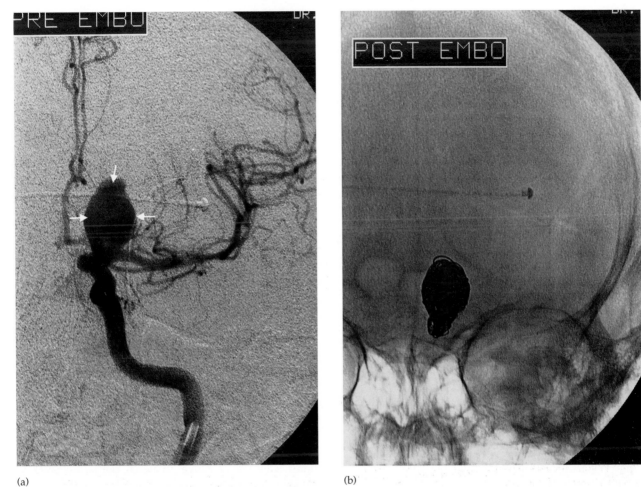

(a) (b)

Fig. 17.10 Aneurysm occlusion. (a) Carotid angiogram showing a large aneurysm (arrows) arising at the termination of the internal carotid artery. (b) Plain film after embolization of the aneurysm which is occluded with metal coils.

successfully used in treating arteriovenous malformations in various organs, most notably the brain and the lungs (Fig. 17.9). Aneurysms on the intracranial arteries can be occluded thus avoiding craniotomy (Fig. 17.10).

Vascular catheterization for infusion purposes

Arterial catheters can be accurately placed for infusion of cytotoxic agents directly into malignant tumours and for the infusion of fibrinolytic agents to dissolve fresh clots from the vascular system — a technique known as thrombolysis.

Vascular stents and filters

Stents are expandable metal cylinders that can be embedded in plastic and collapsed to enable them to be inserted through an artery or vein (Fig. 17.11). Stents are being increasingly used in the treatment of arterial stenosis and occlusion in both coronary and peripheral arterial disease.

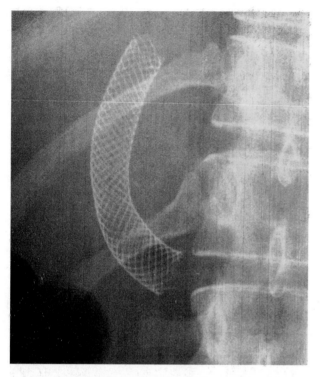

Fig. 17.11 Stent which has been placed in the liver to make a connection between the portal and systemic venous system in the TIPS procedure.

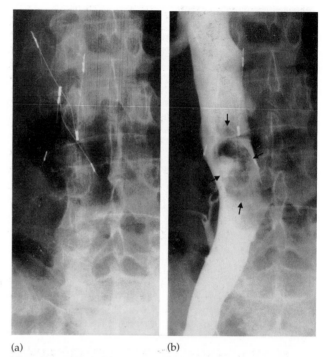

(a)   (b)

Fig. 17.12 IVC filter. (a) Plain film showing the bird's nest filter in place. (b) An inferior vena cavogram shows a large thrombus (arrows) trapped by the filter.

Stents can also be introduced through the femoral vein and placed across a stricture in the superior vena cava to overcome the distressing symptoms of superior vena caval obstruction which is usually caused by a malignant tumour in the mediastinum.

Inferior vena caval filters can be introduced percutaneously through the femoral vein. The filters trap emboli originating from leg or pelvic vein thrombi (Fig. 17.12). They are used in patients who are at risk of pulmonary embolism that cannot be managed satisfactorily with anticoagulation.

Percutaneous needle biopsy

Needle biopsy techniques are particularly useful for the non-operative confirmation of suspected malignancy. Under fluoroscopic, ultrasound or computed tomographic guidance (Fig. 17.13), a needle is passed to the desired site

and a small amount of tissue is removed. Most intrathoracic or intra-abdominal sites can be sampled. With a fine aspiration needle (20–22 gauge), material can be obtained for cytology. This needle can pass through blood vessels, vascular masses, loops of bowel and solid organs with only minimal risk of infection or bleeding. Apart from a small pneumothorax with intrathoracic biopsy, complications are extremely rare. To obtain material for histological study a larger needle (14–18 gauge for soft tissues, 10–13 gauge for bone) is used. The larger needles require specific approaches to avoid damage to intervening structures and require stricter indications than fine needle aspiration.

Percutaneous drainage of abscesses and other fluid collections

Specially designed drainage catheters can be introduced percutaneously into abscesses or other fluid collections. The catheters vary in diameter from 8–14 French depending on

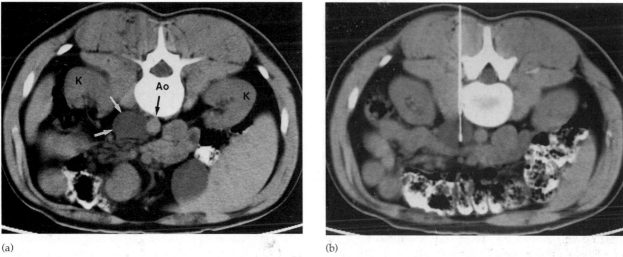

Fig. 17.13 Needle biopsy of an enlarged para-aortic lymph node under CT control with the patient prone. (a) An enlarged lymph node (arrow) is seen to the left of the abdominal aorta (Ao) at the level of the kidneys (K). (b) The tip of an 18-gauge cutting needle has been placed in the enlarged lymph node. The tissue obtained confirmed that the lesion was a metastasis from a germ cell tumour of the testis.

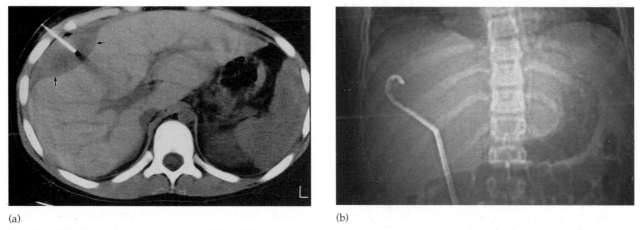

Fig. 17.14 Subphrenic abscess in a 14-year-old boy following acute appendicitis and appendicectomy. (a) An 18-gauge needle has been placed into the subphrenic abscess (arrows) anterior to the liver. A guidewire was passed through this needle and the needle was exchanged for a drainage catheter. (b) Film to show the position of the drainage catheter.

the nature of the fluid to be drained. The larger catheters may have a double lumen to assist with irrigation of an abscess cavity. They are introduced under the control of whichever imaging modality is most convenient; the essential feature is that the operator must know exactly the location of the abscess and must know that the route chosen for the catheter will be safe (Fig. 17.14). Ultrasound, CT and fluoroscopy are the usual methods.

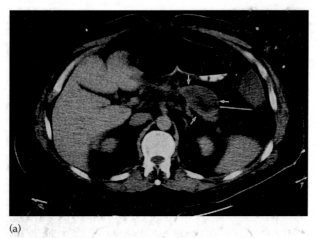 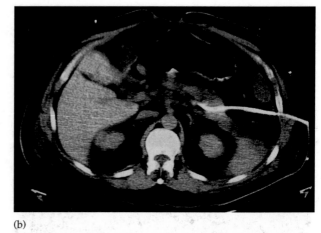

Fig. 17.15 Pancreatic abscess drainage. (a) CT scan showing abscess (arrows) in the body of the pancreas and a fine needle introduced from the left flank, avoiding the spleen, kidney and colon. (b) The needle has been exchanged for a 12 F drainage catheter and the abscess is now smaller. Another abscess is also present (*).

Once the catheter has been placed in an abscess, it is usually necessary to allow the pus to drain for several days. Irrigation of the tube and the abscess cavity is often essential for continued effective drainage. Thus, the placement of the tube is only the first step in successful percutaneous abscess drainage.

The technique is suitable for most abdominal abscesses, though the success with some forms of abscess is considerably greater than with others. For example, percutaneous drainage is usually successful for liver and intraperitoneal abscesses, but much less satisfactory for pancreatic abscesses (Fig. 17.15) particularly if they follow pancreatitis and are multiple or multiloculated.

Drainage of the urinary system

Internal drainage of the urinary system with the use of double-J stents placed into an obstructed pelvicaliceal system with the distal end of the catheter in the bladder has become standard practice. These stents are usually placed via a cystoscope, the catheters being passed into the ureteric orifice under direct vision. Alternatively, the double-J stents for long-term internal drainage catheters may be introduced percutaneously via the loin under ultrasound and fluoroscopic control. Short-term drainage (24–48 hours) can

be achieved by simply puncturing an obstructed kidney under ultrasound or fluoroscopic control, passing a guidewire through the needle and exchanging the needle for a small catheter in order to establish temporary external drainage. This procedure, known as percutaneous nephrostomy, is used almost exclusively to establish drainage in such emergency situations as acute obstruction following extracorporeal shock-wave lithotripsy or to drain an acute pyonephrosis.

Drainage of the biliary system

The last decade has seen an explosion of techniques designed to drain an obstructed biliary system. The methods used can be broadly divided into those in which the drainage tube is introduced endoscopically and those in which it is introduced percutaneously.

The two most common causes of bile duct obstruction are tumours, notably carcinoma of the pancreas or cholangiocarcinoma, and stones in the common bile duct. If the obstruction is due to stones, then endoscopic removal of the stones and sphincterotomy of the papilla of Vater is a frequently chosen option (Fig. 17.16).

The results of surgery for curative treatment of malignant bile duct obstruction are usually most disappointing. Non-

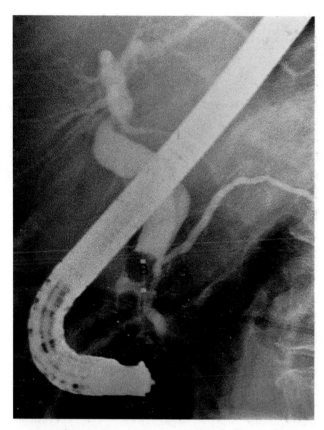

Fig. 17.16 Endoscopic removal of stones in the common bile duct (CBD). A balloon catheter has been passed into the CBD after endoscopic intubation of the papilla of Vater. The stones were then pulled out of the CBD. B, balloon; S, stone.

operative stenting and drainage procedures for patients in whom curative surgery is impossible have therefore become far more frequent in recent years. Patients may live for a considerable time with biliary stents in place, particularly if the responsible tumour is slow-growing, as is the case with many cholangiocarcinomas. Usually the stent is introduced at ERCP by cannulation of the papilla of Vater and passing the stent retrogradely up the common bile duct through the tumour so that bile from the obstructed biliary tree drains into the duodenum. If this approach is not successful, the stent can be placed over a guidewire that has been introduced percutaneously in an antegrade direction following the needle puncture of a dilated bile duct within the liver. The guidewire can be manipulated through the tumour into the duodenum via the common bile duct and the stent can then be passed over the guidewire (Fig. 17.17).

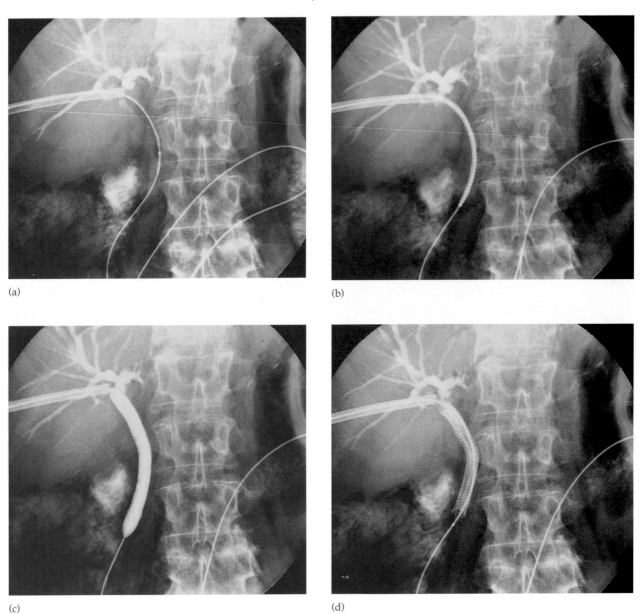

(a)

(b)

(c)

(d)

Fig. 17.17 Percutaneous insertion of a stent to bypass an obstruction in the common hepatic duct. (a) After a biliary duct has been punctured in the liver a guidewire is passed through the stricture and thence through the ampulla into the bowel. (b) A stent over a balloon catheter is threaded over the guidewire to lie across the stricture. (c) The balloon is inflated. (d) The balloon is deflated and the catheter removed leaving the stent in place. The guidewire can then be withdrawn.

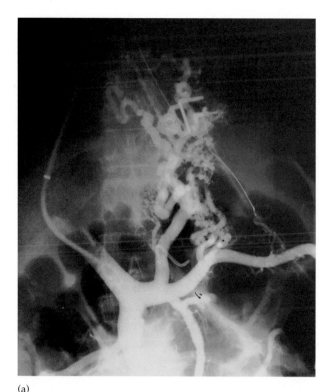

(a)

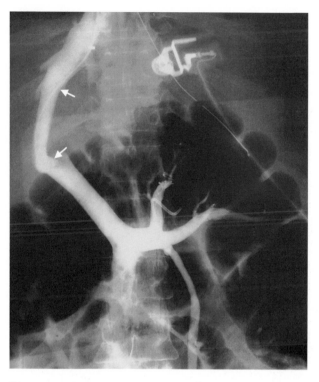

(b)

Fig. 17.18 Transhepatic intrahepatic portosystemic shunt (TIPS). (a) A catheter has been passed from the jugular vein in the neck through the heart into a hepatic vein and then pushed through the liver parenchyma into a portal vein. A retrograde injection is made outlining the portal vein and its tributaries. Note the gastro-oesophageal varices. (b) A connection between the portal vein and a large hepatic vein has been established and a stent inserted. Its position is shown by the arrows. Note the varices no longer fill (in part due to deliberate occlusion).

Transhepatic intrahepatic portosystemic shunt (TIPS)

Patients who have portal hypertension with bleeding gastro-oesophageal varices may benefit from the creation of a communication between the portal and systemic venous system to lower the portal pressure. Nowadays this may be conveniently performed percutaneously under ultrasound guidance. The internal jugular vein is punctured and a catheter passed through the heart into a hepatic vein. Using a special needle introduced through the lumen of the catheter, the catheter can be passed from a hepatic vein into a portal vein. Once this portosystemic connection has been established, it is kept open with a permanent stent (Figs. 7.11, 17.18).

Appendix

CT Anatomy of Abdomen

The normal appearances of the abdomen and pelvis of an adult male are shown in this appendix. The levels of the sections chosen are illustrated in the two diagrams. Each section is 10 mm thick. Gastrografin was given orally twice: 15 minutes and 1.5 hours before-hand. Intravenous contrast was injected during the examination.

Other images from this particular patient were used to illustrate the normal retroperitoneum (Fig. 10.8a, p. 289), and the normal bladder (Fig. 7.10d, p. 228).

Ao   Aorta
D   Diaphragm
Du   Duodenum
D III   Third part of duodenum
GB   Gall bladder
IVC   Inferior vena cava
K   Kidney
Ps   Psoas muscle
PV   Portal vein
SMA   Superior mesenteric artery
SMV   Superior mesenteric vein
Sp   Spine
SV   Splenic vein

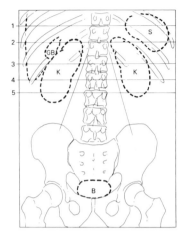

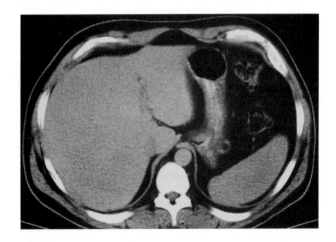

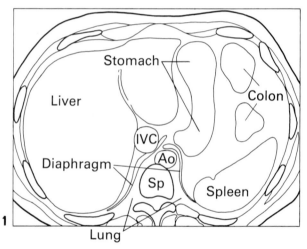

1

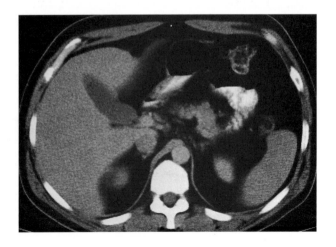

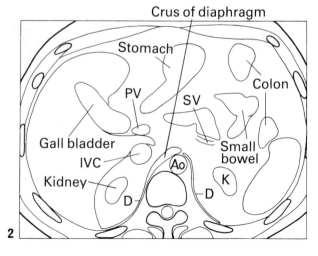

2

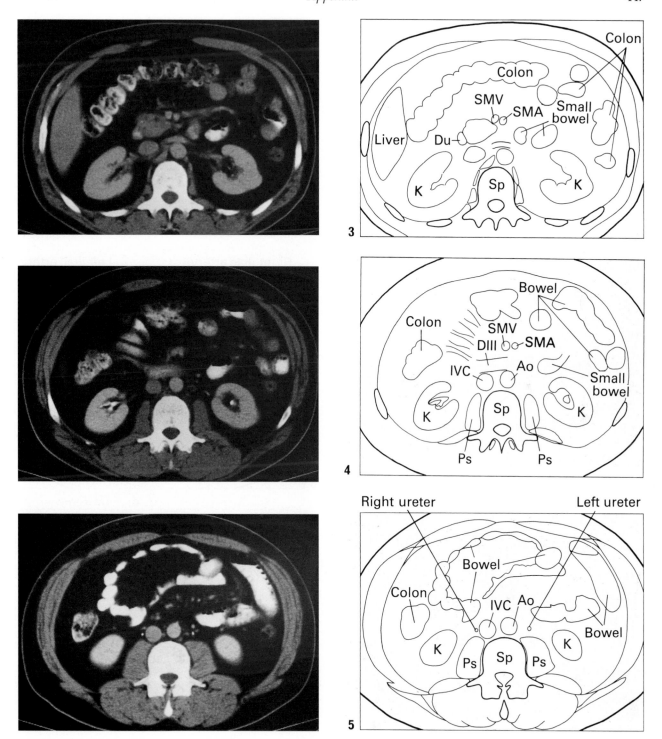

B   Bladder
C   Colon
K   Kidney
Isch. tub Ischial tuberosity
IVC   Inferior vena cava
L. ani   Levator ani
Obt. int. Obturator internus
Ps   Psoas muscle
Sp   Spine
R   Rectum

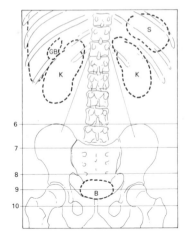

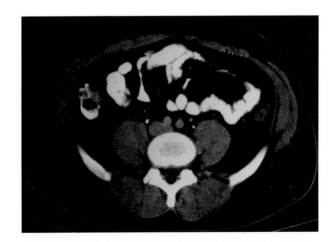

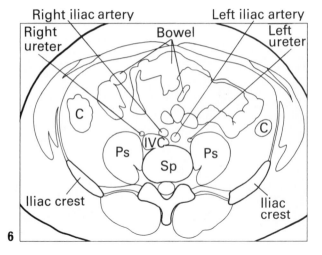

6

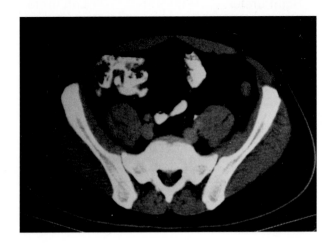

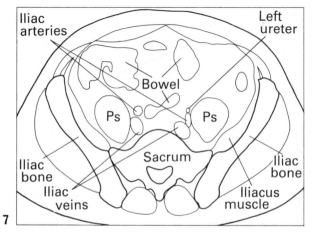

7

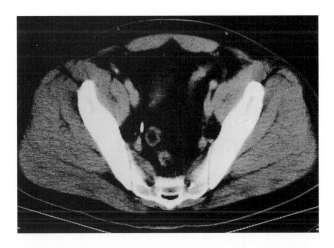

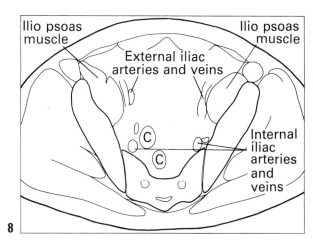

Ilio psoas muscle — Ilio psoas muscle

External iliac arteries and veins

C C

Internal iliac arteries and veins

8

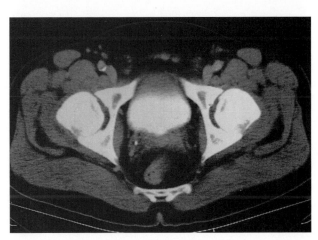

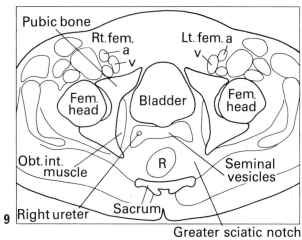

Pubic bone

Rt. fem. — a — v

Lt. fem. a — v

Fem. head — Bladder — Fem. head

Obt. int. muscle

R

Seminal vesicles

9 Right ureter — Sacrum — Greater sciatic notch

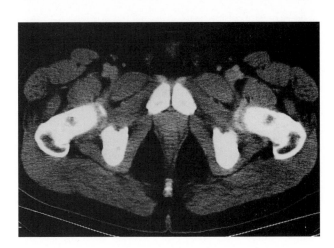

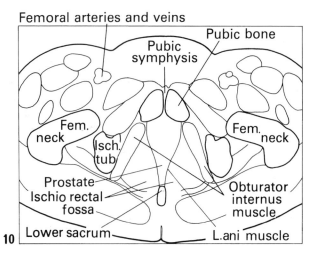

Femoral arteries and veins

Pubic symphysis — Pubic bone

Fem. neck — Fem. neck

Isch. tub

Prostate — Obturator internus muscle

Ischio rectal fossa

10 Lower sacrum — L. ani muscle

Index

Page numbers in *italics* represent figures, those in **bold** represent tables

THE POLITICS AND ECONOMICS OF DRUG PRODUCTION ON THE PAKISTAN-AFGHANISTAN BORDER

For Nargis,

With love and gratitude

The Politics and Economics of Drug Production on the Pakistan–Afghanistan Border

AMIR ZADA ASAD

AND

ROBERT HARRIS

ASHGATE

1004846775

Published by
Ashgate Publishing Limited
Gower House
Croft Road
Aldershot
Hampshire GU11 3HR
England

Ashgate Publishing Company
Suite 420
101 Cherry Street
Burlington, VT 05401-4405
USA

Ashgate website: http://www.ashgate.com

British Library Cataloguing in Publication Data
Asad, Amir Zada
    The politics and economics of drug production on the
    Pakistan-Afghanistan border
    1.Drug traffic - Pakistan - North-west Frontier Province
    2.Drug traffic - Political aspects - Pakistan - North-west
    Frontier Province 3. Drug traffic - Economic aspects -
    Pakistan - North-west Frontier Province 4. Narcotics,
    Control of - Pakistan 5. Pakistan - Politics and government
    - 1988- 6. Pakistan – Foreign relations
    I. Title II. Harris, Robert, 1947-
    363 .4'5'0954912

Library of Congress Cataloging-in-Publication Data
Asad, Amir Zada.
    The politics and economics of drug production on the Pakistan-Afghanistan border:
    implications for a globalized world/Amir Zada Asad and Robert Harris.
        p. cm.
    Includes bibliographical references.
    ISBN 0-7546-3037-4 (alk. paper)
    1. Opium trade--Pakistan. 2. Heroin industry--Pakistan. 3. Narcotics, Control
of--Pakistan. 4. Pakistan--Politics and government. I. Harris, Robert, 1947-II. Title.

HV5840.P18A73 2003
338.1'7375'095491--dc21

2002043697

ISBN 0 7546 3037 4

Printed and bound in Great Britain by MPG Books Ltd, Bodmin, Cornwall.

Contents

Acknowledgements

I would be failing in gratitude if I did not firstly thank Professor Karam Elahi (ex-Dean, Faculty of Social Science, University of Peshawar), without whose support I would not have been able to study in the United Kingdom.

During my stay at the University of Hull many people helped me. Though it is difficult and perhaps unfair to be selective it is also unavoidable, and therefore I especially mention Rahmat Aziz Salik, Minister Hull Mosque and UK Islamic Mission, and his sons (Zia Salik, Abid Salik and Atique Salik), Chaudhry Khurshed-uz-Zaman, Zaheer Iqbal and Suhail Qayyum.

Sher Gul Khan (Lala Jan), Shakeel Ahmad Khan, Asif Khan, Amer Khan and Sajid Khan from Bradford provided me with a UK family-like environment. I am thankful to them.

Dr Eric Gardiner of the Mathematics Department helped me with the statistical analysis, and I am grateful also to Liz Stevenson, Librarian HM Prison Wolds, for her support in providing valuable literature. Mr A.Z. Hilali of the Department of Politics and Asian Studies was a help and support, and Eileen Palphramand and Dennis South of the Social Work Department treated me with courtesy and helpfulness. I am also grateful to Kathryn for proof-reading the draft thesis.

During my fieldwork in Pakistan in winter 1996–7, many people gave me special assistance, financial, physical, moral, and academic, and without their generous support this study would have never been completed. I owe special thanks and indebtedness to my friends Muhammad Shafi Khan of Shah Alam village and the late Muhammad Shah Alam Khan (who passed away in October 1997) of Babuzai village, who accompanied and escorted me throughout my fieldwork.

Malik Hazrat Gul and his sons of Manogai village, Utman Khel, Bajaur Agency made possible my access to Muhamand Agency for data collection by escorting me into this remote area. Similarly, Usmani Gul and Javed Khan of Jolagramm village, Malakand Agency made possible my access to Sharbatai, Bajaur Agency for fieldwork. Muhammad Islam Afridi helped in my fieldwork in Khyber Agency, the most awesome field of all. I am greatly indebted to them all.

Syyed Kamran Shah, Section Officer, Civil Secretariat Peshawar, Arbab Shah Rukh (then Political Agent Bajaur Agency), S. Muhammad Javed (then Deputy Commissioner Dir), Mr. Shad Muhamad Khan, District Social Welfare officer, Dir, Malik Siddique of NAS Peshawar, Mr Simon and Jehgangir Khan of Dir District Development Project, Timargara, Dir, are among the officials who helped me considerably. Again I thank them warmly.

I am naturally thankful to my parents, who constantly remembered me in their prayers and made this study easier for me. I especially wish to mention Nargis, my wife, and my children, Jawwad, Talha, Sara, and Yusra, who gave me their love, and supported my spirit and energy, enabling me to work.

Thanks are also due to George Harris for his expert assistance with the task of producing camera-ready copy.

Amir Zada Asad

List of Acronyms

AMA	(American Medical Association)
ANF	(Anti-Narcotic Force)
ANP	(Awami National Party)
ATT	(Afghan Transit Trade)
BCCI	(Bank of Credit and Commerce International)
CMO	(Comprehensive Multidisciplinary Outline) of Future Activities in Drug Abuse
DEA	(Drug Enforcement Administration)
EIC	(East India Company)
FATAs	(Federally Administered Tribal Areas)
FCR	(Frontier Crimes Regulations)
FR	(Frontier Regions)
JI	(Jamaat-e-Islami), and poppy cultivation
NAS	Narcotics Affairs Section, US State Dept)
NLC	(National Logistic Cell, Pakistan Army)
NNICC	(US National Narcotics Intelligence Consumers Committee)
NWFP	(North West Frontier Province)
PATAs	(Provincially Administered Tribal Areas)
PCSIR	(Pakistan Council of Scientific and Industrial Research)
PIHS	(Pakistan Integrated Household Survey)
PML	(Pakistan Muslim League)
PNCB	(Pakistan Narcotics Control Board)
PPP	(Pakistan People's Party)
PTI	(Pakistan Tehrik-e-Insaf)
TJP	(Tahrik-e-Jafaria)
UNDCP	(United Nations Drug Control Programme)
UNDP	(United Nations Development Programme)
UNFDAC	(United Nations Fund for Drug Abuse Control)
UNHCR	(United Nations High Commission for Refugees)
USAID	(US Agency for International Development)

Preface

This study is mainly about illicit narcotics production in North West Frontier Province (NWFP), Pakistan. Though an area study centrally concerned with development issues, it raises broader dimensions of international relations, political criminology and drugs policy. This should make the book of interest to a wider readership than would normally be attracted to an ethnographic study in a rather wild and, at least until it came to prominence following the events of 11 September 2001, little-heard of region of Pakistan.

The book explains aspects of opium cultivation and its manufacture into addictive drugs – both morphine and, in particular, heroin. Part of the story lies in the character of Pakistan, a country with a troubled history, and today a weak state located in a strategically pivotal position for the western powers. Pakistan has in the past had, and still has today, more than its share of development problems, including political instability, primary poverty, religious intolerance, corruption, illiteracy, health problems and population growth. Accordingly, the bulk of this study comprises a multidisciplinary analysis of ways in which social, economic, cultural, political, historical and geographical forces have together helped create the contemporary problems associated with opium and heroin.

The first author is not only a senior academic but also a tribesman from Pakistan's traditional opium-growing areas in the tribal territories of North West Frontier Province. This is relevant since it was only this that enabled him to conduct his fieldwork in the dangerous and volatile opium growing areas of the tribal provinces, which operate outside Pakistan's federal legal system. Even with this tribal affiliation, however, the majority of the fieldwork had to be undertaken in the company of armed kinsmen, and his life was on several occasions in some danger.[1]

The chief rationale for this study was to establish why, from the 1980s onwards, the production of opium – a crop used for a range of traditional medicinal, cultural and recreational purposes – was transformed into the basis of heroin production. This change had catastrophic consequences for the opium farmers themselves, for the domestic and overseas user population, and for the integrity of government. The first reported case of heroin addiction in Pakistan was as recent as 1979, but today there are probably more than five and a half million addicts, 51 per cent of them addicted to heroin. On average 100,000 people become addicted to heroin annually: a new addict every five minutes.

Chapter I introduces key aspects of opium and heroin production in NWFP, and demonstrates that these opiates are produced there in the face of ineffective and sometimes counterproductive national and international control efforts. In NWFP as well as more generally, socio-economic and political as well as climatic and topographical conditions contribute to drug production. Opium in particular is produced in economically disadvantaged and politically turbulent areas of the globe where it offers a unique remunerative opportunity in the absence of alternative options.

Chapter II briefly introduces aspects of the history and politics of opium, as well as its mode of production, character, uses, biochemistry and forms of imbibing. These latter considerations lead naturally into a brief history of heroin, which gives an indication of its invention and use as a medicine, and its subsequent fall from grace. A brief history of heroin processing in Pakistan is also included.

Chapter III considers the role of national politics in the development of opium and heroin trafficking in Pakistan. Without political patronage and a favourable political atmosphere, drug production would be impossible. Drugs, like the silver in Joseph Conrad's *Nostromo*, however, have the capacity to corrupt the political atmosphere of the producing country, and Pakistan is no exception. The role of political parties in the production and development of opium is discussed, as is politicians' involvement in the drugs trade, an involvement that has fuelled both the specific situation concerning drugs and also the general 'culture of corruption', which permeates Pakistan today.

Chapter IV describes the research strategy: sampling techniques, sources of data collection and why data were collected from different sources. An account is given of the dangers involved in researching in third world countries, particularly in areas where regular state laws are not applicable. Details of the fieldwork and the responses of the different categories of respondent are also presented. We then introduce ethnographic data, which, after etching some more aspects of daily life in the research areas, comprise three case studies. In addition to putting 'flesh on the bones' of why opium is produced, these studies include three balance sheets, drawn up by respondents, highlighting starkly the difference in the financial yield of growing opium against possible alternative crops such as wheat and onion. Finally, we present and analyse some of the empirical data.

Chapter V, which is divided into two parts, first rehearses attempts that have been made at, respectively, national and international level, to control the spread of opium and its derivatives, then discusses the obstacles that have been faced and the extent to which they have been overcome. The second part begins by reflecting more broadly on the whole notion and philosophy of control, raising questions then applied to the subjects of legalization, regulation and medicalization in Pakistan. In politically unstable countries such as Pakistan, laws and rules of governing vary from area to area and person to person. We discuss the legal status of the drugs producing areas as defined by the constitution of the Islamic Republic of Pakistan, giving some idea how the relevant legal systems support the national drug scene.

External political conditions have also played a major role. The revolution in Iran and the Soviet occupation of Afghanistan and the subsequent civil war in that country boosted the drug trade in Pakistan as did, after the study was completed, the support of the western powers for the Northern Alliance in the aftermath of the World Trade Center and Washington attacks. How drugs came to be used as a source of weapon procurement during the Afghan war, the role of the superpowers in drug development in the region, and how heroin was used as weapon during war against the enemy are also considered.

Notes

1   The book is based on the first author's Ph.D. thesis (Asad 2000), where a fuller account of both methodology (including the research instruments used) and findings can be found. As well as being adapted for book form, the thesis has been slightly updated. This is both to take account of new data and to acknowledge the international prominence briefly enjoyed by the tribal territories as a result of the military action following the attacks on Washington and the World Trade Center of 11 September 2001. The first author is responsible for the empirical content and the analysis of events in Pakistan and Afghanistan. The second author, supervisor of the Ph.D., contributed to the development of the analytic framework and to the presentation of the work.

Chapter I

Introduction

Pakistan Introduced

Pakistan is a Muslim country of approximately 134.5 million people (growing by an estimated 3 per cent per annum) and some 530,000 square miles. It is bordered by India to the east, Iran and Afghanistan to the west, China and Russia to the north and the Arabian Sea to the south.

Administratively it is divided into four provinces, Punjab, North West Frontier Province (NWFP), Baluchistan and Sind, plus a federally administered tribal area (FATA) containing seven tribal agencies, six of them on the Afghan border, and the Federal Capital Territory area (Islamabad District). Punjab accounts for some 57.6 per cent of the population, Sind 21.6 per cent, NWFP and the tribal areas 16.8 per cent combined, Baluchistan, though the largest province in area, 3.8 per cent, and the Federal Capital Territory 0.4 per cent. The Federal Capital Territory area is a small area in Punjab, but, as the location of the federal capital, like Canberra and Kuala Lumpur, acquires a special status.

Other than in times of martial law or political crisis, each province is under the administration of a provincial governor and an independent elected provincial legislature led by an elected chief minister and his cabinet. The FATA is situated within NWFP, but tribal people, due to their distinct politico-legal status, are subject not to Pakistan's statute laws but to the hundred year old laws of the colonial era. This system gives immense authority to the political administration but leaves the people largely powerless. Although in theory they live politically as an independent people under *Pakhtoon wali*, their own unwritten laws based on custom and tradition, in practice they are subject to many whims of their rulers, people whom the Pakhtoon people regard as god-like officers.

Topographically and climatically Pakistan encompasses wide variation, from the snow-covered peaks of the north to the deserts of Sind and Baluchistan. Geographically it divides into three regions: the mountains of the north and north-west, the uncultivated tableland of Baluchistan, and the plains of the Indus Basin. The annual rainfall varies from 5 inches in Baluchistan to 30 inches in Punjab, and temperatures, which exceed 50°C in June and July, fall well below freezing in winter, at least in the western and northern areas.

Punjab, the breadbasket of the country, has fertile land irrigated through one of the best networks of irrigation channels in the world. Sind comes second in food production, particularly rice and cane sugar. NWFP has little agriculture and Baluchistan virtually none, so these provinces are dependent on the produce of Punjab and Sind.

Pakistan has been a poor country since independence in 1947. Its economy is underdeveloped, and the country struggles under an external debt of over $40 billion.

There exist extremes of wealth and poverty. In the mid-1990s the national average *per capita* income was officially $420 a year, though some independent critics placed the figure at closer to $120. Certainly with nearly 10 million people known to be earning less than 1,000 rupees (less than $17) a month (assuming an exchange rate of 60 rupees = $1), many Pakistanis were living in primary poverty. Though natural resources abound they are under-exploited as a result of poor technology and a lack of resources exacerbated by political and bureaucratic corruption, including embezzlement and loan sharking by senior administrators and politicians. There are also distinct inequalities within the country itself. Though in theory national resources are distributed according to the population of the provinces, this has never materialized in reality as a result of similar corrupt practices and the political influence of the urban centres in Punjab and Islamabad in particular.

In 1947 Pakistan had not a single industrial establishment, all industry being concentrated in what is now India. Over half a century later, such industry as exists is mainly cottage-based, and the country remains predominantly agrarian, with a surplus labour economy. The rural: urban population ratio is 72:28, and agriculture accounts for 32 per cent of value added in the GDP, against 16 per cent for manufacturing industries and 44 per cent for services.

Social change has been very slow. According to the 1998–99 Pakistan Integrated Household Survey (PIHS), the overall literacy rate for those aged 10 years and above who completed primary level or higher, was 38.1 per cent,[1] a figure that compares unfavourably with the less developed world generally.[2] Pakistan has made especially slow progress in increasing the proportion of school-going children, with 17 million not attending at all, and over 12 million working in factories, sometimes for over 16 hours a day. These figures continue to exist in spite of the fact that the Government introduced an education tax, *iqra surcharge*, in 1980, to increase the literacy ratio, and by 1997 had collected 80 billion rupees.[3] To this day, however, no one appears to know where this money has gone. So primary schools are attended by no more than half of eligible children, largely because of the low enrolment rate, on religio-cultural and economic grounds, of girls. The proportion of children attending secondary and higher secondary schools is a mere 17 per cent and 2 per cent respectively. Pakistan can boast only one teacher for 115 school age children.[4]

In health, too, Pakistan faces major challenges. Life expectancy at birth (currently 51 years) is slightly above the rate of other less developed countries within the region. Nonetheless its infant mortality rate has been estimated at 89 per 1,000 live births – a figure which should, however, be treated with caution, there being substantial problems with birth history data in Pakistan.[5] Thirty-eight per cent of the population have access to safe (not necessarily hygienic) water, there is one doctor per 4,600 population (against 451 in England and Wales), one nurse per 10,030 population (130 in England and Wales) and one hospital bed per 2,200 population (175 in England and Wales).[6]

The Current Research

This study, the first of its nature with respect to Pakistan, addresses illicit narcotics production in North West Frontier Province. This includes the production of raw opium, the mother of addictive and abusive drugs including morphine and diacetyl morphine (heroin). The study gives a description of the causes of the problem, given the complex socio-economic and political conditions prevalent in the country. Although illicit drug production has reduced during the last few years this may prove a temporary phenomenon, as it is difficult to discern any long-lasting alternative means of meeting the demand served by opium cultivation and heroin manufacture or any reason why demand should decline permanently. In this chapter we introduce key aspects of opium and heroin production in NWFP and demonstrate that these opiates are produced there in the face of ineffective and sometimes counterproductive national and international control efforts. As the book continues we argue that in NWFP and generally socio-economic and political as well as climatic and topographical conditions contribute to drug production. Opium in particular is produced in economically disadvantaged and politically turbulent areas of the globe where it offers a unique remunerative opportunity in the absence of similarly attractive options.[7]

We shall show that disparities in national development programmes, which largely work to the disadvantage of NWFP, combined with poor economic opportunities and resources in the poppy cultivating areas in particular, are key predisposing factors to narcotics production. In addition, the Soviet invasion of Afghanistan, exploited by the superpowers for their own interests, blocked the traditional trade routes of the heroin producing areas, creating political as well as economic disorganization and insecurity in NWFP. A similar point can be made about the Iranian Revolution, whose relevance is also analysed.

Since it was, in good part, to overcome these economic insecurities that some people in Khyber Agency shifted to heroin production with foreign technical assistance[8] as an alternative source of livelihood, it is there that we must look to determine the precipitants of opium/heroin production and manufacture. Where large families are combined with small agricultural landholdings in a situation in which expenditure commonly exceeds income, the predisposition to find alternative income sources is inevitably strong. When these factors are combined with the unique income potential from opium cultivation at a time when superpower action in Afghanistan had in some areas a devastating impact on business opportunities, the exploitation of opportunities provided by opiate production and manufacture is yet more likely. This likelihood, in turn, is further increased by Pakistan's unstable political economy and high threshold corruption. Taken together with the cultural tradition of opium use for domestic, particularly medicinal, consumption, these factors make the development of the trade virtually inevitable.

The fieldwork for the book comprised interviews with opiate producers, discussions with academics, politicians and others about policy and legislation, and an analysis of the contribution of narcotics traffic and narco-politics to drug production in NWFP. In addition, historical data, current cultural values concerning drug use, and evidence of the existence of drug sub-cultures are provided to offer a broad appreciation of the nature and evolution of the problem. After all, though the current (and quite recent) explosion of drug production, and Pakistan's involvement in an international network of drug supply was indeed precipitated by politico-economic events, opium production is longstanding. Hence to focus solely on recent events would give only a partial picture.

Inevitably there is much about this study that is provisional, and it is too early to answer definitively such questions as 'What were the respective contributions of the Afghan War and the Iranian Revolution to the development of opium production in NWFP?' Accordingly, we spend more time and space than is probably desirable providing basic (but still frequently new) information, in order both to enrich this study and to prepare the ground for others. We also consider opium and heroin production in Pakistan in relation to geography and economics, current and recent political conditions, history and culture.

In exploring issues raised by these points, the study has the following aims and objectives.

1 To study, from primary and secondary sources, aspects of the historical development of opium and heroin production in NWFP

Opium production has been a part of the agri-economy of the region for more than two millennia. But historically drug production had entirely different social, cultural and economic logics, and only with the beginning of the use of drugs for political purposes during the Mughal period in the early 17th century (a practice perpetuated, adapted and developed by the colonial power) did production become recognizably modern. Because these historical traces drive both production and usage today, it is necessary to consider drug development in the light of policies adopted by the colonial rulers who helped put the drug business on an international footing.

2 To investigate the drug culture in NWFP in order to understand the character, nature and purpose of opium use in the area

Opium has been used not only for euphoric purposes or for processing into heroin (a relatively recent activity) but as a centuries-old part of folk medicine, particularly the *tibbi unani* system of medication. But its social and cultural meaning has changed drastically with the increasing perception and reality of a drug problem, and its contemporary criminal as well as clinical characteristics.

3 To study and analyse production in the area

Economic conditions play an important role in drug production, producing areas normally being characterized by relatively harsh economic conditions and few alternative sources of livelihood for the inhabitants, either through private enterprise or governmental support. Accordingly this study examines the economic conditions in the opium and heroin producing areas. Factors such as *per capita* income and agriculture and employment resources are presented to probe the nature of the relationship between economic conditions and opium and heroin production.

4 To analyse the political factors, national and international, relevant to drug production in NWFP

This includes a geo-political analysis of area, including an assessment of the impact of the Iranian revolution, the Soviet invasion of Afghanistan, and the US intervention in the region, which, while ostensibly intended to defeat communism, effectively stoked the smouldering fire of the drug trade. At a more local level we show the relevance of the existence of different political systems in a single province, and in particular how the involvement of power elites and patronage have facilitated the trade. But narco-politics and political corruption on a national level, and localized poppy politics in the opium producing areas themselves, have interacted not only with each other but with the general culture of Pakistani society to create and sustain the present situation.

5 To consider theoretical issues concerning control

It has been much debated whether attempts to control or suppress a criminal activity that meets widespread demand are worse than the original problem. The arguments are reviewed when we grapple with the policy question of what is to be done.

While it is beyond our scope or wisdom to offer a comprehensive and universal theory of drug production, we identify factors, which, individually and interactively, affect the likelihood of opium, and heroin production occurring and being sustained elsewhere. These, by implication, must be addressed nationally and internationally if production is to be brought to a manageable level, and how this both might and should not be done also feature in the book. It will become clear that for the most part coercion is impractical and likely to be counterproductive, and that Government provision of equally lucrative alternative sources of employment is similarly so, other, perhaps, than as part of a concerted international effort. This, however, is not immediately plausible and could anyway be vulnerable to unintended consequences, as US involvement in the region certainly has been.

The ideal long-term solution may well lie in socio-economic development, including increasing the power of drug producers in the global labour market and removing, by political and economic reform and popular education, the opportunity and incentives for political corruption, including the patronage, nepotism and cronyism prevalent in Pakistan today. It would, however, be utopian to believe this can be achieved in the short to medium term, if indeed it can be achieved at all. Attempts to buck a global market comprising willing producers, huge multinational demand, and the involvement of both national governments and organized criminals are unlikely to be straightforward; and they may, indeed, ultimately prove futile.

This is not to say that nothing can or should be done, and it is in part for that reason that brief reference is also made to issues of rehabilitation (which currently scarcely exists in Pakistan) and market control by localized intervention in the supply-demand nexus. It is, however, important to be realistic, and not to permit personal commitments to get in the way of dispassion. Above all we should disabuse ourselves of any notion that solutions which, if they exist, fall within the remit of international cooperation and intervention can be found at an individual or local level. While palliative interventions may be possible locally (though this study casts doubt on the practicality of even this on anything other than a small scale basis), we should not delude ourselves into believing that palliation is cure, or that to damp the fire is to extinguish it.

The Regional Context

It is impossible to understand the geo-politics of opium and heroin production in Pakistan without locating that country in the geographical context of south-west (and to a degree south-east) Asia. Pakistan is a part of the Golden Crescent, a politico-geographical area comprising Pakistan, Iran and Afghanistan. 'Golden', however, by no means reflects the economic conditions of the region's poverty-stricken opium growing hill tribes. Rather it is a reference to the money to be made by international traffickers. The name was coined by the western media in the early 1980s during the Afghan-Soviet war to designate the mountainous area, which is 'golden' for these opiates. So effectively the Golden Crescent was created by US military engagement in Afghanistan, as was the Golden Triangle by its intervention in Vietnam. The Golden Crescent is important to this study because events in the region led the people of NWFP to commercialize and export their opium production in the late 1970s.

Until the emergence of opium production in the Central Asian States of Tajikistan, Uzbekistan and Turkmenistan, some eastern European countries and Mexico[9] almost all opium cultivation took place in the Crescent and the Triangle, and still today these two regions account for around 90 per cent of world supply.[10] As political, geographical and topographical complexities ensure that no exact figures for the acreage of poppy are available, however, production, consumption and trafficking figures are frequently inflated by western powers for one set of political reasons[11] and deflated by local officials for another.

In Pakistan itself, the Anti-Narcotic Force (ANF) (formerly the Pakistan Narcotics Control Board, or PNCB) is responsible for collecting production and trafficking data. Pakistani data are also gathered, however, by the US Agency for International development (USAID), the US State Department's Narcotics Affairs Section (NAS), the US Embassy Islamabad, the US National Narcotics Intelligence Consumers Committee (NNICC), the UN Drug Control Programme (UNDCP) and the UN Development Programme (UNDP). Unfortunately, if unsurprisingly, figures from these agencies frequently contradict each other.

Where access is possible and production per acre or hectare known, production estimates can be made from ground surveys on a sampling basis; where production areas are known but access impossible they can be based on aerial photography. The problem of measuring the cultivated land remains unsolved, however, as most cultivating areas are geographically dispersed or physically inaccessible, and not included in Government revenue records. Production estimates are also unreliable, as production varies from area to area according to weather, availability of water and the nature of the land.

Politically, the situation is extremely sensitive, and Pakistan and the United States in particular have never agreed production and cultivation figures. Legal production in Pakistan has never been estimated accurately, and the production of illegal drugs is difficult if not impossible to measure. The problem is further complicated by internal political considerations. Inside Pakistan the statistics of opium acreage are underestimated by the political administration of the producing area, in part to show their efficiency in drug control and in part for corrupt purposes discussed elsewhere. Conversely, however, the ANF exaggerates the figures, mainly to support its claims for international aid. The USA, on the other hand, exaggerates *or* minimizes the figures depending on its short term objectives: in a cycle that has continued since the early 1980s, if it wants to pressurize Pakistan it exaggerates the figures, when Pakistan asks for aid to combat production it minimizes them.

The figures, accordingly, are very complex, being subject to macro- and micro-political manipulation and genuine measurement problems as well as price variation due to supply and demand fluctuations and local geopolitical changes which ensure that year on year production figures are liable to dramatic changes. According to the Director of the UNDCP:

> . . . the illicit drug business in the so-called Golden Crescent of Iran, Pakistan and Afghanistan was estimated at $5 billion per year in a global drug trade of $400 billions. Big money is certainly not made in this part of the world. When we take the illicit market or size of business of all these drugs, it has been estimated around $400 billion per year. . . We do estimate that the volume of the drug trade is about $5 billions . . . one kg. of heroin was worth $3,000 in Pakistan's industrial port city Karachi compared with a street value of more than $50,000 in the USA.[12]

Making due allowance for these measurement problems, Pakistan's opium yield fell from around 800 metric tons in 1978–9[13] to 155 metric tons in 1996[14]. In 1999–2000 some 1570 hectares in Khyber Agency alone were cultivated with opium poppies, and in 2000–2001[15] the area of opium cultivation was even greater. This, however, is some 50 times less than the production figure of Afghanistan, now the largest opium producer in the world, which exports up to 90 per cent of its yield to Pakistan for processing into heroin.[16]

This expansion began immediately after the withdrawal of Soviet troops, as leaders of the major resistance parties had, with covert US support, become involved in opium and heroin production, processing and trafficking to finance the war.[17] Whereas in 1995–96 only 38,740 hectares of scarce arable land were estimated as given over to poppy cultivation, with an approximate yield of 1250 metric tons of raw opium,[18] in the following year this figure increased to an estimated 165,000 hectares with a yield of some 2250 metric tons.[19] Probably one million people out of a population of 17 million were directly or indirectly involved in this trade.

Following the Soviet withdrawal Afghanistan became, in effect, a stateless country with no centralized power, as a result, first, of the 12 year conflict with the Soviet Union, and then, after 1991, the fighting between Afghans. So even were the Pakistan Government to eliminate poppy production in Pakistan, this problem of Afghanistan would continue: those responsible for its control are involved in its development, and poppy dollars have become integral to the political economy of Afghanistan.

The other major producer in south-west Asia is India, the world's largest producer of licit opium for its domestic pharmaceutical industry and export to the western market[20] and a considerable producer of illegal opium for processing into heroin. In 1995–96, 800 metric tons of opium were known to have been produced from a cultivated area of 26,200 hectares,[21] though UN/Pakistani sources suggest the real figure is 13–1500 metric tons. Some of this licit production, in addition to an unknown quantity of illicitly produced opium, is processed into heroin. Indian traffickers had already begun experimenting with heroin as far back as 1984 because of the country's high levels of opium production and stockpiles, which at that time were thought by many in the region to pose an international threat.[22] This was underplayed in official western reports, however, probably because of the value of Indian opium to the western pharmaceutical industry as well as for broader political reasons during the Cold War.

In south-east Asia, the Golden Triangle, comprising the north-east border of Myanmar, Northern Thailand and Northern Laos, has traditionally been the largest producer of opium. Of its annual production of 2545 metric tons in 1995–96, Myanmar produced 2340 metric tons from a cultivated area of 154,070 hectares,[23] slightly more than the combined production of Pakistan, Afghanistan and India but from twice the land, the area being less favourable for opium production than the Crescent.

North West Frontier Province: an Overview

> When God had finished making the rest of the world, say Pathans, He took all the odd pieces left over, and threw them down sideways to make the North West Frontier Province.[24]

This local saying exactly reflects the physical nature of NWFP. It is this structure of the land with narrow passes, steep mountains, defiles and unlevelled plains that has made the life of the Pathans so hard. The eastern, northern, north-western and southern parts of the Province are mountainous areas with little agriculture and no other source of livelihood.

Administratively, NWFP is divided into seven Divisions, each under a Divisional Commissioner (This system ceased after July 2001 local bodies elections and transfer of powers to the elected people.) These Divisions are further sub-divided into 19 Districts, each under a Deputy Commissioner (who, since 2001, has served under an elected District *Nazim*). Malakand and Hazara Divisions, in the north and east of the province, are mountainous with very little agriculture; Kohat Division is situated in the arid salt mountain region where no agriculture is possible; Mardan and Peshawar Divisions are the main plains where extensive cultivation and agriculture take place. The dry Bannu and Dera Ismail Khan Divisions are located on the plains and could be irrigated very easily from the Indus river if the proposed 'Right Bank Canal Project' at Dera Ismail Khan, promised since the early 1970s, were executed. But this promise, like so many others, has yet to be fulfilled.

The tribal belt, stretching from north to the west along the 1300-mile border with Afghanistan, is a mountainous area with no significant agriculture or other economic activity. NWFP lags behind Pakistan as a whole in terms of physical and social infrastructure. Some indicators, which, though out of date, continue to offer useful comparative data, are presented in Table 1.1.

Table 1.1 Comparative Socio-Economic Indicators: Pakistan, NWFP and Tribal (Drug Producing) Areas[25]

Indicators	Pakistan	NWFP	Tribal Areas
Area (sq. km):	803,940	74,521 (9.4%)	26,970 (4%)
Population (million):	134	16	Not known
Population density:	106	148	81
Literacy rate:	26.17%	6.70%	6.38%
Children at school (5–9 yrs):	48%	42.7%	30%
Doctor: Population ratio:	1: 4,600	1:7,000	1:19,120
Electric Consumption (kw/capita):	162	129	37
Road length (per 100 sq. km):	28.11	10	3.49
Access to potable water:	8%	40%	1%

Other indicators indicate that the drug producing areas suffer on a number of deprivation indices in comparison with the country as a whole, where standards are themselves poor. Health indicators, reflected in the availability of doctors using western medicine, reflect a similar situation: non-tribal NWFP scores lower than Pakistan as a whole, and tribal NWFP scores lower still – in this case much lower. With medical availability in the tribal areas running at one doctor for almost 20,000 of an impoverished and therefore unhealthy population, one can describe the situation as one of effective non-availability other than (if one is lucky) in case of dire emergencies. The virtual non-availability of electricity (in spite of the fact that it is produced in or very near to the tribal areas) is naturally associated with this problem. Table 1.1 also demonstrates a remarkable lack of potable water in the tribal provinces. Though water is available in abundance in the Province as a whole, it is mostly used for power generation and mainly available in the plains or areas outside the tribal belt. NWFP is the major hydro-electric power producer for the country, but because electricity there is more expensive than in other provinces industrialization has been made difficult for both local investors and domestic users. In the tribal areas not only agriculture but the people are rain dependent for drinking water, often sharing rain water reservoirs (*jowarhs*), which are open to many forms of pollution including animal excreta, with their cattle.

The story is similar with communications and road transportation. While, NWFP being mountainous, it would be costly and difficult to give it equal communications channels with other parts of the country, this is not the whole story, which has more to do with politics and economics than geography and civil engineering. Most roads are in the urban areas, and rural areas are far removed from the centres of political power in the cities. NWFP has had no industrial base since independence, a fact admitted officially for the first time by a Chief Minister of the Province in 1997.[26] Such scattered industry as exists is mainly of a cottage type, and normally non-functional.

In 1986, in a bid to destroy the poppy crop, the government paramilitary forces, under US pressure, massacred the poppy cultivators in Gadoon Amazai area in an intervention which resulted in the deaths of 26 farmers. The US Government responded to the resultant outcry by funding an industrial estate designed to provide alternative sources of livelihood in this poppy-dependent area. In 1988, in the first General Election after 11 years of martial law, the Pakistan People's Party (PPP) came to power. This party, headed and run mainly by feudal lords and the landed aristocracy, established industrial estates which gave such incentives to investors as tax holidays, cheap electricity, and rebates on the import of machinery. Within three years, more than 200 industrial units were in operation. But the inter-provincial politics of ethnic rivalry and the economic dominance of Punjab did not prove conducive to industrialization, and considerable tension with the established industrial class in Punjab and Sind followed. Accordingly, in 1991, when the Pakistan Muslim League (PML) Government under Nawaz Sharif (the biggest industrialist in the country), representing the interests of the urban and industrial classes, came into power all incentives were withdrawn under pressure from the industrialists. So today the industrial estates offer a bleak and deserted picture, all the machinery having been transferred to Punjab and Sind.

Agriculture in NWFP is of a subsistence nature, carried out in the plains of Peshawar and Mardan only. Formerly Swabi District was famous for agricultural production, but since the construction of a dam at Turbela most of the area has been waterlogged and useless. Such agriculture as there is comprises food and cash crops, and, due to the scarcity of land and widespread poverty, cash crops, not only opium but also sugar cane, tobacco, wheat, maize, rice, barley, mustard and vegetables, are given priority. This means that industrial production in the Province is seasonal in nature.

McCoy believed that opium in Pakistan was produced mainly for local consumption.[27] Even in 1972, when he was writing, however, this was unrealistic given the huge quantity of raw opium produced combined with an addiction rate of less than 1 per cent throughout the Province. While the 1972 World Opium Survey showed the licit production of opium in Pakistan as 12 tons it gave figures for illicit production of up to 160 metric tons, twice the present day production of opium.[28] Similarly, in their study of drug addiction in Pakistan, published nine years later, Spencer and Navarathnam observed that 'in spite of extensive cultivation of poppy, the percentage of addiction among the population is negligible'[29] and UNDCP, in its 1994 report on the Dir District Development Project, stated:

> Despite the widespread growing of opium, there does not yet appear to be a serious narcotics abuse problem in the district. . . A subsequent survey by a local voluntary agency identified about 120 heroin addicts within the district.[30]

Given that the population of Dir is some 1.476 million,[31] 120 addicts constitute no more than 0.008 per cent of the population. Further, there exists a hatred for the drug addicts in the country, and areas where an addiction culture exists, such as

Liyari, a Karachi slum, and Kurya, a village in Buner District of NWFP, where some 70 per cent of the male population are said to be addicted,[32] are atypical. In Karachi, a big international seaport and a route for trafficking from South East Asia, people were familiar with opiates much earlier than elsewhere, and Kurya had atypical consumption patterns.

The 1996 report of the Islamabad-based UNDCP regional office for south-west Asia identified the main opium producing areas as Dir District and the Tribal Agencies of Bajaur (Malakand Division), Muhmand and Khyber (Peshawar Division), with only negligible quantities produced in other tribal agencies. According to these sources, 25–50 per cent of the Pakistan poppy crop was grown in Dir District, where, in parts of the main poppy valleys, as much as 80 per cent of crop land, mostly irrigated, is devoted to poppies.[33] Their share of opium gum production is probably even greater as a result of the higher yields than in the climatically less favourable southern agencies. The average dry gum yield in the District is estimated at 12 kg per acre on irrigated lands and 10 kg per acre on rain dependent lands, compared with the average national yield of about 8 kg per acre.[34] Depending on the yield estimates used, the total annual production of dry gum in Dir District is between 70 and 90 tons.

Malakand Division, in the north bordering Afghanistan, and divided into the Districts of Chitral, Dir (now the districts of upper Dir and lower Dir), Swat and Buner, Shangla, Bajaur and Malakand Agencies, is a mountainous area, with such little agriculture as there is limited mainly to terraced fields in the mountains and the river plains. Dir, Swat and Chitral Districts were former princely states ruled by local feudal chieftains given official titles (*Nawabs* in Dir, *Wali-e-Swat* or *Mian-Guls* in Swat, and *Mehtar* in Chitral) by the British in return for loyalty to the Crown.[35] Though Dir, Swat and Chitral were merged into the district administration in 1969 to bring them to a par socio-economically with the other parts of the country, in spite of some improvements mentioned below many things changed very little. The average *per capita* income is about one third of national average.[36]

Dir District, comprising 5,282 square miles and with estimated population of 1.6 million,[37] borders Afghanistan to the west, Swat District to the east, Chitral District to the north and north-west and Malakand and Bajaur Agencies to the south and south-west. Dir is formed by a complex of mountain ranges of 10–14,000 feet above sea level, from the north to the south-west. There are two rivers, the Panjkora and the Swat. The Panjkora's source lies in the permanently snow covered area of the northern Hinduraj mountain range, and flows south, mainly in deep gorges, offering little water for irrigation other than on the plains. The Swat flows on the eastern boundary, again yielding water only to low lying areas. The area between the two rivers is on a high elevation and non-irrigable.

Dir is a narrow mountainous valley or pass, connecting Peshawar Valley with Chitral and Gilgit, through the Lowari pass, 13,000 feet above sea level. This mountainous tract has a rugged surface with deep and tortuous valleys that sometimes become narrow gorges. Mountainous passes along the Panjkora's tributaries are situated on high altitudes, so farming, where it is possible, depends on rain or seasonal springs. These are normally sufficient to the purpose, droughts being rare. Climatically it ranges from sub-tropical to highland, with minimum and maximum average January temperatures between –2°C and 38°C.[38] Rainfall (or snow in winter) also varies widely, with Chakdara recording 32.5 inches and Dir 47 inches.

Turning to employment, the total population of Dir, according to the 1981 census (reported in 1996), was 767,000, some 27 per cent of whom were of working age, with an annual growth rate of 4.5 per cent, a figure that has probably doubled since. The major source of livelihood has traditionally been subsistence agriculture, supplemented by casual labour by one or more members of the family in the urban industrial centres, as well as opium cultivation. Dir was in the past neglected by the Nawab, as it was until recently by the Federal and Provincial Governments. After the merging of Dir State into the District Administration, however, the situation started to change, and so, in the second half of the 20th century, for the first time some schools were opened. At present 2052 educational institutions provide employment for 5080 male and 1135[39] female teachers as well as lower grade employees. Though physical infrastructural and institutional facilities are still lacking this sector has provided relatively more jobs for the locals than other public sector departments. The result has been an increase in the literacy rate, now 10.16 per cent overall, comprising 16.93 per cent male and 2.77 per cent female.[40]

A second opportunity was the opening of the Middle Eastern labour market, where a fairly large number of people have obtained jobs and sent huge sums of money back to the country. This situation continues despite the declining labour market there, 11.6 per cent of people travelling to work in the Middle East between 1971–8. Different valleys have different traditions of labour export to specific locations. So Sultan Khel people go to Middle Eastern countries, Painda Khel Karo Valley people go to Baluchistan to work in the coal mines or to Kashmir and Punjab for physical labour, and Nihag Valley people go to Karachi to work as labourers and in industry.

At census time the District had three industrial units and two flour mills. The Dir Forest Industrial Complex was closed down three years after its inception in 1975. Together, these offered employment to 625 persons. At present three flour mills constitute the total industry of the area. The mean annual income is 6500 rupees ($108) per family. The joint family system is prevalent, with an average family size of 13 persons, giving an average monthly *per capita* income of 500 rupees, or $100 *per annum*.[41]

Bajaur Agency is an area of 1290 square kilometres, which, though it has a lower altitude than Dir and its weather in summer is a bit warmer, is among the most inaccessible of all parts of the Province. Bajaur is surrounded by Dir District to the north and north-east, Malakand Agency to the south-east, Muhmand Agency to the south, and Afghanistan to the west and north-west. The area is an extension of the Hinduraj or Hindukush mountains. The Bajaur and Muhmand area is a transborder communication route to Afghanistan[42] to which it is connected by land routes in the shape of low height mountain passes. Forty per cent of the area consists of rocky mountains crossed by a maze of dry ravines and poor quality forest land. There are two rivers, the Rud and the Khar Khwar. The Rud rises in the Nawagai or Sur Kamar valley and flows west to east. No water is taken from the Rud for agriculture, though the Khar Khwar is utilized for very limited irrigation. Except in the south, water is a far greater problem than in Dir, rainfall being unpredictable but probably (though no records are maintained by the Agency administration or any other official body) ranging between about 470 and 850 mm. The Agency is blessed more with winter than with summer rain, and accordingly has winter *(kharif)*, rather than summer *(rabi)* crops.

In fact no reliable climatic data about Bajaur are available, the nearest weather observatory being some 50 miles away, in Dir. During the hottest months, May-August, however, the maximum daily average temperature ranges between about 32–39°C with high humidity; while in winter (November to February) the maximum average temperature is 18°C, with minimum temperatures around freezing point. The plain can be frosty in winter and snow frequently falls in January and February.

Nor are authentic secondary socio-economic data on tribal areas available to elucidate the economic conditions of the area, and official figures are without doubt highly inaccurate.

Demographic surveys, like most other census information in tribal areas, are based on answers provided by 'leading maliks' and are usually collected and collated at the Agency Headquarters or in Peshawar. The statistical accuracy of such surveys may be gauged from the fact that they are officially labelled as 'estimates' or 'enumerations':

. . . In the first census in 1951, after the creation of Pakistan, the population for the tribal areas was also based on estimates. This remained unchanged for the census of 1961 and 1971.[43]

Any inaccuracies may be largely attributable to the fact that the figures are provided by the political administration. Before 1972, tribes were given subsidized food, so there was an inbuilt incentive for exaggerated figures to be provided by *Maliks* both to the political authorities and to census officials. This would certainly help explain a dramatic decline revealed in the 1981 census figures. But local politics and cultural trends are also involved in this official requirement:

Exaggeration of males and deflation of female number in questions regarding demographic or domestic statistics is a common tribal practice. In the eyes of tribesmen this interconnected formula is explained thus: inflated male number increases political (military) prestige and social status and thus commands that much more attention, and allowances from the political administration. The subject of females is strictly private and information regarding their lives is an infringement of this privacy. . . The inflation of population figures may also have a valid explanation. The two house system that many Muhmands maintain may result in double counting. According to the 1971 census, there should be 432 people per square mile in the Agency. However, a superficial visit to the agency with its vast, desolated area will indicate the considerable inflation in the population figures.[44]

There is no industry, and though transport related employment has yielded a few jobs from time to time (notably on road construction), the main occupation is rain-dependent single-crop agriculture *(rabi)*. The two months of the sowing season (November and December) and the two months of harvest (May and June) are the busiest periods, most people being underemployed for the rest of the year. Though some workers migrate to the urban areas in search of menial jobs, returning home at the harvest time, few are believed to go to the Middle East – though once again, no figures are available.[45]

Another source of income is retail and wholesale business in the local markets. Bajaur has three bazaars, Khar, Nawagai and Inayat Kallay, where the main sale items are food, grain, arms and ammunition, and other items of daily use. Prior to the Soviet-Afghan war the major source of income was transborder trade with Afghanistan, which consisted mainly of exporting food items and importing foreign made electronics, tyres, silk and crockery through the mountain passes. But with the war this business came to an end, as it did in other tribal agencies. In addition, the influx of Afghan refugees led to increased competition: they proved economically very aggressive, quickly coming to dominate the local markets, leaving the locals in economic jeopardy. The result was armed conflict between refugees and local people in several tribal agencies. According to a UNHCR (United Nations High Commission For Refugees) Survey in 1989, there were 194,580 registered Afghan refugees in Bajaur Agency, and of the 591 and 518 shops in the two main bazaars, Khar and Inayat Kallay, 245 and 362 respectively belonged to Afghan refugees.

Employment in public sector departments, where jobs are pensionable, is greatly sought after. The Education Department particularly is a source of permanent employment for more than 1100 people as teachers, in addition to lower grade posts. There are 291 educational institutions in the Agency, with a total establishment of 1197[46] comprising both teaching and lower grade staff. If all teaching staff are from the Agency, education employs some 0.28 per cent of the population.

Muhmand Agency has an area of 2296 sq. km and an estimated population (in 1994) of around 243,000. To the north lies Bajaur Agency, to the north-west and west Afghanistan, to the south-west Khyber Agency, to the south-east Peshawar Division, and to the north-east Malakand Agency. Rainfall is low, being around 13 inches maximum, and weather conditions range from 45°C in summer to below freezing in winter. The Agency mainly comprises glens, valleys and hills, and has little vegetation other than coarse grass, dwarf palm (*mezarai*) and scrubwood.

The Muhmand Hills cross into Bajaur in the transitional zone of the Hindukush range. The Sappar and Illazai ranges and the Malakand Hills are the main mountains. The barren Sappar range lies to the north, forming a divide with Afghanistan, though the Malakand Hills to the east have a thin cover of olive and wild oak. There is a small plain in the Kabul and Swat river basins. The Kabul has a dam and hydro-electric power station, but fertile land is found only where streams have pierced through the valley sides to form alluvial fans. Most of the very limited rain dependent cultivable area is drained by the Swat. As this river flows into a deep gorge, however, little cultivable land is found along its banks, though there is a rich alluvial loam, aided by floods from the upper areas. The bulk of the Agency, however, is stony and infertile.

As with other tribal areas, in Muhmand Agency no reliable supportive data on the socio-economic conditions of the area exist, and figures, which are estimates by the relevant departments, are all too often self-evidently unreliable. In 1961, for example, the population was recorded as 294,215, rising by 30.2 per cent to 381,922 in 1972, but falling by 57 per cent to 163,933 in 1981.[47] Assuming a 3.5 per cent population growth rate, the estimated population for 1998 is around 260,000.

We have already discussed a number of possible reasons for the unreliability of figures of this kind, but in Muhmand Agency they particularly include the inaccessible nature of many areas: in Ambar, for example, no census was even attempted, the Government relying on local elders/leaders for data collection. These elders would almost certainly have exaggerated their clan population for the political reasons already discussed, and would be ignorant of the importance of the census as well as suspicious of the Government. Even with the best will in the world, however, which they certainly did not have, they would not have been technically or educationally equipped to undertake a reliable census.

The dramatic decline in the 1981 figures has a number of possible explanations. These include emigration, the *dwa kora*, or two houses system which leads to double counting, negative attitudes of officials towards tribal peoples, lack of public interest, and the joint family system. This system, which involves maintaining one house in an urban area and another in the native tribal area, entails three to four generations living together and pooling resources, and a mean household size of 23.5 people. For all this system's economic, political and social advantages, it does not exactly aid accurate recording.

Muhmand Agency's literacy rate is 3.61 per cent (males 6.07 per cent, females 0.64 per cent). While officially Muhmand has 307 educational institutions, these include some 'ghost schools' which exist on paper but not in reality, either through administrative incompetence or as a result of corruption. Nonetheless, education offers employment to 1195 people,[48] almost all of them local, as teachers, and many more in lower grade positions. Another source of income is the three local markets at Ghalanai, Gandab and Yakaghund, where daily necessities are sold. No figures exist on any exodus to the Middle East or the economic and social impacts of remittances from there. Some individuals from the Halim Zai area were, however, known to the first author to be working as labourers in the Gulf region. There is no industry. In 1977 a glass and bottle manufacturing factory was officially established, but as a ghost industry only: almost a quarter of a century later it had still to commence production. The mainstay of the people is the migration to other parts of the country, including, most locally, Peshawar and Mardan in NWFP, for menial jobs and agricultural labour.

Khyber Agency has an area of 257,654 hectares, of which only the 5.43 per cent on the banks of rivers and streams is available for cultivation. 87.21 per cent of this cultivable area is irrigated. The average family holding is 8 *jreebs*.[49] Khyber Agency is bounded by Muhmand Agency to the north-east, the Jalalabad or Ningrahar province of Afghanistan to the north-west, Peshawar district to the east, Orak Zai Agency to the south and Kuram Agency to the south-west. As the only northern land route connecting the subcontinent with Europe, the Khyber Pass has had deep historical significance for invaders from Alexander the Great to the Moguls and Afghans. The region is like a palace, fort or castle, and is appropriately named Khyber, for this Hebrew-derived word means just that. The Pass begins at Jamrud, 16 kilometres west of Peshawar cantonment, twisting north-westerly through the hills for 40 kilometres to Toor Kham, 10 kilometres from Landikotal, a checkpoint with Afghanistan.

The terrain is hilly, with many small valleys in the shape of narrow strips. The mountains are steep, rocky and unfit for vegetation; the valleys are situated in deep gorges. The climate is extreme, being cold to extremely cold in winter, with snow common on high altitudes, and warm to hot in summer. Water is scarce, with a precipitation of only 4–5 inches in summer and 10–15 inches in winter. Though two rivers, Bara and Choora, flow through Khyber, they are of little use for cultivation.

No significant industrial units exist: cigarette and marble factories completed by the FATA Development Corporation in 1976 and 1980 respectively both proved loss making and closed within a few years. Only three private factories exist: one gee mill, one ice factory and one cigarette factory.

As for all Pathans, the extended and joint family system provides the basic necessities of life for every member of the family irrespective of earnings. Pakistan is not a welfare state so there is no concept of income support, child benefit, pensions or social security, and all male earners contribute to the family purse, women being economically inactive other than by helping with agriculture at sowing and harvest times. Marriage and other ceremonies are celebrated with pomp and show, often beyond the means of the family concerned. Excessive expenditure is incurred on such ceremonies, as well as on the eve of the two Eids every year. In the opium growing areas this tradition of over-expenditure normally ensures the people stay in debt until the next harvest of opium offers at least temporary solvency.

Pakistan's birth rate is high (3.0 per cent per annum), and in NWFP, where it is commonly believed that the more males in a family the greater the income (and therefore status), the desire for male children extends the reproductive life of married couples, leading to high population growth. Further contributory reasons for this desire include the high infant mortality rate, estimated at 133/1,000 live births (as against 89/1,000 for Pakistan as a whole) and an understandable desire for insurance against poverty in old age.[50]

The average literacy rate is 10.94 per cent, with male literacy 20.18 per cent and female 0.64 per cent. There are 327 educational institutions of which 78 are for females, including 70 primary schools, five middle schools and three girls' high schools. The education department provides employment for about 1500 persons, or 0.9 per cent of the working population.[51] Estimates suggest a youth unemployment figure of 70,000[52] in the Agency, or 41.6 per cent of the eligible population.

Trade is the major source of income. Afridies and Shinwaries characteristically concentrate on the transport and carriage business. Most inland transport, particularly in NWFP, is owned and controlled by them, though yet again no reliable statistics are available. Owing to the long border with Afghanistan and the Khyber Pass, smuggling is a major activity. Some of the big traders from Khyber Agency deal with international business in foreign-made items like electronic goods, cloth, and crockery, an activity which occupies a considerable number of local people.

Ostensibly to support groups such as widows, orphans, the destitute and students of religious schools, a system of *zakah* was introduced by the Zia government in the early 1980s, and more than 28 billion rupees annually are deducted from personal bank accounts under the *zakah* head. The religious text defines the purpose for which these funds may be used in very broad terms, but, according to many, the money has been used for general purposes by whichever party is in government, too little having found its way to the intended recipients.

Drugs, as we have seen, are mostly produced in economically disadvantaged areas where there is absolute poverty, with off-season migration to industrial centres outside the Province being the only realistic economic alternative. In NWFP, both climatic conditions and geography, which are unlike those in other provinces of the country, make these areas perfect for opium cultivation.

Dir District is characterized by great diversity in soil and climate conditions due to altitudes ranging from 1,000 metres to 3,500 metres. Annual rainfall varies between 600 mm in the south and over 1,000 mm in the north. As the area is mountainous and steep most agriculture requires terracing, and accordingly is complex and back-breaking, with yield and income very low. A population of 1.6 million and an average family size of 13 puts tremendous pressure on the *per capita* available land of 0.36 *jreebs* or 0.073 hectares.

Agriculture is the mainstay of the people, 85 per cent of them directly depending on it. It is mostly primitive, and in some parts very old crude implements such as hand ploughs, planks and digging shovels to level and dig the soil and prepare it for cultivation are used to this day. Hand hoeing and weeding are common sights, and there is little use of improved seeds, fertilizers or pesticides. Some 80 per cent of cultivable land is terraced, and the use of high cost machinery is impossible for a people many of whom cannot even afford a pair of oxen for ploughing. Naturally the development of agriculture depends also on infrastructure investment, including roads, educational facilities, availability of expertise, modern agricultural technology and good health provision as well as land holding reform. All of these are lacking in Dir.

Poppy, however, offers many times the income of other crops (some 6,900 rupees per family per year), and covers 80 per cent of the 59,000 hectares of fertile irrigated lands in the eastern valleys.[53] This is probably almost 530,000 hectares, though the cultivated area was officially reported as only 85,885 hectares in 1992–93, plus cultivable waste land of 1,416 hectares, afforested areas of 171,585 hectares, and non-cultivable land of 10,320 hectares.[54]

A UN report on the socio-economic conditions of the area noted that the Pakistan Government was aware that enforcing the poppy growing ban would cause financial hardship. This, combined with the problem of identifying and accessing the valleys themselves, suggested that prohibition alone was not a viable long term strategy. A UN consultant, reporting on the Dir Development Project, observed:

I believe that the project, in conjunction with a government enforcement programme, will achieve the elimination of poppy production in Dir District. However, I am concerned that as the project stands, the result will be a less sustainable economy than presently exists. . . The project area, particularly the area of concentration for the second phase, is characterized by limited arable land and consequently relatively small farms, often poor soil, large and young families with a high rate of population growth, high levels of illiteracy and few options for income generation off the farm. Many of the small farms appear to be incapable of growing sufficient subsistence crops to feed the rather large farm families and are dependent on poppy production, but to date the project has been unable to identify a cropping system that can effectively replace poppy production. With population pressure growing in any event, I fear one of the impacts of the project will be to accelerate the further impoverishment of small farmers.[55]

Bajaur has an area of 129,035 hectares, out of which 56,000 hectares (43 per cent) are available for cultivation. Only 26.3 per cent of the land (14,720 hectares)[56] has thus far been brought under irrigated agriculture, mainly through some 100 tube wells constructed by the Government in the Khar and Mamund *Tehsils* since 1976. Land per family averages 13 *jreebs*. The major crops are wheat, barley and lentils, and mustard is grown on rain dependent lands. Opium cultivation, once a major cash crop on irrigated lands, appears to have reduced following these developments.

Agriculture in *Muhmand*, unlike Bajaur, is very scanty. Of a total area of 229,620 hectares only 13,500 hectares (5.88 per cent of the total land) are available for agriculture, either in the rain dependent lands of Ambar Tehsil or the irrigated land on the banks of the Swat and Kabul rivers in the low lying areas. Swat river basin consists of steep slopes and gorges, though Kabul river basin is open and satisfactory for subsistence agriculture. Topography is the main problem for agricultural development, as the maximum extension of fertile land, involving an additional 17,331 hectares of cultivable waste, would permit a total fertile area of no more than 30,000 hectares. The average family income is approximately 7,500 rupees per family, or 3840 rupees ($64) per person per year. As a result of low productivity and low income, opium cultivation is widespread in the poorest part of the Agency, Ambar Tehsil, where, in the absence of irrigation, only single cropping is possible.

Conclusion: Opium and Heroin in the Indo-Pak Sub-Continent

Drug abuse has doubtless been part of many cultures and societies since time immemorial, but there is little indication that drugs posed significant problems for social well-being until the 18th and 19th centuries. Certainly prior to that time the idea of drugs being a problem appears nowhere in the literature we were able to trace. Around 200 years ago, however, the abuse of opium and its derivatives began to assume alarming proportions in a number of countries, notably – but not exclusively – China and the USA. Indeed it has been said that in the early 19th century drug abuse was known as the American disease, and, during the US Civil War, as the soldiers' disease.

Since that time, the frequently devastating impact of drug addiction on individuals, families and the social structure has become familiar. Narcotic drugs, including opium and its derivatives, present major economic, social and political challenges to many countries, by no means all of which are equipped to manage them. One such country is Pakistan, and our purpose has been to show, from a multidisciplinary perspective, how a combination of social, economic, cultural, political, historical and geographical forces together create seemingly intractable problems. All the more so given Pakistan's status as a third world country with more than its share of development problems, including political instability, primary poverty, religious intolerance, corruption, illiteracy, health problems and population growth. About the economic plight of such countries, Jones has written:

> Poverty is the central problem. Most third world countries are poor and their people subject to many different forms of deprivation, powerlessness, hunger, urban squalor,

landlessness, illiteracy, avoidable ill health, familial deprivation, the exploitation of women and so on. Most of the poverty in underdeveloped countries is concentrated in the rural areas where most of the people live. The various aspects of poverty interact. Inequality in education perpetuates inequalities in status and 'life chances'. Squalid living conditions adversely affect health and life expectancy. Inequality of powers stands in the way of any steps towards greater social justice. The interactions are endless.[57]

Pakistan has existed as an independent nation for over 50 years. For half that time it has been under emergency or martial law. It has fought three wars with India, became a front line state after the 1979 Soviet invasion of Afghanistan and the 2001 US and allied action against the same country, and has been bearing the consequences for 20 years. The politics of ethnicity have truncated it, religious and ethnic violence have taken a huge toll of human lives, and political corruption is the order of the day. 'State' and 'Government' refer in practice to Islamabad, and 'state' and 'society' could scarcely be further apart. Education is a privilege not a right, health facilities are rudimentary, and politics revolves around the accumulation of power, privilege and wealth. Like many post-colonial states Pakistan has inherited many defects in its political structure. As faces change at the top, policies also change and the public suffers from government to government. There is no uniform legal system, particularly in the drug producing areas, and this situation indirectly and directly aids drug production.

International pressure to solve the problems associated with drugs increased considerably in the early 1970s, when the USA declared its first 'war on drugs'. It was also in the 1970s that drug addiction surfaced as a problem in Pakistan, though at that time there was no inkling of how serious a problem it was to become. Heroin was little known, but such psychotropic synthetic drugs as barbiturates and amphetamines and local drugs like opium and cannabis were part of common culture. Though there are reports that some people in Karachi had used heroin, probably having acquired the habit during international travel[58] or as a result of Karachi's international trade and communications links, Pakistan's first case of heroin addiction came to light in Baluchistan in 1979. A year later the first two cases in NWFP were identified in the provincial capital, Peshawar. Since then heroin addiction has spread like a forest fire: for twenty years some 100,000 people annually have become addicted, and the number of addicts is now probably increasing by 7 per cent annually,[59] with no treatment and rehabilitation of addicts at state level.

Notes

1   Government of Pakistan, Pakistan Integrated Household Survey (PIHS), Round 3:1998/
     99 (Islamabad: Federal Bureau of Statistics, October 2000), 151. Table A-2.
2   United Nations, *A Review of Narcotics Related Matters in NWFP* (Peshawar: Drug
     Control Programme, 1984). pp2–7.
3   M. Haq (Former Finance Minister of Pakistan) in *The News* (London: 25 December
     1997).
4   Government of Pakistan, *National Survey on Drug Abuse in Pakistan* (Islamabad:
     Narcotics Control Board 1986). p11.

5 Government of Pakistan, *PIHS 1998–99, op. cit.* p73.
6 M. Haq *op.cit.*; Government of Great Britain. *Health and Personal Social Services Statistics.* HMSO: London, 1994. p82.
7 T.J. Adden, *The Distribution of Opium Cultivation and the Trade in Opium* (Haarlem: Joh. Enschede En Zonen, 1939). p5.
8 L. Tullis, *Beneficiaries of the Illicit Drug Trade: Political Consequences and International Policy at the Intersection of Supply and Demand* (Geneva: United Nations Research Institute for Social Development, 1991). p8.
9 S. Kumar, 'Drug Trafficking in Pakistan', *Asian Strategic Review* (1994–5). pp196–7.
10 UN Drug Control Programme Report in *The News* (London: 27 June 1997).
11 L. Tullis, *Unintended Consequences: Illicit Drugs and Drugs Policies in Nine Countries* (Boulder, CO: Lynne Rienner, 1995). pp37–8.
12 G. Quaglia, *The News* (London: 27 June 1997).
13 Government of Pakistan, *Resource and Reference Manual for Prevention Resource Consultant Network.* Vol. I (Islamabad: Drug Abuse Prevention Resource Centre, 1990). p14.
14 Government of the United States of America, *International Narcotics Control Strategy Report* (Washington DC: Bureau of International Narcotics and Law Enforcement Affairs, 1996). p234.
15 The researcher's visit to the agency opium cultivating areas was in March 2000. See also the press conference of Dr Nusrat Afridi, who brokered an agreement for the elimination of opium poppies. The agency administration backed out of the deal, however, and hence Dr Afridi was made hostage for recovery of the ransom money (*Daily Mashriq*, Peshawar: April 24, 2000).
16 United Nations, *The Illicit Drug Problem in Southwest Asia: Briefing Note* (Islamabad: Drug Control Programme, 1996).
17 J. Cooley, *Unholy Wars: Afghanistan, America and International Terrorism* (London: Pluto Press, 1999). pp126–30; see also I. Haq, *From Hashish to Heroin* (Lahore: Al-noor Publications 1991). p23.
18 Government of the United States of America, 1996, *op.cit.*
19 *The Times* (London: 11 August 1997).
20 D. Miller, *Licit Narcotics Production and its Ramifications for Foreign Policy* (Washington DC: US State Department, 1980). p1
21 United States Government, *International Narcotics Control Strategy Report*, 1996. p222.
22 H. Wemkel, 'Narcotics Trafficking in Pakistan'. Paper delivered to the Workshop on Mass Media Orientation for Prevention of Drug Abuse, 22–27 October. Reprinted in *Reflections on Drug Abuse: a Collection of Speeches.* (Islamabad: Narcotics Control Board, 1984). p95.
23 Government of the United States of America, *op. cit.* 1996. pp249, 278, 300.
24 L.F. Rushbrook Williams, *The State of Pakistan* (London: Faber and Faber, 1962). p62.
25 United Nations, *A Review of Narcotics Related Matters in NWFP* (Peshawar: Drug Control Programme, 1984).
26 M.A. Abbasi, Chief Minister North West Frontier Province in *The Daily Khabrain* (Islamabad: 29 May 1997).
27 A.W. McCoy, *The Politics of Heroin in South East Asia* (New York: Harper and Row, 1972). p9.
28 Government of the United States of America, *World Opium Survey* (Washington: Cabinet Committee on International Narcotic Control, 1972). pp10–12.
29 C.P. Spencer and V. Navarathnam, *Drug Abuse in South East Asia* (Kuala Lumpur, Oxford University Press, 1981). p23.
30 United Nations, *Dir District Development Project, Phase II: Project Document* (Peshawar: Drug Control Programme, 1994). p9.

31 Government of North West Frontier Province, *Agency-Wide Socio-Economic Indicators* (Peshawar: Bureau of Statistics, Planning and Development Department, 1995). p3.

32 C.P. Spencer and V. Navarathnam, *op.cit*. p12. In fact, in the course of his fieldwork the first author visited Kurya and was told that this figure was exaggerated. This view was confirmed by analysis of a PNCB report (Government of Pakistan, *Buner Agriculture Development Project: The Buner Model 1976–86*. Islamabad: Narcotics Control Board, 1986). According to this report just 52 people out of a population of 425 were addicts, an addiction rate of around 12 per cent.

33 United Nations, *Trends in Poppy Harvest* (Islamabad: Drug Control Programme, 1996). p8.

34 United Nations, *Dir District Development Project: Phase II: Project Document* (Peshawar: Drug Control Programme 1994). p3.

35 Government of India, *Imperial Gazetteer of India: Provincial Series, North West Frontier Province* (Reprint of 1903 edition) (Lahore: Sang-e-Meel Publications, Chawk Urdu Bazaar, 1980). The Nawabs of Dir are descendants of a pious person of local fame, Akhun Sahib, whose grandson, Muhmand Sharif Khan, was given the title of Nawab in Delhi Darbar in 1895 by the British. The *Mian-Guls* of Swat were descendants of Abdul Ghafoor, a poor herd boy from *Gujars* who later became known as Saidu Baba. At a time when the local Pakhtoons were in a state of continuous tribal war with each other, the eldest son of Saidu Baba, known as Bach Sahib, was installed as chief of Swat in 1926, with the title Wali-e-Swat or Mian Gul. Mehtar-e-Chitral is also a royal title, given to the rulers of Chitral in 1895.

36 C.P. Spencer and V. Navarathnam, *op. cit*. 1981. p9.

37 *The Frontier Post* (Peshawar: 16 September 1998).

38 M. Faheem, and A. Saeed, *A Profile of Dir with Agriculture Background* (Timargara: Dir District Development Project, 1991). p4

39 There are 2052 educational institutions for males, including 637 mosque/*maktab* schools, 869 primary schools, 76 middle schools, 81 high schools, 6 higher secondary schools, 2 degree colleges and 2 vocational institutes. For females there are 379 separate educational institutions, including 12 *maktab* schools, 327 primary schools, 29 middle schools and 11 high schools.

40 These and (except where stated otherwise) subsequent figures in this section are from Government of North West Frontier Province, 1996, *op. cit*.

41 G. Kruseman, *Socio-Economic Aspects of Poppy Cultivation: Selected Farm Profile of Eastern Dir Valleys and Dir Kohistan* (Peshawar: Special Development Unit, 1985). p viii

42 Government of North West Frontier Province, *Socio-Economic Profile of Bajaur Agency* (Peshawar: Planning and Development Department, 1992). p2.

43 Akbar S. Ahmad, *Pakhtoon Economy and Society* (London, Routledge and Kegan Paul, 1980). p43.

44 *Ibid*. pp44–45.

45 Government of North West Frontier Province, *op. cit*. 1992. p12.

46 Government of North West Frontier Province, *Important Agency-Wide Socio-Economic Indicators 1994* (Peshawar: Bureau of Statistics, Environment, Planning and Development Department, 1994). pp14, 20. Of this number 1037 were males and 160 females. Probably all females were from the Agency, as female education is very low. The male literacy rate is about 6.8 per cent against 1 per cent for females.

47 Government of North West Frontier Province, *Peshawar, Census of Population: FATA* (Peshawar: FATA Development Corporation, 1981). p15.

48 Government of North West Frontier Province, *Important Agency-Wide Socio-Economic Indicators 1995* (Peshawar: Bureau of Statistics, Environment, Planning and Development Department, 1995).

49 *Jreeb* is a local measure of land. Two *jreebs* make an acre and 2.47 acres make a hectare.

50   World Health Organisation, in *The News International* (London, 11 August 1997).
51   Government of North West Frontier Province, 1995, *op. cit.*
52   Haji Khaista Khan, in *Daily Mashriq* (Peshawar: 2 April 1997).
53   M. Faheem and Abu Saeed 1991, *op.cit.* p4.
54   Government of North West Frontier Province, 1992–3, *Land Utilization Statistics for 1992–3 in NWFP* (Peshawar: Agriculture Department). p22.
55   United Nations, *Dir District Development Project. Phase II.* (Peshawar: Drug Control Programme, 1991). p2.
56   Government of North West Frontier Province, *Land Utilization Report 1992* (Peshawar: Agriculture Department 1992). p2.
57   H. Jones, *Social Welfare in Third World Development* (London: Macmillan Education 1990). pp1–2
58   M. Gossop, *Living With Drugs* (Aldershot: Ashgate Publishing, 1993). p33.
59   *The News* (London: 26 July 1996).

Chapter II

Opium: The Poppy, the Drug and Opium Derivatives

The Opium Poppy

Though many medical histories of opium are available, no authoritative history of the poppy is known to exist. While scattered references can be found, based on archaeological, archaeo-botanical and pharmacological findings, these are shrouded in antiquity[1] and the geographical origins of the plant are contested. Terry and Pellin suggest Mesopotamia, while Berridge and Griffith[2] prefer Egypt, from where, they suggest, the plant spread to Asia Minor and onwards to Greece and Europe. Others again[3] claim Asia Minor itself, and Persia in particular. Merrillees[4] opts for Cyprus, from where, he claims, it was exported to Egypt. Similar views are expressed by Neligan[5] who asserts that the Egyptians were not introduced to opium cultivation before the Greek conquest of the area in 300 BC.

Nor is there consensus about the timing of the origins of the plant, though the use of opium has been traced back to the early Neolithic, Mesolithic or upper Palaeolithic periods. The Sumerians, who settled in Mesopotamia around 6–5000 BC, knew about *papaver somniferum*,[6] and their successors, the Babylonians, took this knowledge to the east (Persia) and west (Egypt) of their Empire.

Etymology is equally contentious. According to Watt[7] the Sanskrit name for opium, *ahiphena*, derives from the Arabic *afiun*; Babar, however, says that *ahiphena*, *afiun* in Urdu, Persian and Arabic, and *afim* in Pashtu are derivations or distortions of the ancient Sanskrit word *ahiuphena* or *ohifaus*.[8]

Even botanists, from whom one might expect greater scientific precision, are uncertain about the plant's origins and ancestry, and its internal taxonomy is similarly controversial. While some plants can be traced to their original geographical ranges of distribution and identified with the real, natural-growing progenitor, in the case of the poppy the true wild ancestor is obscure. While it is generally agreed that *papaver somniferum* belongs to the order *papaverales* or *rhoedale*,[9] an order of flowering plants of relatively primitive evolutionary development, one botanist, Campbell suggests there are four families in the order while another, Hutchinson, believes there to be only two. The number of *genera* and species is similarly contested, Porter claiming to have identified 24 *genera* and 450 species[10] while Core has found 28 *genera* but only 250 species.[11] These taxonomic disputes, though we address them only briefly here as they are tangential to our theme, contribute to the ancestral uncertainties to which we have already drawn attention.

If the history of the poppy is obscure to scholars, the contemporary conditions of poppy growing are equally misunderstood by laymen. It is not true, for example, that the poppy grows almost anywhere irrespective of climatic conditions. In fact great skill and experience are required if the crop is to succeed. Though it is indeed a drought resistant crop which can grow on as little as 15 inches annual rainfall[12] the poppy requires particular soil and climatic conditions, as variations affect morphine content, and heavy rains can ruin a crop. So while in irrigated areas where soil is rich production is relatively straightforward,[13] in rain dependent locations such as Bajaur and Muhmand Agencies, 3–4 manual or bull ploughings are required for propagation, followed by carefully prepared manuring. In such areas the small size and irregular shape of the plots would make tractor ploughing impractical even if tractors could be afforded. And after harvesting the *kharif* (November–May or winter/spring) crop (normally the only crop on rain dependent lands) the whole process begins again.

Poppies with high morphine content have been cultivated in tropical, subtropical and temperate climates all over the world.[14] *Papaver somniferum* has a number of geographical strains, and transplantation of one geographical race to another weakens plants, rendering them susceptible to disease. For centuries the poppies of the southern form, those of Afghanistan, Iran and India, best grown in a dry and warm climate and requiring a shorter vegetative period, have been cultivated in NWFP. In fact two main varieties of opium poppy are currently cultivated there, one with white, the other with red or purple flowers, normally at elevations of 2–6,000 feet. While a poppy normally requires a temperature of 3–6°C to germinate, once established it can withstand temperatures below freezing.

Nor is the poppy as amenable to different soil types as is sometimes imagined. Clays are unsuitable because of their higher moisture content, since under heavy rains where the soil remains saturated for several days, the poppy will wither and die. Conversely sand is too drought-prone and infertile, while soils lacking good tilth are unsuitable because the small seed lacks strength to break through the crust. The ideal texture is a sandy loam augmented by heavy manuring. In NWFP the crop is usually sown during mid-October to end-November, when rain dependent land has been watered by the late monsoon or early winter rains. By the end of December the plant is normally 1–3 inches high, with two or three leaves, and can resist the cold.

December and January are the months for weeding, hoeing and thinning, normally by women and children. These are labour intensive tasks, and often only a part of even a small field of size 35 × 10 feet can be cleaned in a day. Proper thinning and weeding create 3–4 additional branches and hence capsules. By March–April the plant attains its maximum height of 35–55 inches. Soon afterwards blossoming starts, and for 2–3 weeks the area is a colourful sight of white, red and purple flowers. The anthers crack open and expose the sticky pollen, which enables wind as well as insect pollination (though the latter is more important for fertilization). By mid-April the pod is exposed, and when the petals finally drop it is ready for lancing/incising. At this point the third and last but most difficult stage of labour begins. With the help of a small 3–5 bladed knife (*panja*) the incision of the corona starts. As the corona is incised, a white milky liquid oozes out and coagulates in 5–8 hours. This coagulated juice, which turns deep brown, is opium resin. Incision is normally done on alternate days in the afternoon, the gum being collected next morning with the help of a blunt scraper.

At this point, rain can destroy the opium resin, so the heavy rains characteristic of spring in Pakistan constitute the main risk. The opium gum, moistened by nocturnal dew, must be scraped off before the sun gets warm and the gum dry and hard. Incising or lancing is a skilled and delicate job: up to 6 incisions are needed, and if any incision is too deep the yield is damaged. Normally, in a one-acre field, six persons lance and then collect the gum. Following lancing the capsule dries on the plant for 10–15 days when the capsules are harvested by hand, sun dried and beaten and broken with a club. When more seeds exist in the capsules they are separated by filtering through a sieve.

To collect 1 kg of raw opium, 40–50 man hours' work are needed, so remunerative production is dependent on the existence of poverty, large families and low wages. Opium is not produced by big landowners, but by peasants who possess or rent as much land as they can work manually with their families. Production is further aided by the custom of *ashar*, under which, in times of need, relatives or local people must help their kinsmen in return for rich food arranged in their honour. The beneficiary of *ashar* then reciprocates when he in turn is needed.

Opium's significance cannot be measured only in sales, however, for it represents a whole domestic economy, culture and way of life, its significance being akin to that of the banana or coconut elsewhere. Every part of this plant has its use. The seeds and broken capsules are packed separately for market; the dry stalk is used as fodder, for fencing the fields or as fuel; dry capsules are kept in private homes as medicine. Growing and harvesting opium are skills passed down the generations, and, as we shall see, not always substitutable by alternative activities devised by international organizations or national governments.

Opium the Drug

I would order poppies to be sown in all fields of Portugal and command *afyum* [opium] to be made . . . and the labourers would gain much also, and the people of India are lost without it.[15]

The history of opium itself, as medicine and source of euphoria, stretches back before recorded history. The first written record of opium occurs around 800 BC when Homer mentions a city near Corinth named Mekone (Poppy Town), the name signifying that opium poppies are cultivated in the area. Hippocrates (460–377 BC) makes frequent mention of poppy as a medicine; Theophrastus and Aristotle (384–322 BC) similarly make many references to it.

Though opium is the name of the coagulated juice or latex of the poppy plant obtained by the incision of the unripe but mature capsule of the plant, such importance now attaches to the word that in English the plant as a whole is popularly called opium. This is not the case in every language: Pashtu in particular has a richer vocabulary, using different words for the seeds (*khash khash*), the plant (*koknar*), and the capsule or corona (*doodha* or *ghootai*).

The circumstances of the introduction of opium to the sub-continent are obscure.[16] Some scholars believe the plant originated there, whereas Kritikos and Papadaki say it originated in the west and spread to India.[17] Many non-Muslim writers[18] argue that opium was introduced to the East by Arabs,[19] a number of Indian scholars believing that as their sacred books, *Vedas*, do not make any mention of the plant it must have come late into India, probably with the Muslims or Arabs.[20] Muslim scholars conversely, say that such mention does occur: Babar, for example, quotes *Regveda* of 500 BC as saying 'drug plants preceded even the Gods'. Many authors, however, believe the Arabs of the Mohammedan era or Muslims took opium to the area around the 7–8th centuries AD. Anslinger goes further, saying (controversially for many Muslims) that the rise of Islam provided a stimulus to the spread of opium use through its concept of the separation of the spiritual and physical nature. In particular, as Islam forbade the use of wine, people switched to opium and other sources of intoxication.[21] Sharma[22] suggests that the earliest mention of opium as a product of India is found in the memoirs of Barbosa in AD 1511. Certainly opium was used as a medicine and to pacify infants under Muslim rule, and cultivation and usage spread so rapidly that by AD 1000 it was widely used throughout the social spectrum and was, though for unclear reasons, banned by Emperor Allauddin Khelji in AD 1310.[23]

According to one oral tradition, *Chandu*, a form of smoking opium, was introduced by a Hindu Prince. Chandan Kumar alias *Chandu* took to opium smoking in China and on his return introduced it among his close aides, before the practice filtered down to lesser folk.[24] It is certainly possible that during the British opium trading period influential individuals had access to opium and introduced the habit. According to oral tradition in Muslim NWFP and Eastern Afghanistan opium was introduced by the Greeks, and records certainly suggest that Alexander the Great introduced it to India and that his army used it *en route*.[25] In view of the medicinal value of opium as an analgesic, anaesthetic and anti-diarrhoea preparation this is plausible, particularly as the areas most extensively cultivated for centuries have been Persia, Turkey, India, Afghanistan and Central Asia, all of them on Alexander's route to India in 334 BC.[26] Certainly Greek physicians, later to be popularized by the Arabs as *unani hakeems*, have extensively described the medical use of opium, and in Swat, then a Graeco-Bactirean valley, and the adjoining districts of Dir, Swabi, Chitral and Bajaur, opium was extensively used for medical purposes – in winter for colds, influenza and coughs, in summer for diarrhoea, pain relief and inducing sleep.

Zaheerud Din Babar conquered India in AD 1526 and founded the Mughal dynasty, giving opium Government patronage for revenue generation purposes. Poppy cultivation then became a state monopoly, and opium was not only an important article of trade with China and other countries[27] where usage was much greater than in India, but an elite recreational drink used by Akber the Great himself, in a form called *charberga*, or four leaves.[28] In imitation of him ordinary people also started to use it:

> Although they take it in small quantity, it is a merchandise in great demand everywhere it is consumed, for if they do not take it they are in danger of death, and this is the reason why in the countries I am talking about it is very expensive. They always try to keep a supply of it (as they keep wheat for May). Those who take it go about sleepy, and they say they take it so as to dispel cares.[29]

Before the western occupation of the Indian sub-continent all governments depended on land revenue for wealth and power.[30] Trade had little importance compared with what was to come later, for example in the lucrative trade in spices, particularly pepper. The focus of the imperial administration was the accurate assessment of agriculture revenue and its transfer to the centre of power in coins. This agrarian base supported courts, army and administration. Agricultural production was mainly directed to self-sufficiency, so priority was given to food crops, and while the revenue collected from opium was at this time higher than revenue from food crops, opium is mentioned in records as but one of the agricultural goods thus taxed or monopolized by Government. No special position was given to it, either as a drug crop or a dangerous commodity, nor were special measures taken to control it.

The greatest development in drug production, and the one with the deepest repercussions, took place during the colonial era. All colonial powers benefited from opium trading in the East, and every stage of opium development has been shaped and formed by the rise and fall of the western empires. The present massive opium production in South Asia is the culmination of 400 years' western patronage of opium: opium smoking was introduced by the Portuguese and Dutch in 1500, and by the 18th and 19th centuries every European colony had its official opium dens.

The British involvement at this time is especially notorious because of its involvement at state level in superintending a trade declared illegal by China, patronising smugglers and waging war on the pretext of impeding the business in opium. The British did not, however, enter the opium trade until the middle of the 18th century, when, following the battle of Plessey (1764) Bengal, the richest province in the continent, fell to Robert Clive's East India Company (EIC). Assuming control of the area, the EIC leased out the trade to Patna traders and ordered farmers to give up food production and convert their lands into a mono-culture of opium poppies:

> It was impossible to get them to continue producing opium except by compulsion; either legal, as in those districts where it could be claimed that tenancies would be forfeited unless poppy was grown (as the company's agent was also the magistrate he could also lay down, as well as enforce the law), or financial through the manipulation of advances in order to get the cultivator into debt and keep him there, so that jail and eviction would face him if he disobeyed.[31]

In 1773, as Governor General of the EIC, Warren Hastings brought the opium trade under the direct control of the Company, abolishing the Patna syndicate and giving the EIC or its agents exclusive rights to purchase opium from Bengali farmers and auction it for export. In Bengal over 500 square miles were cultivated with opium, involving over one million registered farmers, 500,000 acres of prime land[32] and 2,000 agents employed by the Company to collect the crop.[33] The commercial attractiveness of opium led to conflict within India, and it is sometimes said that Britain's first opium war was as early as 1818, when attempts by Marhatta State to export opium to China in direct competition with British traders were suppressed.

Partly as a result of the supply of narcotics by the EIC, opium addiction had become a social problem in China by the 19th century. Between 40 million[34] (27 per cent of the adult male population) and 100 million[35] Chinese were addicted, enabling Great Britain to export 6,000 tons of opium annually to China by the late 19th century.[36] In order to check the growing menace of addiction the Chinese authorities planned to stop smuggling and ordered confiscation. In 1839, 20,000 chests of opium worth £2,000,000 owned by British and American companies[37] were confiscated by the Chinese authorities. This led to the first Opium War of 1839–42, the cession of Hong Kong and the payment of heavy compensation in the Treaty of Nanking. In 1858, China lost the Second Opium War, opening other Chinese ports for opium trading by Britain.

But concern about the situation in China and America combined with public unease in Britain about the morality of the Opium Wars to trigger a change in official attitudes. The Quaker William Storrs Fry asked in 1840, for example:

> What would happen if French wines were banned in Britain and the French government, holding a wine monopoly, had proceeded deliberately to make wine to the British taste; established depots ships off the English coast; corrupted the English customs services by bribery; when warned, taken no notice; and when intercepted, employed armed crafts to fight their way through with the contraband wine. Would this not inevitably have led to war?[38]

A report published in *The Times* after the First Opium War in 1842 reads:

> . . . we think it of the highest moment that the Government of Great Britain should wash its hands once for all, not only of all diplomatic, but of all moral and practical responsibility for this (the Opium) traffic; that we should cease to be mixed up with it, to foster it, or to make it a source of Indian revenue. . . We owe some moral compensation to China for pillaging her towns and slaughtering her citizens in a quarrel which never could have arisen if we had not been guilty of this national crime.[39]

Such resistance effectively shamed the British Government into agreeing to restrict opium supplies to China[40] by 10 per cent annually, ceasing to trade entirely by 1916, and heightened international awareness that drug use was potentially a far-reaching problem. But, then as later, efforts to curtail or, ideally, eliminate it were unsuccessful. Opium was a legal drug when today's powerful anti-drug countries were involved in its trade and development, but when the trade passed into the hands of less powerful countries it became a forbidden substance, publicized so as to induce horror and fear.

In spite of the political impact in Britain of popular unease about the Opium Wars, it is naive to assume that international politics and finance can be driven by humanitarian concern. This is well illustrated by the case of India, where by 1869 the Bengal Government was taking active measures to increase the supply of opium to the Chinese market, including advancing interest-free loans to producers. By 1875 Bengal's production of 4,000 tons of raw opium was generating about 1/6th of India's total revenue, and by 1879 exports to China reached a peak of 105,508 300 lb chests. The war against drugs being fought by the Chinese was subjugated by the gunboat diplomacy of the British in order to continue to profit from the opium trade, confirming the primacy of economic over social or moral considerations. Perhaps not surprisingly, therefore, Buddenberg observes caustically that 'Politically, the British Raj was as addicted to opium as any twenty-pipe-a-day coolie in China'.[41]

Britain consolidated its opium monopoly following the quelling of the Mutiny (or, depending on one's perspective, War of Independence), by the Opium Act 1857. This Act prohibited the cultivation of opium poppies except under licence, and provided for Government procurement of the entire supply at prices determined according to quality and morphine content. Illegal crops were destroyed and cultivators prosecuted. The law, administered by the Opium Department, was supplemented by another Opium Act in 1878, which regulated not only trading but also possession for personal use.

Opium in Pakistan

Bengal was partitioned into Muslim and Hindu Bengal in 1947. The former comprised East Pakistan until the foundation of Bangladesh in 1971; the latter became a part of India. Opium is still officially cultivated in West Bengal, and though cultivation in East Pakistan was not permitted, illicit cultivation was rife until the mid-1950s, when jute production, for which the Korean War created a market, largely replaced it. So opium was cultivated with little control in Punjab, including the part abutting Peshawar and Dera Ismail Khan, and the hill territories west of the Indus under the control of the Punjab Government[42] (now NWFP) even before the colonial era. Hence the present NWFP is the only territory in Pakistan where opium cultivation has been in practice even since pre-colonial times.

Post-independence, opium policy/poppy production in Pakistan can be divided into five stages: 1947–53; 1954–56; 1957–72; 1973–78 and 1979–present.

Stage 1: 1947–53

On independence, in order to meet demand, the Government imported opium from India, selling it through the century old vend system. This involved shops, which received licences from the Excise Department which were auctioned annually on a district basis, selling opium to registered users (private smoking having been made illegal in 1950) and *hakeems*. On independence these shops numbered 328, of which 267 were in Punjab, with only a handful in NWFP, where opium was abundantly available.

There were at this time 260,000–280,000[43] users. These included a few *kasabgars* (artisans), who supposedly used opium to increase their working efficiency, and landlords or members of ruling elites, who occasionally used the most potent form of the drug (*chandu* or *madak*) for recreational purposes. In addition, the *unani hakeems* and other practitioners such as the 68,000 herbal practitioners, homeopaths and *ayvervedics* met the medical needs of over 80 per cent of the population.[44] It would be an error, however, to exaggerate the place of opium in these medication systems. Chopra and Chopra[45] note that out of 200–250 stock preparations of traditional medicines in the main dispensary of Ayuervedic and Tibbi college of Delhi only a few contained opium, and these were sparingly used. Indiscriminate use occurred rather in the household, as a remedy for diarrhoea, dysentery, coughs, bronchitis, asthma, colic, piles, neuralgia, fevers, rheumatism, diabetes and similar complaints. As a folk medicine, opium was administered to infants in NWFP, both in the belief that it protected them from such common viral diseases of dehydration as vomiting and diarrhoea (the major causes of infant mortality) and to lull them to sleep, freeing mothers to do domestic and agricultural work. A tragic consequence of this mistaken belief, however, was a rising incidence of child mortality.[46]

Stage 2: 1954–56

Under the International Opium Protocol of 1953 the UN permitted production in Pakistan. As a result, importation ceased and the Government, reinvoking the 1857 and 1878 Opium Acts, permitted cultivation in Punjab (though not NWFP), initially using seeds imported from India.[47] An opium factory was established in Lahore to supply opium to the vend shops, but this was not a success. Though the Punjab is famous for cotton and wheat, opium cultivation failed through weather problems, labour intensiveness (which, in the different social structure there, made it uneconomic), and lack of farming expertise.

Stage 3: 1957–72

As a result of this failure of the Punjab experiment the Government allowed poppy cultivation in NWFP in 1956–7. Licences were issued to farmers in Swabi, Mardan and Peshawar Districts, and regulated cultivation started in these settled areas in addition to the traditional unregulated cultivation in the tribal areas. Under the 1956 Constitution, responsibility for opium production passed to the Provincial Government whose responsibility it became to procure the gum from licensed farmers. This system increased production, and by 1958 the number of vend shops had increased to 789.

Individual licences were issued to farmers directly but joint licences, specifying the acreage permitted to be cultivated, were issued to villages, under the administration of the headman (*lamberdar*). The *lamberdar*, in return for 2 per cent commission, was charged with dividing the quota according to farmers' land holding size, and ensuring that all the opium was procured. Opium purchase depots were established and farmers informed in advance of the venue and date of procurement.

Though contravention of the law was punishable by a fine, imprisonment or both, it was widely flouted by officers as well as farmers: bribery was common, with licensing officers extracting money from licensees under threat of reporting over-cultivation. When, in response to this, the Federal Government sent in the PNCB in 1974, bribery actually increased, officials taking bribes from licensees and non-licensees alike. The extent of the enforcement problem can be judged from the fact that by 1977–78 an acreage of 8,960 was recorded[48] whereas licensed acreage was only 2,500 acres.

Stage 4: 1973–78

While this stage is characterized by increased control efforts it was, paradoxically but significantly, a period of massive expansion. Administratively this was facilitated by the undefined role of PNCB, instituted under Article 13 of the UN Single Convention of 1961. Opium and poppy cultivation remained a provincial responsibility, and anomalies appeared in the respective roles of PNCB and provincial opium officers, causing ambiguity as to the respective responsibilities of Federal and Provincial Governments. The ensuing confusion provided opportunities for corruption, and with both PNCB and Opium Department officials extracting money from farmers, enforcement failure ensured that opium production was effectively unmonitored.

Stage 5: 1979–Present

Prior to 1970, some 24 per cent of the world's total illicit opium production, estimated at 1400[49] tons a year, had come from the whole of south-west Asia. By 1978–9 NWFP alone was producing some 800 metric tons, of which only 4.77[50] metric tons were legal. The illicitly produced crop was either locally processed into heroin or transported to Iran or Turkey to be processed there. Realizing the bumper crop for the season 1978–9, the UN and some western countries pressurized Pakistan to outlaw opium production. As a result, in 1979 the military Government promulgated the Hudood Ordinance, an Islamic law banning the use, traffic and production of all intoxicants, including opium, and abolishing the vend system. Though presented as an Islamic provision the Ordinance was probably motivated less by Islam than by American pressure.[51] Certainly it misinterpreted Islamic law, for Islam does not forbid agricultural produce, whether poppies or the barley, grapes and apples which are processed into beer, wine and cider. Though in fact the law said nothing explicit about poppy cultivation[52] it was interpreted by the bureaucracy as doing so until, in 1995, a Presidential Ordinance clarified the situation.[53]

Also in 1979, following the Iranian Revolution, opium production was declared unlawful there too, a situation which opened a substantial new market for Pakistani and Afghan opium. In the same year Soviet troops entered Afghanistan, and a hitherto unprecedented influx of Afghan refugees fled to Pakistan, with NWFP in particular becoming in effect a reinforcement camp for Afghan resistance fighters. Lawlessness in Afghanistan led to opium cultivation on a large scale, as no other crops could resource the fighters and their families to the same degree. Since 1979, therefore, opium production has been a political issue not only in Pakistan but internationally.

Opium, then, was used first as medicine and a euphoric, then as an economic and political commodity. Its medicinal value is undeniable, and in the Indian sub-continent it has been used for treating complaints including insomnia, nervous irritability, dyspepsia, diarrhoea, dysentery, neuralgia, neuritis, rheumatic pains, influenza and coughing, apparently with no problems of addiction. Whole communities in the late 19th century were known to take a small amount of opium daily, apparently without exhibiting addictive characteristics. It has been variously, if immoderately, described as the world's great pain-killer, God's own medicine, the most hypnotic and the most potent of all drugs in the pharmacopoeia,[54] the oldest narcotic, the stone of immortality[55] and a remedy for 700 problems.[56] The medical attractiveness of opium lies chiefly in its special analgesic action, which makes it a master anaesthetic.[57] References to its pharmacological benefits have existed at least since the 5th century BC, when it was described as a drug that numbs the senses and induces deadening sleep. In Paranoiac times in Egypt, it was used much as we use aspirin today.[58]

In Europe, opium was once so heavily prescribed that the Dutch physician and chemist Sylvius de la Boe declared that without it he could not practise.[59] Among the educated class it was believed to increase the intellect and stimulate the imagination. In Britain it was cultivated in Buckinghamshire, Somerset and Edinburgh, and in the United States in Virginia, Tennessee, South Carolina, Georgia, Vermont, New Hampshire and Connecticut. US research on its medicinal value began around the time of the War of Independence, and it came to be used for spasms, dyspepsia, violent hysteria, hypochondriasis, dropsy, tetanus, typhus, venereal diseases, nervous headaches, fractures, palpitation, asthma, stomach problems, vomiting, dysentery, diarrhoea, rheumatism and fevers.[60]

In NWFP opium was traditionally used mainly by two groups: lower class labourers and artisans, and a relatively rich group of the petty land owning class. Among the former, opium consumption had economic logic. Housewives gave infants a little opium to make them sleep during the peak season of work, and their husbands took the drug to avert tiredness and do more work, the cost being more than recovered by the additional income. Among the latter group, the situation was quite different. Opium was taken hedonistically, and frequently proved a serious drain on resources, with many small landowners selling their possessions to buy drugs. A couplet in the shape of a dialogue between a husband and wife portrays the situation:

Husband: O poppy you are really nice to my heart. I wish to cultivate your plant all over the world. You cost little, but you give swing worth a million.

Wife: O poppy, I wish to eradicate your plant because you made us sell all our belongings and gave us the beggar's bowl in hands.

This cultural trait of disapproval has helped keep consumption to manageable levels. It occurs elsewhere too: an opium user is called an *amali*, a derogatory word meaning an idle and absurd daydreamer. Another indication of disapproval refers to opium's constipating properties: a man who spends a long time defecating is called an *afimi*. This is both a joke and a medically proved fact: opium abusers do indeed spend a long time defecating, producing stools which are dry and hard, and ejected, with considerable strain, in the form of *scybala*.

Stories exist about opium's power to increase sexual potency and reduce the likelihood of premature ejaculation. It is also often said that opium is not bad for the wealthy who can afford a rich diet. The older generation used opium orally and prepared it differently, and even today some affluent old people who use it for euphoric purposes boil it in milk, believing this reduces the morphine and codeine content, rendering it less dangerous. In our research areas, opium is still taken orally in Dir, Bajaur, Swat, Buner, Chitral, Swabi, Muhmand, Peshawar and Charsadda.

Patterns of usage have, of course, changed in the 50 years since independence, as they have in most parts of the world. Up to the mid-1960s raw opium (and also cannabis and its local derivatives), and a country-made alcohol, *tarra*, were mainly used, *tarra* in particular being attractive to low income people, as well as to non-Muslims permitted the use of alcohol. The elites who patronised imported alcohol, held local drugs in contempt, and opium remained primarily the province of the two categories of user already discussed. Subsequently Pakistan was by no means unaffected by changing patterns of drug use elsewhere. In the 1960s many Pakistani youths smoked cannabis, albeit mainly in a crude form, in imitation of their western counterparts, and subsequent years saw increases in the use of synthetic drugs. As elsewhere, barbiturates, stimulants, depressants and hallucinogens or pills had a deep cultural impact, and many people now take sleeping pills to sleep, and amphetamines, diazepam, seconal and ativan to keep awake.

There are three main methods for the preparation and smoking of opium or its derivatives: *chando*, *madak* and *dhoda*. These were demonstrated to the first author in the course of fieldwork and are reported briefly here. They all have side-effects and are all, to a degree, dangerous. We hint, in discussing the first of these three methods, *chando*, at anthropological significance, and a similar point could be made about *madak* and *dhoda*, but as this is not part of the analytic framework we do not pursue it here.

First, *chando* is a particularly notorious method of preparation and consumption. The method arranged for observation during field work in a feudal village guest house simply entails raw opium being boiled in water to remove impurities until smooth, brown paste is obtained, of a consistency which sticks to the end of a metallic needle. The apparatus for smoking this manufactured opium comprises a specially designed smoking pipe, a needle normally made from the spoke of a bicycle wheel and a lamp (*dewa*) filled with mustard oil or butter oil (*ghwari*). Finally there is a wooden bowl with a bulb at the lower end to cover the lamp and an aperture at the top, through which the needle is passed. The smoker lies on the floor with a brick or stone beneath his head. He places the wooden bowl on the lamp, holds one end of the pipe in his mouth and places the other end of the pipe on top of the bowl. He passes the needle through the aperture and holds it over the flame of the lamp with the other hand. As the opium burns it produces smoke inside the bowl, which is inhaled with the help of the pipe. Another person may help the smoker by holding the needle over the flame, and periodically more opium is taken on the tip of the needle and inserted it into the hole over the lamp. This process goes on until the smoker becomes benumbed or can no longer hold the pipe.

To anthropologists, the way in which this drug is administered has symbolic as well as functional meaning.[61] Lying on a hard floor with a hard brick or stone pillow has ritualistic meaning, invoking the idea of passing on to another world, since when a dead man is buried he is laid on hard ground with a raised portion under the head. And, as the dead belong to another world, so does the opium smoker take flight to another world of fantasy.

Chando is restricted to a few people. Whereas once *chando* was prepared and smoked in isolated locations like deserted water mills or ruins, nowadays this occurs in the guest houses of feudal villages to which law enforcement personnel cannot gain access. In NWFP *chando* smoking is known to take place in Charsadda,

Mardan, Peshawar and Mansehra Districts, all fertile areas with productivity far above subsistence level, a fact that probably led to the development of hedonistic psycho-cultural activities. This form of opium smoking is very dangerous, however, and even a small overdose can be fatal.

A second method of preparation and consumption is *madak*, the history of which is also uncertain. *Madak* seems to be the invention of the poor who could not afford *chando* (in which pure opium is smoked) or who were addicted to opium smoking but who were not such hard smokers as *chandobaz*. *Madak* is also a type of prepared opium for smoking but less dangerous to the nervous system. The preparation is similar, though the paste is more dilute and charred rice or barley husk is mixed with the opium solution until the solution is absorbed and pills can be made of it. These pills are normally smoked in a hubble bubble, though the event witnessed during fieldwork involved a tobacco pipe not a hubble-bubble, apparently to make it appear that they were smoking not *madak* but imported tobacco. The users observed also kept the *madak* pills in the imported tobacco containers to maintain secrecy.

Thirdly, a few individuals, like beggars and mendicants or the poor and disabled, use *dhoda*, the unlanced or lanced dry capsule, ground to a powder and taken with water. In NWFP *dhoda* is a commonly used remedy for complaints such as coughs, diarrhoea, headache, dysentery, asthma and digestive troubles in children; if administered to pregnant women it is said to cause an abortion. Its symptoms and effects are generally milder and less long lasting than those of opium. A few minutes after taking the potion the user feels a sense of relaxation and well-being, and a marvellous change in attitude and behaviour can be observed. From a condition of lethargy, fretfulness, moroseness and peevishness the user passes into one of gaiety and talkativeness. This lasts for 1–2 hours, after which he begins to appear depressed and drowsy, and may indeed fall asleep. In many cases menial workers like *kochwans* (horse-buggy drivers) and *malangs* (mendicants) use *dhoda* both to avoid tiredness and for subsequent sleep. Habitual use of *dhoda* makes the abuser forgetful. He may sit in one place for hours doing nothing, a habit which well suits beggars or, conversely, go throw himself into extended periods of physical work, feeling no strain.

Opium Derivatives

Opium's alkaloids have made it a source of many other products, most significantly heroin. It is this complexity – opium's simultaneous potential for good and harm and its strong attractiveness to users – that explains its importance in the history of medicine, the criminality and corruption associated with it, and its capacity to generate immense wealth. Wherever it has been cultivated it has produced both benefits and dangers – medicinal, economic, ritualistic and, significantly, political, primarily through its use as a source of state finance, a weapon against enemies, and a tool of international terrorism and political blackmail of individuals and nations.

Opium comprises gum (25 per cent), resin (4 per cent), rubber (6 per cent), oils (2 per cent), water (10 per cent), meconic acid (1 per cent), morphine (10–15 per cent), codeine (1–2 per cent), pigments and other extraneous matter (24 per cent). Its seeds contain 50 per cent oil, and some 32 alkaloids have been extracted from it, including narcotine, narcerine, laudanine and papaverine (15 per cent) of which morphine and codeine are the most commonly used. Morphine, opium's major alkaloid, was isolated in 1804, but commercial production began in 1827, gaining popularity in the United States as a self-prescribed medicine during the Civil War and becoming the first source of heroin manufacture in Great Britain. It is so powerful that it is believed that the versatility of opium is largely due to this single constituent's analgesic, anaesthetic, narcotic, stimulant and depressant properties. It can be extracted by a chemical process involving ammonia or directly from the poppy heads and stalk before the poppy goes into the opium stage. Morphine is addictive, causing physical and psychological dependence, but was in the past used therapeutically for pre-surgical anaesthesia and post-surgical analgesia.

Its other major licit use is in conversion into codeine, the second important alkaloid of opium, with up to 90 per cent of licit morphine being converted into this and other anti-tussives.[62] Codeine is less addictive, stimulant and depressant than morphine. It causes no euphoria but stimulates the spinal cord and the lower part of the brain. Small doses are soporific, large doses cause restlessness and increase reflex excitability. Its major illicit use is for conversion into heroin.

In 1874, an English chemist, Wright, accidentally synthesized diacetylmorphine by heating morphine and acetic anhydride, known as AA. The drug was subjected to further experimentation, but after careful analysis and experiments on dogs it was identified as producing such negative somatic effects that further experimentation ceased. In 1890, however, a German chemist, Dankwortt, synthesized diacetyl morphine by heating anhydrous morphine and acetyl chloride, and soon the medical profession accepted the drug as an effective, non-addictive anaesthetic and analgesic, as well as a treatment for morphine addiction (rather as they had previously seen morphine as a treatment for opium addiction). With the approval and encouragement of the medical profession, therefore, the Bayer Pharmaceutical Company started commercial production in Germany in 1898, giving it the market name heroin.

Heroin soon outstripped both penicillin and cortisone in the treatment of respiratory diseases, which, in the cold western world, were major causes of fatality, particularly among the old. Heroin soon came to be regarded as a super drug, demand being stoked by an aggressive campaign promoting it as a 'respiratory, stimulant, sedative, expectorant and analgesic in the treatment of cough, bronchitis, laryngitis, pneumonia, whooping cough, asthma, colds etc.' which dissolved on the tongue.

The USA and Austria declared heroin an official drug in 1906, the American Medical Association (AMA) recommending it as an effective substitute for morphine and codeine. There was, however, a cautionary note even at this stage, the AMA warning that, while safe in small doses, in large doses heroin could induce 'dizziness, nausea, and occasionally constipation and in poisonous amounts, twitching of the extremities, great exhaustion and dimness of vision.' In particular, an overdose 'cripples the body's central nervous system, plunges the victim into a deep coma, and usually produces death within a matter of minutes'.[63] Official support for heroin was short lived, its manufacture and import being outlawed in America in 1924, around the time that, as we shall see in the next section, the League of Nations was beginning its attempts at eradication.

Heroin addiction became a problem in China, where 27 per cent of all male adults were addicted to opium in the early years of the century.[64] The Government had banned opium smoking, and the compulsory registration of opium addicts encouraged users to discover the potency of heroin and morphine instead. This occurred to such an extent that in 1934 the Shanghai Municipal Council reported that heroin consumption had overtaken opium smoking in popularity. Though the Government declared the production and trafficking of heroin a serious crime, political factors were to thwart the anti-drug policy. Chief among these was the outbreak of the Sino-Japanese war in 1937, when Japanese occupying forces were so aggressive in their sales of opium and heroin that some estimates suggested that one in eight of the population of Nanking were being poisoned.[65]

Iran, too, is a traditionally heavy user of opium derivatives. According to US estimates, by 1949 11 per cent of the adult population were addicts, a number outstripped only by China.[66] In 1955, however, the Shah peremptorily banned opium production, causing demand to be met by supplies from Turkey, Afghanistan and Pakistan – a significant early step towards expanding the opium market of the Pak-Afghan cultivators. The lifting of this ban in 1969 was associated with compulsory registration, but few addicts registered, the majority continuing to obtain supplies smuggled from Afghanistan and Pakistan. The World Opium Survey of 1972 reported that the Afridi Pathans of Khyber Agency controlled and dominated the opium trade and traffic in Pakistan. To meet increased demand in Iran, the Afridi either transported their produce through Afghanistan or, through tribal relationships, passed their opium to the Shinwaries (a big tribe across the Afghan border around Landi Kotal, still in Khyber Agency) and the Ghilzais (a nomadic tribe from Afghanistan who travel to the plains in Pakistan during the winter and return in summer) for onward transportation.

As with China, Hong Kong and Laos, in Iran the sequence of prohibition leading to regulation promoted the rise of heroin, which, by 1972, was feeding some 30,000 local opium addicts who had avoided registration. By 1974 Iran was a heroin exporting country, production increasing to an estimated 200–400 metric tons by 1988–9 and the heroin addicted population numbering some two million.[67]

In Pakistan the first step towards heroin manufacture, morphine synthesis, started in the early 1970s, when the Pakistan Council of Scientific and Industrial Research (PCSIR) developed techniques of morphine sulphate synthesis from raw opium cultivated by farmers as well as by various research organizations. In 1972, in spite of the fact that the processing of this alkaloid was illegal, PCSIR Laboratories Peshawar sold the formula for morphine sulphate manufacture to a pharmaceutical company, Sharex, of Sadiqabad in Punjab Province. The Government banned production, and court action followed, and in 1973 the High Court decided in favour of the Government, and processing ceased altogether.

Like previous prohibitions, however, this one drove the technology underground, clandestine manufacture beginning in inaccessible areas such as Swat, Gadoon and Amazai, where opium cultivation was heavily concentrated. The first clandestine morphine sulphate laboratory, owned and operated inside his house by Ataullah Choohan alias Wakeel Sahib, an official of the then Wali-Swat,[68] was unearthed and demolished by the PNCB in Swat in July 1975. The second such laboratory was destroyed in Zulfiqar Garhi, Khyber Agency in 1976, to be followed by six more 'busts' during the next year. The International Narcotic Control Board expressed concern that this would lead to the promotion of local heroin manufacture.

This apprehension proved correct, and the first heroin laboratory, owned by the biggest opium vend contractor in the country, Shahwas Khan, was unearthed by PNCB in Gadoon, Swabi district, in 1978. This laboratory was, however, described as a morphine sulphate manufacturing laboratory as a result of political pressure and corruption. By this time opium production in North West Pakistan was probably over the officially quoted 800 metric tons, since drought conditions had caused production in the Golden Triangle to fall from 600 to 200 tons per annum[69] forcing up prices in Pakistan so that production became financially attractive.

When the PNCB expanded its efforts to locate such laboratories of heroin manufacture, the drug barons moved into the tribal areas in NWFP, which, with their different political and legal status were the safest locations. The first heroin laboratory in a tribal area was established by the Afghan Muhmand tribesman Haji Umar, in Lakarho, Muhmand Agency, in 1978. Haji Umar had a base in the heroin processing Herat province of Afghanistan, and when PNCB officials raided the laboratory Haji made his escape back there.

There is disagreement as to who introduced the technology of synthesising heroin from opium manufacture in the tribal areas. Some attribute the discovery to a nomad from Afghanistan known as a *kochai*, though this was probably Haji Umar himself. The origins of heroin manufacture in Khyber Agency, however, can be more confidently ascribed. Research at Quid-e-Azam University Islamabad reveals that heroin processing in the Gadoon area was first introduced by German chemists,[70] supporting a popular belief in Khyber Agency that this was so.[71] Germans had been entering the area for many years to trade in *hashish*, and had introduced the technology of THC, or *hashish* oil, and later imparted heroin knowledge to local people.

By 1978 brown (No 1) heroin was being manufactured in the area. This is not water-soluble, but smoked over a tin foil with the help of a pipe, *panne* ('chasing the dragon'). The higher grade China White (No 4 and 5) heroin manufacture started in Khyber Agency in 1979. Haji Ghilzai was the first to start, using a clandestine 'bath tub laboratory', but now the business has spread to the industrial centres. The quantity of heroin manufactured in the tribal areas is unknown. The extent of production can, however, be estimated by the number of laboratories detected and destroyed, and their output capacity. In 1982, the US Drug Enforcement Administration reported that 15–20 such laboratories[72] had been demolished. In 1985, the *Daily Telegraph*[73] reported that 47 had been demolished in the first nine months of that year in the tribal areas, of which some 90 per cent were located in Khyber Agency. Each of these had a production capacity of over 50 kg a month, with 65–80 per cent purity for brown, and up to 90 per cent purity for white, heroin powder.

The Hudood Ordinance 1979 was to become, effectively, a licence for heroin. Pakistan's rapidly increasing opium using population provided a considerable heroin market[74] which pushed opium production to far flung areas in the tribal belt. In the late 1970s the introduction of heroin production led to a marked increase in opium cultivation, as the crop offered infinitely the most attractive yield among the few crops that were cultivable on non-irrigable land. Pakistan, therefore, is now a producer, a major transit country and consumer of heroin. Thereafter heroin usage spread rapidly from the 1980s, and by the mid-1990s the number of addicts has been estimated as standing at around 2 million out of a total addicted population of 3.7 million. Interestingly these figures included an increasing proportion of females.

Expansion brought problems of theft, burglary, family violence and trafficking, and in particular the increasing criminal involvement in the trade of politicians and influential people. This involvement helped create a *nouveau riche* class who were to use drug money to pursue personal power, sometimes in the national political arena. The association between drug production and supply and political corruption which this nexus heralds makes finding a solution especially difficult: how does one tackle corruption when members of the legislature and the executive are themselves beneficiaries of this lucrative crime? When there is no recourse to the law making process because that process is itself undermined?

By 1981 Pakistan was a fully-fledged production country, its authorities seizing some 400 kg of indigenous heroin in 1981 against less than 10 kg a year earlier. By the end of 1981 Pakistani heroin accounted for 73 per cent of all heroin seized in Europe, the Mid-East, Africa and Central Asia, including 90 per cent of that seized in the United Kingdom, 56 per cent in the Netherlands and 24 per cent seized in Italy.[75]

Conclusion

We have dealt in this chapter with a number of key features of poppy cultivation, and reviewed the main literature on the history of the poppy and its usage. In terms of early history the main data are archaeological or archaeo-botanical descriptions of fossils and objects, and little is certain about these origins, either globally or in the sub-continent. Subsequently, colonialism left a deep impression on the politics and economy of Pakistan, and it is impossible to understand poppy production today other than in a post-colonial context. Nonetheless it would be wrong to pursue this as a main explanatory framework for current problems in Pakistan. Five of the six historical stages of production identified occurred after independence, and present an interesting political case study, with policies designed first to develop, patronise and extend opium production, and then to control and, ideally, eliminate it.

Analysis can reveal the contemporary significance of ancient tensions. These include tensions between Muslims and Hindus or Pakistan and India; the impact of colonialism in the partition of Bengal; the role of the United Nations and the superpowers. At other times the inferences are there to be drawn, as in the generational transmission of cynicism, exploitation and greed from the former colonial masters to the generation of corrupt officials and politicians familiar in the Pakistan of today. How do we apportion the blame for the human misery associated with poppy production? The former colonial powers, today's leaders of Pakistan and the developed countries which not only permit but, when it suits them, encourage the spread of drugs and the dependence of cultivators on their production all share responsibility; but all are liable to blame each other.

These political questions naturally require political answers, though our more limited aim in this book is to raise the issues and assemble the knowledge necessary for these answers to be provided. This is, therefore, a preliminary and not a definitive study. The history of these matters is not so well documented that we can fillet our discussions so ruthlessly as to omit materials not of demonstrable relevance to our areas of concern, or even broader questions posed for consideration. So some of the history is simply there because we cannot know our topic without it. The fieldwork too was undertaken in such a spirit. The *chandos* session does not necessarily enlighten us about poppy politics, though it is, as it happens, an interesting, though implicit, case study in the social stratification of drug use, as well as an intriguing metaphorical anthropology of death as a transcendental, euphoric moment. It does, however, offer a unique insight into the lives of the people smoking opium by this dangerous method, and is included because we believe the book would be the poorer without it.

Notes

1   C.E. Terry and M. Pellin, *The Opium Problem* (New York: Bureau of Social Hygiene, 1928). p53.

2   V. Berridge and E. Griffith, *The Opium and People* (Harmondsworth: Penguin Books, 1981). p xxiii.

3   G. Watt, *A Dictionary of the Economic Products of India*; Vol VI, Part I (London: W.H. Allen, 1893). p102; see also A.F. Hill, *Economic Botany: A Text Book of Useful Plants and Plants Products* (New York: McGraw Hill, 1937).

4   R.S. Merrillees, 'Opium Trade in the Bronze Age Levant', *Antiquity* Vol. 36, 1962. pp287–92.

5   A.R. Neligan, *The Opium Question with Special Reference to Persia* (London: John Bales Sons and Danielson, 1927). p2.

6   For further elucidation of these points see D.H. Campbell, *The Evolution of Land Plants,* (Stanford, CA: Stanford University Press, 1939); M.M. David, *Cultural Geography of Opium: Its Cultivation and Spread through the Bronze Age* (Ph.D. Thesis. Hawaii: University of Hawaii, 1979); and F.E. Zeuner, *Cultivation of Plants: A History, 1.* (Oxford: Oxford University Press, 1954).

7   Watt, *op. cit.* p150.

8   K. Babar, 'Pakistan's Narcotics Problem'. *Journal of Rural Development and Administration*, XXI, 4 (Peshawar: Pakistan Academy for Rural Development, October–December 1989). p119.

9   J. Hutchinson, *Families of Flowering Plants. Vol. I: Dicotyledons Arranged According to a New System Based on the Probable Phylogeny* (Oxford: The Clarendon Press, 1959). pp422–3.

10   C. L. Porter, *Taxonomy of Flowering Plants* (Englewood Cliffs, NJ: Prentice Hall, 1967). p267.

11   E. Core, *Plant Taxonomy* (Englewood Cliffs, NJ: Prentice Hall, 1955). p320.

12   N.I. Mian *et al.*, *Causes, Effects and Remedies of Poppy Cultivation in Swabi-Gadoon Areas: A Survey of Opium Cultivation* Volume II (Peshawar: University of Peshawar, 1979). pp12–20.

13   S.A. Cheema, 'Implications of Growing Alternative Crops For Poppy in the Northern Region of Pakistan' in Anwar-ul-Haq and Umar Farooq (eds) *Drug Addiction and Rehabilitation of Addicts in Pakistan*, (Faisalabad: Agriculture University, 1979). pp134–5.

14   T.J. Adden, *The Distribution of Opium Cultivation and the Trade in Opium* (Haarlem: Joh. Enschede En Zonen, 1939). p5.

15　D. Owen, *British Opium Policy in China and India* (New Haven: Yale University Press 1934). p2.

16　M. C. Sharma, 'History of Narcotics Control in India', in M. Desai, H. S. Sethi *et al.* (eds) *Current Research in Drug Abuse in India* (New Delhi, 1981). p274.

17　*Ibid.*

18　Government of Great Britain. *The First Report of the Royal Commission on Opium 1893–4.* Appendix II (London: Eyre and Spottiswoode, 1894). p148; Watt, *op. cit.* 102–5; United Nations, *Piami*. Vol. 6 (Karachi: UNESCO/Hamdard Foundation, 1982). p2; seminar paper by G. Sonnedecker, 'Emergence and Concept of Addiction Problem', in *Proceedings of the Symposium on History of Narcotics and Drug Addiction Problem* (Mar Bathesda, 1962). p16; G.H.M. Batten, 'The Society of Arts'. In *The First Report of the Royal Commission on Opium 1893–4 with Minutes of Evidence, op. cit.* p144; D. E. Miller, *Licit Narcotics Production and its Ramifications for Foreign Policy,* US State Department, 1980). p5; R.H. Blummer, *Drugs, I: Society and Drugs* (San Francisco, CA: Jossey-Bass, 1974). p100; D.T. Machete, 'The History of Opium and some of its Preparations and Alkaloids'. *Journal of American Medical Association,* 6 February 1915, cited in Terry and Pellin, *op. cit.* 5); A.F. Hill, *Economic Botany: A Text Book of Useful Plants and Plant Products* (New York: McGraw Hill, 1937). p290; and J. Rowntree, *The Imperial Drug Trade* (London: Methuen, 1905). p116.

19　Sharma, *op. cit.* 274–83; see also C.P. Spencer and V. Navarathnam, *Drug Abuse in South East Asia* (Kuala Lumpur: Oxford University Press, 1981). p10.

20　S.C. Dwarkanath, 'The Use of Opium and Cannabis in the Traditional System of Medicines in India', in *UN Bulletin on Narcotics* (New York, 1965). 17, 1. pp15–19; R.N. Chopra and I.C. Chopra, *Drug Addiction with Special Reference to India* (New Delhi: Indian Council of Scientific and Industrial Research, 1965). p184; U.O. Dutt, 'Materia Medica Sanskrit', in Watt, *op. cit.* p150.

21　Miller, *op. cit.* 5.

22　Sharma, *op. cit.* pp274–5.

23　Government of Pakistan, *Resource and Reference Manual for Prevention Resource Consultant Network.* Vol. I (Islamabad: Drug Abuse Prevention Resource Centre 1990). p4.

24　Interview with Khan Sultan Khan of Tangi, 22 May 1997.

25　P.G. Kritikos and S.P. Papadaki, 'The History of the Poppy and of Opium and their Expansion in Antiquity in the Eastern Mediterranean Area', in *UN Bulletin on Narcotics.* XIX, 3 (New York, 1967). p38.

26　I.H. Qureshi, (ed.) *A Short History of Pakistan* (Karachi: University of Karachi, 1987). p91.

27　D. Buddenberg, *Illicit Drug Use in Afghanistan and Pakistan* (Islamabad United Nations Drug Control Programme, 1992). p1 and p275. See also Government of Pakistan, *Resource and Reference Manual for Prevention Resource Consultant Network* (Islamabad: Drug Abuse Prevention Resource Centre, 1990). p5; Spencer and Navarathnam, *op. cit.* p10.

28　Blummer, *op. cit.* p47. See also Chopra and Chopra, *op. cit.* p182.

29　Government of Pakistan, *op. cit.* 5.

30　D. Buddenberg, *op. cit.* p1992.

31　D.E. Owen, *op. cit.* pp3–10.

32　J. Stratchey, *India: Its Administration and Progress* (London: Macmillan, 1903). pp133–42.

33　A.W. McCoy, *The Politics of Heroin: CIA Complicity in the Global Drug Trade* (New York: Harper and Row, 1994). p81

34 R. Stevenson, *Winning the War on Drugs: to Legalize or Not?* Hobart Paper 124. (London: Institute of Economic Affairs, 1994). p76; US Department of Commerce, Statistical Abstract 1915. p713 (Cited in A. W. McCoy, 1994 *op. cit.* 88).
35 A. Jamieson, *Global Drug Trafficking. Conflict Studies* 234 (London: Research Institute for the Study of Conflict and Terrorism, 1990). p2.
36 A. Masood, *Esi Bulandi Esi Pasti* (Rawalpendi: Ahsan Publishing House, 1981). p19.
37 Stevenson, *op. cit.* p75. Also see McCoy, *op. cit.* p86
38 Buddenberg, *op. cit.* pp12–13
39 *Ibid.*
40 R. Stevenson, *Winning the War on Drugs: to Legalize or Not?* Hobart Paper 124. (London: Institute of Economic Affairs, 1994). p76.
41 Buddenberg, *op. cit.* p11.
42 Government of Great Britain, *First Report of the Royal Commission on Opium with Minutes of Evidence and Appendices* (London: Eyre and Spottiswoode, 1893–4). p349.
43 United Nations,1991, *op. cit.* p6.
44 Spencer and Navarathnam, 1981, *op. cit.* p60.
45 Chopra and Chopra, 1965 *op. cit.* pp184–88.
46 M. Imran and T.B. Uppal, 'Opium Administration to Infants in Peshawar Region of Pakistan'. *UN Bulletin on Narcotics*, XXXI, 3 and 4 (1979). pp69–75.
47 Interview with Sardar Sajjad Hussain Zahid, 16 December 1996.
48 Extracted from Opium Officer Peshawar and Tehsildar Swabi Office Records.
49 Government of the United States of America. *The World Opium Situation* (Washington DC: Bureau of Narcotics and Dangerous Drugs, 1970). p10.
50 Government of Pakistan, *Narcotics Production Report 1987* (Islamabad: Narcotics Control Board/UNFDAC, 1987). p3.
51 McCoy, 1994, *op. cit.* p447.
52 R.A.K. Sahib Zada, Poppy Cultivation in North West Frontier Province (NWFP): Its Present, Past and Future. (Islamabad: Department of Agriculture and Rural Development, 1991). p6.
53 Government of Pakistan. *The Gazette of Pakistan: Extra Ordinary: Ordinance No XLVI of 18 April 1995.* Ch. II, Prohibition and Punishment Section 4 (Islamabad: Ministry of Law, Justice and Parliamentary Affairs, 18 April 1995). p2.
54 A.D. Wright, 'The History of Opium Transaction'. *Studies of the Royal College of Physicians of Philadelphia*, 29, 1, 1969. pp22–7.
55 V. Berridge and E. Griffith, *Opium and the People* (Harmondsworth: Penguin Books, 1981). p xxii.
56 Terry and Pellin, *op.cit.* 1928. p53.
57 D. Bingham, *Opium Addiction in Chicago* (Montclair, N.J.: Smith Paterson, 1970). pp18–19.
58 R.S. Merrillees, 'Opium Trade in the Bronze Age Levant' (*Antiquity* XXXVII, 1962). p287.
59 Berridge and Edwards, *op. cit.* p xxiii.
60 V. Seaman, 'On Opium'. M.D. Thesis (Philadelphia, 1792). Cited in Terry and Pellin, *op. cit.* pp59–60.
61 K. Elahi, 'A Profile of Drug Abuse and Addiction in Pakistan'. Paper read at the International Narcotics Conference, Quetta, Pakistan, 8–10 August 1982. *Conference Proceedings,* pp11–12.
62 Chopra and Chopra, *op. cit.* pp26–7.
63 McCoy, 1972. *op.cit.* p7
64 R.D. Ranara, *Socio-Economic and Political Impacts of Production, Trade and Use of Narcotic Drugs in Burma* (Geneva: United Nations Research Institute For Social Development, 1992). p24.

65 S.K. Ghosh, *The Traffic in Narcotics and Drug Addiction* (Delhi: Ashis Publishing House, 1987).
66 McCoy, 1994, *op. cit.* p443.
67 Jamieson, *op. cit.* p11.
68 Interview with Rahim Shah Khan (Lala) of village Garhi, District Swat. He reported that this man came from Punjab and was an official of the Bacha Sahib (The First Wali-Swat) and then became private secretary to Mian Gul Jehanzeb, the second and last Wali-swat. According to Rahim Shah Khan, the children of this man are now among the biggest industrialists in the country.
69 Government of Pakistan, 1990, *op. cit.* p21
70 M. Asif, 'Heroin Addiction in Rural Society' (Islamabad: Quaid-e-Azam University, 1985). p49.
71 Interviews with Hakim Khan Afridi (Assistant Director Social Welfare Department, Government of North West Frontier Province) 8.5.97 and with Khalid Khan Shinwari, on 16.3.97. Hakim Khan is the nephew of the late Chief of Kokikhel, Wali Khan, whose house and village were bombarded by Government forces in 1984 on charges of running a heroin laboratory in the village. Khalid Khan is a dealer in auto-tyres who, before the Afghan war, was doing business in Kabul and Jalalabad. He has also been personal secretary to the drug baron Haji Ayub Afridi, who was subsequently extradited to USA and imprisoned for five years and fined $100,000. The first author is grateful to Kokikhel and Shinwari for their detailed and frank discussion about drug manufacture in the area.
72 US Drug Enforcement Administration Report 1982. Cited in Government of Pakistan, 1990, *op. cit.* p21.
73 *Daily Telegraph* (London: 5 October 1985).
74 United Nations, 1994, *op. cit.* p1.
75 Government of Pakistan, 1990, *op. cit.* p23.

Chapter III

The Politics of Drugs in Pakistan

The politics of drug production in Pakistan has both internal and external dimensions. Internal factors include the divergent administrative systems in North West Frontier Province, arguably a main cause of drug production there, the role of politicians and political parties, and narco-politics, as a result of which laws are corruptly flouted by those who make and administer them. External factors include the Soviet invasion of Afghanistan and the unending civil war there, which was originally in good part financed by narcotics with the support of the western powers, and the Iranian revolution.

Internal Factors

1 Divergent Administrative Systems in NWFP

NWFP has a divergent administrative structure. Originally part of the Punjab during the British Raj, the present Province was created in 1901 as a result of political problems stemming from its 1200-mile border with Afghanistan and the freedom loving nature of its inhabitants. Three distinct administrative systems were put in place. These were the *settled administration*, comprising the conquered areas, the *tribal areas* outside British control, and the former *aristocratic states* of Dir, Swat, and Chitra (now Malakand Division), whose rulers received annual subventions from Britain in return for loyalty to the Crown.

   The laws of British India were applicable to the settled administration, with the Frontier Crimes Regulations (FCR), widely known as the black law and still in force today, applicable to the tribal areas. Tribal areas were divided into Agencies, subject to no formal laws and under a political agent with wide discretionary powers to represent the British interest. This duality was preserved under the Act of India 1935, when the Provincial Governor was given dual responsibility as constitutional Head of the Province in the settled districts and agent to the Viceroy/Governor General (now to the President of the Islamic Republic of Pakistan) in the tribal areas. The administrative structure of these seven areas, now, with the exception of Malakand Division which is a Provincially Administered Tribal Area or PATA, called Federally Administered Tribal Areas (FATAs), remains substantially unchanged. Until 1993–94 the Agencies were a Federal responsibility, subject to only those state criminal laws prescribed by the President himself. Hence, Article 247 section 3 of the Constitution affirms that:

> No Act of Parliament shall apply to any Federally Administered Tribal Areas or to any part thereof unless the President so directs, and no Act of Parliament or a Provincial assembly

> shall apply to a Provincially Administered Tribal Area or any part thereof unless the Governor of the Province in which the Tribal area is situated, with the approval of the President, so directs.

and section 7 that:

> Neither the Supreme Court nor a High Court shall exercise any jurisdiction under the constitution in relation to a Tribal Area unless Parliament by law otherwise provides.[1]

In 1993–4, following an uprising among the tribal peoples demanding Islamic Sharia as a panacea for their problems with the corrupt central administration, the administration of PATAs was transferred to the Provincial Government. Legal matters in the tribal areas are for the most part settled by unwritten customary laws, *pukhtoon wali*, administered in FATAs through a network of trusted *maliks* linked to the political agent, who effectively run affairs on the basis of treaties with the administration.

This complexity and tenuous character of Government control do not permit a uniform approach to narcotics. These warlike areas[2] have guarded their freedom for over a century, and armed intervention, which would be costly in money and lives, could not be successfully undertaken without heavy US military support.[3] Blood was shed in 1986 in Gadoon Amazai, where many opium cultivators were killed by law enforcers; and in 1989 NWFP's Inspector General of Police observed ruefully 'It's very difficult fiddling around with the tribes – the British and the Russians found that out to their cost'.[4] In addition, until 1979 the laws regulating opium production were more than 150 years old. The Hudood Ordinance of that year, according to a senior official in the Ministry of Narcotics 'penalised everything from production and possession to transportation and conversion, but planting of opium poppies did not fall under it.[5] This point was initially unclear, however, and the Ordinance was widely used to control poppy cultivation until 1995, when a presidential ordinance brought poppy cultivation under state law.[6]

Under such conditions the Government could only fulfil its international obligations at the cost of its own people. Government attempts to be seen to be accelerating efforts to suppress opium production has brought income in the shape of foreign aid, but heroin production is such a source of corruption, and so easily secured by exploiting Afghan opium, that such attempts seem likely to continue to be ineffective.

2 The Party System

In addition to the fact that, in Pakistan, drugs are produced in areas where Government control is limited or non-existent, and where fierce local communities depend on the income, the political party system also supports drug production. It is scarcely too cynical to say that every Opposition party criticizes the ruling party's drug policies and supports growers and producers, but only until it acquires power. Conversely, a Government party may try to eradicate poppies, but only until it enters Opposition. Though Pakistan has more than 50 political parties, there are only four in the drugs producing areas – the Awami National Party (ANP), the Pakistan

People's Party (PPP), the Pakistan Muslim League (PML), and Jamaat-e-Islami (JI). All these parties have supported drug production at different times; indeed one official said 'No one can win elections in the area without the poppy farmers' support'.[7]

Like all political parties in the area, ANP, a party seldom in government but known for pleading ethnic politics for Pashtu speakers, has the slogan *khpala khawra khpal* 'our land, our choice'. This has brought it strong support in the poppy growing areas, particularly Dir, where previously it had a very limited foothold. Commenting on Government policies regarding narcotics production in the area, ANP Leader Khan Abdul Wali Khan has said:

> We tell the farmers that unless the government comes to an honourable agreement it is their right to grow poppy. No such decision could be made without reference to Kabul. Approval from Kabul is required under international treaty. . . There is nothing wrong in growing opium but it is wrong to refine it into heroin. The raw material is not harmful. It has been eaten for many years.[8]

Locally, no politician of any party can afford to upset poppy farmers, and even MPs from districts not directly involved with narcotics are sometimes obligated to the Deputy Commissioner and project officials.[9] More significantly, in Sultan Khel and Painda Khel areas, where opium is cultivated to the maximum, there is widespread support for the Jamaat-e-Islami, a religio-political party whose candidates and members in the provincial assembly are themselves cultivators, opposing any ban on religious grounds. In 1995 a former JI member of the Provincial Assembly[10] led a march both against the ban and against senior officials' misuse of the Narcotics Fund. In 1997 another distributed poppy seeds free of charge.[11] Another JI activist said:

> None of the crops fetch even one-third the price of what we receive from poppy. How can the US ask us to stop poppy cultivation? Have we ever asked them not to produce guns, tanks and bombs, which also kill people? We prefer to die fighting, rather than to die from hunger.[12]

During the 1997 election campaign, which took place during the poppy seasons, the Government sprayed herbicide on a few standing poppy crop fields in Usherai Dara, part of Sultan Khel, during the night, causing local people to block the main road and stone official vehicles the following day. The ruling party candidate quickly opened negotiations with the Deputy Commissioner, and finally the officials were accused of interfering with the election campaign of the Pakistan Muslim League and threatened with dire consequences. The matter was resolved, and the rest of the crop harvested.[13]

3 Causes of the Narcotics Boom

It is widely accepted that three main events led to the present narcotics boom in Pakistan: General Zia's Hudood Ordinance, the Soviet intervention in Afghanistan and the Iranian revolution, though there is less agreement as to which was the prime cause. CIA reports point to the Iranian revolution, but inside as well as outside

Pakistan opinion is divided, some experts favouring the Afghanistan-Soviet war others the Hudood Ordinance.[14] In our view internal laws, particularly the Hudood Ordinance, and the Afghanistan problem are interrelated. The Iranian factor, though less relevant to drug production in particular, has been of wider general political significance, and may have impacted indirectly on drug production and supply. Further, sectarian terrorism between the Iranian backed Tahrik-e-Jafaria Pakistan (TJP), Shia, and the Saudi Arabian and Kuwaiti backed Sipah-i-Sahaba (Sunni) groups,[15] involving an annual toll of 1,000 lives in the Punjab alone, inevitably contributes to the political instability so nurturing of drug production and supply.

In our view the ill-timed and ill-planned Hudood Ordinance[16] promulgated on 10 February 1979, was the main cause of Pakistan's drug problem. The Ordinance was possibly enforced under US pressure, though this has yet to be established definitively, some believing it was imposed by Pakistan's rulers to affect a monopoly of the drugs trade. Certainly, after the Ordinance the drug trade came to be confined to a few hands at the helms of affairs and their accomplices. On the other hand superpower pressure and responsibility are, truthfully or not, held responsible by General Zia himself in his assertion that his Government 'did not harbour the scourge of drug trafficking and so it was not his problem. It was America's doing and she should handle it'.[17]

Drug development has three dimensions: financing, logistics and political patronage.[18] In Pakistan, all three have been and still are readily available. The existence of bureaucratic and political patronage, the logistical support of the CIA and the National Logistic Cell (NLC) of the Pakistan Army during the Afghan war, and the money laundering of Pakistani and foreign banks, of which the most notorious was the Bank of Credit and Commerce International (BCCI), are well attested.[19] Describing the *modus operandi* of the NLC, McCoy quotes a monthly magazine *The Herald of Pakistan* of September 1985 which claims that NLC trucks, '. . . arriving with CIA arms from Karachi often returned loaded with heroin protected by ISI papers from police search. . . they come from Peshawar to Pepri, Jungshahi, Jhimpir where they deliver their cargo, sacks of grains, to government godowns. Some of these sacks contain packets of heroin. This has been going on now for about three and a half years'.[20]

4   Some Problems with the Statistics of Addiction

The best available figures purport to show that Pakistan had 3,005,649 drug addicts in 1993, of whom 50.7 per cent, or 1,524,000, used heroin.[21] By mid-1997 the number of drug addicts had risen to about 3.7 million, of whom some 2 million were heroin addicts. Cautiously assuming an annual increase of 7 per cent[22] and a static relationship between the numbers of opium and heroin users, by mid-2001 the addicted population would total 5.7 million,[23] including over 2.5 million heroin addicts.

The National Drug Abuse Survey of 1986 reported an average daily consumption of 0.9 grams of heroin per addict.[24] Combining the two reports, it can be calculated that, in the mid-1990s, the total daily consumption of heroin in Pakistan was around 2,250 kg. In terms of opium equivalent, 1 kg of heroin is made out of 10 kg of raw opium, so Pakistani heroin addicts were consuming 22,500 kg of raw opium daily, or almost 8.21 million kg (8212.5 metric tons) annually. This is in addition to the amount consumed by 315,000 opium addicts, each of whom, on average, was consuming 1.3 grams a day, or 150 metric tons annually.[25]

These are remarkable figures given that Pakistan produces only about up to 120 metric tons against Afghanistan's 2500 metric tons. And since UNDCP reports suggest that in 1999 only 578 metric tons of heroin were manufactured from 5780 metric tons of raw opium[26] Pakistanis appear to consume more opium than the total world production. So what is going on? In fact the figures are obviously exaggerated, and for three possible reasons.

Exaggerating consumption by officials who attract more foreign aid, a good part of which goes into overseas numbered bank accounts.

Underestimating production by the administrative authorities of the opium producing areas. None of the opium producing areas have been measured precisely, so we do not know exactly how much land is cultivated with opium. The concerned administration, in order to show their efficiency, might submit low figures: in addition, as none of them ever bothers (or dares) to visit these areas they must depend upon local informants or community elders, who may give biased estimates or fail to understand the measuring units. The main reason for any local understatement, however, is corruption. Almost certainly many deputy commissioners and political agents in charge of development projects financed by foreign governments embezzle large sums, submitting low figures and selling the hidden surplus privately. Similarly at least some NGOs are headed or owned by political figures who, to secure more grants-in-aid, give false area based addiction figures, which then form a basis of national statistics.

Defective survey methodology There are a number of technical problems that vitiate the value of much of the survey work undertaken, though this is not the place to detail them at length. In particular, however, National Drug Abuse Surveys in Pakistan employ snowball sampling, which dispenses with a sampling frame, using known respondents to identify unknown ones, 'obtaining a sample by having initially identified subjects who can refer you to other subjects with like or similar characteristics'.[27] Parker, Bakx and Newcombe used snowballing to establish the number of unknown drug addicts in USA, and they detail a number of quite fundamental problems with the approach. These include biases in the knowledge of known users, the uncertain ratio of known to unknown users, the size of the total heroin user population, the questionable generalizability of data established by this means, the problem of double counting and the impact on reliability of researchers depending and relying on personal relationships with users.[28]

5 Corruption

Pakistan is a post-colonial, overdeveloped bureaucratic state, where economic and political institutions are weak but bureaucrats strong, and where state and society are far apart. Normally the social and economic position of bureaucrats is lower middle or middle class, though their aspirations are considerably higher, and many rely for upward mobility on exploiting their position to take kickbacks in contract procurement and other forms of corruption.[29] Institutions responsible for eliminating drugs are among those that offer the most lucrative postings, and these are normally sold to the highest bidder by federal ministers/Secretaries. Naturally an employee who has spent a hefty sum to secure employment will have to earn sufficient to pay this off before his investment becomes profitable. It follows that, on the Indian sub-continent as well as among other newly developing and less developed countries, it is widely accepted that a predatory rather than public service approach to bureaucratic duties is unavoidable.[30]

Pakistani politics have traditionally been dominated by landed aristocracy and feudal lords. By the 1960s, the urban commercial and industrial class had entered the political scene, but in the 1980s, a new class entered politics, with few political aims other than accumulating wealth and political power. This class emerged under the patronage of strong leaders with dictatorial tendencies, and continues to affect contemporary politics. Drug money has increasingly come to play an important role in these politics, financing political parties irrespective of changes of government or leadership, and capable of destabilizing Government when business is threatened. Many of those concerned are elite figures, including politicians, industrialists, sportsmen, businessmen, army officers, publishing magnates and philanthropists. Unsurprisingly in such an atmosphere, febrile political rumour and gossip among both educated and uneducated classes is ubiquitous.

Widely suspected, rightly or wrongly, of being one such by being involved in heroin smuggling in his official plane[31] was General Zia-ul-Haq himself, then Martial Law Administrator and President of Pakistan. In 1983, when Raza Qureshi was arrested in possession of heroin at Oslo Airport, he named Hamid Hasnain, zonal chief of the Habib Bank and the person handling General Zia's family accounts[32] and two others as leaders of a heroin smuggling cartel. Under diplomatic pressure from Norway he was arrested, and, when sentenced to 15 years imprisonment and a heavy fine by the Federal Shariat Court in 1989, his solicitor claimed he had been made a scapegoat for the misdeeds of more powerful others. Similarly General Zia's close friend, and Governor NWFP, (late) General Fazal Haq, patron of such anti-narcotics NGOs as the Green December Movement Peshawar, is alleged by many[33] to be actively involved in the business, raiding his rivals' heroin factories to secure a monopoly.[34]

The election to the National Assembly of Salim Khan, an unemployed law graduate with a poor family background from Peshawar, is believed by many to be attributable to support from drug interests such as that of Seth Saifullah, a drug dealer arrested in Karachi. Similarly, Haji Ayub Afridi, a heroin manufacturer and drug dealer subsequently imprisoned in the United States, was elected to the National Assembly in 1990, after which, in spite of being under suspicion by law enforcement agencies, he had immunity from arrest as a Member of Parliament.[35]

Most if not all governments, civil as well as military, are widely believed to have been the beneficiaries of drug money. Benazir Bhutto, who is popular in the west, announced a war against drugs, repeatedly claiming that drug money was being used to destabilize her Government. But to many of her detractors this was mere propaganda. Allegations were widely circulating concerning her foreign minister and a former minister of narcotics, who had allegedly smuggled 400 kg of narcotics in rice bags from his rice mills in Pakistan. These suspicions extended to Benazir's own husband, Asif Ali Zardari, also a minister in her Cabinet, who, according to evidence from undercover operations, used the Prime Minister's residence as a base from which to sell drugs to western traders and others.[36]

A defendant in a drug trial, Haji Iqbal Baig, claimed to have financed the 1985 election of Prime Minister Nawaz Sharif, and the 1988 election campaigns of at least five PPP candidates who went on to become ministers. He further claimed that his surrender was negotiated by the Speaker of the National Assembly and the Prime Minister, Meraj Khalid.[37] A 1992 CIA report was reported as listing Nawaz Sharif, President Ghulam Ishaq Khan, his personal secretary and a senior civil servant, then a minister, Roidad Khan, four National Assembly members from Khyber Agency and the Baluchistan representatives as beneficiaries. The same report claimed that the campaign of Nawaz's Islami Jamhori Ittehad Party was financed by drug money, used specifically by Nawaz to buy the loyalty of the military.[38]

A more recent entrant to the political scene has been the former cricketer Imran Khan, head of the Pakistan Justice Movement (Pakistan Tehrik-e-Insaf or PTI), under a political slogan proclaiming social justice for the Pakistani people and the punishment of those who amassed wealth unethically. Surrounding Imran there are many confusions and controversies. Many ordinary Pakistanis believe his late British father-in-law's wealth combined with his own fame have been – and will be – sufficient to help him in Pakistani politics, where success is unattainable without wealth. On the other hand it has been very strongly alleged that Imran was himself financed by the drug Mafia and traffickers in northern Punjab,[39] while others still believe he is a political plant, placed in politics by the Pakistani intelligence agencies.

But whatever the details of individual cases it is beyond dispute that drug money fuels the political system. A list of drug barons issued by the Benazir Bhutto's Pakistan People Party (PPP) contains 353 civil and military personnel. These include an air chief, colonels and brigadiers, a president, prime ministers, governors and chief ministers of NWFP, ministers and MPs, bankers, owners of influential newspapers, leading political families, and heads of intelligence and law enforcing agencies including the Head of the Anti-Narcotics Force itself.[40] While this kind of list is clearly attractive as political propaganda, its publication indicates the gravity of the situation. When power elites are involved, a political solution is inevitably elusive: corruption becomes the norm, and the norm filters down to every social stratum.

Money laundering is another aspect of narco-politics. In 1993 the Government declared a *jihad* – holy war – against drugs, saying that their production, processing and trafficking posed a national threat of immense proportions. Five weeks later the Industrial Development Bank of Pakistan publicly invited citizens to open foreign currency accounts or 'step-in with 100,000 rupees and allow the bank to do the rest', prospective depositors being assured that 'no question will be asked by any authority about the source of acquisition of Foreign Exchange'.[41] Subsequently advertisements have appeared which effectively invite narco-barons to invest in various sectors, particularly property, as, because of widespread corruption in Pakistan's Land Revenue and Registry System, no proper documentation of sale and purchase is needed and transactions can be conducted under different names. Many also believe the Government's privatization programme is designed to launder narco-money and bring it under Government control. The army is similarly suspected of involvement, as is the Intelligence Branch (ISI), which conspired with the CIA to deploy drugs as a weapon against Soviet forces in Afghanistan in the 1980s. There have also been reports of major heroin syndicates inside the Pakistan army itself. In June 1986, for example, Pakistan police arrested an army major driving from Peshawar to Karachi with 220 kg of heroin. Two months later police arrested an air force lieutenant carrying an identical amount – an indication, perhaps, of a tidy military mind organizing uniform deliveries. Before the two could be interrogated both escaped from custody under what Pakistan's Defence Journal called 'mystifying circumstances'.[42] This political involvement has had many repercussions, particularly economic, on Pakistan society. Experts believe the drug trade penetrates every aspect of the economy, and though it is not measurable directly, the indicators most liable to be affected are 'inflation, money supply, interest rates, traditional contrabands, foreign exchange reserves, black market currency, property value, wages and the cost of goods and services'.[43] While some forms of petty corruption are culturally comprehensible in Pakistan, where it is not considered shameful to give or receive bribes and kickbacks in spite of legal and religious laws which may prohibit them, cultural analyses of this kind offer an insufficient and superficial picture of the situation as a whole. A CIA report analysed it thus:

> Pakistan is at a stage in its development wherein corruption is simply the norm. Those who have any kind of influence or access to the corridors of political powers flout the laws of the land with impunity. . . . the country's elite leaders, politicians, industrialists, generals, bankers, landlords with few exceptions use their positions to enrich themselves, their families, their relatives . . . jobs in the country's bureaucracy are literally purchased: those moving up or laterally to more lucrative position buy it from those above. And, if the highest bidder lacks the capacity to honour his bid right away, he simply takes the money out of the salaries of those below him.[44]

In June 1996 the Anti-Narcotics Force (ANF) seized two tons of heroin, the biggest seizure in the country's history, in Baluchistan, and invited foreign diplomats to watch its destruction and analyse the haul. But, according to the *Times*, 'with that Pakistan's credibility also went up in flames'[45] since, according to US analysts who denounced the drama as a hoax, the ashes contained only traces of heroin. It is not difficult to detect what happened to the heroin. Nearly every month a Pakistani is executed in Saudi Arabia for drug smuggling, and how they manage to carry the drugs can possibly be understood from the claim of a smuggler that he was helped by an FIA (Federal Police) officer to board a Copenhagen-bound flight with a false passport. He was arrested on the German border with 1.5 kg of heroin, and sentenced to five years imprisonment.[46] Drug power, therefore, has come to infect the body politic of Pakistan. Heroin trafficking, one of the many scourges gifted to Pakistan by the Afghan *jihad*, is now a fully-fledged industry[47] which has spawned drug barons with such enormous fortunes as to render them effectively above the law. As a result, narco-barons have now infiltrated a number of social and political elites, including those offering them access to the highest offices in the land. Narco-money funds political parties, finances election campaigns and vote buying, and purchases the favour of the generals who frequently determine which politicians remain in power and which fall from grace.

Of all these indicators, the devaluation of the currency and the existence of a black economy have been the most dramatic. During the first ten months of 1997 the Nawaz Government devalued six times, and the Finance Minister admitted to the Senate that a black economy to the tune of 1,500–2,000 billion rupees existed.[48] Inevitably this encouraged currency speculation and a flight from the rupee, and widespread political and bureaucratic rent-seeking[49] followed, inhibiting long-term investment in the industrial sector and encouraging officials to offer incentives to foreign investors on terms favourable to themselves rather than to the national economy.

The Prime Minister claimed in 1997 to have washed away the label of 'the most corrupt country in the world' from the face of Pakistan, claiming 'Pakistan is now number 5 in corruption in the world'.[50] It would still, however, be difficult to overstate the significance of institutionalized corruption in any study of drug production and supply in Pakistan. To suggest, as some have, that corruption brings economic benefits[51] could scarcely be more wrong, and more recent evidence shows that in addition to upsetting markets it does fundamental corrosive damage:

> The effects of corruption are especially disruptive in democracies: by attacking some of the basic principles on which democracy rests. . . corruption contributes to the delegitimation of the political and institutional systems in which it takes root. It is for this reason that political corruption is rightly a central focus of concern in contemporary democracies.[52]

Particularly in countries such as Pakistan, in the absence of transparent procurement procedures corruption damages inward investment by reputable international corporations. The market imperfections created by rent-seeking entail investing in unproductive political capital rather than in economically or socially productive public goods. They reduce the volume of international trade, and, by leaving the door open for less fastidious companies to provide inferior services at high prices, diminish the possibility of such countries forging mature trading relationships of longer term collective benefit. So whatever benefits may accrue to the corrupt parties themselves, the process of diverting policy objectives away from the public and towards the private good creates a major impediment to free trade, creating hidden costs for the countries concerned.

External Factors

1 The Iranian Revolution

Iran, which has been producing opium for centuries, has a large addicted population whose need is satisfied by heroin from neighbouring countries. Iran thus serves as a market for heroin manufactured in the region, a transit country for opium to Turkey and elsewhere and as an opium producer. Like Pakistan Iran has tribal areas (including Irani Baluchistan and Kurdish territory) where opium is cultivated, but its magnitude has not been widely reported since the 1979 Revolution. Given the number of users and the corruptibility of law enforcers, however, there is a strong likelihood of heroin processing occurring on a substantial scale in the remote border areas with Pakistan and Afghanistan.

The western media believe, as do many Pakistani experts,[53] that the Iranian Revolution was a significant cause of drug development in Pakistan. Though opinion differs as to detail, there is broad agreement that the strict anti-narcotics laws that followed the toppling of the Shah contributed to the problem. Certainly in the year following the Revolution opium production increased, but, after the country had stabilized, the Government ordered the persecution of traffickers.

As a result, the Mafia in Iran left the country, some coming to Baluchistan to establish their business there. They also introduced Pakistani smugglers, who had previously sold opium solely or mainly to Iranians, to the international market. When Iranian experts came to Pakistan they not only established heroin laboratories and made advance payments to farmers in Helmad Province, Afghanistan, but were already familiar with the international Mafia. The contribution of the Revolution to drug production in Pakistan was certainly not minimal, therefore, but while it impacted most directly on Baluchistan it had less impact on NWFP's tribal areas. The migration of Iranian drug barons, however, contributed to the internationalization of Pakistan's production and to its increasing involvement in organized distribution networks.

2 The Afghan-Soviet War

Afghanistan is the second most important factor in drug development in Pakistan after the Hudood Ordinance. Afghanistan's impact on the drug situation in Pakistan can be divided into three stages: 1978–1979, 1980–1989, and 1989 to the present.

The impact of the *first stage* of the Afghan crisis on the drug situation in Pakistan began immediately after the pro-Communist coup which, in April 1978, toppled the kingship and Sardar Daud Khan's Government, replacing the latter with a pro-Moscow regime. In the same year the US ambassador was killed in dubious circumstances. The Americans were watching the situation carefully, and created and sustained anti-Communist insurgence groups inside Afghanistan, masterminded from Peshawar. The Americans knew the strategic importance of Pakistan for anti-Soviet activities and were creating financial resources for the long expected anti-Communist war. In April 1979, events began when CIA and Afghan resistance groups started working together, eight months before Soviet troops entered Afghanistan.

Afghanistan had been an opium producer from time immemorial, exporting raw opium to what is now Pakistan for both medicinal and recreational use. When opium production began in Pakistan's non-tribal areas following the 1953 UN Protocol, Iran quickly became Pakistan's main market, with a 1955 ban fuelling demand, until 1969, when the Iranian Government again permitted opium production. This new crop was largely destined for Turkey and other western countries for processing into heroin; accordingly Pakistani and Afghani cultivators were encouraged to increase production. Following the 1978 coup, internal unrest, disorganization and a blockade of the traditional opium smuggling route led to a fall in production, while the Hudood Ordinance was disrupting business in Pakistan. In response to this market disequilibrium, smugglers had for some time been stockpiling opium at Turkham, a border town between Pakistan and Afghanistan. Now they began introducing heroin processing to the area to maximize profit by exporting heroin rather than the bulkier and less valuable raw opium.

The *second stage* of the influence of the Afghan war, from 1980–1989, saw the central involvement of the CIA. Though Mark Mansfield, a CIA spokesman, told a press conference that 'the CIA neither engages in nor condones drug trafficking'[54] later incidents and official reports indicated that this was far from the case. In the words of a State Department official, 'We are not going to let a little thing like drugs get in the way of the political situation'.[55] It is now widely acknowledged that drug money financed resistance to the Soviet forces,[56] and that over half US economic and military aid during the Afghan-Soviet war was channelled through the guerrilla commander Hikmatyar, who was running six heroin laboratories in Helmand Province[57] and south west Pakistan.[58]

The details are startling.[59] According to Cooley, soon after his inauguration in January 1981, President Reagan met the head of the French Secret Foreign Intelligence Service, Count Alexandre de Marenches, in the Oval Office. The Count had a suggestion for a Franco-American venture to counter the Soviet threat in Afghanistan. Operation Mosquito entailed using confiscated drugs precisely as the Vietcong did with the US army in Vietnam: secretly supplying the Soviet forces with illicit drugs in order to demoralize them and dissipate their fighting ability. The Count claimed to be in contact with 'bright young journalists' who could facilitate this at a cost of just $1 million. The President agreed, and instructed the Head of the CIA, William Casey, to pursue the idea. Two days later the Count met Casey, who 'loved' the idea and sought France's assistance in return for the Agency putting up the cash. The Count agreed, but only on condition that Casey would guarantee that his own name and that of France would not be mentioned in published articles. Casey could not give this guarantee because Washington 'leaked like a sieve', so France, having provided the original idea, withdrew.

Three years later Casey raised the issue with the Pakistan President, General Zia-ul-Haq, who was hesitant. He (Casey) then reportedly contacted a leading Mujahideen leader through the offices of French journalists where he received a more enthusiastic response, as a result of which funds and technical expertise were provided to facilitate the establishment of heroin factories.

The hollowness of the denials was further exposed by Senator Kerry's statement to the US Senate, in the wake of the Iran-Contra scandal, that:

> . . . it is clear that individuals who were involved in drug trafficking, the supply of the Contras network was used by drug trafficking organizations and elements of the Contras themselves knowingly received financial and material assistance from the drug traffickers. In each case, one or another agency of the US Government had information regarding the involvement either while it was occurring or immediately thereafter.[60]

In its assault on communist imperialism US inspired covert operations were crucial, but:

During the 1980s the CIA's two main covert operations became interwoven with the global narcotics trade. The agency's support for Afghan guerrillas through Pakistan coincided with the emergence of southern Asia as the major heroin supplier for European and American markets. Although the US maintained a substantial force of DEA agents in Islamabad during the 1980s, the unit was restrained by US national security imperatives and did almost nothing to slow Pakistan's booming heroin export to America.[61]

In 1986, a report to the US Congress on the American contribution to the anti-drugs effort reflected the resultant dilemma nicely:

In this region, as in Central America, the CIA and drug enforcement officials are in effect against each other. The CIA wishes to maximise Mujahideen war efforts against the Russians in Afghanistan. This includes assistance in weapons procurement . . . The Mujahideen are, however, undersupplied with armaments, as recent Western news reports have indicated. Unless the US increases military aid, the only other real source for arms funding is the drug trade in hashish, heroin and opium.[62]

But the CIA and the *Mujahideen* not only sought to finance the war through drug money but also meant to use drugs to undermine the Red Army morally and physically. One Afghan freedom fighter was quoted as saying:

We try to poison the Russians with it. . . they sell opium and hashish mostly but now also heroin to the Russian soldiers in exchange for guns and to poison their spirit.[63]

This was confirmed in fieldwork conducted for this study. In an interview in 1997 Rahmat Gul Shinwari indicated a building in Landi Kotal Bazaar, where he claimed US, Pakistani and Saudi Arabian intelligence agents filled cigarettes with hashish and heroin for the political administrator to give to Pakistani and Afghan drivers, with instructions to offer them to Soviet soldiers in Afghanistan as they crossed the frontier.

Another report of the then UN representative on the Soviet-Afghan issue, Diego Cardoviez, discussing the American efforts to demoralise the Communists, writes:

. . . some reports indicated that half of the men in certain combat units were ill at any given time . . . In January 1987, out of six people in Moscow surveyed in a government sponsored opinion poll openly criticised the war, blaming it for widespread drug addiction and juvenile delinquency.[64]

This second stage, then, covered the 1980s, when heroin processing became widespread in both Pakistan and Afghanistan. In Afghanistan opium production began on an unprecedented level under the patronage of the guerrilla leaders, and the country was converted into a mono-culture. In Pakistan, heroin became almost an 'ordinary-daily-use' commodity, sold openly and cheaply in markets like Jamrud, Bara and Landi Kotal, with free samples distributed to potential users in and around Peshawar University.

The *third stage*, the post-Afghan War era, will have far reaching impact on drugs the world over. Afghanistan was under Soviet occupation for nearly 12 years, and the subsequent and protracted civil war and lack of centralized authority or government aggravated the narcotics situation, with Afghans facing a militarily self-sufficient superpower while being dependent on others even for small assault weapons. Soon after the Soviet invasion, however, the Afghans began to realize the value of their opium crop, and 'drugs for arms' became the business of the day. Though they received arms supplies from many western countries this was never going to be sufficient to fight a superpower. This tremendously increased opium production, which came increasingly to be converted into heroin inside both Pakistan and Afghanistan.

Another important factor was that the war had provided most of the male population with jobs. Their families were looked after properly inside Pakistan with the help of the international community, and they were free of the pressure of earning their livelihood. With the Soviet withdrawal, western aid began to dwindle, eventually drying up completely. Pakistan could no longer afford to feed five million people out of its own resources, and consequently repatriated the Afghan refugees. This repatriation, undertaken without international aid or pre-arrangement, brought more misery. The Soviet Union had destroyed the infrastructure: the lack of roads, irrigation channels or dwellings in which to hide from extreme weather conditions, the millions of land mines, and above all a lack of any centralized authority led the repatriated people to look towards sure and prompt sources of survival. The obvious source was opium cultivation on lands available for agricultural purposes. Accordingly, opium cultivation escalated, and by 1998 official sources in Islamabad were claiming that Afghanistan was for the first time on target to outstrip Myanmar in opium production, so becoming the largest opium producing country in the world. Virtually all the warlords ran heroin processing laboratories and were procuring arms through its sale.[65]

The period 1996–7 witnessed another wave of political changes, this time in the shape of Taliban, whose uprising had been encouraged by the US, Saudi Arabia and Pakistan under Benazir Bhutto.[66] Taliban legalized opium production by imposing the *ushr* tithe, with the result that, by 1999, to international concern Afghanistan was producing over 5000 metric tons of opium. Suddenly, however, in 2000, Taliban banned opium production, and strong indications exist that poppy cultivation was indeed largely eradicated in Taliban-controlled areas. In fact the first author visited Afghanistan twice between July 2000, when the edict was passed, and late 2001, and was unable to find a single poppy plant in the entire Nangrahar (Jalalabad) area, where the crop is normally extensively harvested. This view has been confirmed in an as yet unpublished report by Paoli, of the Max Planck Institute (with which the first author was involved), which found that following the edict the 2001 harvest had shown a 95 per cent reduction over 2000. Yet further confirmation was received from the then Taliban Minister of Agriculture, who, in an interview with the first author, stated that opium cultivation had been banned not because it was un-Islamic but because Afghanistan had also to bear world opinion in mind.

It appears, therefore, that Taliban did indeed prohibit drug production, and probably did so much more successfully than any other country in history. One reason for this was certainly Taliban's ambition, subsequently to be dramatically aborted, to secure international recognition of their regime. Though some western commentators have also suggested that supply side reductions were introduced to force up prices, no evidence of this has as yet come to light. Whatever the motivation for the edict, however, it is certain that, following it, there was a dramatic reduction, and in some areas eradication of the crop. Equally it is clear that the fall of Taliban in late 2001 means that the 2002 harvest will involve an unprecedented increase in supply.

The reason for this is that the Northern Alliance, supported by Russia and the major western countries, continued to produce drugs to procure arms to aid in its armed struggle against Taliban,[67] and this situation has not changed with the interim government in place at the time of writing (March 2002). Northern Alliance cultivation was admitted by the US Drug Enforcement Administration's Asa Hutchinson, who conceded that 'we are not naïve (in thinking) that the Northern Alliance does not have their own interests and history in poppy cultivation and trafficking'.[68]

Reporting on the involvement of the Northern Alliance, a German journalist returned from Afghan–Tajikistan border revealed widespread drug smuggling among named Northern Alliance and Russian personnel even prior to September 11 2001, claiming that helicopters were making daily sorties carrying huge quantities of narcotics destined for the European market.[69] It was Opposition-controlled areas that were licensed to cultivate opium, with the proceeds from this being deployed for arms procurement. A UNDCP report of 5 December 2001 confirms that, following September 11, opium production and heroin processing recommenced throughout Afghanistan, and identified ten mobile heroin factories.[70] Inevitably production will continue unchecked in the future as long as it remains consistent with superpower *Realpolitik*.

The Impact of the Afghan War on the Local Economy of NWFP

Examining the family income of the four main drug producing areas gives an indication of the poverty of the people of Khyber Agency, with a mean family income of 11,500 rupees, or 469 rupees ($10) *per capita* per month. For centuries in Khyber Agency there has been no sure source of livelihood, and people had three main ways of surviving. Some were migratory, descending in winter from the cool uplands of Tirah, bringing their flocks and herds to graze in low country round Peshawar; secondly, the poorer people carried firewood into Peshawar to sell there as a principal occupation (a surprising and difficult activity since the rocky land is in capable of sustaining flora). The third occupation was raiding the neighbourhoods in order to survive.[71]

In a region characterized by extensive cross-border smuggling, trade in guns and ammunition has also been a major source of livelihood for the Afridies in particular.[72] In the inhospitable arid belt along the border no other gainful occupation is possible. To local people smuggling is a meaningless concept. Laws are not applied and smuggling is perceived simply as a form of trade – in firearms, electronic and luxury goods of foreign make and, now, narcotics. It has been thus for centuries, regardless of shifting national boundaries; and since the 1950s it has been carried out in *Bara* markets designed almost exclusively for merchandising smuggled goods.

Initially this trade was conducted only in Landi Kotal, but by the 1960s *bara* markets extended to other parts of the Agency under government patronage. Because luxury goods were available there at much lower prices than in the settled areas business flourished, in a short time bringing prosperity to the local people, no outsider being permitted to trade without their permission. These markets spread into Government controlled areas, their main supply source being Afghanistan, from where such items were imported and being sold on to Pakistani businessmen.

Another source of income was Pak-Afghan transit trade. Afghanistan is a landlocked country and access to developed countries is mainly through Pakistan or Iran. Accordingly imports into Afghanistan were channelled through Pakistan ports and transported through Khyber Agency, the shortest and safest route into Afghanistan. But Afghanistan, a poor country with widespread availability of electricity only in Kabul, did not need imported electronics and other luxury goods, which, in consequence, were intercepted in Khyber Agency and found their way into the *bara* markets.

The Afghan-Soviet war blocked this trade in three ways. Firstly, most traders had left Afghanistan at the start of the war, so there was no importer. Secondly, the Soviets marketed their own goods at very cheap rates, though they were not popular due to low quality and negative public attitudes. Thirdly, the routes were at the mercy of Soviet troops who demanded heavy bribes for permitting trading. Since the Afghan fighters also levied heavy taxes on such imports–exports the business in the Pakistani tribal areas came to a standstill, compelling the locals to seek alternative sources of livelihood, most notably heroin processing.

More recently, the Government of Pakistan has limited the Afghan Transit Trade (ATT) to just a few items. Inevitably this will eventually have a negative impact on the income level of the tribal people of Khyber Agency.

Drugs and United States' Politics

Internationally drug politics can constitute an effective propaganda tool for defamation and blackmail. This fact has political consequences for aid-receiving countries such as Pakistan as it has been used as a pretext to interfere with the internal affairs of other countries. Pakistan has been engaged in controlling drugs through eliminating opium production and combating trafficking since 1979, but these efforts never gained recognition in the United States. As we have seen, attempts have been made to eliminate opium crops both by herbicide sprayed from US-supplied thrush air crafts flown by Pakistan army pilots and normally supervised by DEA officials from the US Embassy in Islamabad and, with more constructive intent, by crop substitution programmes. These latter, however, have generally offered such meagre benefits that their impact has been negligible; but anyway, as US official documents acknowledge that crop substitution is not a promising strategy for reducing drug production even in the Andes, how could it be suitable for Pakistan?

It is very doubtful whether successive US wars on drugs have achieved their objectives or have simply had the counterproductive effect of increasing the number of addicts inside America. And, it must further be asked, is the war on drugs primarily to be waged inside or outside that country? In 1971 the USA had 560,000 heroin addicts;[73] by 1988 this number was much the same but the number of cocaine addicts had risen to almost 6 million, with 18 million marijuana users – figures that give the USA the world's largest user population.[74] So the wars on drugs have scarcely been a great success at home, and it must be asked whether they were mainly a ploy to trap economic and politically weak countries that the US wanted to manipulate for political purposes. Whereas in Pakistan Zia-ul-Haq's regime was almost certainly responsible for the spread of drugs through high level corruption, on his death the State Department called General Zia 'a strong supporter of anti-narcotics activities in Pakistan', expressing the fear that his death 'would slow the fight against drugs'.[75]

Inside Pakistan there has been widespread suspicion that, in the guise of a war against drugs, American drug agents and other diplomats are interfering with the internal affairs of the country. But such interference has been justified first by the fact that historically Pakistan is an aid-dependent country vulnerable to US pressure and liable to lose international aid or loans unless a certificate of good conduct and support of American interests, required under 1986 US law, is obtained. Since 1971 the United States has used diplomacy as well as financial and military assistance to deal with producer countries like Pakistan, but her efforts have had no discernible impact on availability. This is because her anti-drugs policies frequently conflict with her foreign policy, a contradiction at the heart of US policy, and, such are the size and influence of the only remaining superpower, of international control efforts also.

The second American justification for intervention is the corruptibility of Pakistani officials and politicians. They receive massive aid for drug control in Pakistan with one hand, but with the other, invest it in western countries[76] where, according to some reports, Pakistani politicians – including Benazir Bhutto who is alleged to have US $1 billion in Swiss bank accounts – have up to US $140 billion.[77]

How Americans are using drugs as political propaganda against Pakistan can be understood from the US role during the Afghan war. Both the United States and the Afghan resistance fighters financed the war effort by drug money. Of Afghans it can be said they had no resources, and were using every available means of fighting a powerful enemy. But why did Americans not stop them, or at least report the drug business? Until the end of the war in 1989 even the western media did not mention the unholy alliance between Americans and the Afghan leaders or drugs dealers.[78] Yet the day after the Soviet withdrawal was signed, the Afghan *Mujahideen* (holy fighters), hitherto saluted as heroic freedom fighters, were branded fundamentalists and terrorists.

In relation to Pakistan, American policies change repeatedly. During Zia's regime, when the CIA and the intelligence branch of the Pakistan army were working hand in glove to finance the Afghan war, the issue of drugs was never raised. When Nawaz was elected Prime Minister, the CIA report mentioned earlier cited him as a protector of a relative involved in the drugs trade. But still the Americans announced their support for Nawaz's policies during his second tenure as Prime Minister, and the relative concerned was received as a state guest during Nawaz's visit to USA in 1998. However, the US International Narcotics Control Strategy Report for 1995–6 felt able to claim that no 'senior official of the government encourages or facilitates the illicit production or distribution of narcotics or psychotropic drugs or other controlled substances, or the laundering of proceeds from illegal drug transactions.'[79]

Nonetheless, during Benazir Bhutto's Government (1993–1996), while the Americans insisted on the extradition of some unimportant drug barons, they never mentioned that both her husband and foreign minister (ironically a former minister of narcotics control) were allegedly involved in the trade inside the Prime Minister's own house. When Scotland Yard police officers pointed this out, US officials are said to have replied that they did not want to destabilize Pakistan.[80] Shortly after Bhutto's fall in 1997, however, the US Government blamed Pakistan for supporting drugs trafficking and money laundering.[81] How the United States tried to use narcotics for political blackmailing can be judged from the stage-managed arrest of an Officer of Pakistan Air Force in possession of 2 kg of heroin at Dallas International Airport. On investigation it came to light that this appeared to be a pre-planned operation designed to malign and embarrass the Pakistan Army, DEA agents in Islamabad having trapped some officers in order to defame the Pakistan army and give a pretext for American blackmail. But Pakistani intelligence agencies were smart enough to foil this US plot, and protested over the matter. As a result, for the first time in the 50 years of Pakistan's history, the US formally apologized to Pakistan over the DEA agents' conduct.[82] More recently, reports have suggested, reliably or not, that US and British intelligence agencies played an important role in drug production and supply, and that in doing so they were in fact giving succour to separatist groups whose political agenda was to make separate states out of such opium producing areas as Dir, Bajaur, Gadoon, Buner and Muhmand Agency.[83]

Conclusion

Drug production and supply in Pakistan have internal and external causes. Internally the country is unstable: institutions are weak, bureaucrats strong. There is a multiplicity of laws and administrative arrangements in different parts of NWFP, and the resulting confusion benefits politicians, government officials and drug producers. Political parties oppose drug production when in power, but in opposition support and even encourage it to attract farmers' votes. External factors include the political conditions of the region and international narco-politics. Pressure from neighbouring countries is unlikely to diminish in the medium term, and the use of narcotics-related issues against Pakistan by western powers will continue to have an impact as the Pakistani public's attitude towards some such countries is becoming increasingly hostile generally. Regionally the problem has no foreseeable end, as more countries are becoming involved in production.

The role of the United States in drugs development in Pakistan and Afghanistan has been that of an active, if sometimes hypocritical, collaborator and protector, condoning or supporting the trade depending on the *Realpolitik* of the moment.

Notes

1   Government of Pakistan, *The Constitution of the Islamic Republic of Pakistan* (Islamabad: Ministry of Law, Justice and Parliamentary Affairs, 1973). pp101–2.
2   Dir is the most formidable of these areas, with its population of 1.6 million thought to possess between them over four million AK-47s as well as other heavy armaments.
3   I. Haq, *From Hasheesh to Heroin* (Lahore: Al-noor Publications, 1991). p19.
4   M.A. Khan, Ex-Inspector General Frontier Police (Now Minister of NWFP) in *NewsLine* (Karachi: December 1989). p25.
5   R.A.K. Sahibzada, *Poppy Cultivation in North West Frontier Province (NWFP): Its Past, Present and Future* (Islamabad: Ministry of Agriculture and Rural Development, 1991). p6.
6   Government of Pakistan, *Gazette of Pakistan: Prohibition and Punishment*, Chapter II section 4 (Islamabad: Ministry of Law, Justice and Parliamentary Affairs 1995). p359: 'No one shall cultivate any cannabis plant, coca bush or opium, or gather any portion of a cannabis plant, coca bush or opium plant.'
7   *NewsLine* (Karachi: May 1993). p41.
8   M.K. Jalal Zai, *The Drug War in South Asia* (Lahore: Institute of Current Affairs, 1993). 64. See also *NewsLine* (Karachi: December 1989). p25.
9   Bakht Baidar Khan MPA of the Pakistan People's Party claimed in an interview with the first author that the Deputy Commissioner Dir gave him a foreign-made handgun paid for out of the Narcotics Fund.
10 Malik Bahram Khan, alias Dogram Malik, a cultivator himself, is an aggressive supporter of other cultivators, and led a march of local people in December 1995 to press their demands. See the *Daily Jang* (London: 16 December 1995).
11 *NewsLine*, December 1989, *op. cit.* p28.
12 M. K. Jalal Zai, *op. cit.* p41.
13 The first author was undertaking fieldwork in the area on 28 January 1997 when he observed PML candidate Malik Jehanzeb supporting the local people and assuring them that the Government would not destroy their crops. He secured their support on the basis of this assurance and is now a member of the Provincial Assembly and Minister for Narcotics Control in the provincial cabinet.
14 C. Spencer and V. Navarathnam, *Drug Abuse in South East Asia*, 61; see also A. Masood, '*Esi Bulandi Esi Pasti*', 57; *Ajrak Monthly* (Karachi, May–June 1994). p18.
15 These two groups were banned by General Musharaf's Government in January 2002.
16 Hudood, plural of the Arabic Hadd, means penalties under the Islamic system of criminal justice.
17 *The Frontier Post* (Peshawar: May 7 1997). p2.
18 A.W. McCoy, 1994, *op. cit.* p11.
19 *Ibid.* p457. Also see Victor Mosquera Chaux, Colombian Ambassador to USA in *International Herald Tribune* (New York: 12 January 1989).
20 A.W. McCoy, 1994, op. *cit.* p454.
21 Government of Pakistan, *National Survey on Drug Abuse in Pakistan 1993* (Islamabad, Narcotics Control Division, 1994). pp21–22.
22 This is no more than a guesstimate based on the fact that the sources of these figures reported an increase in heroin addiction of 12.1 per cent during 1982–88 and 6.8 per cent during 1988–93.
23 Muhammad Atif and Shaheen Hasan. *Daily Jang* (Rawalpendi: 26 June 2001).
24 Government of Pakistan, *National Survey on Drug Abuse in Pakistan* (Islamabad: Narcotics Control Board, 1986). 150 (Table 5.13).
25 *Ibid.* pvii. The 1993 survey shows 171,322 persons addicted to opium.

26 Muhammad Atif and Shaheen Hasan, 2001, *op. cit.* See also Government of the United States of America, *International Narcotics Control Strategy Report* (Washington DC: Bureau of International Narcotics and Law Enforcement Affairs, 1996). p217 and 222.
27 G.R. Adam and J.D. Schevaneldt, *Understanding Research Methods* (New York: Longman, 1985). p182.
28 H. Parker, K. Bakx and R. Newcombe, *Living with Heroin* (Buckingham: Open University Press, 1988). pp69–72.
29 S.H. Alatas, *Corruption: Its Nature, Causes and Functions* (Kuala Lumpur: S. Abdul Majeed and Co, 1991). pp78–80.
30 See for example S. Das, *Public Office, Private Interest: Bureaucracy and Corruption in India* (New Delhi: Oxford University Press, 2001).
31 'Heroin was smuggled in Zia's aircraft', *The Frontier Post* (Lahore: 7 May 1997).
32 I. Haq, 1991, *op. cit.* pp12–14.
33 A.W. McCoy, 1994, *op. cit.* pp454.
34 A. Gohar, 'Are We Going Down the Central American Route?' *National Policy and Public Awareness Conference on Drug Abuse* (Islamabad, PNCB, 17–19 May 1993). p185; *NewsLine*, (December 1985). p29.
35 J. Cooley, *Unholy Wars: Afghanistan, America and International Terrorism* (London: Pluto Press). pp138–141. Haji Ayub Afridi voluntarily surrendered to the US authorities, but his surrender is an interesting story. The husband of the then Prime Minister, Benazir Bhutto, Asif Ali Zardari, notorious for his alleged corruption, is believed to have asked him for 100 million rupees to remove his name from the list of drug barons, and subsequently to have demanded more money. Haji sent a message that Zardari should send a reliable person to collect the money. Zardari sent his brother-in law, Habib, but Haji Ayub allegedly kidnapped him, holding him in Afghanistan for three months and then demanding twice the original sum back as a ransom. His house was raided by the army several times, but he avoided arrest. After this incident, apparently to avoid giving credit to Benazir Bhutto, he surrendered to the American Embassy in the United Arab Emirates.
36 'Bhutto's husband was targeted in a US drug sting'. *Sunday Times* (London: 23 February 1997). Zardari's assets in UK and Switzerland were subsequently investigated on suspicion of his having acquired his properties through drug money.
37 *NewsLine, op. cit.* pp14–16. Iqbal Baig's statement was supported by the then Prime Minister Meraj Khalid in an interview with the *Khaleej Times*, in which he alleged Benazir Bhutto had sought support from the Drug Mafiosi in 1989 (quoted by the *Daily Kasooti*: Peshawar: 4 March 1997). On the other hand Benazir Bhutto denied to gave a ticket to Meraj Khalid, as he was very close to Iqbal Baig and other drug Mafia members.
38 CIA report on Heroin in Pakistan: 'Sowing the Winds', in *Friday Times* (Lahore: 26 March 1992). p3.
39 Interview with Mr Hussain Shah, a Pakistani British citizen serving an eight year sentence in England (HM Prison Wolds, Everthorpe, East Yorkshire) for his involvement in heroin import into UK. He claimed in interview to have spent hundreds of thousands of rupees on Imran Khan's General Election campaign in the belief that Imran was a sure winner, and that he was promised that in return his name would be removed from the United Kingdom drug smugglers' list.
40 Rahmat Shah Afridi, owner of Peshawar's only English language daily newspaper, was arrested by the Pakistan Anti-Narcotic Force (ANF) on 1 April 1999 for involvement in the drug business. See also 'PPP releases govt's list of 353 drug barons: civil and military bigwigs among the accused'. *Frontier Post* (Peshawar: 25 May 1998).
41 A. Gohar, *op. cit.* p183.
42 A.W. McCoy, *The Politics of Heroin: CIA Complicity in the Global Drug Trade* (New York: Lawrence Hill Books, 1991), p456.

43   R.B. Craig, 'Illicit Drug Traffic: Implications for South American Source Countries'. *Inter-American Studies and World Affairs,* 29,2 (Summer 1987). pp1–34.

44   Cited in the *Friday Times op. cit.* p17.

45   'A Skirmish Over Drugs', *The Times* (London: 2 June 1997). p55.

46   Javed is from Dir and lives in hiding, as three attempts have been made on his life for his allegation to the Central Intelligence Agency that the head of the Mafia was a former federal minister from the Punjab.

47   *NewsLine,* May 1993, *op. cit.* p13.

48   I. Dar (Pakistan Finance Minister) reported in *Daily Jang* (London: 28 May 1999).

49   Rent-seeking is normally defined as the 'use of resources to obtain through the political process special privileges in which the injury to other people arguably is greater than the gain to the people who obtain rents' (G. Tullock, *Rent Seeking.* The Shaftesbury Papers, 2. Aldershot: Edward Elgar, 1993). p22.

50   *Daily Jang* (London: 27 May 1997). pp26, 144. Pakistan was 79th out of 91 countries in Transparency International's 2001 Corruption Perceptions Index (http://www.transparency. Org/documents/cpi /2001/cpi2001.html#cpi).

51   See for example G. Myrdal, *Asian Drama: an Inquiry into the Poverty of Nations.* Volume II (New York: Pantheon, 1968); R. Tilman, 'Emergence of Black-Market Bureaucracy: Administration, Development and Corruption in the New States', *Political Administration Review,* XXVIII, p5, 1968; and J. Nye, 'Corruption and Political Development: a Cost-Benefit Analysis', *American Political Science Review,* p61, 1967.

52   P. Heywood (ed.) *Political Corruption* (Oxford: Blackwell for the Political Studies Association, 1997). p5.

53   'Asia's "Golden Crescent" Heroin Floods the West', *Christian Science Monitor* (9 November 1982). p12; I.L. Griffith, 'From Cold War Geopolitics to Post Cold War Geonarcotics' *International Journal.* XLIX (Winter 1993–4). p6; A.W. McCoy, 1994, *op. cit.* p446; R.A.K. Sahib Zada *op. cit.* p2.

54   C. Lausane, *Pipe Dream Blues: Racism and the War on Drugs* (Boston: South End Press, 1991). p116.

55   *New York Times* (10 April 1988).

56   A. Gohar, *op. cit.* p185. Also see I. Haq, *op. cit.* pp16–19; A. Jamieson, *Global Drug Trafficking. Conflict Studies* (London: Research Institute for the Study of Conflict and Terrorism, September 1990). p11; I. L. Griffith, *op. cit.* p5.

57   A.W. McCoy, 1994. *op. cit.* p454.

58   *The Washington Post* (13 May 1990). p1.

59   J. Cooley, *op. cit.* pp126–133; see also Muhammad Yousaf, 'Drugs and Destruction' in Daily Dawn (Karachi: 24 June 2001).

60   Muhammad Shafiq Khan (Maj. Retd). 'TAs Socio-Economic Structure-III', in *The Frontier Post* (Peshawar: 7 April 1997).

61   A.W. McCoy, 1994, *op. cit.* p491.

62   I. Haq, *op. cit.* p20.

63   J. Cooley, *op. cit.* pp126–130 ; see also *Christian Science Monitor,* 1982, *op. cit.*

64   D. Cardovez and S. Harrison, *Out of Afghanistan: The Inner Story of the Soviet Withdrawal* (New York: Oxford University Press, 1995). pp151, 161.

65   J. Cooley, *op. cit.* pp126–139. See also *The Frontier Post* (Peshawar: 25 March 1998).

66   Sir Martin Ewan, 'Afghanistan: A New History'. *The Daily News* (Islamabad: December 16, 2001).

67   'US Concerned Over Afghan Opium Surge'. *The Frontier Post* (Peshawar: November 28, 2001).

68   *Ibid.*

69   *The Frontier Post* (Peshawar: August 1 2001). See also J. Cooley, *op. cit.* pp126–40.

70 *The Frontier Post* (Peshawar: December 5, 2001). See also *The Daily Mashriq* (Peshawar: December 12, 2001) and the *Chicago Tribune* as cited in *The Frontier Post* (Peshawar: December 28 2001).
71 R.T. Ridway, *Pathans* (Calcutta: Government Printing Press, 1910). p51
72 A. Kepple, *Gun Running and NWF of India*. Cited in R.T. Ridway, 1910, *op. cit.* p16.
73 A.W. McCoy, *The Politics of Heroin in Southeast Asia* (New York: Harper & Row, 1972). p1.
74 D. Scott, 'Spread of Drugs, Crack-down or Crack-up' in *The South* (London: August 1988). pp9–10.
75 *The New York Times* (7 September 1988).
76 Victor Mosquera Chaux (Colombian Ambassador to USA) in *International Herald Tribune*, (New York: 12 January 1989).
77 *The Nation*, (London: 12–18 September 1997).
78 A.W. McCoy, 1994, *op. cit.* p453.
79 'Today's News on Afghanistan' in *The Times* (London: 9 March 1997).
80 'Bhutto's Husband was targeted in US Drugs sting' in *Sunday Times*, *op. cit.*
81 *Daily Pakistan*, (Islamabad: 3 March 1997). See also Daily Khabrain (Islamabad: 4 March 1997).
82 'US apologise over DEA agents' conduct' in *The News* (London, 8 July 1997). The story led to the arrest and execution of a DEA Pakistani agent, Ayaz Balooch. But the Air Force officer arrested in USA was never handed over to Pakistan for trial, and is believed to be currently enjoying political asylum there.
83 *Daily Mashriq* (Peshawar: 5 December 2001).

Chapter IV
Methodology, Ethnography and Data Analysis

This chapter falls into three parts. The first part explains the basis and structure of the study; the second part comprises an ethnography deriving from the empirical work; the third part comprises the data analysis.

˙ Executing this study involved a number of unusual features. The research offers a multidisciplinary framework buttressed (but not wholly driven) by the empirical data. It offers, by definition, new knowledge since no other study of this kind exists, and it could have been undertaken only by a very small number of people. The fieldwork involved danger to life and liberty; and it was conducted with few resources, so much resourcefulness was necessary. My[1] blood ties with many of the subjects enabled me not only to survive the fieldwork (itself not a foregone conclusion) but also to produce data of a kind which would not have been available to other researchers, or to NGO, Federal Government or UN officials.

The research is, therefore, a path-breaking study, predominantly exploratory in focus, which, as well as offering a unique empirical contribution, draws together data from a number of distinct areas of knowledge (official, governmental and UN data, and scholarship in a number of disciplines) as well as newspaper reports. This combination of sources offers an insight into the actual context in which the research was conducted – a context of political instability and corruption, some of it inherited from colonial times, much of it, however, post-colonial. The picture is of life in territories outwith state law and largely uninfluenced by social developments elsewhere. In addition, therefore, to offering an account of methodology, this chapter has some of the characteristics of a narrative. This, anyway, is the view of western audiences who have been exposed to drafts of this book. It follows that certain allowances need from time to time to be made by the scientifically positivist reader, but it is hoped that a certain generosity of spirit there will be rewarded by an account which is (certainly) original and (one hopes) accurate.

Part A: Description and Methodology

Gaining Access

Theoretically, gaining access to the tribal areas for this fieldwork should not have been problematic. This was an overt study involving open access; the researcher was a university teacher and respect for teachers is a religious obligation; and he belongs to the area and has tribal blood as well as reciprocal social relations with people from the opium growing communities. These factors certainly helped him gain access to areas where local administrators did not dare venture. But in fact things were not so straightforward.

Firstly, access was far from simple or safe. Tribal society is closed, and the entry of an outsider, even from a neighbouring village, is immediately noticed. Every male member of the village who meets a stranger (and any lone stranger would be male) outside or even inside the village asks about his host or asks whom the guest (*melma*) wants to meet. The outsider must reveal the purpose of the visit and name the person he wishes to meet; the visitor is then led to the guesthouse (*hujra*) whereupon he becomes a guest of the whole village. Access to information collection depends, therefore, upon the cultural value of *melmastia* (hospitality) which:

> . . . involves a set of conventions whereby the person on the home ground has obligations towards the outsider to incorporate him into the local group, temporarily be responsible for his security and provide for his needs. The obligation is brought into play by the visitor presenting himself in the alien setting.[2]

Secondly, the continuing conflict between poppy cultivators and Government made access to these inaccessible mountainous areas, outwith the jurisdiction of federal law[3] and accessible only by foot,[4] difficult and dangerous. Most poppy areas are remote, involving travel by foot for 8–12 hours in steep mountains, sometimes in temperatures well in excess of 40°C, to reach the sampled villages. This caused health problems and hyper-exhaustion. In addition, the law and order situation during 1996–7 made it unsafe to travel to these areas without a proper escort or without prior contact with influential members of the communities concerned. The journey itself brought many dangers, an example of which is *baramta*, by which an innocent outsider is confined as a *baramta* hostage in order to recover disputed money. If a person from one part of the tribal area owes money to someone from another part and the money cannot be reclaimed, the aggrieved party takes as a hostage a person of status from the debtor's village. He then sends a message to both the debtor and the hostage's family that the hostage will be kept in *baramta* unless the debt is repaid or the debtor comes to a *Jargah* tribal council to negotiate settlement. In the common event of non-cooperation, the relatives, family, tribe or village of the hostage pay the kidnappers and then take over the role of creditor. A number of people from my own community were known to me to be debtors, so I was obviously at risk of becoming a *baramta* hostage. In the event, however, blood ties elsewhere in the tribal areas proved helpful in enabling me to walk into the poppy fields, albeit escorted by armed kinsmen, and to have frank discussions with the cultivators.

Thirdly, the need to secure sufficient trust to discuss the tribesmen's problems, the causes of opium poppy cultivation, the output and the role of Government officers meant that the perils of access were but the first of many challenges. Government functionaries were at that time destroying poppy crops with herbicides in nocturnal raids, and cultivators were actively trying to identify Government agents. In a climate where any stranger was a possible agent, cultivators could all too easily have misinterpreted my necessary research questions. Nonetheless, the farmers are not organized criminals who protect their crops from outsiders, but are perfectly happy to talk to anyone who can help them. Hence once access had been achieved and trust secured I faced problems of evasion and dissimulation only where there was suspicion of the involvement of Government agents.

Fourthly, there were dangers from Government officers guilty of embezzling foreign aid intended for developing the poppy growing areas, and naturally less than anxious to have outsiders probing their activities. Such officers were known within the community to have had strangers kidnapped in order to keep them away from the scenes of their crimes; so capture by renegade officials was also a possibility.

Opium and Heroin Production Areas and Sampling Methodology

NWFP's tribal area is geographically and ethnically part of the Province, but under the control of the Federal (FATA) or Provincial (PATA) Government. Our concern is with the drug producing parts of Malakand (PATA) and Peshawar (FATA) Divisions. According to international reports, in NWFP as a whole in 1995–6, 1,038 hectares[5] were cultivated with poppies, of which 1,027 hectares were in Dir (474 hectares), Bajaur (400 hectares), Muhmand (114 hectares) and Khyber (39 hectares). Heroin is processed mainly in Khyber Agency. Other Divisions are largely drug free.[6]

Malakand, the largest Division, is sub-divided into Dir, Buner, Swat and Chitral Districts, and Bajaur and Malakand tribal Agencies. Peshawar Division comprises Peshawar, Charsadda and Nowshehra Divisions and Muhmand and Khyber Agencies as well as special areas called Frontier Regions (FRs), which are effectively FATAs. Since the Hudood Ordinance in 1979, apart from negligible quantities in South and North Waziristan tribal Agencies, drug production has occurred only in Khyber and Muhmand, so I selected these agencies for this study.

Samples were selected on a representative basis to establish the circumstances that led to opium cultivation and heroin manufacture in these areas. With only insignificant exceptions, therefore, the study embraced the entire opium growing and heroin manufacturing parts of NWFP. While they have the common characteristic that they lie on the border with Afghanistan, are mountainous in nature and inaccessible, they are in other respects very diverse, being occupied by different sub-tribes of one ethnic group, *Pathan*s or *Pakhtoons* (Pushtu speaking people), and being part of different administrative units.

Samples were drawn from different areas, not for comparative study (for practical and resource reasons a systematic comparison of producing and non-producing areas would have been impossible) but to represent key characteristics of the drug producing areas. It was clear from available statistical information, however, that producing areas have a greater preponderance of poverty, lack of alternative subsistence income sources, inaccessible geographical location and ambiguous political status than opium free areas. According to official reports in 1986, poppy yielded 46 per cent of the gross value added in agriculture and 40 per cent of the total income of the communities concerned. The gross value added per unit of cultivated area for poppy was more than twice that of the next crop, and constituted 82 per cent of the total sale.[7]

Data were collected from three strata: farmers/opium cultivators in Muhmand, Bajaur and Dir Agencies (stratum 1), tribal leaders and opinion formers in Khyber Agency (stratum 2), and opinion formers and intellectuals in NWFP generally (stratum 3). The main method of primary data collection was the semi-structured interview, which combines open and closed questions, with data recorded in field notes, tape recordings and photographs. Questionnaire use is impossible in illiterate societies and participative observation would have been dangerous and inappropriate. While the interview method is imperfect[8], overall the approach worked well, permitting respondents from strikingly different backgrounds to offer their own perspectives; and problems associated with cross-cultural interviewing were obviated by my own ethnic and tribal background. The open questions made it possible to achieve a rich understanding of local socio-economic conditions and their relationship with drug production, while the closed questions clearly facilitated the quantification and coding necessary for securing hard information. Interviews focused on cultivators' socio-economic circumstances, their acquisition of knowledge for heroin manufacture, the creation of the local market, the Government's suppression policy, poppy's impact on the local economy and agriculture, the relation between national politics and drugs and respondents' views about foreign involvement.

Stratum 1: Farmers and Opium Cultivators

Forty cultivators from the poppy cultivation areas in Dir District, Bajaur Agency (Ghar Utman Khel area) and Muhmand Agency (Ambar Tehsil) were selected for interview on a proportional basis reflecting production levels. Though randomization was attempted it was not invariably achieved: for example the status of some of those providing advice and support was too high for their opinions to be ignored. Nonetheless, it was decided to obtain an official list of all poppy cultivating communities, villages and cultivators from the appropriate senior official. It was quickly established, however, (both from the Deputy Commissioner of Dir and the political agent of Bajaur) that none of the official bodies concerned (either governments themselves or the Anti-Narcotic Force for NWFP) had any such list. Accordingly personal visits had to be made to the areas before data collection began, and complete lists of the villages/communities and cultivators were compiled with the aid of local community leaders such as school teachers, and other personal contacts and kinsmen. This list constituted the sampling frame. Interviewees were questioned about their economic circumstances, why they cultivated poppies, the role of area development projects (such as agriculture development, crop substitution and job creation) and about opium production's religious implications.

Fieldwork commenced at the beginning of December 1996 when crops were ready for weeding and hoeing, and cultivators would be at home to look after them. The provincial Home Department was approached to seek permission to enter the tribal areas. Personal relations and my status as a university teacher were of great assistance here, as it is very difficult to approach senior officials for such help. In the event, the Home Department kindly requested the Deputy Commissioner of Dir, the Political Agents of Bajaur, Muhmand and Khyber Agencies and the Director of the Anti-Narcotic Force (ANF) to extend every assistance. Of these only the ANF proved uninterested and uncooperative. Obtaining access to Dir and Bajaur Agencies was further aided by personal as well as blood relations, as I had been a teacher at the Agency Headquarters High School at Khar Bajaur Agency from 1976–1980, and my former students were now responsible and respected members of their communities.

The most difficult area to penetrate was *Muhmand Agency (Area A)*, as I knew no influential people there, the political administration lacked information and the terrain is remote and barely accessible. Eventually access was gained through the good offices of blood relatives in Bajaur Agency, who were asked to identify opium producing villages. Some ten villages in the Ambar Tehsil of the Agency were listed, of which one, Pai Khan, was selected randomly for data collection, the same relatives contacting key people in Pai Khan. Completing the fieldwork in Muhmand Agency was a priority because the opium crop is harvested there first, after which the local people migrate to the urban areas.

After two weeks I was informed that the mother of Pai Khan's village chief had passed away, and if possible I should go with them to offer *fatiha* (condolence). This was a God-sent chance, as sharing and participation in *Pakhtoon* grief are always remembered and reciprocated. I accordingly travelled to Khar Bajaur by road, and from there on foot for six kilometres to my relatives' village, Manoogai, in Utman Khel. The next day, at 6.00 am, we set off for Pai Khan on an eight-hour journey through Mount Kohimoor, the highest mountain in Bajaur. After offering *fatiha*, we were invited to stay overnight, as it was too dangerous to go back in the dark. We walked through the poppy fields with our host (Mohammed Yar Khan), who inquired about my tribe, occupation, residence and other such matters, and my relatives told him that I wanted to talk to his people for my thesis. After dinner, arranged for all the guests by another villager (according to both culture and religion a family in mourning does not cook food for three days), we discussed the crop and the problems of the area. The next day our host told us he would invite us back when the rituals of *fatiha* had been completed.

On 5 January 1997 my relative informed me that an invitation had been received. On 6 January I reached Bajaur, and the next day we crossed the mountain, again on foot, to reach Pai Khan. After dinner in the guesthouse (*hujra* or *dera*), all the males of the village gathered to welcome and converse with us. Most of the time the villagers talked about their problems, presumably in the hope that one of us would convey them to the authorities and that they would get help. During the conversation a list of opium cultivators was made. Of 23 cultivators, five were selected for interview. Our host asked these five people to stay at home the next day, to be at our service. On that day, 8 January, we were invited by another villager, the first cousin of our host, for tea, and in a sense this was our first interview. It took some three hours, as more than the scheduled questions were asked and both participation and general observation for orientation purposes were involved. On that day three persons were interviewed, leaving two for the next day.

The following day, after completing the interviews we again walked through the poppy fields and saw a ruined house-like dwelling. I was told that the villagers wanted to educate their children but could not do so due to lack of the required facilities. This dilapidated house had once been a school, which the villagers had run on a self-help basis, paying the teacher 'in kind' – $^{1}/_{4}$ seer ($^{1}/_{2}$ lb) of opium per house, irrespective of the number of children, bringing the teacher some 30 kg of opium annually. However, due to the uncertain future of opium and constant pressure from the political administration to destroy opium poppies the teacher left, and no school now exists within eight kilometres for the children of the near 120 families of the area.

Pai Khan is a small village of about 30 households. It is in the jurisdiction of Muhmand Agency, but populated by *Aseel Utman Khel*, Bajaur people. It is on sloping land surrounded by mountains on three sides, the fourth leading to the main road, ten kilometres away. The village lacks all facilities, with no electricity, roads, market, school or dispensary. The main means of communication is by foot or pack animal; the nearest market is 20 kilometres away; water is carried by women or pack animals; though in winter some is available from springs and streams, in summer there is insufficient for drinking. Bathing is rare, and the used bath water is kept in a pit for cattle. In medical emergencies villagers put the patient on a stretcher or *kat* and carry him or her for 25 kilometres across the steep mountains to hospital in Ghalanai. Many, including women in labour, die *en route*.

The soil is sandy, made by the torrential rain from the nearby mountains. There is little visible economic activity except for opium production. Agriculture is single cropped, and, apart from opium, mainly comprises barley and mustard, neither of which even begins to offer the economic benefits of opium. Barley is harvested as a grain but, during the severe months of November to February when grass is scarce, is used for fodder, as are mustard husks; though mustard leaves are used as a vegetable, and the seeds crushed to extract oil.

The opium growing areas of *Bajaur Agency (Area B)*, mainly Salarzai on the Pak-Afghan border, Arang and Barang Tehsil, are also mountainous and inaccessible. Salarzai and Arang grow fewer opium poppies than Barang Tehsil, where seven opium villages were identified, of which two, Amankot and Sharbatai, at opposite ends of the Tehsil, were included in the sample. Amankot, like Pai Khan populated by *Aseel Utman Khel*, is 20 kilometres from Agency headquarters, but accessible by means of a non-metalled road. The area has been used for opium growing for a long time, opium being the only possible crop due to the non-availability of irrigation water. Land is scarce, and, overshadowed by Mount Kohimoor, receives little sunshine, particularly in winter. There is a primary school, but no health care, drinking water or electricity. Electricity poles have been erected but local people are pessimistic about getting electricity in the near future. The existing road has been constructed with the help of USAID/NAS, but local people believe the Government's main objective in building it was not welfare but to increase the area's accessibility for its own atrocities.

The Provincial Home Department wrote to all the heads of administration of the poppy growing areas about my visits and asked for every possible help. In mid-March the Political Agent arranged our visit to Amankot. The village elders were informed in advance and the political *Tehsildar Barang* was assigned the duty of escorting me to the village. The *Tehsildar* and I were accompanied by a dozen local levy personnel, and official vehicles were provided by the Agent. This was a very formal visit, the locals having been briefed in advance what to say about poppy production. Eight respondents had been preselected for sampling and were present on the spot. Interviews started in the presence of the *Tehsildar* but it quickly became apparent that the answers were prompted and pre-planned. Many farmers praised the local administration and Pakistani Government for solving their problems, though some implausibly exaggerated and others understated the income from opium production. Often the *Tehsildar* answered on behalf of the respondent. Due to his official status and mine as a guest it was impossible to request him not to represent the farmers, although intervention was clearly detrimental to the study. Accordingly, after the fourth interview I thanked the *Tehsildar* and asked to go back. He was co-operative and sincere, but did not understand research, so I had to make other arrangements.

After three days, on 19 March 1997, I went into the village without escort, heading straight for the school, where a teacher was known to me through friends. I introduced myself as an ex-teacher of the Government High School in Khar and a university teacher at present, and explained the purpose of my visit. We made another list of cultivators, and new respondents were selected, this time from three adjoining sub-villages, Aseel Targhao, Tar and Anjokai. By the evening we had conducted two interviews. The next day we interviewed three more people in the poppy fields while they were hoeing. A further three agreed to come to Khar Bajaur for interview rather than be interviewed that day, and by 21 March two of these interviews had been successfully completed.

Sharbatai, also selected for data collection, is away from Bajaur Khar, being closer to Malakand Agency, across the River Swat. Two students of the University of Peshawar, Usmani Gul and Javed Khan, of Jolagram village, Malakand Agency, had relations in Sharbatai and they accompanied me there. It was the second week of May, very hot and with a temperature of over 40°C. Sharbatai is surrounded by steep barren mountains on all sides, and, due to its closed location, is very hot and suffocating in summer. Recently, with the help of USAID, the Government has started a road from the bank of the Swat to the village, which, however, will be of no use unless a bridge is constructed, only one person at a time being able to cross the present suspension bridge. The village has no electricity, hospital or dispensary. There are separate primary schools for boys and girls and a new middle school. Water is scarce: irrigation water is not available and spring water is for drinking only. The springs are owned by local people, the biggest spring being in the lands of the village chief who, because he stores the water for agricultural purposes, has the best crops.

Nine respondents were selected, with the help of Karim Khan, the son of the village chief and himself an interviewee. The interviews took three days only, but the near unbearable heat made this the most difficult part of all the fieldwork.

In *Dir District (Area C)* opium is cultivated in the eastern valleys of Karo, Nihag Dara and Usherai Dara. There was no problem of access to the area as I belong to one of the local tribes, Sultan Khel. Two of these valleys, Nihag and Usherai, were selected randomly to yield the necessary 19 interviewees, one village from each, Aligasar and Badalai, being selected by lot.

Arrangements for data collection from Aligasar, Usherai Dara, were made for February 1997, immediately after Ramadhan and the month of the General Election which followed the dissolution of the Assemblies and termination of the Government in November 1996. On 15 February, known local elders were contacted for help in gaining access to Aligasar, eight miles from the main Usherai road, itself only jeepable. But by grave misfortune that night herbicide spraying had occurred by, it was locally believed, agents of the Narcotics Affairs Section (NAS) of the US Embassy in Islamabad, and farmers had blocked the main road in protest. District officials were there to quell trouble, and paramilitary forces and a heavy contingent of police were deployed, while the heavily armed local people had occupied strategic positions on the surrounding mountains. A campaigning candidate from the ruling party came to negotiate – a long and tortuous process – and though on the assurance of the authorities that no further crops would be destroyed the blockade was ended, data collection would have been not only dangerous but against local conventions. Hence no data could be collected.

The next step, on 8 March, was to go to Badalai, an isolated area of Nihag Dara, high in the mountains, about 6,000 feet above sea level, by an irregular jeepable road constructed by local people themselves. Badalai, the largest village of the area, with 380 households and a population of 5,000, is isolated and lacks all amenities except two recently constructed primary schools, one of them constructed by the then Provincial Assembly member from his quota of development works,[9] and a middle school for boys. There is no electricity, though ample snowfall ensures abundant water. While most people go to urban areas of the country in search of livelihood, the major occupation of those who stay behind is logging. Hence, aided and abetted by the new road, the destruction of forests has accelerated. Nine to ten respondents were required from Badalai. A local elder, Mulvi Muhammad Sherin, alias Baba, a scholar and former member of the District Council, was our host and resource, and with his support, and by going to interviewees' houses, data collection was completed in two days.

As our friends in Usherai Dara advised us not to go into Aligasar, the locals being still in search of those who had sprayed their crops, data were collected instead from the Karo Dara area, close to my own village. The area is typical of opium growing areas, with its lack of basic facilities other than primary schools, isolated location and absence of all sources of livelihood except subsistence agriculture. A visit was made and five villages with opium poppies identified, from which one, Manai, was selected by lot. A list of cultivators was easily prepared as most residents were known to me personally. Nine respondents were selected by lot, and data collection was completed in three days.

Stratum 2: Tribal Leaders and Opinion Formers in Khyber Agency

This stratum comprised ten respondents, five active in local politics (as members or supporters of a political party, market committee leaders or *khel* [lineage] leaders), and five educated persons, mainly civil servants in the Provincial or Federal Government. The latter were selected purposively, preference being given to those who were indigenous and who had knowledge of all the changes that had taken place in the area. Because educational levels are very low, Government servants are few and widely known. Interviews sought to establish details of heroin production, its impact on the local economy and the role of the political administration in the drug business.

Access to Khyber Agency was achieved through an ex-student of the Social Work Department at Peshawar University, Muhammad Islam Afridi, presently a senior official with the Narcotics Control Division of the Federal Government. Afridi belongs to the Zakha Khel tribe, which comes from an area famous for heroin processing and for containing international drug traffickers. He introduced us to many elders, of whom five were selected. The remaining five persons, including our resource person, were interviewed in Peshawar and Islamabad.

Except for a metalled road leading from Peshawar to Afghanistan, the entire area except Jamrud and Landikotal lacks basic necessities. Water in Landikotal is scarce, and people bring it from springs near the border check post, about six kilometres from the main bazaar. The existing water supply is only meant for officers of the political administration.

Because no authoritative work exists on the history and politics of drug production in the Province, or indeed Pakistan as a whole, *Stratum 3* comprised 16 Opinion Formers and Intellectuals in NWFP. These comprised two each of rural sociologists, anthropologists, economists, historians, serious journalists, political scientists, psychologists and law enforcement personnel.

Part B: Some Ethnographic Data

The sampled area is occupied by *Pukhtoon* (whose language is *Pukhto*), *Pushtoon* (*Urdu, Baluchi*), *Pathans* (English) and Afghans (Persian, *Pushto*). The main tribe is divided into many sub-tribes, *qam* or *qaum*, the largest social unit (now each one a tribe by themselves). Each occupies a specific territorial area and has a distinct dress and dialect of the *Pukhto* language. The *qam* is further divided into sub-tribes or *Khels*, a collection of a few extended families. An extended family is called a *Koranai or Khandan*. *Pukhtoons* mostly live in joint families, where parents and their married sons and their children live together under the same roof so long as compatibility permits.

They live a tribal life, largely unchanged over the centuries, and behaviour is largely governed by formal and traditional laws and tribal codes, *Pukhtoonwali*. Various cultural practices keep the *Pukhtoons* always indebted to each other. A *Pukhtoon* will keep a good gun before having good food; he will keep and save money to feed his guest and reciprocate his social obligations before having a good life himself; he will sell land before allowing his women to work for money. Federal laws are contrary to such cultural practices but a corrupt judicial system encourages the people to decide their matter themselves either through a *Jargah* or a rifle. An outsider may initially think *Pukhtoon* society lawless and disorganized, but these unwritten laws in fact keep it generally peaceful and organized.

The central concepts are *Gherat* (honour, associated with bravery or defending one's ego), *Nang* (associated with sacrifice, unconditional support or obligation) and *Izzat* (respect associated with the ego of a person). If a *Pukhtoon* utters the words '*Khabara da Izzat da*' his words of honour, he will not change his position even if his initial decision was unwise. The greatest insult to a *Pukhtoon*, and for which he will kill, is to be called a '*Begherata*' (a person who lacks courage to take revenge) or '*Dala*' (a person dependent upon others), as these signify someone acting against, or failing to respect, social norms. *Pukhtoonwali* has specific features, including *Jargah* (tribal council), *Melmastia* (hospitality or the honourable use of material goods), *Hujra* (men's guest house), *Badal* (vendetta, revenge or exchange), *Toor* and *Peghoor* (stigma and sarcasm), *Tarboorwali* (kinship, lineage system or power blocks within a *Khel* competing for power and prestige) and *Nanawati,* (arrangements for an apology through mediators by a wrong doer).

These concepts have deep meaning and embody feelings of social stratification and adherence to custom and tradition. *Pukhtoons* are patriarchal, patrilineal and patrilocal. They claim their descent to a common ancestor in Afghanistan, and in theory all *Pukhtoons* are equal: everybody with his name on the genealogical chart of the *khel* has a right to inheritance, no matter how small. The village area encompasses all lands over which *Khels* have ownership rights. These are defined in terms of measurement units like '*Motai*', '*Rupai*', '*Piasa*' and '*Nimakai*'. The total number of shares relates to the whole of the village area. Each type of arable land, whether annually or seasonally irrigated or rain fed, is geographically divided. Communal land, *Shamelat*, is normally left for pasture, graveyards and mosques, as well, more recently, as for schools and other official buildings. *Shamelat* areas are not divided.

The joint family system gives strength to the family, and having a large number of males in a *Khel* family is socially desirable. All earners contribute to the family purse, kept by the head of the family, the father or the elder brother, and each obtains according to his needs, irrespective of earning status. Differences between father and sons and between elder and younger brother are observed. Marriages are arranged, and preference is given to marriage within the family as this does not involve the transfer of the daughter's or sister's property share and can settle outstanding feuds, as the exchange of girls in marriage bringing two parts of the family closer. Marriages and other ceremonies are celebrated with pomp and show promoted by a sense of competition, and excessive expenditure is always incurred.

Pukhtoon society is highly stratified. *Khans* are the most powerful people, with most of the lands in the area and other sources of wealth in their possession. *Maliks* are second to *Khans* and possess political as well as economic power. Ordinary *Pukhtoons* are those who have their names on the *Khel* genealogical chart and have inherited nominal lands but have no other sources of income than their labour on the small family lands. Land ownership groups with rights often consist of more than one *Khel.* The division of the village into groups to whom rights or shares are given takes place on the basis of kinship, place of living in the main village, or on a *Khel* basis, normally to give each *Khel* access to the same class or quality of land.

The lower classes are *Kasabgars* or professional people, including *Nai* (barbers), *Shakhel* (sieve and thorn makers) *Dam* (musicians), *Jola* (weavers) and *Chamyar* (cobblers). *Kasabgars* are paid in kind at each harvest and have no rights of property unless the Pukhtoon do not want to buy from each other. Outside these two groups is another class of sacred or religious people, *Astanadar*. These consist of a number of sub-groups – *Sayyeds* (the highest religious class who are the descendants of the holy prophet Muhammad through his daughters Fatima and cousin and son-in-law Ali), *Miagans* (the descendants of a recent saint who may or may not be a Sayyed) and *Akhunzadas* (religious people descendants of a pious person of local fame). Even more than in Pakistan as a whole, religion is a pervasive influence in *Pukhtoon*, who introduced Islam to the area around AD 1,000. Members of the *Ulema* religious scholars are called *Mullahs, Mulvis, Maulanas, Mufti* and *Imams.*

Mulvi Sahib or *Maulana Sahib* and *Mufti Sahib* are titles given to those who have acquired command in religious matters and have graduated from a *Madrasa* or seminary, and who can interpret religious laws and related matters. A *Mullah* belongs to a *Mullah* family and may or may not be a scholar; the term *Imam* has many meanings but can be a person who leads the daily prayers in the mosques or a paid official in charge of the mosque. The incomes of *Imams* and *Akhuns* are not secure and may be paid out of voluntary funds or just at the time of harvest.

Political groups within a community are called *Dhala* or power blocs. The creation of a power bloc leads immediately to the creation of rival blocs. To take a village decision the two parties have to agree, but one party will always oppose initially if the other is in favour. Each other's positions are approached with suspicion, though cooperation can be achieved, for example by the creation of joint interest. As *Pukhtoons* are always in conflict, either with each other or with an outside body, these situations maintain unity for collective defence.

Political issues are decided by a *Jargah*, the grand assembly of local men. The composition and nature of a *Jargah* varies. Among the Afridis and Shinwaries of Khyber Agency and Muhmand Agency, people sit in a circle, with no head of the council, arguing out the matter in hand until resolution. Among the Yousafzai in Dir, a *Jargah* is a temporary body comprising the representatives of the major power blocs, and with a universally acceptable composition. *Jargahs* have the two main tasks of problem solving and regulation, to prevent problems from happening or from getting out of hand if they do.[10]

Turning to hospitality, *Melmastia*, 'wealth is not for amassing, but for use and basically without importance, that only the weak man is attached to property and makes himself dependent on it.'[11] Hospitality is reciprocal, and though its appropriate form varies it normally involves allocating publicly accessible space, normally a special men's house or sitting room. *Melmastia* involves conduct that can be publicly judged – for example the host can exhibit competence in management, resources and status, particularly the reliance others place on him – and it facilitates the conversion of wealth into political influence. A *Hujra* or men's house is where all the men of the community gather and entertain themselves and their guests, and where they spend their free time. Unmarried youths confine their activities to the *Hujra* and mostly sleep there; outsiders go straight into *Hujras* to visit their hosts without knocking on the door. A *Hujra*, is a symbol of great political power. It may be maintained by the *Khan* or *Malik* of the village, or collectively. If the *Hujra* is maintained by the lineage, on the visit of a guest the surrounding people bring in prepared food and share it.

Badal, or vendetta, requires retaliation when physical or social injury is done to the prestige of a family. If a family member is killed it is the responsibility of the larger family to take revenge. As a result feuds and factions continue for centuries – *Pukhtoons* say it is not too late to take revenge after a hundred years. *Badal*, however, is not solely negative, and also entails reciprocity of help and support at times of need: food, shelter, physical help or money offered when a person is away from his group and village is remembered and reciprocated to people of that area.

Pukhtoons are very sensitive to their code of honour and tolerate no transgression. Women are kept in *Purdah*, which normally restricts them to housekeeping, though they may also work on the family land if supervised by a male relative, and unprotected women may work in other's households as domestic servants. Women and landed property are the two symbols of honour and shame: insult to a woman is *Toor*, shame and stigma. *Toor* is interpreted very widely, so a stranger cannot ask a young woman about his host or even for travel directions. Any hint of sexual relations between a male and female is a great stigma for the woman's family and can only be expiated with the blood of both those involved. Often, however, only the woman is killed, the man escaping but becoming an absconder for life, unable to return home unless agreement is reached between the two families, often by *Swara*, whereby a woman from the aggressor family marries into the aggrieved family.

In terms of food, wheat, maize and rice are the three most important foodstuffs, extensive agriculture being possible only in Peshawar and Mardan, where cash crops including tobacco and sugar beet and cane are preferred. Maize, once the food of poor people is today the food of farmers only. Rice is common, being quick to prepare and relatively cheap. Broken rice is mostly used in poor families: boiled and salted it is eaten with any *Shoorva* or *Khoorva* (curry) or *Masta* (curd), or butter oil if that can be afforded. Wheat, customarily served as bread – *Dodaii* or *Nan* depending on the language – and served with meat curry or vegetables is the staple diet. Spices are liberally used in food preparation, or used independently as chutney; chillies are crushed and normally eaten with bread.

Only limited quantities of food crops are grown, and local people mainly buy food from markets, spending up to 58 per cent of their income on food. In many rural areas meat eating is exceptional, and people have a diet of spinach, vegetables and buttermilk. Tea is especially common: tea leaves and sugar are boiled, and milk if available is poured into the teapot and boiled again, and then sipped. In many remote households tea and bread are eaten instead of curry; spinach and dried vegetables are staple, pulses and meat being unavailable or costly. Most households keep livestock for milk, either to put in tea or for curd and buttermilk. Buttermilk, especially popular in summer, is the favourite food of farming people, often taken with maize bread wrapped in an onion leaf. Poultry are kept mostly for guests and social occasions; slaughtering a chicken for a guest is both common and important.

Livestock farming is undertaken by up to 90 per cent of households to meet the demand for milk, buttermilk and curd. Cows, oxen and a few sheep and goats are kept in mountainous areas, though most farmers avoid goats and sheep, which are associated with Gujars, a nomadic people who travel with large flocks from high mountain pastures at the end of summer and return at the start of summer. Cows, oxen and buffaloes are kept in the plains for ploughing and breeding, the dung being used for fuel and manure. Land is allocated for fodder production, though the by-products of other food crops like wheat *Bhoos,* and rice *Proorha* or *Palala* are the main winter fodder.

The common dress is *Kamees* and *Partoog* shirt and shilwar or baggy pants, stitched by tailors in the villages or big markets. This shirt is longer than its western counterpart, and generally made with buttons extending only part way down the front. It must be pulled over the head and is not tucked in at the waist. *Swati* or *Chitrali pakool* hats and turbans serve as headgear, though younger people increasingly go bareheaded. *Saplai* are the commonest footwear, though among educated and well off people the use of boots is common. In poor communities people use low quality and non-durable plastic footwear, continuous use of which, it was reported by some respondents, caused chapped heels and skin problems. Women's dress consists of *kamees* and *Partoog* and, outside the house, a big embroidered sheet, *parhoonai*, or tent-like *Burqa*, usually made of light cloth, coloured black, white or tan. The *Burqa* is worn over other garments, completely concealing the wearer's body, but with a square of loose netting in front of the eyes to permit some vision. *Burqa* is normally worn by women of high status and by those women who observe *Purdah* or who prefer to remain inconspicuous in public places. Women in rural areas who work in the fields do not use *Burqa*.

Housing consists of stone walls around a courtyard, followed by a veranda and the rooms, each normally occupied by a family. Inside the house a room is often specified for cattle and fodder, though often people and cattle live in the same room. The walls are of stone, with no cement or mud. Within them are pillars and log beams, so a room of five square yards will have two to three logs. Over the logs are crossed small logs, then leaves covered with earth. There are no windows, but in the roof is a smoke hole. Some people have metal sheets on their roof to avoid water running down during winter rain or snow. There is no concept of a bedroom or living room, though a separate room for guests serves as a sitting room *Bhetak* when guests are present.

Case Studies

Case 1 Mulvi Muhammad Sherin (Baba) of Badalai, Nihag Dara, Dir District

Mulvi Muhammad Sherin alias Baba (elder man), in his fifties, a *Pukhtoon* land owner, is a well known and highly respected political and religious figure in Painda Khel. He belongs to the *Mubarak Khel* clan of the *Painda Khel* tribe. His father was illiterate but sent him to a *Madrasa* (religious school) to get education. He is a very vocal person, and even in official circles is considered someone who can arbitrate any problem. He was elected as a district counsellor in 1990 but encountered difficulties with the other elected members whose sole or main purpose was to amass wealth by any means, and resigned in protest at the attitude of the Chairman of Dir District Council.

Mulvi Sahib lives in a joint family of 12 persons comprising his four sons, four daughters, one daughter-in-law and a grandson and his wife. His two elder sons are illiterate, but he sent his two younger sons to school in the village. The family owns two *jreebs* of terraced land, half cultivable and half cultivable waste (land which only human labour can cultivate, even a bullock being unsuitable). Hence the only possible crop is opium.

No family member has been able to secure a government job in spite of his membership of the District Council – a fact which stands testament to Mulvi Sahib's incorruptibility. The other source of family income is a watch repair shop in the Bazaar Wari, where he and his sons work, but he reported that this yields only about 3,000 rupees ($50) a month. I asked him why he cultivated opium in the face of Government prohibition, and he replied that in March 1996 officials came to discuss substitute crops, but never returned. He said that the officers had claimed the area was opium free, but that foreign governments had proof of cultivation and that the next step would be troop deployment, with the worst possible consequences. Asked about the Islamic position on opium cultivation, Mulvi Sahib said that Islam prohibited no land production. Opium had been cultivated in his village for 100–150 years and was widely used as a medicine, though commercial production began only in the late 1970s. He said the people could not understand how it was that in an Islamic country alcohol could be licensed but opium banned. Since Islam allows believers to eat even the flesh of a dead animal to avoid starvation, even if opium were forbidden growing it would be legitimate where, as was the case in his village, no alternative existed, a view shared by many other scholars as well as the Afghan Government.

Mulvi Sahib described the economics of opium as shown in Table 4.1. The figures include a notional production cost based on the necessity of hiring labour and the 'actual' production cost which assumes labour costs and seeds saved from last year at zero. This is economically incorrect as clearly opportunity costs were involved (Mulvi Sahib and his family would otherwise have been available for hire). It does, however, reflect the perceptions of the cultivators, and these perceptions, not the analysis of western economists, constitute the basis for the decision as to whether to cultivate.

Table 4.1   Mulvi Muhammad Sherin: Production Costs (per *jreeb* of opium poppy)

Costs	
Seeds	75 rupees (used from last year)
Fertilizers (two applications)	550 rupees (purchased)
2 man days ploughing	100 rupees (family labour)
4 man days levelling and breaking clods	200 rupees (family labour)
2 man days sowing	100 rupees (family labour)
12 man days hoeing and weeding	600 rupees (family labour)
10 man days repeat hoeing and weeding	500 rupees (family labour)
10 *punja* (lancing knives)	60 rupees (purchased)
50 man days lancing and gum extraction	3,000 rupees (family labour)
6 man days capsule plucking and breaking; Seed collection	300 rupees (family labour)
Two man days tidying, collection of stalks etc.	100 rupees (family labour)
Net production costs	5585 rupees
Actual production costs	610 rupees

Income	
7 kg gum sold	33,600 rupees
50 kg seeds	600 rupees
3 bags dhoda	150 rupees
Total gross income	34,350 rupees
Net income per jreeb	28,765 rupees
Actual net income per jreeb	33,740 rupees

Case 2   Karim Khan of Sharbatai, Barang Tehsil, Bajaur Agency

Muhammad Karim Khan, the son of the village headman, is in his early twenties and lives in a joint family with his three elder brothers, father, mother, paternal uncle, uncle's wife, five cousins and the family of his elder brother – 30 people in all. The family belongs to the *Aseel* sub-clan of *Utman Khel*. The family has a strong educational tradition and Karim is himself an undergraduate at Government College in Bajaur Agency. The family lands are the most extensive in the village – 27 *jreebs*, of which seven are irrigated by springs, the remaining 20 being rain dependent. Karim's eldest brother and uncle are employed by the political administration and earn 2,000 rupees a month each. His second brother works as a labourer in Karachi in the off season; four men of the family are engaged in agriculture. In terms of grain they are self sufficient other than for rice which they purchase from the local market, their irrigated land producing adequate vegetables, maize, green fodder such as Persian clover, and wheat. Most of the rain-dependent land is cultivated with opium poppies.

Asked why his family cultivated opium, Karim replied by asking innocently how he could otherwise go to college. When asked whether they would continue opium cultivation he nodded affirmatively, but was visibly upset by the question. When further probed he said they did not want to give up opium poppies, but that his brother and uncle would lose their jobs if the family did not comply with the prohibition. Family members would then have to work as labourers somewhere in the country, as he could not afford to buy a government job for himself or his younger relatives.

Regarding the activities of the developmental projects he said they hoped to have a bridge on the river to connect the area with Malakand Agency, and a road to connect them with Agency headquarters, but that no other benefits were anticipated. The nearest electricity was three miles away in Malakand Agency, and the Government would probably make cessation of opium production a condition of extending electricity to *Sharbatai*. Asked how optimistic he was about his future, he said the tribal people had no hope of a good life if the present political system, whereby the rich could obtain anything they wanted by corruption, continued to prevail.

To assess the comparative economic benefits of opium and alternative crops, Karim was asked about the economics of wheat, which on his family's land was grown in close to optimal conditions (see Table 4.2).

Table 4.2   Karim Khan: Production Costs (per *jreeb* of wheat)

Costs	
Seed	75 rupees (stored from last year)
Fertilizers	500 rupees (purchased)
4 man days ploughing/planking/clod breaking	240 rupees (family labour)
2 man days sowing	160 rupees (family labour)
3 man days weeding (used as fodder)	180 rupees (family labour)
2 man days threshing with bulls	120 rupees (bulls borrowed)
Miscellaneous costs	150 rupees (spent)
3 man days irrigating (3 times)	180 rupees (family labour)
Net production costs	1605 rupees
Actual production costs	650 rupees
Income	
Wheat	3,500 rupees
Hay and straw	1,500 rupees
Total gross income	5,000 rupees
Net income per jreeb	3,395 rupees
Actual net income per jreeb	4,350 rupees

Case 3   Salamin Khan, Manrai Village, Karo Dara (Karo Valley)

Salamin Khan, a *Pukhtoon*, belongs to the *Himmat Khel* branch of the *Hussain Khel* clan of *Painda Khel* tribe in Manrai village. He is 30 years old, illiterate like all members of his family, and the youngest brother. His father, an octogenarian, mostly stays in bed, and Salamin is responsible for all family affairs, his other brothers working as miners in Baluchistan. They live in a joint family of 25 people, his step-brother living elsewhere because of strained family relations. Salamin's two *jreebs* of land are segmented into five (*pati* or *barhai*) and jointly cultivated. All the land is irrigated by water channelled by the village people from two miles distant.

Salamin's crops, opium and onions, are the only ones of which he has had experience, and he works alone. His father cannot work, his brothers are away, the women are not allowed to work and there is no one else to help. While wheat does not grow well he can manage onion because (he claims – though the following figures appear to belie this view) it is not labour intensive and yields a reasonable income (which the following figures confirm). Opium, however, is by far the most lucrative cash crop, bringing money for marriage feasts and other celebrations. When told that because opium is banned his family is breaking the law, he said that the head of the village had told him that too, but that the headman cultivates more opium than he, and the villagers take their lead from him. If the Government banned production effectively, people would resist strongly unless they were compensated. His calculation of the economics of one *jreeb* of onion was as shown in Table 4.3.

Table 4.3   Salamin Khan: Production Costs (per *jreeb* of onion)

Costs	
2 man days ploughing/planking/clod breaking	120 rupees (family labour)
2 man days preparing beds	120 rupees (family labour)
Fertilizers	500 rupees (purchased)
Seeds	500 rupees (from last year)
1 man day sowing and irrigation	60 rupees (own labour)
12 man days weeding	600 rupees (family labour)
10 man days preparing land for transplantation	500 rupees (family labour)
10 man days transplanting saplings	500 rupees (family labour
10 man days hoeing, etc.	600 rupees (family labour)
10 10 man days harvesting/cleaning/ sorting	600 rupees (family labour)
Net production costs	4100 rupees
Actual production costs	500 rupees
Income	
1 sale of 50 maunds onions	10,000 rupees
2 sale of onion saplings	1,200 rupees
Total gross income	11,200 rupees
Net income per jreeb	7,100 rupees
Actual net income per jreeb	10,700 rupees

Part C: Data Analysis[12]

Two clusters/areas were identified: areas opium was cultivated, and those where heroin was processed. For Cluster 1 Dir District and Bajaur Agency were selected; and for Cluster 2 Khyber and Muhmand Agencies. These areas are not significantly different ethnically or geographically, but administratively they may be under either Provincial or Federal Government control, and were sampled on this basis.

The first area of enquiry related to family size. For opium cultivation areas, of the 40 respondents 14 (35 per cent) had 1–12 members in their families, 19 (47.5 per cent) had 13–24 and 17.5 per cent had 25 and more members in their families, giving a mean family size of 15.4. When the enquiry was extended to include both clusters, however, significant variations were found to exist, with Dir District having an average family size of 13, Bajaur having 21, Muhmand Agency 23.2 and Khyber Agency 23.8. This variation is probably attributable to geographical remoteness, lack of infrastructural facilities and services, and the local cultural features of revenge (*badal*), inter-family and inter-tribal vendettas (*ghalimi*) and high economic familial interdependencies. Such phenomena increase the need for family strength and cohesion and point to large joint and extended families as a logical response, family members combining their material and non-material resources for survival. Overall, 26 per cent of families had a family size of up to 12 persons, 50 per cent of up to 24, while 24 per cent of respondents had families of more than 25 persons. The average family size of 16.9 in all the drug producing areas and 15.4 in the opium cultivating areas, is well over the average for the country as a whole – 7.8 according to the 1981 census.

Nonetheless, of the 40 respondents in these areas only 31 were (or admitted to being) opium cultivators, and the study does not support the hypothesis that there is a direct correlation between production and family size within these areas. In fact opium cultivation was more common among respondents with small families of 1–12 (92.3 per cent) than among those with more than 13 (of whom 70.2 per cent were cultivators). The numbers were, however, very small, (only 13 respondents had a family size of 1–12) and should not be taken as definitive. A larger scale study might consider using more complex definitions of small and large and creating a more sophisticated typology which takes account of such variables as the gender and ages of the children.

Notwithstanding these findings, both categories of family are, as a result of the joint family system, large by western standards, and large families are necessary for drug production in the area to exist. Opium is a labour intensive crop, needing readily available labour at all stages. In Pakistan, where basic facilities like education are lacking, it is possible for children to labour on small opium farms. In fact, in the absence of alternative industry and other income generating sources the entire family, male, female and children, are available to work on the land at sowing and harvest times. Thus, large families with no other jobs and economic activities actually suit the demands of poppy cultivation very well.

Sixty per cent of the 40 respondents had no education in their families, and in half of those that did the respondent or his children were educated only to primary level (5–6 years schooling). Thus, only eight households had members with more than minimum education such as to give them a chance of securing skilled employment.

Of these, four had completed high school or higher secondary school education (known as Metric or Intermediate level) which qualifies people for government white-collar jobs like school teaching and clerical work, three had first degrees and one a postgraduate qualification.

Education has the latent function of expediting social adjustment and social and geographical mobility. In its absence most people remain at their ancestral villages throughout their lives, never venturing out of the area. They know little or nothing of the external world, its opportunities and challenges, nor about respect for the law – or even what the law is. They remain unquestioningly loyal to their customs and traditions, inclining to fatalism and resistance to the social changes that would inevitably accompany improved facilities. In terms of development, the major negative consequence of the lack of educational opportunity is child labour. Male children in particular are an economic asset and culturally obligated to help their parents earn their bread. Consequently they are kept busy working on their farms, and, other than in Khyber, which is close to the provincial capital Peshawar, where higher education is available, never press for schooling.

In terms of *income*, 36 of the 40 respondents in the drug producing areas (90 per cent) fell in the lowest income category of less than 10,000 rupees per month. Three families had a monthly income of 11,000–20,000 rupees, with only one family's income exceeding 20,000 rupees. The mean monthly income was 6,300 rupees ($102). The monthly *per capita* income level was similar throughout the drug growing areas, at 6500 rupees per family or 500 per head in Dir District, 6,125 rupees per family or 330 per head in Bajaur Agency, and 7500 rupees per family or 320 per head in Muhmand Agency. In Khyber Agency, where there is currently no agriculture at all, the local people depending on transborder trade, people had a comparatively higher level of income at 11,500 rupees per family per month or 469 rupees per head. The figures for Dir, Bajaur and Muhmand areas are broadly consistent with estimates by independent foreign experts.

Of the 31 opium cultivators 24 (77 per cent) had a family income of no more than 6,000 rupees against 70 per cent of all respondents (28/40), and the p value of the chi-square test (0.05) supports an association between low family income and opium cultivation. Further, 85.7 per cent of low income families cultivated opium, against 58.3 per cent in the high income group; expressed differently, of those who did not cultivate opium, 55.6 per cent were in the high income group, even though the high income population was smaller.

Turning to *expenditure* levels, 31 of the 40 respondents in the drug producing areas (77.5 per cent) spent up to 10,000 rupees while the remainder spent no more than 20,000. Average family expenditure was 7,362 rupees as compared to the average family income of 6,300, a significant mean deficit of 1,062 rupees per family, likely to result from the practice of lavish expenditure on major social occasions. Accordingly debt and poor living are endemic. In Dir District and Bajaur Agency almost all respondents belonged to the first expenditure group (94.7 per cent and 93.8 per cent respectively); in Muhmand the figure was 80 per cent. In the non-drug producing Khyber Agency, however, the percentage of respondents (50 per cent) in the first group was much less, with 30 per cent spending up to 20,000 rupees and 10 per cent spending more than this.

The hypothesis that high expenditure is associated with opium cultivation is supported with a p value of 0.05: a majority (58.1 per cent, or 18/31) families in the low expenditure group were cultivators, against 13/31 or 41.9 per cent high income respondents. Of non-cultivators, 22.2 per cent were in the low expenditure group and 77.8 per cent in the high expenditure group. The probability value of the chi-square test therefore supports an association between family expenditure and opium cultivation.

Landholding size is a crucial determinant of status in NWFP: the greater a man's landholding the greater his social and political influence. Conversely, according to local custom a landless person, even though he may speak *Pushtu*, is not a true *Pakhtoon*. Eight out of 40 respondents in the drug producing areas owned less than one *jreeb* of land, almost half (19) owned 1–10 *jreebs*; 13 had more than 10 *jreebs*, of whom eight possessed more than 21 *jreebs*. The mean *jreebage* per family was 9.8, or 0.6 *jreeb per capita*, and though this varied between 4.7 *jreebs* in Dir District (where irrigation was normally possible) and 19.5 *jreebs* in Muhmand Agency (where it was not), everywhere the mean *per capita jreebage* was less than one. On average the total irrigated land per family was 0.85 *jreebs*, and rain dependent land was 9.75 *jreebs*.

Nonetheless, in this very small-scale study the chi-square shows no relationship between the size of land holding of the family and opium cultivation. Though 71 per cent of the opium cultivators were in the small land holding group, this simply reflects the fact that the majority of respondents as a whole owned no more than 10 *jreebs*. Of the nine respondents who did not cultivate opium, five were among the small land holding group.

Why Opium?

Without unrealistic, probably ecologically damaging and, in some areas, impracticable mechanization, in most of the drug producing areas the quantity of cultivable land cannot be increased or improved. Its usage, too, is very limited – it is, for example, unsuitable for cereals – so it will inevitably remain at a premium, and opium cultivation will continue to be uniquely economically attractive. Climate is also crucial, opium being a drought resistant crop needing little irrigation and offering the highest yield in the cold temperatures of the mountainous regions. Hence many factors combine to create a predisposition to opium cultivation. Of these, the main ones are land scarcity, poor land quality, large families, ancient cultivation traditions, favourable climatic conditions, lack of alternative income sources, physically inaccessible location near the national borders, the tribal areas' legally ambiguous status and the corruptibility of officials at all levels. On the other hand, people in the plains areas, where the prohibition of opium cultivation is accepted, do not face the same set of circumstances, their lands being vast, irrigated, and fertile, with landholding sizes considerably larger and adequate to feed a family. Literacy levels are also higher and there is access to such urban benefits as jobs, government employment, education, other sources of livelihood and health facilities. The other key inhibitor to opium cultivation in these areas is that they are visible and accessible to law, and any illegal activity can therefore be easily detected. Both because opium cultivation is labour intensive and because most farmers lack the resources for additional land or labour, production is almost always small scale. All but one of our respondents were owner cultivators, though a very small number of tenants and share croppers (who cultivate another's land in return for equal distribution of the yield) do exist.

Faced with a multiple choice question about the reasons for opium cultivation, 29 of the 31 respondents in the drug growing areas who were themselves cultivators gave soil and climatic conditions as the main reasons why opium was cultivated there. The land is hard and stony, and inhospitable to other, particularly summer, crops as it cannot retain moisture. Poppy, on the other hand, as a highly drought resistant plant, can cope with mainly rain dependent conditions in the absence of widespread irrigation. Similarly the mountainous terrain influences the size and shape of the small poppy fields which cannot be mechanized or levelled to produce other crops: human labour and bull-ploughs are the only sources of power that can cultivate these lands. In the high mountainous areas in Dir District, some tracts which receive insufficient sun are termed 'cold' lands, capable only of producing poppy. In more hospitable areas, because poppy has the advantage of an early harvest and is believed not to deplete the soil, it leaves the land available for summer crops such as maize. If such lands were cultivated with cereal crops such as wheat, the lateness of the harvest (in late July) would be such that the land could not be cultivated a second time.

In Bajaur Agency all respondents cited land structure and climatic conditions as reasons for opium cultivation. Whereas in Dir rainfall is reasonable, in Bajaur the cultivating areas are totally dry and rain dependent. The only possible means of irrigation is tube-wells, an unrealistically costly process as these need electricity, which is unavailable, and which, even if it were not, could not be afforded by farmers many of whom cannot even afford a pair of bullocks. In parts of Muhmand Agency there is no water at all for drinking and washing, and respondents here were unanimous that poverty, remoteness, lack of infrastructure and the sandy nature of the land were the main problems they faced.

In addition and unsurprisingly, in every area, all respondents pointed to opium's uniquely remunerative return and, from the fact that respondents' average income from opium is 10,375 rupees per crop, it is clear that this is the main reason for opium cultivation. While the absolute per *jreeb* figures from the case studies of gross returns of 34,350 rupees for opium, 11,200 rupees for onion and 5,000 rupees for wheat are much higher than 'guesstimate' data provided in response to less precise questioning, the relativities are unlikely to mislead seriously.

Geographically there were differences in income from opium. In Dir District, where average landholdings were smaller than the rest of the drug producing areas, the average income from opium was 6842 rupees, while in the rest of the areas the income was two or three times more than that of Dir. In Bajaur Agency it was 12,183 rupees, and in Muhmand Agency 18,000 rupees. In Khyber Agency, where the people have given up agriculture as unprofitable, or at least less profitable than heroin, no opium has been grown for the last 10 to 15 years. Nine of the 31 respondents, however, advanced reasons other than these. These reasons included political justifications such as official corruption in relation to overseas development aid, the hypocrisy of Pakistani governments which, when in power, oppose opium cultivation but support it when in opposition, and hostility towards consumer countries seen as attacking Muslim morality by exporting alcohol to Pakistan. Proponents of the latter view basically regarded narcotics export as a well-deserved *quid pro quo*.

This question was designed to test the attitude of opium cultivators toward government policy on opium cultivation. Attitudes are contagious and can help determine the future of opium production. The Government targeted 1997 as the year by which poppy cultivation would be eradicated, but according to a US Government report, by that year cultivation was actually occurring in areas that were free from cultivation just a few years previously.[13] Respondents expressed various attitudes: over three-quarters were rebellious, openly rejecting the law (or claiming, acerbically, never to have heard of it), saying they were masters of their own lands and cursing government officers for accepting money from western countries for themselves in return for prohibiting cultivation. All but one of the 31 respondents said the law was against the interests of the people, saying they grew opium as a sure source of survival. If the Government could not provide them with the basic necessities why should it take their own bread out of their mouths? Sixteen respondents believed that in the tribal area where Pakistan's regular or criminal law is not applicable the Government was not legally empowered to ban opium, and that the 1979 Hudood Ordinance was therefore *ultra vires*.

These responses combine the economic and the political, illustrating all too clearly the distance and, in particular, the lack of trust, between rulers and ruled in Pakistan. The people expect their public representatives to be instrumental in helping them with 'private' problems such as securing a job, but the politicians and government functionaries consider the public as subjects not citizens, often treating them with ill-concealed contempt. Law-making seldom proceeds with public consent, and is often against the public will.

Finally, eight of the ten respondents in the non-opium cultivating Khyber Agency were of the opinion that heroin was being processed there. Six of these eight respondents attributed this to the impact on local businesses of the Soviet-Afghan conflict, which had led many local businessmen to switch to drug production; though two respondents believed the two phenomena to be unrelated. Two respondents also said that the war had had no effect on the drugs business in Khyber Agency, or on their own business either. The probability value of 0.42 does not provide evidence that those interviewed believed that the Afghan war led to increased drug production in the area.

Conclusion

Most of NWFP is occupied by a large ethnic group, *Pukhtoons*, who live in both settled and tribal areas, with a code of life based on *Pukhtoonwali*, unwritten customary laws prevalent for centuries, and including the concepts of vendetta, guest house, lineage system and hospitality.

Pukhtoons have a rigid social differentiation based on a class (but not caste) system. The dominant class comprises landowners, of whom the most senior are the *Khans*, followed by the *Maliks*. There is also a class of sacred people with religious responsibilities, the *Astanadars*, comprising *Sayyeds*, descendants of the holy prophets, *Miangan*, descendants of a *Sayyed* or non-*Sayyed* saint of great fame, *Mullahs* and *Akhunzadas*. The *Astanadars* have the use of land, *Serai*, given to them by the *Pukhtoons* for their sacred services.

The *Khel*, the centre of all social and political activities, controls all inter village and supra-village activities and politics, and is also the nucleus of interpersonal relations. The *Hujra* or guest house is the place where all the male activities take place. It is an entertainment centre for the younger people and a dormitory for many unmarried men. *Hujra* is maintained by a *Khan* or *Malik*, or collectively by the *Khel* or *Cham* or *Kandai* or *Palo* depending on the socio-economic and political status of a person or persons. *Melmastia*, another salient feature of the *Pukhtoons* of NWFP, means the honourable use of material goods and space, implying the offer of food and shelter and meeting any other need of a visitor by the host. Hospitality and *Hujra* are also used for gaining political influence. *Badal*, though having mostly the negative sense of taking revenge or vendetta, also has a positive dimension, signifying reciprocity or exchange. An insult or loss to some one or a good at a time of need is always remembered and reciprocated. The *Jargah*, or grand council, is the forum where all males have equal rights and are allowed to present their viewpoint.

These features of *Pukhtoon* culture keep the people busy and alert, co-operative and submissive to fellow people. While social changes mean that the practice of *Hujra* is giving way to drawing rooms and guest rooms, the remaining customs still exist, particularly in rural areas where change is slow.

Wheat, barley, maize, mustard, onions and opium are the major crops. Land possession is very small; grain is seldom economic, particularly in high altitude farms, though wheat is a staple food in the plain, and wheat and maize are popular in many rural areas. Other crops are sown either for food or fodder. Opium yields three to ten times more income than other crops, and the case studies, for all their technical limitations, offer at least an approximation of the comparative yields from opium, wheat and onion. Given that the mean annual family income is around 6,300 rupees and expenditure 7,362 rupees, opium's economic importance becomes clear, and the solution to the 'problems' it appears to present ever more elusive.

But is opium cultivation properly seen as a 'problem' and if so, of what kind and for whom? In the next chapter we address these questions, and whether the solution does in fact lie in prohibition, or whether an alternative approach, ranging from, at one extreme, legalization through decriminalization to regulation involving licensing and inspection, is more practical, and indeed desirable. Attempting to eliminate a global trade involving impoverished suppliers, affluent, determined and sometimes clinically addicted consumers, internationally organized criminals and, when it suits their *Realpolitik*, first world governments, is a heroic endeavour; indeed, one which has about it, perhaps, a slight hint of tilting at windmills. But prohibition may also be damaging, to the suppliers themselves obviously, but also to the political process in supplier countries. This is both because drugs become as much a focus for the corruption of government officials and a pollutant of the polity itself as was the silver mine in a fictitious Latin American country in Joseph Conrad's epic novel *Nostromo*. And, because the act of suppression can destabilize internal peace and security, the 'drug problem' can, and frequently does, create civil unrest among producers, contributing to their further alienation from the political process and to the increased involvement of organized international criminals.

Notes

1   Where the first person is used in this chapter it invariably refers to the first author.
2   F. Barth, *Political Leadership Among Swat Pathans* (London: Athlone Press, 1953). p120.
3   S. Sen 'Heroin Trafficking in the Golden Crescent'. *Police Journal* (July–September 1992). pp251–6.
4   *Far Eastern Economic Review* (Hong Kong: 13 June 1995). p97.
5   United Nations, *Poppy Cultivation in Pakistan: Briefing Note* (Islamabad: Drug Control Programme, 1996). p1.
6   I. Haq, *From Hashish to Heroin* (Lahore: Al-noor Printers and Publishers, 1991). p27. See also Government of Pakistan, *Resource and Reference Manual for Prevention Resource Consultant Network* (Islamabad: Drug Abuse Prevention Resource Centre, 1995).
7   Government of Pakistan, *Buner Agriculture Development Project: The Buner Model 1976-86* (Islamabad: Narcotics Control Board, 1986). p22.
8   The limitations of the methodology are discussed in Asad 2000 *op. cit.* and are not rehearsed in detail here.
9   Construction of such institutions in tribal areas is made under an agreement with the Government, whereby the seller of the land either becomes the contractor or two members of his family are employed on the project. Consequently, most constructions are substandard, and buildings meant for schools or dispensaries are considered more the personal property of the family than public buildings.
10   F. Werter, *Cultural Values, Land Management and Land Degradation* (Saidu Swat: Malakand Social Forestry Project, November 1994). p10.
11   F. Barth, *op. cit.* 1953. p121.
12   This is an abbreviated account of the data analysis only. In the original thesis (Asad 2000) (*q.v.*) the discussion is supported by 19 tables. Except where otherwise stated, this analysis refers to Stratum A (opium farmers and cultivators) only.
13   *Daily Jang* (London: 22 February 1998).

Chapter V

Dilemmas of Control

This chapter is divided into two parts. The first rehearses attempts made at, respectively, national and international level to control the spread of opium and its derivatives, and discusses the obstacles they have faced and the extent to which they have been overcome. The story is not encouraging, these attempts having all too often been subverted by national *Realpolitik* and personal corruption. In cases such as crop spraying the cure may have been worse than the disease, leading as it has to breakdowns in civil order and political trust. Further, artificially disrupting the market in opiates in one part of the world often leads only to market distortion elsewhere. Such is the global nature of the trade that a change of policy in Iran impacts directly on the political economy of drug production in Pakistan and Afghanistan. The ripple effect of civil strife in one country, funded by drug money, can have a transformational effect on the geopolitics of production and supply elsewhere.

In the second part of the chapter we reflect more broadly on the notion and philosophy of control. Are the problems encountered in this case study insurmountable? Is there, within a national or international control policy, a set of options that would do more good than harm? Or is an entirely different framework necessary? 'Control' carries different meanings: it can be, and in this field often is, synonymous with suppression, even prohibition. But an alternative meaning is regulation – bringing the production and supply of opiates within an expanded legal sphere. Control in this regulatory sense already exists in many countries at an individual level by registration; is it necessary, feasible or desirable for this principle to be extended to production and supply at a national or even international level? These are questions we apply to the situation in Pakistan.

It is fair to say that our conclusion as to the recommended way forward for Pakistan, while it gains support from the fieldwork, reported in the last chapter, does not derive from it. The fieldwork offers illumination and explanation, but it is of itself insufficiently wide in scope or sophisticated in method to justify major policy proposals. Such proposals are nonetheless buttressed by the empirical data.

Part A: Control Attempts at National and International Levels

The National Effort: Pakistan

Pakistan is signatory to all UN conventions on drug production, trafficking and addiction, accepting an obligation to check illicit opium and heroin production within her territorial jurisdiction and to check heroin addiction. In particular, following the introduction of the Hudood Ordinance in 1979, Pakistan embarked on a two-pronged strategy to combat addiction through demand side reduction involving improvements in treatment and rehabilitation and criminal sanctions, as well as a range of control measures on the supply side. So far as demand side reduction is concerned, there is an almost complete lack of treatment and rehabilitation facilities, with only 200 treatment centres for three million addicts[1] (one per 15,000 addicts), and detoxification the only approach nationally available. As a result, sepsis due to scars and wounds made by begging addicts to arouse public sympathy, unhygienic living conditions among beggars who live on or near garbage dumps and other unclean places, hepatitis and other liver diseases contribute to high premature death rates among addicts. Corruption among politicians and law enforcement agencies has deterred the widespread use of criminal sanctions, though these would, anyway, have little impact on the problem other than as part of a coordinated effort including also treatment and rehabilitation. But there is a great scarcity of health resources, and such resources as do exist are unevenly distributed between and within provinces. Further, rehabilitation needs training, job placement and employment, but, with a youth employment rate of 46 per cent and a basic education rate of 26 per cent, the scope for funding rehabilitation is slight. Nor is there any political capital in diverting resources into drug rehabilitation, and since rehabilitating more than two million heroin addicts is well beyond the capacity of the state anyway – attempting to do so would simply cause embarrassment by bringing the problem into international focus. Accordingly, Pakistan lacks rehabilitation programmes[2] in spite of the speed with which addiction is increasing: there is said to be a new addict every five and a half minutes[3] on the face of the CNS Act (Control of Narcotics Substances) 1997.

NWFP has just ten public sector detoxification units and six private sector maintenance clinics for an addicted population of 589,000, which includes 223,000 heroin users. Public sector drug treatment centres have 120–140 beds, but official statistics show very low admission rates, figures indicative of a striking lack of commitment to addressing the problem. Even if used to the maximum, however, 140 beds would be grossly incommensurate with the number of addicts; as it is, their impact is minimal. Detoxification is also carried out through outdoor treatment, however. This can involve conventional western medicine as well as *tibbi unani*, homeopathy and acupuncture, though no figures exist as to their rehabilitative efficacy. In addition, many patent anti-drug medicines, marketed by both genuine and fake firms and *hakeems*, some themselves laden with opium, have flooded the market.

So far as supply side control is concerned, on a national level supply itself fuels demand.[4] So whereas demand side measures, punitive or therapeutic, would, even if effective, merely hold the problem at bay, effective prevention requires supply side attrition. Two quotations illustrate the point:

> . . . the greater the availability of a drug in a society, the more people are likely to use it, and the more they are likely to run into problems with it[5]

> Availability affects the degree of use and acceptance into the culture. . . Production and cultivation of the substance is commonly a consequence of the cultural influence, but may

also influence the rate of acceptance. As availability increases, use tends to increase. Further, when it is difficult to obtain one drug, another drug may be substituted.[6]

Four kinds of availability have been identified: *physical, social* (the extent to which drug use is socially sanctioned), *psychological* (an individual's personality, characteristics, beliefs) and *economic* (whether drugs are affordable). All four are present in Pakistan. In the early days, heroin was sold in shops in the tribal area as an everyday commodity, but today it is readily available in all major cities, small towns and even rural areas and villages.[7] In 1982, US Attorney-General William French Smith was surprised when one of his aides saw heroin samples displayed in a public market near Peshawar,[8] and in similar vein a Pakistani expert spoke of:

> . . . its easy availability on stops on national highways from Peshawar to Karachi and other connecting routes as well as in cities and towns in Pakistan . . . producers and manufacturers for their economic profits operate to promote the spread and continued use of drugs. The skills and intelligence they bring to task of promoting the spread of drugs in opposition to law enforcement agencies successfully impair the effectiveness of control system.[9]

Economically, Pakistan probably has the world's cheapest heroin, the street price reaching an all time low till 2000. When, in the early days of production, free samples were distributed in and around Peshawar University to attract youths to the drug, prices were so low that a gram of heroin with 80–90 per cent purity cost only ten rupees.

For a long time the preferred means of combating the problem was crop elimination and destruction. This, however, was naturally resisted by the growers, and a theoretically more acceptable alternative, crop substitution, emerged, in furtherance of which some 4–5 foreign and UN assisted projects were introduced to provide alternative means of livelihood. This was welcomed in many communities, but corruption meant that the projects did less for local development than for the administrators and politicians whom they enabled to amass huge illicit fortunes. When the public raised voices against the corrupt practices of those in power, the policy switched again to eradication, with disastrous personal, social, political and economic consequences. Law enforcers killed many farmers to show their efficiency to donor countries and the international community; helicopters and land forces were used to eradicate the crops in areas easily conquered. Where armed resistance was feared, overnight spraying was undertaken without concern for toxicity. To the researcher's personal knowledge, for example, dichlorophenoxyacetic acid and paraquat were sprayed in spite of the fact that most land sprayed with such herbicides cannot produce any other crop for at least four years. The damage to soil, water, plants and animals, as well as to the farmers themselves and their families, has never been fully assessed, but some experts claim that paraquat causes irreversible lung fibrosis, dermatitis, eye injury and severe nose bleeding.

So why cannot production and addiction be brought under control? What has hindered the law in eliminating these drugs? Is it socio-economic conditions in the drug producing areas, national politics or both that have maintained opium and heroin production? And if politics are involved, are they internal or external? Are there solutions that can overcome these problems?

Clearly economic factors are often crucial in paving the way for a thriving parallel drug market. Drug producing countries have low *per capita* incomes, with numerous people living in poverty, economic resources being available only to those with political power, and widespread corruption and instability:

> Political instability is a major factor in the growth of the illicit drug trade and is one of the biggest obstacles to combating it. In the last twenty years the drug producing countries of Latin America and of southern Asia have all experienced one or more of the following – coup d'etat, revolution, tribal tensions, violent ethnic and/or religious protest, invasion, intensive guerrilla warfare. In materially impoverished, politically turbulent parts of the world, drugs have become the principal currency for the purchase of weapons and[10] as has been proved, the human and organizational structure for the one illicit trade has come to overlap or coincide with the other.

Geography plays a dual role in the production of opium in Pakistan, not only constituting a permanent barrier to land development but also keeping cultivation areas inaccessible to control. The only economic resource of communities in such areas is their small, poor quality land holdings:

> It is a fact the world over that those areas which produce narcotics often lack any government support and basic social services like health, education, communicational infrastructure and security. As a result of these insecurities they make the best use of the only resources available, the land. Poverty is their main cause of all other social problems. They are socially and geographically isolated from the mainstream of the society.[11]

Subsistence agriculture is the main economy of poppy producing areas such as Dir and Buner Districts and Bajaur and Muhmand Agencies, in most of which the lands are dry, rain dependent and single cropping. Agriculture cannot be mechanized and fertilizers and pesticide are beyond farmers' purchasing power:

> It is precisely these countries which have been disadvantaged in the new international global political economy, in part because they have not developed an indigenous industrial or financial commercial class and now rely on whatever agriculture product they can produce with minimal technology. The really powerful demand and highest market price, are for drugs.[12]

In these circumstances it is difficult to detect even a glimmer of light for national control efforts. Demand is fuelled by supply, and supply is created by the economic position of the farmers, the political position of the tribal peoples and geographical inaccessibility. It is then sustained by low and high level corruption, which ensure respectively that local control is ineffective and that finances intended for policies which integrate eradication with substitution are diverted for personal use. But even were they not, such is the economic attraction of drug production and supply that it must be questionable to what extent substitution is a feasible policy.

We have shown that the proposition that opium and heroin are largely produced for local consumption is wrong. Though Pakistan's problems of addiction are increasing exponentially, the main demand for Pakistan's drugs is from first world countries. Without this demand supply would diminish and Pakistan's own addiction rate would begin to decline. So in a global transaction involving an exchange relationship between a powerful first world country and an impoverished, unstable third world country, the financial benefits accruing to the latter from its merchandise come at a high price. Much of the gain is private, public funds being diverted into the pockets of politicians and administrators, but the cost is public: the co-existence of international development funding and drugs has brought organized, international crime and national politics into close proximity. Pakistan's high threshold political corruption has had negative consequences among both the international political and financial communities and potential inward investors. The financial resources of such investors are badly needed if Pakistan is to escape from the vicious circle of daunting social and political problems and inadequate resources to solve them in which it is currently trapped.

Towards an International Framework: Control Efforts in an Historical Context

Drug production is international in character, and it has long been recognized that any solution to it must also, therefore, be internationally conceived and implemented. International control efforts were accordingly initially coordinated by the League of Nations following the First World War. Even under this generally lacklustre and ineffective body, the situation was, at least initially, better than at present, world opium cultivation actually falling from 41,600 to 7,600 tons, and heroin production from 20,000 to 2,200 kg between 1906 and 1934.

However, the *Realpolitik* of later years, particularly the Cold War, effectively protected and developed the business, with control strategies proving subservient to the foreign policies of a developed world community willing to support drug production when drug money funded the military efforts of anti-communist freedom fighters. The potential for poppy locations to be internationally mobile furthered US foreign policy objectives, and poppy power increasingly became a tool in Cold War geopolitical strategy. Hence, while the mid-1960s saw the European heroin industry served predominantly by Turkish opium, by the end of that decade production had shifted to Iran and south-east Asia. The latter shift in particular was caused in good part by US military support for anti-communist guerrilla commanders, notably in South Vietnam, whom they knew to be heroin dealers and manufacturers.[13]

Following the Vietnam War policies changed again and opium production shifted to south-west Asia, particularly Afghanistan, Pakistan, Myanmar and Iran, from where heroin flooded western markets. Again US foreign policy took precedence over any war on drugs it might be inclined to fight, and today's drug boom in Pakistan is largely the product of superpower confrontation, and addiction therefore a by-product of international politics. And though the Soviet withdrawal from Afghanistan heralded a decline in opium production in Pakistan, the anarchy unleashed in Afghanistan precipitated historically unmatched levels of drug production and processing, at least until Taliban eliminated production in those parts of the country which were, relatively briefly, under its control.

Fundamentally, however, international efforts have consistently failed to manage the unintended consequences of attempts to suppress any market where virtually unlimited demand chases elastic supply. These consequences include health problems brought about by lack of product control and user education, and high prices. The nexus of illegality, seemingly limitless demand, low risk of apprehension and high prices offers the promise of profit beyond avarice, ensuring that organized international criminals become active in the supply chain. Accordingly, drug-dependent users become vulnerable to intimidation and blackmail, with many themselves co-opted into the criminal supply chain to feed their habit by recruiting and maintaining new consumers in a business whose logic presently appears relentlessly expansionist.

Historically, these phenomena most obviously occurred in early 20th century USA. As is well known, prohibition, while achieving reductions in narcotic and alcohol usage and creating cultural disapprobation in many parts of the country, did so at the price of paving the way for mass abuse, particularly of black market heroin. This led suppliers to develop codeine as a substitute, but since up to six times more codeine than heroin is required to achieve the same effect, demand for opium, far from declining, actually increased. Opium, a legal drug when today's powerful anti-drug countries were involved in its trade, was prohibited (and publicized so as to induce horror and fear) only when trading passed into the hands of less powerful countries. In the florid language of two observers:

> Governments who capitalise on public shock-horrors have a splendid means of diverting public attention and anger from real issues and for interfering in the affairs of other nations, even to the extent of sending spies and troops.[14]

In February 1909, the United States, which then had no domestic laws regarding narcotics use (though in a face-saving measure, it was quick to pass one), convened a conference in Shanghai, termed the Opium Commission. This Commission, comprising the main countries with interests in the Far East[15], passed resolutions aimed at the gradual suppression of opium smoking, limiting the uses of opium to medical purposes and restricting international trade in opium and its derivatives.[16] US motives for convening this conference were, however, primarily to protect its financial interests and domestic welfare. In the depression of the 1890s Chinese labourers, with whom opium smoking was popularly associated, who had been imported as railroad construction workers in the boom years of the 1870s, were increasingly adjudged an economic threat, and came to experience antagonism and attempts at expulsion. During this period, however, US economic interests in China were increasing, on the ground that 'a pair of shoes sold to each Chinese would keep American shoe factories busy for years'. Accordingly, any expulsion of Chinese labourers would have impacted negatively on its Far Eastern policy, which included increasing its own market share in narcotics. China, however, angry at the treatment of its nationals in the USA, heightened diplomatic tensions between the countries, and the United States hoped to use the Shanghai Conference to soften attitudes.

In fact the Shanghai Conference was less significant for its own activities than for spawning another more important conference in The Hague in 1912. Though this Convention was to lay the foundations for contemporary global attempts at drug control, it saw major differences emerge between the leading players. The US wanted The Hague Convention to lead to official commitments, but the Netherlands and Great Britain, which had no wish to put on the table the lucrative Sino-Indian opium trade which it saw as solely between London and Peking, insisted it be mandated only to make recommendations. In the event The Convention placed heroin in the same category as morphine and cocaine. It imposed an obligation on contracting members to use their best efforts to limit its manufacture, sale and use to medical and scientific purposes, and operationalized 1909 Commission resolutions dealing with international co-operation, trade, law and statistical exchange. In the United States the pace of domestic legislation was also increasing and the Hague Convention was followed two years later by the Harrison Act of 1914, which prohibited doctors from prescribing heroin, morphine and cocaine. The Act was, however, widely ignored, a single illicit New York 'dope doctor' apparently prescribing 68,282 grains of heroin, 54,097 grains of morphine and 30,280 grains of cocaine in a month.[17]

Since World War II, the United Nations has had the main international responsibility for drug policy. Largely funded by powerful consumer countries, however, it is not empowered to exercise independent authority, so, in drug control as in much else, it will remain ineffective unless the western powers extremely improbably choose to pool sovereignty and give it a decisive role. The UN began by instituting a Commission on Narcotic Drugs, and the Commission's attempt, in 1946, to bring all new drugs under full control led to the Paris Protocol of 1948. This extended the control efforts of international organizations to any drug not covered under previous legislation, an approach which, however, failed to address the technological and commercial advances perpetrated by the criminal underworld. A 1953 Protocol again sought to restrict poppy cultivation, production, use and international trade to medical and scientific purposes, and empowered the Permanent Central Opium Board, with the consent of the government concerned, to impose an embargo on the opium trade. The Protocol permitted only India, USSR, Bulgaria, Iran, Greece, Turkey and Yugoslavia to export opium, and Pakistan to cultivate it for domestic use. However, it was widely believed that the international machinery so established was 'more showy than efficient'.[18]

Between 1912–1960 international narcotic laws had grown haphazardly and become unwieldy, and a plenipotentiary meeting was called to discuss all previous international laws on drugs control. This led to the Single Convention of 1961, implemented in 1964, which unified all previous laws and formulated new ones. The Permanent Central Opium Board was renamed the International Narcotic Control Board; emphasis was placed on the treatment and rehabilitation of addicts; opium, coca-leaf and hashish use for non-medical purposes was prohibited; and all narcotics, including cannabis, were put on the control list. A new Schedule IV was created for dangerous drugs such as heroin, deemed devoid of therapeutic benefits, and member states were recommended to prohibit dealing in them. The Convention specified conditions under which cultivation should be banned, but left implementation to national legislation. It prescribed import and export certificates for the transportation of poppy straw, authorised all countries to produce and export up to five tons of opium annually and added new countries, including Afghanistan, Vietnam and Burma, to the exporting countries list.

The Convention's ineffectiveness can be judged from the US refusal to ratify it for six years, largely on the ground that it was more permissive than its predecessors – a step backwards not forwards. In shifting responsibility for control from the UN to national governments, the Convention adopted an approach akin to letting suspected criminals decide whether to be tried, and one which constituted a microcosm of the problem that international organizations (IOs) can move only with the consent of the most reluctant member states. Even sympathetic member states may be reluctant to permit the erosion of national sovereignty in case they are in future forced to accept measures contrary to their national interest, and since the legitimacy of IOs stems from inclusivity, expulsion can be used only in the most extreme circumstances.

It was 11 years before political circumstances changed and the UN was able to replace the 1961 Convention with the 1972 Protocol. This came into force in 1975, with more enthusiastic American support, expanding the powers of the International Narcotic Control Board to limit the illegal traffic, production, cultivation and use of drugs, and providing for treatment and rehabilitation. The Protocol was signed a year after the 1971 Convention on Psychotropic Drugs, which placed psychotropic substances like amphetamines, sedatives, hypnotics and hallucinogens under international control for the first time, so considerably expanding the international drug control system.

Nonetheless, further increases in drug trafficking in the late 1970s led the General Assembly to ask the Commission on Narcotic Drugs to prepare a comprehensive and workable control strategy. This resulted in the 1981 International Drug Abuse Control Strategy. This was a five year plan dealing with every aspect of drug control, including the establishment of a new balance between legitimate drug supply and demand, the eradication of illicit drug production and trafficking, demand reduction, and the treatment, rehabilitation and social reintegration of addicts. The Strategy called for increased inter-governmental co-operation, the participation of non-governmental organizations (NGOs) and intra-UN co-ordination to support member states in law enforcement, crop substitution and preventive education. The General Assembly asked the Commission to consult other interest groups and establish a task force to review, monitor and co-ordinate implementation, and to report annually.

Nonetheless, 1984 saw another wave of trafficking, and the UN responded in two ways. First, the General Assembly resolved that a new international instrument was needed to address aspects of illicit trafficking inadequately covered by existing treaties, and instructed the Commission on Narcotic Drugs to produce a draft convention, which duly appeared in 1985 and was implemented in 1988. It contained 14 Articles, addressing issues ranging from illicit production to narco-money laundering, and was designed both to strengthen international co-operation and institutional co-ordination and to provide effective legal guidelines. Further, terming trafficking and abuse a collective responsibility and an 'international criminal activity demanding greater and urgent attention and maximum priority', the General Assembly adopted the 1984 Declaration on the Control of Drugs Trafficking and Drugs Abuse which declared:

> The illegal production of, illegal demand for, abuse of and illicit trafficking in drugs impede economic and social progress, constitute a grave threat to the security and development of many countries and peoples and should be combated by all moral, legal and institutional means, at all national, regional and international levels.[19]

Reflecting the perceived magnitude of the problem the Secretary General's 1985 report to the General Assembly addressed drug abuse and illicit trafficking, urging the international community to eliminate this 'peril' and proposing a world conference to deal with it. The International Conference on Drug Abuse and Illicit Trafficking in Vienna mandated the UN 'to generate universal action to combat the drug problem in all its forms at the national, regional and international levels'.[20] This led to the Comprehensive Multidisciplinary Outline of Future Activities in Drug Abuse Control 1987 (CMO). Not a formal legal instrument, the CMO was a handbook for nations and interested organizations to be used as a source of ideas, and translated into action in accordance with local circumstances.

What impact did these developments have on Pakistan? First, it had come to be increasingly accepted by the late 1960s that punitive measures could not succeed unless cultivators were offered alternative sources of income[21] and accordingly the United Nations Fund for Drug Abuse Control (UNFDAC) was established in 1971. UNFDAC is a voluntary fund which finances projects designed to put an end to the illegal and uncontrolled production, processing, manufacturing and marketing, through approaches such as crop substitution and law enforcement.

In 1973 the Pakistan Government requested UN assistance in tackling drug production and devising a developmental intervention programme. UNFDAC granted $3.3 million and Pakistan contributed $2.4 million for an initial period of three years, later extended to five. The programme was executed by the UN Division of Narcotic Drugs in association with the Food and Agriculture Organization, the World Health Organization, the International Labour Organization and PNCB.[22] Two strategies were adopted – an agriculture development project in the Buner area and a countrywide network of treatment facilities. The first component reflected the fact that rural areas had been seriously neglected since independence, with strong political preference given to urban areas in spite of a rural:urban population ratio of 72:28. As far as treatment is concerned, addiction was not then a problem in the drug producing areas:

> At the time of the 1974 study, except for Kurya village where there were 52 hard-core opium addicts out of a total village population of 425, addiction was negligible in the area. In the other five villages, there were only eight reported cases of addiction. Among the 52 cases from Kurya, 30 were over 45 years old, including two women over sixty. The remaining were between 20 and 45 years of age, and eight were dependants of their parents. . . Poppy was extensively cultivated for its profitability, which was almost 70 per cent higher than the next crop. Cultivators thought that a ban on poppy would ruin them. But the fact remained that poppy cultivation had done nothing for the uplift of the community. Hence high yield substitute crops would willingly be accepted.[23]

The Government, however, was more interested in securing the UN money than in Buner or treatment, and police and paramilitary forces were used to prevent cultivation and destroy standing crops by aerial sprays and land forces. The project was revived in 1978 by a joint UN/Pakistan Government evaluation mission, emphasizing upgrading crops such as wheat and maize, already known to farmers, and developing irrigation techniques. Ten years and 115,237 million rupees later, however, the project had led to the destruction of 10,000 acres of opium through aerial sprays and paramilitary forces. Its more positive achievements, however, amounted to little. There were 17 irrigation schemes, 8 tube wells, 93 kilometres of road (reported by local people to have been constructed unpaid in spite of the funding allocation), 12 water supply schemes, 1855 acres of land levelling, 380 tons of wheat and maize seed, 60 tons of cane sugar seed (wasted, as sugar does not grow in Buner) and 520 acres of fruit orchards.

After the Buner area development project, UNFDAC, now the United Nations Drug Control Programme (UNDCP)[24] offered assistance in the elimination of poppy production from Dir. The Dir District Development Project started in 1985, for a five-year period under UNDCP control, but because the original agreement was unacceptable to the Government of NWFP the project was transferred to the Federal Government in 1987.

Since 1985, over $30 million has been spent by UNDCP[25] on infrastructure and green sector development in the area, particularly road construction, more to open up areas inaccessible to law enforcement agencies for crop destruction than for developmental activities. Only around 367 developmental projects have been completed in ten years. These include 39 drinking water schemes, a few bridges, electrification of 35 villages, and 744 small schemes such as culverts, flood protection dikes, road improvements and land levelling schemes.[26] In addition, several projects in the tribal Agencies of Bajaur, Muhmand, Khyber and Malakand, and Kala Dhaka area have been undertaken with US support, though few or no details have been made public. It is widely believed by local people, to many of whom these developmental projects are little more than political bribes, that all that has been achieved is the construction of non-metal roads in parts of the region hitherto unknown to the Government. In some, probably many, cases these roads were constructed by local communities, as in Badalay Nihag Dara, Dir, but fraudulently claimed to be project financed. Similarly foreign aid has been fraudulently claimed to cover non-existent electrification costs in rural areas.

Part B: Drugs as Global Enterprise: Thinking the Unthinkable?

The Possibility of Legalization: the Global Picture

> Repressive anti-drug legislation in the US has contributed to one of the major social disasters of the country's development. . . such a situation as has developed in the States should be avoided in other countries at all costs. . . prohibition of intoxicants in a free society does not work. When such a policy was applied to alcohol in the USA, it failed dismally, applied to heroin the outcome has been a disaster on national and even international scale. Why should a counterproductive measure be pursued in the face of the evidence?[27]

Prohibition has failed before in America, and many believe that the war on drugs has failed.[28]

Simply stated, legalizing cocaine, heroin, and other relatively dangerous drugs may well be the only way to reverse the destructive impacts of drugs and current drug policies.[29]

The two main aspects of the drug problem are production and consumption. As will already be clear, the many efforts, national and international, at supply-side control have failed: production is still rising and the various counter-measures have served mainly to change the locations of production. In the West, where numerous drugs are consumed but only cannabis is produced on a commercial scale, much emphasis is put on reducing drug abuse, and eliminating drug production and producers is the main thrust. Accordingly, economically poor and politically unstable countries, vulnerable to US pressure on a number of fronts, typically pursue drug control policies in accordance with US dictates. But when cannabis production is included in the equation, the United States is one of the world's largest drug producers, with cannabis said to be the fourth largest cash crop in the country and the largest in California[30], internal production meeting 25 per cent of domestic demand.[31] And, though its own supply-side control efforts have failed, the US continues to press others to eliminate drug production.

The negative experiences of almost a century of attempted supply-side enforcement suggest a need for alternative models:

> The attempt to eliminate drugs from our civilization has failed. The demand for drugs has lingered despite all efforts, and everything points to the fact that we will have to continue living with drugs and drug users in the future.[32]

Immediate full legalization would be an extreme, unrealistic and probably reckless possibility, with medicalization or restricted decriminalization more realistic steps along the way. Since, however, as *The Lancet* points out, more harmful and addictive drugs than opiates, such as alcohol and tobacco (which, according to WHO, causes 10,000 deaths a day globally),[33] are not only legal but socially respectable.[34] Why one drug is an illegal violation of social norms and another not justifies consideration.[35] The USA alone has some 10 million known alcoholics[36] and almost five million deaths annually from alcohol and tobacco[37], but only 200,000 for injecting drug abusers.[38]

The idea of legalization is not new, nor are calls for it restricted to liberal psychiatrists and reforming or reformed addicts. Historically, drugs and their prohibition have been the subject of arguments between the absolutists, or conservatives, who call for strict penalties and the relativists, or liberals, who advocate greater tolerance.[39] The conservative group includes most US policy makers, who adopt a deviance model of drug abuse, an approach which received formal ratification in the years following the 1914 Harrison Act when drug abuse came to be deemed a crime and all hard drug users criminals. The liberal group on the other hand has drawn its support from European countries that have liberalized drugs since the early 20th century, either on libertarian grounds or by adopting a disease model reflecting a need for treatment among addicts. The disease model is by no means absent from American thinking, of course, and is hegemonic in the case of *legal* drug abuse, publicity associated with high profile alcoholics such as Betty Ford having done much to support the idea of alcoholism as a respectable illness. Indeed lucrative private practices have emerged to provide psychological and medical therapy for people struggling with addictions.

With illegal drugs, however, the position is more complex. While by definition curing clinical addiction is likely to be beyond personal will-power, the illegality of the substances and the involvement of criminal elements create a conjunction between health and criminality on which widely differing ideological stances are inevitably taken. In particular, the oversimplified popular distinction between 'pushers' and 'users' reflects a model of addiction which perceives 'criminals' and 'victims' co-existing within an overall framework of illegality: 'victim' users may be contaminated by 'criminal' pushers, but, for reasons of deterrence, both require condign punishment. Hence has emerged the 'victim-to-criminal-to-victim' approach which has operated in the United States for the last century, with, on the whole, negative consequences.

The Harrison Act, the first major step towards contemporary American internal drug policy, involved taxing opiates and licensing and registering all the importers, manufacturers, distributors, physicians, and pharmacists involved in distribution, with records of all transactions scrupulously maintained. The Act did not, however, seek to deny addicts legal access to narcotics or to spell out what was meant by 'legitimate medical practice', which it assumed physicians were best placed to define. And the Act appeared to satisfy everyone: international commitments, including efforts to control the narcotics trade and American relations with China, had been met; criminal groups found it difficult to acquire opiates without going through a physician (which pleased the public); physicians and pharmacists were given distinctive recognition and authority; addicts, though not mentioned in the Act, had been reassured that they would not be cut off from their supply[40]; and physicians, for the time being anyway, were permitted to maintain addicted patients on constant dosage.

This latter practice was, however, prohibited by the Bureau of Internal Revenue the following year. Because it made the possession of more narcotics than prescribed an offence, this prohibition constituted the next step towards the criminalization of addiction. A third step occurred in 1919, when the Supreme Court ruled that maintenance was not a legitimate medical practice, a decision which led to the prosecution of physicians who, fearing the consequences for patients, continued to prescribe. Possession of narcotics by unregistered addicts was criminalized, so addicts who lacked a prescription for the drugs they possessed were liable to prosecution, a move which firmly lodged the association between crime with addiction in the public mind. Next, during the 1920s, NGOs and other anti-narcotic groups, lodges and civic clubs fed public anxiety by launching massive propaganda campaigns against the evils of narcotics, associating violent crime particularly[41] with drug abuse. In the words of a contemporary critic:

> The narcotics laws have made a crime out of a weakness in order to protect persons from the consequences of this weakness and, as a result, many of the weaklings have of necessity been sent to prison.[42]

Although in 1925 the US Supreme Court declared drug addiction a disease not a crime, the Government continued with the enforcement approach[43] and the prosecution of addicts. In 1951, the Boggs Amendment provided for a mandatory minimum prison sentence of two years on first conviction of drug addiction, raised to five years by the Narcotics Control Act 1956, when addiction became officially and constitutionally a crime. In 1962, however, an era when drugs were praised in songs like Bob Dylan's 'Everybody must get stoned', a more liberal Supreme Court reverted to regarding addiction as a disease, deeming punishment for addiction as cruel and unusual.[44] The following year the Presidential Commission on Narcotics and Drug Abuse recommended that the mandatory minimum imprisonment be reduced, with, as far as possible, decisions left to the medical profession. By this time, if we include alcohol and nicotine among drugs, much of the western world in general was indeed getting 'stoned'.

In a further twist, however, in 1967 the Presidential Commission on Law Enforcement and Administration of Justice, concerned about the impact of drugs on US soldiers in Vietnam and increasing evidence of drug addiction and associated crimes at home, again recommended harsher penalties. This reflected President Nixon's belief that drugs were responsible for increases in street crimes, and it was Nixon who launched the first US 'war on drugs' in 1972[45], highlighting global drug production and trafficking as domestic political issues. The Drug Enforcement Administration (DEA), was created in 1973 to augment the 32 federal agencies already co-operating in the field, with the task of eliminating drugs as close as possible to their source, and disrupting supply.[46] While the United States was by no means inactive in attempting to depress internal demand for drugs, policies concentrated primarily on supply, on the logically slightly dubious assumption that the less each source country produced the less would be exported to the USA.

In fact history has shown, on the contrary, that even major variations in production, for example reductions in Pakistan and Turkey and increases in Afghanistan and Myanmar, have little impact on levels of export to the United States. In international commerce between first and third world countries the balance of the market is determined by the former, so the greater the demand the greater the supply, the lesser the demand the lesser the supply. Commenting on the demand for drugs in the USA, the Colombian President Bentançuo, admittedly not an entirely dispassionate observer, was reported as saying:

> In the world war against narcotics, we need the commitment of the consumer nations to attack the demand with the same vigour we have shown. We can make all sacrifices possible, but if there is enormous demand, production will never be completely eradicated.[47]

Since 1973, however, direct US intervention in foreign countries has been predicated on controlling narcotic supply. Since the time when President Carter, who himself supported the decriminalization of marijuana[48], ordered the DEA to eradicate opium in Mexico, successive US administrations have been aware of the importance of drugs, particularly during the Reagan presidency, when Vice President Bush, a former CIA head, was especially well-informed. During the Reagan era the United States and Pakistan were very close, though in spite of huge amounts of US dollars, accompanied, naturally, by DEA agents, coming to Pakistan in the name of drug control, production and consumption both increased exponentially.

In 1986, President Reagan declared a second war on drugs, as part of which 26 farmers were killed in Gadoon Amazai in a battle over a crop destruction operation planned by the CIA and DEA. The US gave compensation for the killings and offered to help establish an industrial estate to offer alternative resources to opium growers. Still this did not reduce overall production, as the tribal areas and Afghanistan were able, under CIA patronage during this intense period of the Afghan war, to make good any shortfalls in supply. Five years later, in 1991, President Bush declared a third war on drugs.

Arguments for and against Legalization

Anti-criminalization voices had been heard in the United States at least as far back as the 1940s, when it was suggested that a medical model, then not entirely accurately termed 'the British model', be adopted. In 1961 a joint report of the American Medical Association and the American Bar Association argued for the legal availability of drugs to addicts, pleading that if addiction could not be cured it could be managed, much as diabetes was managed, by maintenance doses. Debates about legalization and decriminalization were especially lively in the early 1960s, and in 1964 experts started looking at the economics of legalization.[49]

The more recent campaign started when, in April 1988, Baltimore's Mayor Kurt Schmoke publicly urged law-makers to consider the legalization of illicit substances. In 1993, the US Surgeon General also called for legalization, and since then, many politicians, including former Secretary of State George Shultz, prominent economists and law enforcement officers including Ralph Salerno (an expert on organized crime) and former New York City Police Commissioner Patrick Murphy have called for a change in policy. Objections to legalization are not mainly geared to defending the *status quo*, and some opponents of legalization have been very blunt as to the nature of present problems: it is less in their analysis of the present than in their proposals for reform that they differ from the legalization lobby. For example, among the opponents of legalization Aker argues that prohibition has a number of negative impacts, including the creation of a crime tariff whereby a profitable black market for drugs is promoted, which in turn supports criminal organizations.[50]

The main objections have to do with distinct kinds of fear. There is a *social fear* of broader social damage being created by decriminalization. There is a *moral fear* that legalization is an unacceptable surrender to criminals. There is a *tactical fear* that such surrender will have a domino effect, leading to pressure to bring about other undesired social changes. And there is a *utilitarian fear* that legalization, by creating an imbalance between pleasure and pain, will increase the rate of addiction further, as well as leading to increased criminality.

Of these objections, the last in particular certainly cannot be dismissed lightly. In support of it opponents of legalization can point to the high proportion of current crimes committed under the influence of (legal) alcohol, as well as to road accidents and other causes of increased personal social, health and medical costs. The legal status of alcohol may well mean that insufficient attention is addressed to it, with the illegal status of heroin leading to exaggerated emphasis on the dangers associated with it. If this is indeed so it suggests that the approval implicit in legalization might divert public and political attention away from concern with addiction, returning a public issue to being a private sorrow.

Modelling the impact of legalization on health economics is inevitably speculative. While savings would accrue in areas such as dealing with the effects of adulterated substances and needles, any expansion in usage might impact negatively on the health budget and insurance premiums. Certainly these social costs suggest strongly to opponents of legalization that the issue is far more complex than a matter of private choice: in a complex society the conduct of one person affects others in many ways.

The main arguments advanced by the legalization lobby are:

- current policies are simply repeating the mistakes associated with alcohol prohibition in 1917 and are therefore counterproductive. In particular, just as the huge profits to be realized from prohibition generated powerful and wealthy criminal organizations which diminished in influence when alcohol was legalized by 1933, so will legalization today undermine the corruption prevalent in the drug world;
- legalization would improve public safety by reducing the numbers of violent and property crimes committed in order to obtain drugs;
- legalization would save the exchequer the huge sums currently spent on law enforcement, as well as increasing revenue by taxation;
- while legalization might not reduce the problem of drug abuse and some addicts would continue to lead chaotic lives, cheaper and more available drugs would reduce the pressure to commit crimes to obtain these drugs. Addicts would be better integrated into their families and society at large, and would be more likely to be employed, and more amenable to treatment. All this would help them restore their health, lost due to adulterated street drugs;
- legalization would lead to improved quality control: the fact that many drugs are currently adulterated means that health risks associated with consumption are high;
- while drug addiction and abuse are already on the increase, there is little reason to believe that legalization would create an epidemic. The end of Prohibition saw reductions in alcohol-related organized crime, while production and consumption fell by 60 per cent;[51]
- a victimless crime (or, in John Stuart Mill's phrase, a self-regarding act) such as drug use does not warrant application of the coercive power of the state to suppress freedom of choice, as long as this freedom does not impinge excessively upon the freedom of others. In a democratic society it is not the responsibility of government to make all decisions for the people;
- legalization would eliminate the personal stigma and social consequences experienced by otherwise law-abiding citizens criminalized for drug use alone, who therefore experience the social exclusion (and secondary deviance this can spawn) associated with a criminal record. One of the arguments of the Dutch system is that labelling and embarrassing an abuser is more dangerous than being an addict;[52]
- the unintended consequences of prohibition are unpredictable and therefore unmanageable by Government. For example, research shows that tighter

policing of marijuana imports has stimulated domestic production by raising potency from 1 per cent to 18 per cent, increasing supply, encouraging the introduction of new dangerous drugs to the market, and prompting the creation of marijuana syndicates in place of the small, disorganized growers which had dominated the market before the eradication campaign.[53]

Addiction and Control in Pakistan

When, prior to the Hudood Ordinance of 1979, there was abundant opium production in Pakistan, there was almost no addiction problem, with no more than 315,000 opium abusers[54] out of a population of 100 million – around 0.3 per cent. When opium was banned and production reduced, heroin took its place in such an alarming way that in less than 20 years two million people became addicted. Here, we discuss how a classic moral panic was created to serve vested interests.

In the early 1980s, when heroin was introduced into Pakistan, it was little known. The state-controlled print and electronic media played a vital role in creating a moral panic about opium and heroin, but not other drugs, including cannabis and alcohol, the latter, manufactured in Pakistan in spite of religious prohibition, being the preferred intoxicant of the upper classes. But the more intense the movement against opiates became, the more addiction spread. The actors in this panic were the print and electronic media, officials of the Narcotics Control Board, politicians, and government and foreign funded NGOs. The media exaggerated and distorted the facts, created stereotypes and sensationalized and dramatized events. Local newspapers over-reported minor domestic problems, attributing them to heroin addiction. Violence against women, a common characteristic of Pakistani society, and theft and burglary were increasingly reported as resulting from the desire to satisfy the cravings of addicts.

In the printed media opium crops and poppy capsules were portrayed as cobras devouring youths. Well to do people were dramatized as opiate victims, both involuntarily causing and helplessly witnessing the destruction of their families. Heroin seized from addicts was reported as destined for international trafficking, and addicts came to be associated with the international drug Mafia. The value of seized drugs was exaggerated and glamorized, being reported in millions of dollars rather than in Pakistani currency, creating an impression of large-scale smuggling. The arrests of Pakistani traffickers in many foreign countries and their execution in some so-called Islamic countries was widely and graphically reported. Governors and Chief Ministers who spoke against drugs were given heavy media coverage. New and well-funded anti-drug NGOs exaggerated the situation for their own ends, organizing street corner meetings to which addicts' parents were encouraged to report, tearfully, their children's plight. The Narcotics Control Board organized symposia in five star hotels, with international speakers. But when asked about the production statistics, officials deflected questions or became rude.[55] In fact 60 per cent of Pakistan's heroin addicts are literate, and a similar percentage were employed when their drug use commenced.[56]

Why was this moral panic created? Experts have identified three models of moral panic – grass-roots, elite-engineered, and interest group.[57] In Pakistan, the panic about drugs comes closest to being elite-engineered; though it does not entirely comfortably match the following formulation:

> An elite group deliberately and consciously undertake a campaign to generate and sustain concern, fear, and panic on the part of the public over an issue. . . Typically this campaign is intended to divert attention away from the real problems in the society, where solution would threaten or undermine the interest of the elites. . . Elites have immense powers over the other members of the society – they dominate the media, determine the content of legislation and the direction of law enforcement, and control much of the resources on which action groups and social movements depend.[58]

In Pakistan at this time far more serious internal and external problems than drugs existed. There was a military government. The civilian political leadership was disorganized and had been driven underground. Civil rights were ignored and the constitution suspended. The Supreme Court had deployed the Theory of Necessity to justify the imposition of Martial law. The Islamic Code was selectively deployed so as to strengthen the powers of the military regime. An elected Prime Minister had been executed. Extremists engaged in terrorist atrocities. Corruption was widely deployed, even among student activists, to buy loyalty to the Government. State institutions were in disarray. New and inexperienced politicians were promoted on a non-party basis. Corruption was fuelled by every MP being given development funds of not less than five million rupees a year in a manner which made embezzlement simple. Well organized religio-political parties which threatened the ruling *junta* were weakened. New parties such as MQM in Sind[59] were created and patronized on an ethnic basis.

Following the Soviet intervention, the Afghan problem was gaining momentum, and many people had already fled to Pakistan. As a result, terrorist activity spread, bomb blasts being a daily occurrence in bazaars and other public places. The situation in Iran, where anti-Shah demonstrations were culminating in bloody clashes between law enforcers and the people, had led to many Iranians also coming to Pakistan, some as refugees. Meanwhile many donor countries had halted foreign aid programmes following the suspension of democracy. The attitude of the Carter Administration was cold, if not entirely negative, and the military authorities, aware that US support constituted their only possible bail-out, were doing everything within their power to court them. Pakistan and the United States were both mindful of the dangers resulting from the Iranian and Afghan situations, particularly the threat to US containment policy of the Soviet intervention in Afghanistan. So the fact that Islamabad needed US support while the USA needed Pakistani land as a front line against Russian designs brought the two countries into common cause against communism. The inevitable bargaining process began with General Zia branding a US aid offer 'peanuts'[60] and ended with Pakistan receiving a more than satisfying package. But:

> . . . the aim of US foreign aid, despite predictable protests to the contrary, has never been to eliminate poverty or to expand democracy. . . US foreign aid – whether economic, developmental or military – has always served the dual purpose of politically rewarding our perceived friends and forcing US capital into foreign markets.[61]

Since 1970, drug control has often dominated US–Pakistan relationships[62] and in 1979 the second war on drugs was extended to Pakistan. Soon after this, the Reagan administration was generous in its aid package, and the person in charge of the anti-narcotics task force, Vice President George Bush, was, as a former CIA head, well aware of the importance of narcotics in furthering US interests in the area.

While a moral panic was created officially, however, it lacked many of the indicators of such a panic identified by Goode and Ben-Yahuda, including *concern, hostility, consensus, volatility,* and *disproportionality.* For example, *concern* is possibly best measured by the availability and success of treatment facilities throughout in the country, but there were and are no rehabilitation services.[63] Heroin supply was under the patronage of the law enforcement agencies, particularly police and customs;[64] officials of the national airline, PIA, used food trolleys to smuggle heroin out;[65] prison officials openly sold heroin, brutalizing anyone who reported them;[66] Members of Parliament have been involved in drug trafficking, and some of them have been awaiting trial for many years. The latest list of drug traffickers reported by the Press includes the name of God-like politicians and officials[67] and some uniformed officials.[68]

Nor has there been great public concern about these matters, characteristic responses being:

- Drugs are no problem, leave these poor people alone, they haven't caused any harm.
- Didn't you know people have been smoking these drugs, what is new about it? Are you a foreigner?
- We manufacture and process drugs primarily for export because people abroad need these drugs. Have the people of the west closed down their breweries and pharmaceutical factories?
- How many are the addicts? What percentage of the population? How many thousands? You don't have a significant number of people addicted to drugs.[69]

These responses reflect the traditional attitude of indifference prevalent among the majority of the population. It is not without reason. People have known opiates for ages and believe that drug use is still fairly moderate except among small sub-groups where there is, no doubt abuse, which is, however, of little interest to them.

As government functionaries and international experts on narcotics know well, religion and religious leaders have a profound influence in Pakistan in general and the tribal areas in particular. Accordingly they tried to use them to speak against opium, but with little success, most religious scholars being largely indifferent to opium production.[70] In 1997, the United Nations tried to persuade the then Taliban Government in Afghanistan to reject opium production[71] but at this stage the Taliban declared opium production (as opposed to heroin manufacture) not against Islam.[72] Few religious leaders in Pakistan were willing to speak out against opium, and even politico-religious leaders close to government, who were invited to meetings to speak against drugs, while willing to oppose intoxicants, were seldom willing to proscribe opium cultivation.

Nor is there great hostility towards addicts or addiction. Poor addicts may be despised and pitied, but they are seldom perceived as being involved in organized crime, this being assumed to be the province of elite groups above the law and above criticism. Officials and official figures are routinely disbelieved, and state institutions are widely seen as breaching state law. Indeed the notion that customs and police officials in particular are illicit beneficiaries of the drugs business is so widely held that ordinary people no more debate it than they debate whether the sun rises in the east.

The Case for Controlled Legalization

Pakistan has had no indigenous drug policy since independence, initially adopting former colonial policies of 1858 and 1878 other than that it produced its own opium instead of importing it from India. The system of licensing opium consumption (opium being the only significant drug available at that time) was otherwise largely unchanged and broadly satisfactory until 1979. As a result of the Hudood Ordinance Pakistan lost a source of revenue, thousands of Pakistani people lost a source of livelihood, addiction emerged as a problem and the way became clear for India to become the world's largest licit opium producer.

It is not too late, however, for Pakistan to emulate India and formulate a new and balanced drug policy to suit its own interests. The problems lie not with opium production but with the Government's institutional corruption and inefficiency, and with the propaganda and exaggerations that made it appear one. Politically motivated donations and assistance to eliminate opium production will not serve the long term national interest. If US drug priorities were to change, where would Pakistan stand?

There are voices inside Pakistan now favouring controlled cultivation in order to produce enough opium for use by the pharmaceutical industry. Doctors such as Sher Muhammad Khan, a cancer specialist from NWFP, have repeatedly stressed the need for controlled use of opium and its derivative as a pain killer, particularly for patients suffering from cancer.[73]

There is much to be said for creating a balanced and controlled policy of drug production involving medicalization and decriminalization in a way which integrates the European model with Pakistan's traditional model prior to 1979. Reuter's 'risk and price' approach suggests that all enforcement efforts thus far, including eradication, refinery destruction and intensified policing, by increasing risk, have led simply to price increases. Controlled legalization, involving licensing or regulating opium production combined with the medicalization of its derivatives is the only means of reducing the real risks posed by hard drugs, particularly heroin. Pakistan should therefore revert to its pre-1979 policy, permitting opium cultivation, and making prescription heroin available for addicts, but bolstered by more serious attempts at rehabilitation.

In drug treatment, opiates are used as a substitute. After all, what is Methadone? Is raw opium not used for heroin addiction treatment in Pakistan? Why should the use of one opiate be legal while another is not? Why cannot sale through pharmacies and hospitals instead of the traditional vend system be adopted? Opium has had legitimate uses, for example as a cough depressant and painkiller, for more than two millennia and still there is a large and apparently controlled legal production of opium in countries including India and France.[74] In India, opium is a traditional folk medicine, a raw material for export and a basis for semi-synthetic and synthetic medical products inside the country. Pakistan could deploy the same model for the pharmaceutical industry and export. But for this to happen the Government would have to allow production.

Pakistan is a poor and loan-dependent country with an international debt of $40 billion. Opium production is some 70 per cent more profitable than the next crop[75] and local people are dependent on it in lieu of any other source of livelihood. When opium cultivation was banned the state deprived its own people of a hitherto legitimate source of livelihood and added to their already severe economic burdens. Controlled legalization would allow these communities to earn their livelihood as they did before the ban. The major role for Government would be to procure opium according to the market price to eliminate competition from the illicit market.

The Government's internationally funded crop substitution programme cannot offer long-term solutions and is almost certainly a waste of resources, not least because, as the Senate Committee on Interior and Drugs pointed out, so much funding has been embezzled.[76] Similar programmes were tried for almost three decades in some South American countries, notably Bolivia and the Andean nations, where they too deprived many farmers of their livelihood until the Andean governments switched to non-coercive programmes.[77] In Pakistan, where such evidence as there is in the effectiveness of crop-substitution programmes is so discouraging,[78] the Government switched back to coercion, allocating ever more resources to this doomed policy whose main effect was further to destabilize the polity by turning the military on the people. At present Pakistan's enforcement agencies have been maintained by foreign funding, but should international donations dry up, maintaining these forces would be difficult for the Government.[79]

Such a policy as is here proposed would help the national exchequer in another way. In Pakistan the bureaucracy is already oversized and Pakistan has faced demands from the IMF and World Bank to downsize the service sector to reduce the need for further loans. Legalization would free up resources currently devoted to the enforcement policy, opening the door for the serious development of such scandalously neglected demand side reduction strategies as therapy and rehabilitation.

Black money is a big problem in Pakistan, leading to many other economic problems. At present its volume is said to be 1,500 to 2,000 billion rupees,[80] of which 96 billion are profits for drug traffickers. Drugs bring immense profits, which in turn increase susceptibility to corruption. With medicalization there would be no more profits for drug pushers, enabling the Government to overcome a major source of corruption and black money. Heroin would no longer be disproportionately profitable, so there would be less chance of uncontrolled drug availability, permitting the Government to concentrate on suppressing illicit trafficking. What is true in the US is logical in Pakistan:

> If you take the profit out of drug trafficking, you won't have young children selling drugs on behalf of pushers for $100 a night or wearing beepers to school because it makes more sense to run drugs for someone than to take some of the jobs that are available. I don't know any kid who is making money by running booze.[81]

Drugs would be available to addicts legally and more cheaply. At present stringent enforcement means higher prices, and, according to the US Surgeon-General, the costs of prohibition include violence among drug traffickers, crime caused by addicts having to pay inflated prices, overdosing and poisoning from contaminated illegal drugs, and the spread of HIV and other infections through contaminated needles.[82] It would be preferable for the public health system to be given the lead role in preventing and treating substance abuse, with Government not criminals controlling price, distribution, purity and access. Such a policy would generate revenue which could be spent on other aspects of drug related problems. Pharmacologically unadulterated heroin causes little physical damage to the human body: it is the uncontrolled nature of street heroin that causes poisoning and leads to overdosing. Addicts, currently at the mercy of traffickers and smugglers, should no longer be termed criminals but sick people in need of drugs. Legitimate provision would reduce costs and hence the need to commit crimes to satisfy their addiction. In Amsterdam, where only 0.4 per cent of the population are heroin addicts, experiments along these lines have been associated with dramatic reductions in addiction.

This approach would not mean that drug addiction would come to an end, of course, and the fact has also to be faced that addiction and production might increase temporarily. The probability is, however, that it would subside with time, much as many of the problems associated with Prohibition did in the United States of the 1930s. But addiction would at least be controlled, and knowledge as to the numbers and distribution of addicts would, in stark contrast to the prevalent statistics, be of epidemiological value, and constitute a necessary basis for coherent demand side policy development.

Four main types of drug-related crimes are committed, but such are the limitations of statistics that it is impossible to mount even a 'guesstimate' of the numbers involved.

- *Drug trafficking*, which involves mostly the intelligence agencies of the major countries[83] and their clients elsewhere, has not been effectively controlled for 90 years. Vast sums of drug money are used by smugglers, narco-politicians and narco-guerrillas to produce ever more illegal drugs and for non-monetary but seditious purposes. Ethnic violence in southern Pakistan and the sectarian violence that takes a heavy toll of lives every year, particularly in Punjab, are said by western intelligence reports to be financed by drugs trafficking. Legalization could attenuate this source of terrorist money.
- *Crimes committed to obtain drugs or money to pay for them.* The number of crimes committed to obtain drugs represents neither a significant threat to public order nor a significant proportion of crimes in the western world.[84] In Pakistan, crimes to obtain drugs are surprisingly low given that an addict spends on average 2,000 rupees annually on drugs,[85] though, as we have seen, 60 per cent of addicts are educated and employed at the time of initiating drugs.[86] The main crime committed by addicts is begging, which is prohibited under the 1958 Vagrancy Ordinance, but no steps to implement the law or help beggars not to beg have yet been taken. Naturally addicts who are cast

out by their family members have a miserable life. They live on or near garbage dumps, waiting rooms of railway stations and bus terminals, in the shades of shops and other unhygienic places. They ultimately fall prey to infectious diseases, dying in miserable conditions, their bodies devoured by dogs and other animals. In the face of such circumstances we might enquire which is more humane: leaving addicts to the mercy of their addiction or meeting their needs at a low price? Legalization would also eliminate the trend of addicts to become suppliers and peddlers, mixing with, and becoming, smugglers, to satisfy their need.

- *Crime committed under the influence of drugs* (alcohol) because judgement is impaired. Such crime may be violent, even fatal.
- *Corruption* is a serious problem, and drugs have great potential to corrupt. If drugs were regulated and legalized, incidents of corruption would decrease because drug dealing would no longer be profitable for police and other law enforcers. At present the forces of corruption are too often stronger than the anti-narcotic force.

Pakistan's present addiction problem stems largely from the Hudood Ordinance, whose enactment, and therefore disastrous consequences, are popularly attributed to US influence. While there is public resentment at US interference in domestic affairs, such interference is perpetuated by the ruling classes. If the Government adopted its own model of drug management, even by reverting to the system in use for more than a century, it could return most addicts to opium, which would be regulated, and permit heroin of known purity to be medically prescribed. This would give the public a sense of independence, eliminate US pressure and dictates, and create a sense of psychological liberation within the country. US pressure is, however, the major problem: there is a saying that 'Three As rule Pakistan: America, Allah and the Army', and how, given the size of its current debt, Pakistan is to address this problem is far beyond our scope in this book.

Politicians in government normally oppose liberalization of narcotics legislation. In Pakistan, however, the most vocal politician, Khan Abdul Wali Khan, Leader of the Awami National Party, has termed opium production the right of the growers,[87] suggesting that Government should buy from the farmers. The overall political climate is not hostile to opium production, and it would not be hard for Government, with its strong executive and weak legislative branch, to revert to previous policies. Law making is, after all, by decree or Presidential Ordinance, with Parliament, elected members and experts never taken into the executive's confidence, so serious opposition to reversion is improbable.

Nor can prohibition be defended on moral or religious grounds, or at least any such argument needs to be very selectively deployed. The Hudood Ordinance was not directed only at opium. General Zia was equally against alcohol, having many drinkers arrested and whipped publicly to implement his brand of Islam. But there was only one alcoholic beverage factory in the country before 1979. Today, though alcohol use, manufacture and transportation are still prohibited under the Constitution, that factory has developed into a major cartel with half a dozen branch factories in different parts of the country, and two further companies licensed to manufacture wine, beer and spirits. In Punjab, 25,000 vendors are licensed to sell alcohol, in Lahore the figure is 15,000. So it can be safely claimed that alcohol use is on the rise inside the country, but that alcohol is treated entirely differently from opium.[88]

This change, however, took place very quietly. Initially the prohibition was relaxed for non-Muslims who, in the second phase, were permitted to import wine. Gradually many Muslims became permit holders, licensed to sell wine and other alcoholic drinks. Smuggled wine was confiscated by the authorities and auctioned to five star hotels and other influential places, often at nominal prices. Wine is enjoyed by many parliamentarians: for example, in 1997 a sweeper in the MNAs' (Members of the National Assembly) hostel threatened to disclose the names of the many Members who had purchased wine from him unless they paid him the 500,000 rupees outstanding on their accounts.

Conclusion

In this chapter we have shown how, in criminalizing drugs in Pakistan in 1979, politicians, officials and the state-controlled media combined to create a moral panic of a particular kind. At this time heroin was almost unknown, the main drugs of the day being opium and hashish, but the 'panic' glamorized heroin in particular, which duly became a drug of choice in Pakistan.

This was, in Goode and Ben-Yahuda's formulation, close to an elite-engineered model of moral panic. It was created to divert public attention from the political issues facing the country at a time of Martial Law and the suspension of civil governance, and to secure approval from the United States, Pakistan's major donor country. But we have also shown that this panic lacked many of the indicators identified by Goode and Ben-Yahuda, in particular public concern, public hostility towards drugs, and drugs dealers and consensus. The Government as well as the international community tried to obtain the support of the clergy in Pakistan in the drugs field, but they failed, and in Afghanistan the Taliban Government, though it was later to ban production, declared opium production not against Islam.

Given the concerted media campaign and the diversionary intent of the introduction of the panic including the demonization of the crop itself, however, there seems little doubt that this was an attempt to create an élite-engineered moral panic. But a two-fold theoretical lesson from this incident is, first, that the attempt, though unsuccessful in creating public support for the Ordinance and the military Government, was not necessary for the Ordinance to do its job. This suggests that the model of moral panic developed by these authors requires revision in a country ruled by a military dictatorship. Secondly the campaign had another, entirely different, consequence, in that it contributed to genuine changes in behaviour, but not those intended by the authors of the panic. While we cannot know whether, without the campaign and the Ordinance, heroin would anyway have gained in popularity, there is no specific reason to believe it should have done. A twin effect appears, therefore, to have occurred: the criminalization of a hitherto popular product fuelled demand for a related but new product, and glamorization resulted from misjudged propaganda: what was intended as a threat was interpreted by its target audience as a challenge. Such an effect is plausible, and recognizable to many drugs professionals in the west.

The topic of drugs remains one of high politics and propaganda. The picture is changing slowly, however, as more people become disenchanted with repressive policies. The movement for liberalization is gaining momentum, with politicians, police and other law enforcement officers, medical professionals and legal experts increasingly regarding legalization as the only way to tackle drugs and drug related problems. This lobby bases its arguments on the historical, economic, political and sociological experience of drug policies: basically prohibition has failed, the war is lost, the fight hopeless; and pursuing failed policies has become counterproductive in terms of political stability, health and criminality. Legalization would reduce the burden on the national exchequer and permit the reallocation of resources to more constructive ends. It would lead to improvements in health for the addicted, reducing such drug-related harms as adulterated drugs and overdoses, the major causes of drug-related deaths, and lead to significant reductions in the crime rate.

On the other hand, opponents of legalization believe that cheaply available drugs would increase yet further the rate of addiction, particularly the abuse of hard drugs such as heroin and cocaine. Proponents respond that addiction is already on the increase and legalization of itself would, after uncertain short-term consequences, facilitate longer-term management of the problem. The major source of opposition, however, is moral, with legalization regarded by many as a surrender to criminals and drug pushers of a kind which does not behove a civilized society. The proponents' riposte is that what is being sought is hardly more than already applies in the case of alcohol.

Though these arguments may seem to be being played out like a tennis match, the legalization lobby appears to be gaining ground. Nevertheless, the gap between winning an argument and securing radical policy change in the face of strong opposition from both powerful Muslim interests and developed world creditors is vast; but come the right political moment the rational way forward is clear.

Notes

1   South Asian Association for Regional Co-operation, *Proceedings of Workshop on Effective Utilization of Indigenous Methods for Treatment of Drug Dependants: Pakistan Country Paper.* (Islamabad: 1996). p3; see also *The News* (London: 31 March 1999).
2   Government of Pakistan, *Resource and Reference Manual for Prevention Resource Consultant Network*, Vol. II (Islamabad: Narcotics Control Board, 1990). p170.
3   *The Dawn* (Karachi: 26 June 1997).
4   As we show later, the market operates by a different mechanism in the case of first world imports from developing countries, where the purchasing power of consumer countries is sufficiently strong to generate an adequate supply by switching markets as necessary. This point has, we believe, been insufficiently grasped by the United States, especially in the work of the DEA post-1973.
5   M. Gossop and M. Grant (eds) *Preventing and Controlling Drug Abuse* (Geneva: World Health Organization, 1990). p2.
6   R. H. Blummer, *Drugs I: Society and Drugs* (Francisco, CA: Jossey Bass, 1974).

7   L. Tullis, *Unintended Consequences: Illicit Drugs and Drugs Policies in Nine Countries* (Boulder, CO: Lynne Rienner, 1995). p120.
8   R. Reeves, *Passage to Peshawar* (New York: Simon and Schuster, 1984). p159.
9   K. Elahi, 'Factors Affecting Drug Addiction'. Paper read at International Mass Media Conference, Karachi, 10–12 May 1984, *Conference Proceedings*. p2.
10 A. Jamieson, *Global Drug Trafficking, Conflict Studies 234* (London: Institute for the Study of Conflict and Terrorism, September 1990). p4.
11 M. L. Smith, *Why People Grow Drugs* (London: Panoos Publications 1992). p18
12 M.J. McConohy and R. Kirk, 'Over There: American Drug War Abroad', *Mother Jones*, 14, 2, 1988. p9.
13 T. Clarke and J. Tigue, Jr. *Dirty Money: Swiss Banks, the Mafia, and White Collar Crime* (London: Millington Books, 1976). pp103–105.
14 R. Porter and M. Teich (eds), *Drugs and Narcotics in History* (Cambridge: Cambridge University Press, 1995). p199.
15 Those attending were Russia, China, France, Japan, Persia, Britain, Germany, Siam, Italy, Austria-Hungary, Netherlands and Portugal.
16 D. Buddenberg, *Illicit Drug Use in Afghanistan and Pakistan* (Islamabad: United Nations Drug Control Programme, 1992). p18.
17 D.F. Musto, *The American Disease* (New Haven: Yale University Press, 1973). pp3–40.
18 A.S. Nane, 'UN Activities in International Drug Control'. In I.R. Simon and A.A. Said, *Drugs, Politics and Diplomacy* (London: Sage, 1974). p261.
19 United Nations, *Declaration on the Control of Drug Trafficking and Drug Abuse* (New York: United Nations, 1984). p8.
20 Government of Pakistan, *Resource and Reference Manual for Prevention Resource Consultant Network Vol. II* (Islamabad: Pakistan Narcotics Control Board, 1990). p122.
21 C.P Spencer and V. Navarathnam, *Drug Abuse in South East Asia* (Kuala Lumpur: Oxford University Press, 1981). p23.
22 United Nations, *Dir District Development Project. Phase II: Planning Report.* (Peshawar: Drug Control Programme, 1992). p1
23 Government of Pakistan. *Buner Agriculture Development Project: The Buner Model 1976-86.* Islamabad: Narcotics Control Board, 1986. pp24–5.
24 The United Nations Division on Narcotic Drugs (UNDND), the International Narcotics Control Board (INCB) and UNFDAC (the United Nations Fund For Drug Abuse Control) work as a team of UNDCP.
25 United Nations, *Poppy Cultivation in Pakistan: Briefing Note, February 1997* (Islamabad: UNDCP, 1997). p1.
26 *The Frontier Post* (Peshawar: 25 October 1997).
27 'Management of Drug Addiction: Hostility, Humanity and Pragmatism', *The Lancet*, I, 8541 (9 May 1987). Editorial. pp1068–9.
28 J. Elders (Surgeon General USA), in *The Economist* (22 January 1994). p44.
29 E.A. Nadelmann, 'Drugs Prohibition in the United States: Costs, Consequences and Alternatives' in *Science*, 245 (Washington DC: American Association for the Advancement of Science, 1989). pp939–47.
30 *'Marijuana Update'* Editorial Research Reprint, February 12 1982. pp114–5
31 R. Stevenson, *Winning the War on Drugs: To Legalize or Not?* (London: Institute of Economic Affairs, 1994). 35; see also *British Journal of Addiction*. 84, 9, 1989. p995.
32 'Your Heroin, Sir' *The Lancet*, 337, 8738 (16 February 1991). p402.
33 World Health Organization Report in *The Dawn* (Karachi: 1 June 1999).
34 K. Leech and B. Jordan, *Drugs for Young People: Their Uses and Misuses* (Oxford: The Religious Education Press, 1967). p24.

35 J. Young, *The Drugtakers: The Social Meaning of Drug Use* (London: MacGibbon and Kee, 1971). p9; M.D. Lyman and G.W. Potter, *Drugs in Society: Causes, Concepts and Control*, 2nd Ed (Cincinnati: Anderson Publishing, 1996). p 371.

36 J.H. Reiman, *The Rich Get Rich and the Poor Get Prison* (New York: John Wiley, 1979). p32.

37 J.A. Cercone, *Alcohol-Related Problems as an Obstacle to the Development of Human Capital: Issues and Policy Options* (Washington DC. World Bank Technical Report No. 219, 1994).

38 J. Fischer, *Substance Abuse Related Mortality: A Worldwide Review* (Washington DC: World Bank, March 1994). p4.

39 M.D. Lyman and G.W. Potter, *op. cit.* 365; J. Young, *op. cit.* p49.

40 D.F. Musto, *The American Disease* (New Haven: Yale University Press, 1973). p 64.

41 D.F. Musto, 'Opium, Cocaine, and Marijuana in American History'. *Scientific American.* 265, July 1991.

42 L. Kolb, 'Drug Addiction in Its Relation To Crime', *Mental Hygiene* (9 January 1925). pp74–89.

43 T. Duster, *The Legislation of Morality* (New York: Free Press, 1970). p18.

44 J. Platt and C. Labate, *Heroin Addiction: Theory, Research and Treatment* (New York: John Wiley, 1976). p28.

45 A.W. McCoy, *The Politics of Heroin: CIA Complicity in the Global Drug Trade* (New York: Harper and Row, 1994). p xvi.

46 M.D. Lyman and G.W. Potter, *op. cit.* p297.

47 *The Los Angeles Times* (Los Angeles: 1 December 1985)

48 G. Fine, *Talking Sociology* (Newton, MA: Allyn and Bacon, 1985). p222.

49 H.I. Packer, 'The Crime Tariff', *American Scholar*, 33 (Autumn 1964). pp551–7.

50 R.L. Aker, *Drugs, Alcohol and Society: Social Structure, Process and Policy* (California: Wadsworth, 1992). pp154–5; see also H. Kalant, 'The Great Legalization Debate', in E. Griffith *et al.* (eds) *Drugs, Alcohol, and Tobacco: – Making the Science and Policy Connection* (Oxford: Oxford University Press). 1993 pp276–77.

51 Some of these arguments are summarized in R. Stevenson, *op. cit.* pp53–82.

52 E.L. Engelsman, 'Dutch Management of the Drug Problem', *British Journal of Addiction*, 2, 84 (July 1989). p211.

53 E.A. Nadelmann, 'Drugs, Prohibition in the United States: Costs, Consequences and Alternatives', *Science*, 245 (Washington DC: American Association for the Advancement of Science, 1989); R. Stevenson, *op. cit.* pp52–61.

54 Government of Pakistan, *National Survey on Drug Abuse in Pakistan* (Islamabad: Pakistan Narcotics Control Board, 1986). p vii.

55 In July 1985, in a seminar organized by the Pakistan Narcotics Control Board, Mr Taha Qureshi, a senior PNCB official, presented implausibly high addiction figures. When the first author drew his attention to the high number of addicts and the limited quantity of opium produced in Pakistan and asked where the rest of the supply came from, Qureshi simply said 'Don't be defensive on the part of NWFP'.

56 *South Asian Association for Regional Cooperation (SAARC) Workshop* on 'Effective Utilization of Indigenous Methods For Treatment of Drug Dependence'. Country Paper, Pakistan (Islamabad, 1–2 October 1996). p1.

57 E. Goode and N. Ben-Yahuda, *Moral Panics: The Social Construction of Deviance* (Oxford: Blackwell 1994). pp124–41.

58 *Ibid.* p135.

59 *The News* (London: Internet Edition, 12 July 1999).

60 A.W. McCoy, 1994, *op. cit.* p448.

61 C. Lausane, *Pipe Dream Blues: Racism and the War on Drugs* (Boston: South End Press, 1991). p112.

62 P. Reuter, 'The Limits and Consequences of US Foreign Drug Control Efforts', *Annals of the American Academy of Political and Social Sciences*, 521 (London: Sage, May 1992). p152.

63 Government of Pakistan, *Resource and Reference Manual for Prevention Resource Consultant Network*. Vol. I (Islamabad: Drug Abuse Prevention Resource Centre, 1990). p170.

64 'Customs Patronising Drug-Trafficking', *The Frontier Post* (Peshawar: 11 March 1997)

65 *Takbeer* Weekly, Vol 18 No. 12 (Karachi: Ummat Printing Press, 15–21 March 1996). pp4–5

66 *The Frontier Post* (Peshawar: 19 May 1998).

67 'Heroin was smuggled in Zia's aircraft', *The Frontier Post* (Lahore: 7 May 1997).

68 'PPP releases Government's list of 353 Drug Barons; Civil and Military big wigs among the accused', *The Frontier Post* (Peshawar: 25 May 1998).

69 K. Elahi, 'A Profile of Drug Abuse and Addiction in Pakistan'. Paper read at the *International Narcotics Conference* (Quetta, 8–10 August 1982). p3.

70 Government of Pakistan, *Buner Agriculture Development Project: The Buner Model 1976–86,* (Islamabad: Pakistan Narcotics Control Board, 1986). p23.

71 *The Times* (London: 11 August 1997).

72 'Taliban say poppy cultivation is not against Islam' in *The Frontier Post* (Peshawar: 8 November 1998).

73 'The Case for Opium', *Daily News* (Islamabad: 25 June 2000).

74 P. Reuter, 'Eternal Hope: America's Quest for Narcotics Control'. *The Public Interest*, 79 (1985). p82.

75 Government of Pakistan, *Buner Agriculture Development Project: The Buner Model, op. cit.* p25

76 *Daily Jang* (London: 29 April 1999).

77 P. Reuter, 1992, *op. cit.* p158.

78 *Ibid.*

79 2001 saw a resurgence of poppy cultivation in Dir, Khyber and Muhmand Agencies. An observation visit in December of that year amply demonstrated that, with the Army busy watching the western as well as eastern borders, farmers had an excellent opportunity to cultivate their choice crop – a situation that created a degree of political turmoil in the country.

80 I. Dar (Pakistan Finance Minister) reported in *Daily Jang* (London: 28 May 1999). p1 and Editorial.

81 M.D. Lyman and G.W. Potter *op. cit.* p369.

82 *The Economist*, 22 January 1994.

83 Notably US Intelligence Services, Britain's MI5, France's SDEC, Germany's Gehlen Organisation, Italy's SUFFERS and India's RAW.

84 P. Gordon, 'Why Drugs Must be Made Legal', *Police Review* 100, 28, February 1992. pp388–9.

85 *Daily Jang* (London: 28.6.99)

86 South Asian Association for Regional Cooperation (SAARC) Workshop, *op. cit.* p1.

87 M.K. Jalal Zai, *The Drug War in South Asia* (Lahore: Institute of Current Affairs, 1993). p25.

88 *Daily Jang* (London: 5 May 1999).

Chapter VI

Summary and Conclusion

Pakistan is an underdeveloped south Asian country. Mismanagement and political corruption since independence in 1947 have led to its current dependence on foreign loans and donations. Recent international reports put the average national *per capita* annual income at around $420[1], but the *per capita* income in NWFP in general and in the opium producing areas in particular is far less than this: empirical data showed it to be around $136. Even on World Bank figures, however, the average income would be no more than $1.15 a day.

Politically the country is weak and riddled with contradictions, for example between political ideology and political culture, and between the Constitution and the legal system. Constitutionally the country is an Islamic Republic, but its legal practices are often anti-Islamic and anti-democratic, many laws and practices of the colonial era which favour the rulers and politicians remaining in force. Pakistan's federal system concentrates power in a few hands and greatly favours Punjab. Administratively the country is divided into four provinces – Baluchistan, Punjab, NWFP and Sind – the Federal Capital Territory (Islamabad District) and the Federally Administered Tribal Areas (FATAs) and Provincially Administered Tribal Areas (PATAs) of NWFP, which have different legal and political systems. Pakistan has been under martial law for half of its 50 years of independence, but some of the so-called elected democratic governments have proved, if anything, even more corrupt and less competent than the military ones. Externally, Pakistan's weakness derives from its economic vulnerability, which means that it can seldom withstand pressure of any kind from western powers.

In education, Pakistan cannot compete even with many other third world countries. Even today, more than 17 million children do not attend school, and the under-resourced health system does not begin to meet demand. The drug producing tribal areas are the worst affected economically and politically, lacking the opportunity for honourable survival. Development is affected by inequity in Pakistan's Five Year Development Plans, and areas which produce opium and heroin are virtually compelled to do so by a combination of internal socio-economic conditions and external geopolitics.

According to a World Bank report, NWFP is the most backward administrative part of the country. Despite fragmented attempts by successive provincial governments, with foreign assistance, to establish industrial estates in opium growing parts of the province it has no industrial base, something that many political and economic analysts see as ethnically-based discrimination by a government dominated by urban Punjabis. Ethnically, the majority of the people of NWFP are *Pukhtoon* or *Pushtoons*. *Pushto* speaking people in general and the people of the tribal areas in particular migrated from Afghanistan in the 15th and 16th centuries.

They still live a tribal life governed by the unwritten, customary laws of *Pukhtoonwali*. This embraces:

- *Melmastia* (the honourable use of material possessions)
- *Hujra* (guest house, the centre of local political and social activities)
- *Badal* (the reciprocity of conduct, good and bad)
- *Jarga* (an assembly which resolves interpersonal and intertribal disputes)
- *Tarboorwali* (patrilineal descent to a common ancestor as the basis of property and political alliances)
- *Toor* and *Peghor* (jeering at someone for his own or his family's socially disapproved conduct).

Agriculture is subsistent and confined to the plain areas in Peshawar and surrounding districts. The only significant source of revenue is a royalty on hydro-electric power generation, which is, however, never fully paid by central government. Tobacco, cane sugar and wheat are the main crops of the plains, while wheat, barley, maize, mustard and onions are the crops of the hilly areas. The agronomic practice of opium cultivation is probably the oldest in the area.

The Opium Poppy and Opium

The origins of *papaver somniferum* or the poppy plant probably lie in Mesopotamia, the eastern Mediterranean or Europe, though evidence as to its origin and history is speculative. Botanists are as unsure about its progenitors as they are about its internal taxonomy. It is clear, however, that opium was used by the Romans and Greeks as an analgesic and anaesthetic, and there is broad consensus that opium was the world's first medicine, being popular in the west in 500–400 BC.

Within the sub-continent, discussions as to origins have been affected by tensions between Muslims and Hindus, and between Muslims and western experts. The predominant western view is that Arabs took the plant not only into the sub-continent but to the entire east, including China.[2] This, however, may refer to Arabs of antiquity, since some experts mention that Arabs before Islam[3] appreciated the value of opium and took it to the east.[4] Indian scholars say that it was Muslims who introduced opium into the area and that their own sacred books do not mention the plant, though Muslims argue that the sacred Hindu text *Vedas* mentions opium in 500 BC[5] and make other claims calling the Hindu version of history into question.

In the early 16th century, with the arrival of the Mughals, opium assumed the status of a political commodity, being taxed and so becoming a source of state revenue. But the Mughals, being mainly concerned with self-sufficiency in food crops, the only source of their strength and richness being income from land, did not give opium special status or interfere with farmers' decisions as to how much of their land to cultivate with opium.

With the advent of British rule in the 18th century, however, the British East India Company rapidly monopolized production and supply, converting much of Bengal and some other parts of their domain into a poppy mono-culture, destroying other crops and penalizing the farmers responsible. The British fought three opium wars to monopolize the business and its smuggling into China, and the weight of historical evidence suggests that it was their supervision of the trade rather than the legacy of the Mughals which spread the drug in India.

The recent history of opium began in 1953, when a UN Protocol allowing Pakistan to produce opium led to official efforts to produce opium for medical and non-medical purposes. But then policies changed, efforts formerly put into producing opium being devoted to prohibiting it, a policy change to be influential in the spread of heroin addiction in particular.

The medicinal value of opium has been known since pre-historic times, and advances in biochemical science enhanced its importance during the early 19th century, when morphine, the most natural alkaloid and in medical use ever since, was isolated from opium. Heroin was synthesized accidentally in 1874 but found to be dangerous; when, in 1890, it was synthesized in Germany by a different method, however, it was considered a medicine. Bayer accordingly commenced commercial production in 1898, and the drug obtained recognition from the Austrian and American Medical Associations in 1906. By 1910–12, however, its addictive potential had led to efforts to contain its use, and it was finally prohibited in the United States in 1924. The League of Nations imposed bans on manufacture, transportation and international trading, but these led to production going underground. Since then the world has witnessed this outlawed drug being used politically against individuals and states, to finance wars and terrorism, as a source of survival in producing countries, and as a source of affluence and might by politicians, criminals and predatory states.

Heroin was introduced to Pakistan in the late 1970s, and by the early 1980s Pakistan was an exporter, increased production being linked with local political and economic conditions, and stemming in particular from US deployment of heroin both to finance the Afghan War and to undermine the Soviets. This legacy is plaguing Pakistan's youth, and Pakistan has done almost nothing by way of rehabilitation or care.

The Political Economy of Opium: The Research Outlined

The politics of drug demand and supply has assumed a special place in international politics and diplomacy. While narco-politics has become a tool of both overt and covert US security policy, narcotics consumption at home has presented enduring problems for domestic policy, particularly health and law enforcement. This awkward conjunction has led to an opportunist approach by the United States to the politics of drugs. Three successive wars on drugs at home, waged while producers overseas were receiving covert CIA support, have done nothing to diminish the deep cynicism about the US approach felt in many producer countries. US drugs policies have done little to promote stable or honest government in such countries, and have done damage to the social, economic and political fabric there.

In Pakistan these policies have contributed to creating a situation in which heroin addicts now constitute 25 per cent of the world's total.[6] Heroin addiction was first reported by a hospital in Baluchistan in 1979, and the next two cases were reported in 1980 in Peshawar. Since then addiction has spread like a contagious disease.

Today there are reported to be more than five million addicts, of whom almost 51 per cent are addicted to heroin, with some 100,000 new addicts annually.

The Government, meanwhile, under US pressure, took steps to reduce production by an eradication and substitution programme on which it embarked in the knowledge that any reductions in exports would simply be made good by Afghanistan. This situation began in 1979 immediately after the ban on opium production and sale through the century old vend system. This almost precisely reflected the experience in south-east Asia, where anti-opium laws proved a boon for heroin: until opium was banned usage was widespread but limited, and addiction almost unknown; thereafter heroin took its place with disastrous consequences.

The study reported in this book was conducted in the opium and heroin producing tribal areas of North West Frontier Province: the provincially administered District of Dir, and the federally administered Agencies of Bajaur, Khyber and Muhmand. The study answers the question of why and how drugs are produced in Pakistan: to what extent and how are economic, political, historical and geographical factors responsible? In what ways are the political considerations national, regional or international?

History has played an important impact in the development of drugs and drug culture in the area, and we have traced the history of opium in the sub-continent in general and the area under study in particular. Many experts are of the opinion that poor economic and turbulent political conditions in some areas of the globe predispose the production of drugs.[7] Although our study is not comparative we have been able to demonstrate that poor economic conditions, political instability and poor administration are indeed associated with drug production; and we have shown some of the cultural facilitators of opium production, such as family and tribal structures. We have also proposed a solution to the drug problem, involving a qualified return to the pre-1979 situation, with the addition of a rehabilitative framework to cope with the problems of the last generation.

The research universe was divided into two clusters: Peshawar Division in the west and Malakand Division in the north. From these clusters two areas each were selected for data collection. In the first cluster the tribal Agencies of Muhmand and Khyber were selected, where, respectively, opium and heroin are produced. In the northern cluster, the District of Dir and Bajaur Agency, which have been very famous for this crop internationally, were selected. Sampling size was determined proportionally: the greater the area cultivated with opium the greater its representation. Opium growing communities were sampled in all three areas and personal contacts used to gain access. During visits to the research areas, lists of opium cultivators were constructed as a sampling frame, from which, no list of opium cultivators being available from administrative or developmental offices in the areas, respondents were randomly selected. Semi-structured interviews were then conducted.

A second interview schedule was used to study heroin production in the non-producing Khyber Agency. Educated local people were interviewed about the historical development of heroin in the area, the economic conditions of the people and the impact of the Afghan war on the local economy. Ordinary people such as market committee representatives and political activists were asked about the supply structure, and their views about the involvement of administrators and politicians were discussed.

Prior to this study, little information existed about the history of opium and heroin, the addiction situation, the Government's role in the development of poor communities, the economic and political causes of opium and heroin production, and possible solutions to the various problems that arose. These issues were therefore discussed in a third interview schedule[8] with intellectuals, including law enforcement officers, development economists, politicians, anthropologists, historians, psychiatrists and political scientists.

To determine the political causes of production we discussed the political systems operating in drug producing areas, the regional impact of the Iranian revolution and the Soviet intervention in Afghanistan, the consequences of superpower involvement and the roles of political corruption and the political atmosphere in the opium producing areas.

The Afghan conflict may have triggered the trade, but its perpetuation has mainly economic and political causes. The drug producing areas have common economic characteristics. They:

- are geographically inaccessible, with minimal communication sources
- lack economic opportunities, including private and public sector industry
- are characterized by large families
- have subsistence farming based on small and irregular land holdings, normally on top of mountains and hills, and without irrigation
- have surplus labour, due to the opportunity structure
- are characterized by widespread poverty of all kinds.

Dir is mostly mountainous, inaccessible, with no industry and nominal agriculture but a population of 1.6 million, an average family size of 13 and an average family land holding of only 4.7 *jreebs* (less than 1 hectare). Its economics revolve round off-season migration. Only 16 per cent of the land is available for agriculture, and, even it could be afforded, mechanization would be technically impossible. Eighty per cent of agricultural land is devoted to opium. Among poppy growers the average annual *per capita* income is around 6,000 rupees, much more than would otherwise be available.

Bajaur is mountainous, inaccessible, dry and rain dependent for even a single annual crop. No industry exists, the people migrate to work, and conditions have worsened through the presence of some 200,000 Afghan refugees. The average family land holding is 13 *jreebs*, the annual average *per capita* income is 3,960 rupees and the average family size is 18.

Muhmand, the most backward area, is mostly mountainous, but the mountains are barren and void of vegetation. Water is scarce even for drinking so most people migrate in summer. Agriculture is backward due to scarcity of land (only 5.88 per cent of the total land is available for agriculture) and increased provision is geologically impossible. *Per capita* annual income averages 3,840 rupees, the average family size is 23.2 and the average family land holding is 19.5 *jreebs*.

Khyber, an inaccessible mountainous area, lacks agricultural activity due to shortages of land and water. The main economic resource, the trans-Afghan border trade, flourished for 20 years, bringing some alleviation of poverty, but was halted by the Soviet intervention, which encouraged people to switch to drug production as a prompt and sure source of survival. *Per capita* annual income is 5,682 rupees and average family size is 23.8.

Politics of Opium and Heroin

The economic value of opium has probably been known since the Bronze Age,[9] when it was exported from Cyprus to Egypt as a commodity of revenue generation. In the Indo-Pakistan sub-continent the use of opium during the 16th century by the Muslim rulers became the basis of the later development of opium for more aggressive purposes during the Raj, when opium's economic importance overrode humanitarian and political considerations, leading to the Opium Wars with China. Paradoxically these wars became the basis of international but unsuccessful and sometimes counterproductive control efforts for almost a century.

Pakistan is still in good part run on the basis of colonial laws, which originally reflected not traditional indigenous legislation but the determination of foreign rulers to dominate an area which they could not incorporate into their administration. In particular drugs laws are seldom applied fairly: impoverished traffickers are fined and imprisoned while powerful traffickers are seldom brought to justice at all. As well as the law, politics in the drug producing areas favours production. Even in the context of legal prohibition all political parties and politicians support the cultivators – at least until they secure power, when external political pressures lead them to support attempts at eradication. Moreover, the poppy dollars donated by western nations are a source of wealth for many politicians, and in order to attract more foreign donations the Government has in the past presented exaggerated figures of addiction.

The Hudood Ordinance prohibited opium production and sale, whether to addicts or for medicinal purposes. Though there seems no logical or religious basis for the Ordinance, two political purposes existed at the time: a desire to convince the people that General Zia's Government was trying to implement Islam, and to eliminate opium and heroin meant for the US market. It is now believed by many western experts that the latter was the real objective, the Ordinance being promulgated as part of the US war on drugs, and merely coated with the name of Islam in order to ensure domestic compliance. After all, if the aim was to develop an Islamic legal system forbidding intoxication and intoxicants, why was opium alone selected for prohibition, whereas alcohol production enjoyed official acquiescence?

There is a widespread belief in Pakistan, then, that the Hudood Ordinance was enacted under US pressure, and was a symptom of political uncertainty, subservience and dependence. To justify it, an elite engineered form of moral panic was created in the state controlled media, with propaganda reminiscent of that associated with US prohibition in the early quarter of the last century. These tactics brought in millions of dollars but did nothing for the welfare of addicts or opium growers, not least because so much of the revenue was embezzled.[10]

Today drug addiction is therefore associated in the minds of many Pakistani people with US domestic policies; and was in particular fuelled by US *Realpolitik* associated with the Afghan war. The suppression of the opium farmers is part of the political culture of a country whose rulers have embarked on a path that gives them no alternative to force. Political corruption and the involvement of the 'bigwigs' who patronize drug trafficking are also strongly associated with drug production and addiction. This corruption is not merely low-level activity on the part of ordinary state servants, but involves the top echelon of politics, including successive presidents, prime ministers, generals, parliamentarians, ministers. It also includes senior officials such as the Head of the Anti-Narcotic Force himself, facts that demonstrate all too clearly that, in Pakistan, the forces of corruption are greater than the anti-narcotics forces ranged against them.

The external factors associated with the drug boom are the Soviet-Afghan war and the Iranian revolution, both of which occurred in 1979. The former is widely believed to have been financed by drug money under the patronage of the CIA, which not only turned a blind eye to the activities of the Afghan leaders but actively participated in trafficking, even after the withdrawal of Soviet forces. Today, many Pakistani leaders known to have benefited from drug money are welcome visitors in USA and remain immune from prosecution.

The Iranian revolution caused many Iranian traffickers to flee to Pakistan and establish heroin factories there and in Afghanistan, using their contacts to introduce Pakistani traffickers to international *Mafiosi*. The revolution also heralded an increase in religious sectarian conflict in Pakistan. In Iran, mostly *Shiaism* is practised, while followers of this sect inside Pakistan, where most Muslims are *Sunnies*, are in a minority. As a result of Iranian support for *Shias* in Pakistan this sect has become militant and sectarian intolerance is now prevalent, with the *Sunnies* blaming the *Shias* and Iran for using narcotics to terrorize the non-*Shias*. This has led to further violence, which continues today.

The study contained quantitative as well as qualitative data. On the whole, however, the quantitative findings were inconclusive, and as the study proceeded they became of less significance than had originally been anticipated. While inconclusive chi-squares give no reason to reject the original hypotheses, more substantial investigation is required for levels of confidence to be such that the data can be described as authoritative.

Towards Controlled Legalization?

In the preceding pages we have discussed the economic and political conditions of Pakistan in general and the drug producing areas in particular. We began with the assumption that poor economies and weak politics would be the prime causes of drug production the world over, but this study has highlighted many more relevant factors: it is clear, for example, that political might and economic invincibility also promote production and trafficking. US patronage of drugs production and trafficking the world over is extensive and well known, and its successive wars on drugs collectively comprise a slogan and a tool to pressurize weaker, debtor, countries, and interfere with their domestic policies. In Pakistan, US pressure has led to efforts to eliminate poppies from areas where opium has been cultivated for at least one and a half centuries. As a result, opium production is surely reduced, but the supply from Afghanistan, which has accordingly emerged as the biggest opium producer in the world, remains uncontrolled, and this has led to a massive expansion of heroin manufacture in Pakistan. This follows the pattern the world over: variations in drugs production in particular countries have little or no impact on world drug abuse, with the result that in Pakistan drug addiction is increasing faster than the population, and Pakistan's population of 134 million now includes three million heroin addicts.

The reintroduction of a version of the pre-Hudood system of control, combined with even modest improvements in rehabilitation, would yield many of the benefits normally associated with regulation, and would certainly be less harmful than the present system of repression. As we have shown throughout, even the best regional, national, international and transnational control efforts have been not only ineffective but also counterproductive. Controlled legalization would offer a middle ground between the present war on drugs and complete legalization, within the boundaries of an international prohibitive approach.

Drug treatment is a long process requiring resources, patience and planning at state level. At present there is a lack of medical resources, and treatment programmes last, on average, only 12 days. This is clearly a waste of resources since the first thing a discharged addict will do on his discharge is 'score' from a dealer, who may well be waiting for him as he leaves the rehabilitation centre. Legalization would not mean the harmful physical effects of drug use being ignored: in fact health would be of prime concern. But a gradual process of controlled integration of drugs in society would both acknowledge the unavoidable reality of the situation and teach its members to cope better with it. Addiction would continue to exist but it could be scaled down from a public issue to a private grief. After all, the law is only one tool in dealing with drugs problems, and discouraging usage need not entail criminalizing users. Regulation would put opiates on a par with tobacco and alcohol, where policies can be adjusted according to developing scientific evidence of harm and changing public attitudes. It would also mean that:

- product quality could be assured and drug related deaths diminished. Pure heroin is less dangerous than heroin adulterated by substances such as quinine, talcum powder, white chalk and gluten in brown heroin, many of which are more dangerous to inhale than the original heroin;
- criminal involvement would be reduced. When a commodity is prohibited, black marketeering (which is growing exponentially in Pakistan) is the natural partner of prohibition. Addicts often finance consumption by selling their own and other's possessions, or by dealing on behalf of drug syndicates. Legalization might not prevent them remaining addicts but it would reduce the side effects of hustling, damage to properties and organized criminal involvement;
- because drugs would be brought within the fiscal system, recycling the revenue raised would fund new resources which could, if the political will to do so were there, be hypothecated for rehabilitation and health education. By the same token, legalization would save money currently spent, to little or no positive effect, on enforcement – police, prisons, courts, military – by reducing the scale of drug-related criminality.

Drug abuse cannot be simply a matter of policing and prohibition; it must also be one of health and welfare, the aim being to return to addicts the dignity and independence currently denied them. But the problems entailed in embarking on such a programme are daunting indeed. Any move towards controlled legalization on the part of a country whose debtor status inevitably diminishes its practical exercise of sovereignty would inevitably provoke superpower controversy and hostility. Its likely consequences would require immensely sensitive negotiation internationally. Since, however, the United Nations lacks the authority as well as the ability to control the drugs trade it is more likely that bilateral discussions with the superpower, either involving Pakistan alone or a consortium of producer countries, would be a more probable first step. Though such a discussion might seem improbable, US efforts to draw Pakistan into its anti-Taliban alliance following the terrorist attacks on Washington and the World Trade Center of September 11 2001 serve as a reminder that at the right political moment weaker powers can exercise a surprising degree of leverage over stronger ones.

In addition, those who plead for strict control and penalties for addicts and drugs production should remember that some people will always take drugs. Indeed history shows that societies that have been too strict about drugs are often the worst affected by them, their politics being instrumental in the expansion of production, trafficking and the black market. Pakistan has lost much in a foreign war on drugs fought on its own land against its own people: it has lost the economic resource of a large population, the health of its people, a source of state revenue and political sovereignty. It has gained in return poppy dollars (largely embezzled), increased political corruption, a loss of confidence among the people, and wholesale drug smuggling.[11]

Activities such as creating panic through the state controlled media and exaggerating addiction statistics to attract foreign aid will not work in the long run and are not in the national interest. To curtail corruption and black money it is necessary to regulate drugs. This would mean Pakistan would need to produce its own opium, which would of itself help solve the problems of communities dependent on opium production. It is not a perfect solution, but it is certainly a less bad one than exists at present. How much good it would do we cannot say with confidence, though if backed with resources recycled into treatment and rehabilitation the answer could be 'an awful lot'. But it would at the very least do less harm: *primum non nocere* (above all do no harm) is the prime duty of the physician, and it is, we believe, a respectable and possibly attainable objective for nation states too.

Notes

1   World Bank, *World Tables* (Baltimore: Johns Hopkins University Press, 1995). pp525–6.
2   Government of Great Britain, *The First Report of the Royal Commission on Opium 1893–4* (London: Eyre and Spottiswoode, 1894). p148. See also G. Watt, *A Dictionary of the Economic Products of India*. VI, 1 (London: W.H. Allen, 1893). pp102–5.

3   C.E. Terry and M. Pellin, 'Drug Addiction' in *Encyclopaedia of Social Sciences*, V (New York: Macmillan, 1931). pp242–51. Also see D.F. Musto, *The American Disease: The Origin of Narcotics Control* (London: Yale University Press, 1973). p1.
4   G. Watt. *op. cit*. pp102–5.
5   K. Babar, 'Pakistan's Narcotics Problems'. *Journal of Rural Development and Administration*, Vol. XXI, 4. p.119 (Peshawar: Pakistan Academy for Rural Development, October–December 1989). p119.
6   Pakistan Senate Committee on Interiors and Narcotics. *Daily Jang* (London, April 29, 1999).
7   A. Jamieson, *Global Drug Trafficking. Conflict Studies* 234 (London: Institute for the Study of Conflict and Terrorism, September 1990). p4.
8   These schedules are reproduced in Asad 2000, *op. cit.*
9   R.S. Merrillees 'Opium Trade in the Bronze Age Levant', *Antiquity* Vol. XXXVI (1962). pp287–92.
10 *Daily Jang* (London: 29 April 1999), *op. cit.*
11 S. Hamid, (Governor of Punjab), quoted in the *Daily Jang* (London: 20 March 1999).

Bibliography

Adam, G.R. and Schevaneldt J.D. *Understanding Research Methods*. New York: Longman, 1985.

Adden, T.J. *The Distribution of Opium Cultivation and the Trade in Opium*. Haarlem: Joh. Enschede En Zonen, 1939.

Ahmad, A.S. *Pukhtoon Economy and Society*. London: Routledge and Kegan Paul, 1980.

Aker, R.L. *Drugs, Alcohol and Society: Social Structure, Process and Policy*. California: Wadsworth, 1992.

Alatas, S.H. *Corruption: Its Nature, Causes and Functions*. Kuala Lumpur: Majeed, 1991.

Allan, N. *The Opium Trade*. Boston, Massachusetts: Milford, 1973.

Asif, M. *Heroin Addiction in Rural Society*. MA Thesis. Islamabad Quaid-e-Azam University, 1985.

Babar, K. 'Pakistan's Narcotics Problem'. *Journal of Rural Development and Administration*. XXI, 4, 1989.

Barth, F. *Political Leadership Among Swat Pathans*. London: Athlone Press, 1953.

Berridge, V. and Griffith, E. *Opium and the People*. Harmondsworth: Penguin Books, 1981.

Bingham, D. *Opium Addiction in Chicago*. Montclair, New Jersey: Smith Paterson, 1970.

Blummer, R.H. *Drugs, I: Society and Drugs*. San Francisco, California: Jossey-Bass, 1974.

Buddenberg, D. *Illicit Drug Use in Afghanistan and Pakistan*. Islamabad: United Nations Drug Control Programme, 1992.

Campbell, D.H. *The Evolution of Land Plants*. Stanford California: Stanford University Press, 1939

Cardovez, D. and Harrison S.S. *Out of Afghanistan: The Inner Story of the Soviet Withdrawal*. New York: Oxford University Press, 1995.

Cercone, J.A. *Alcohol-Related Problems as an Obstacle to the Development of Human Capital: Issues and Policy Options*. Washington DC: World Bank Technical Report No. 219, 1994.

Cheema, S.A. 'Implications of Growing Alternative Crops For Poppy in the Northern Region of Pakistan'. In Anwar-ul-Haq and Umar Farooq (eds.) *Drug Addiction and Rehabilitation of Addicts in Pakistan*. Faisalabad: Agriculture University, 1978.

Chopra, R.N. and Chopra, I.C. *Drug Addiction with Special Reference to India*. New Delhi: Indian Council of Scientific and Industrial Research, 1965.

Clarke, T. and Tigue, J., Jr. *Dirty Money: Swiss Banks, the Mafia, and White Collar Crime*. London: Millington Books, 1976.

Cooley, J. *Unholy Wars: Afghanistan, America and International Terrorism.* London: Pluto Press, 1999

Core, E. *Plant Taxonomy.* Englewood Cliffs, New Jersey: Prentice Hall, 1955.

Craig, R.B. 'Illicit Drug Traffic: Implications for South American Source Countries'. *Journal of Inter-American Studies and World Affairs* 29, 2, 1987. pp1-34.

Das, S. *Public Office, Private Interest: Bureaucracy and Corruption in India.* New Delhi: Oxford University Press, 2001.

David, M.M. *Cultural Geography of Opium: Its Cultivation and Spread through the Bronze Age.* Ph.D. Thesis. Hawaii: University of Hawaii, 1979.

Desai, M. and Sethi, H.S. *et al.* (eds) *Current Research in Drug Abuse in India.* New Delhi, 1981.

Duster, T. *The Legislation of Morality.* New York: Free Press, 1970.

Dwarkanath, S.C. 'The Use of Opium and Cannabis in the Traditional System of Medicines in India'. *UN Bulletin on Narcotics.* 17, 1. 1965.

Elahi, K. 'A Profile of Drug Abuse and Addiction in Pakistan'. *International Conference on Narcotics.* Quetta, Pakistan, 8–10 August 1982.

Elahi, K. 'Factors Affecting Drug Addiction'. *International Mass Media Conference.* Karachi, 10–12 May 1984.

Engelsman, E.L. 'Dutch Management of the Drug Problem' *British Journal of Addiction.* 2, 84, July 1989. pp211–18.

Faheem, M. and Saeed A. *A Profile of Dir with Agriculture Background.* Timargara: Dir District Development Project, 1991.

Fine, G.A. *Talking Sociology.* Newton, Massachusetts: Allyn and Bacon, 1985.

Fischer, J. *Substance Abuse Related Mortality: A Worldwide Review.* Washington DC: World Bank, March 1994.

Ghosh, S.K. *The Traffic in Narcotics and Drug Addiction.* New Delhi: Ashis Publishing Co, 1987.

Gohar, A. 'Are We Going Down the Central American Route?' *National Policy and Public Awareness Conference on Drug Abuse.* Islamabad: PNCB, 17–19 May 1993.

Goode, E. and Ben Yahuda, N. *Moral Panics: The Social Construction of Deviance.* Oxford: Blackwell, 1994.

Gordon, P. 'Why Drugs Must be Made Legal' *Police Review* 100, 28, February 1992. pp388–9.

Gossop, M. *Living With Drugs.* Aldershot: Ashgate, 1993.

Gossop, M. and Grant, M. (eds) *Preventing and Controlling Drug Abuse.* Geneva: World Health Organization, 1990.

Government of Great Britain. *The First Report of the Royal Commission on Opium, 1893–4.* London: Eyre and Spottiswoode, 1894.

Government of Great Britain. *Health and Personal Social Services Statistics.* HMSO: London, 1994.

Government of India. *Imperial Gazetteer of India: Provincial Series: North West Frontier Province (NWFP)* (Originally 1903). Lahore: Sange-Meel Publications, 1979.

Government of North West Frontier Province. *Census of Population: FATA.* Peshawar: FATA Development Corporation, 1981.

Government of North West Frontier Province. *Socio-Economic Profile of Bajaur Agency.* Peshawar: Planning and Development Department 1992a.

Government of North West Frontier Province. *Land Utilization Statistics for 1992–3 in NWFP.* Peshawar: Agriculture Department, 1992b.

Government of North West Frontier Province. *Important Agency-Wide Socio-Economic Indicators.* Peshawar: Bureau of Statistics, Environment, Planning and Development Department, 1992c, 1995 and 1996.

Government of Pakistan. *The Constitution of Islamic Republic of Pakistan.* Islamabad: Ministry of Law, Justice and Parliamentary Affairs, 1973.

Government of Pakistan. *National Survey on Drug Abuse in Pakistan (1982, 1986, 1993).* Islamabad: Narcotics Control Board, 1982a.

Government of Pakistan. *Survey Report on Drug Production.* Islamabad: Narcotics Control Board/UNFDAC, 1982b.

Government of Pakistan. *Buner Agriculture Development Project: The Buner Model 1976-86.* Islamabad: Narcotics Control Board, 1986.

Government of Pakistan. *Resource and Reference Manual for Prevention Resource Consultant Network.* Volume I. Islamabad: Drug Abuse Prevention Resource Centre, 1990.

Government of Pakistan. *The Gazette of Pakistan: Extra Ordinary: Ordinance No XLVI of 18 April 1995.* Ch. II, Prohibition and Punishment Section 4. Islamabad: Ministry of Law, Justice and Parliamentary Affairs, 18 April 1995a.

Government of Pakistan. *Master Plan for Drug Abuse Control in Pakistan.* Islamabad: Narcotics Control Board, 1995b.

Government of Pakistan, Pakistan Integrated Household Survey (PIHS), Round 3:1998/99 (Islamabad: Federal Bureau of Statistics, October 2000).

Government of the United States of America. *The World Opium Situation.* Washington DC: Bureau of Narcotics and Dangerous Drugs, 1970.

Government of the United States of America. *World Opium Survey: Cabinet Committee Report on International Narcotics Control.* Washington DC: State Department, 1972.

Government of the United States of America. *International Narcotics Control Strategy Report.* Washington DC: Bureau of International Narcotics and Law Enforcement Affairs, 1990, 1996.

Griffith, E. *et al.* (eds) *Drugs, Alcohol and Tobacco: Making the Science and Policy Connection.* Oxford: Oxford University Press, 1993.

Griffith, I.L. 'From Cold War Geo-Politics to Post Cold War Geo-Narcotics'. *International Journal,* XLIX, Winter 1993–94.

Haq, A. and Farooq U. (eds) *Drug Addiction and Rehabilitation of Addicts in Pakistan.* Faisalabad: Agriculture University, 1979.

Haq, I. *From Hashish to Heroin.* Lahore: Al-Noor Publications, 1991.

Heywood, P. (ed.) *Political Corruption.* Oxford: Blackwell for the Political Studies Association, 1997.

Hill, A.F. *Economic Botany: A Text Book of Useful Plants and Plant Products.* New York: McGraw Hill, 1937.

Hutchinson, J. *Families of Flowering Plants.* Volume I: *Dicotyledons Arranged According to a New System Based on the Probable Phylogeny,* I. Oxford: The Clarendon Press, 1959.

Imran, M. and Uppal, T.B. 'Opium Administration to Infants in Peshawar Region'. *UN Bulletin on Narcotics*. XXXI, pp3 and 4, 1979.

Jalal Zai, M.K. *The Drug War in South Asia*. Lahore: Institute of Current Affairs, 1993.

Jamieson, A. *Global Drug Trafficking. Conflict Studies*. p234. London: Institute for the Study of Conflict and Terrorism. September 1990.

Jones, H. *Social Welfare in Third World Development*. London: Macmillan Education, 1990.

Kalant, H. 'The Great Legalization Debate', in E. Griffith *et al.* (eds) *Drugs, Alcohol, and Tobacco: Making the Science and Policy Connection*. Oxford: Oxford University Press, 1993.

Kolb, L. 'Drug Addiction in Its Relation to Crime'. *Mental Hygiene*, 9 January 1925. pp74–89.

Kritikos, P.G. and Papadaki, S.P. 'The History of the Poppy and of Opium and their Expansion in Antiquity in the Eastern Mediterranean Area'. *UN Bulletin on Narcotics*. XIX, p3, 1967.

Kruseman, G. *Socio-Economic Aspects of Poppy Cultivation: Selected Farm Profile of Eastern Dir Valleys and Dir Kohistan*. Peshawar: Special Development Unit, 1985.

Kumar, S. 'Drug Trafficking in Pakistan'. *Asian Strategic Review* 1994–95.

Lausane, C. *Pipe Dream Blues: Racism and The War on Drugs*. Boston, MA: South End Press, 1991.

Leech, K. and Jordan, B. *Drugs for Young People: Their Uses and Misuses*. Oxford: The Religious Education Press, 1967.

Lyman, M.D. and Potter, G.W. *Drugs in Society: Causes, Concepts and Control*, 2nd edn. Cincinnati: Anderson, 1996.

McConohy, M.J. and Kirk, R. 'Over There: American Drug War Abroad'. *Mother Jones*, pp14, 2. 1984. pp9-13.

McCoy, A.W. *The Politics of Heroin in Southeast Asia*. New York: Harper & Row, 1972.

McCoy, A.W. *The Politics of Heroin: CIA Complicity in the Global Trade*. New York: Lawrence Hill Books, 1991.

McCoy, A.W. *The Politics of Heroin: CIA Complicity in the Global Trade*, 2nd edn. New York: Harper & Row, 1994.

MacMahon, A. *The Tribes of Dir, Swat, and Chitral, With Epilogue on Utman Khel and Sama Ranezai*. Peshawar: Saeed Book Bank, 1980.

Machete, D.T. 'The History of Opium and Some of its Preparations and Alkaloids'. *Journal of American Medical Association*, 6 February 1915.

Masood, A. *Esi Bulandi Esi Pasti*. Rawalpendi: Ahsan, 1981.

Merrillees, R.S. 'Opium Trade in the Bronze Age Levant'. *Antiquity* 36, 1962. pp287–92.

Mian, I.N. *et al. Causes, Effects and Remedies of Poppy Cultivation in Swabi-Gadoon Areas: A Survey of Opium Cultivation*. Peshawar: University of Peshawar, 1979.

Miller, D. E. *Licit Narcotics Production and Its Ramifications for Foreign Policy*. Washington DC: US State Department, 1980.

Musto, D.F. *The American Disease: Origins of Narcotic Control.* New Haven: Yale University Press, 1973.

Musto, D.F 'Opium, Cocaine, and Marijuana in American History'. *Scientific American.* 265, July 1991. pp20–27.

Myrdal, G. *Asian Drama: an Inquiry into the Poverty of Nations.* Volume II. New York: Pantheon, 1968.

Nadelmann, E.A. 'Drugs Prohibition in the United States: Costs, Consequences, and Alternatives'. *Science*, p245, 1989. pp939–47.

Nane, A.S. 'UN Activities in International Drug Control'. In I.R. Simon and A.A. Said, *Drugs, Politics and Diplomacy.* London: Sage, 1974.

Neligan, A.R. *The Opium Question with Special Reference to Persia.* London: John Bales Sons and Danielson, 1927.

Nye, J. 'Corruption and Political Development: a Cost-Benefit Analysis'. *American Political Science Review.* p61, 1967.

Owen, D.E., *British Opium Policy in China and India.* New Haven: Yale University Press, 1934.

Packer, H.L. 'The Crime Tariff'. *American Scholar.* 33, Autumn 1964. pp551–7.

Parker, H. Bakx, K. and Newcombe R. *Living with Heroin.* Buckingham: Open University Press, 1988.

Platt, J.J. and Labate, C. *Heroin Addiction: Theory, Research and Treatment.* New York: Wiley, 1976.

Porter, C.L. *The Taxonomy of Flowering Plants.* Englewood Cliffs, New Jersey: Prentice Hall, 1967.

Porter, R. and Teich, M. (eds) *Drugs and Narcotics in History.* Cambridge: Cambridge University Press, 1995.

Qureshi, I.H. *A Short History of Pakistan: Books I-IV.* Karachi: University of Karachi, 1987.

Ranara, R. D. *Socio-Economic and Political Impacts of Production, Trade and Use of Narcotic Drugs in Burma.* Geneva: United Nations: Research Institute for Social Development, 1992.

Reeves, R. *Passage to Peshawar.* New York: Simon and Schuster, 1984.

Reiman, J.H. *The Rich Get Rich and the Poor Get Prison.* New York: John Wiley, 1979.

Reuter, P. 'Eternal Hope: America's Quest for Narcotics Control'. *The Public Interest*, p79. 1985.

Reuter, P. 'The Limits and Consequences of US Foreign Drug Control Efforts'. *The Annals of American Academy of Political and Social Sciences*, 521, May 1992. pp151–62.

Ridway, T I., *Pathans.* Calcutta: Government Printing Press, 1910.

Rowntree, J. *The Imperial Drug Trade.* London: Methuen, 1905.

Rushbrook Williams, L.F. *The State of Pakistan.* London: Faber and Faber, 1962.

Sahibzada, R.A.K. *Poppy Cultivation in North West Frontier Province (NWFP): Its Present, Past and Future.* Islamabad: Department of Agriculture and Rural Development, 1991.

Schery, R.W. *Plants for Man*, 2nd edn. Englewood Cliffs, New Jersey: Prentice Hall, 1974.

Scott, P.D. 'Spread of Drugs: Crack Down or Crack-Up'. *The South*, August 1988. pp9–10.

Sen, S. 'Heroin Trafficking in the Golden Crescent'. *Police Journal*, July–September 1992. pp251–6.

Sharma, M.C. 'History of Narcotics Control in India' In. M. Desai, H. S. Sethi *et al.* (eds) *Current Research in Drug Abuse in India*. New Delhi, 1981.

Simon, I. R. and Said, A.A. *Drug Politics and Diplomacy*. London: Sage, 1974.

Smith, M. L. *Why People Grow Drugs*. London: Panoos Publications, 1992.

Sonnedecker, G. 'Emergence and Concept of Addiction Problem'. *Symposium on History of Narcotics and Drug Addiction*. Marbathesda, 1962.

South Asian Association for Regional Co-operation. *Proceedings of Workshop on Effective Utilization of Indigenous Methods for Treatment of Drug Dependants. Pakistan Country Paper*. Islamabad: SAARC, 1996.

Spencer, C.P. and Navarathnam, V. *Drug Abuse in South East Asia*. Kuala Lumpur: Oxford University Press, 1981.

Stevenson, R. *Winning the War on Drugs: To Legalize or Not?* Hobart Paper 124. London: Institute of Economic Affairs, 1994.

Stratchey, J. *India: Its Administration and Progress*. London: Macmillan, 1903.

Terry, C E. and Pellin, M. *The Opium Problem*. New York: Bureau of Social Hygiene, 1928.

Terry, C.E. and Pellin, M. 'Drug Addiction'. In *Encyclopaedia of Social Sciences*. New York: Macmillan, 1931.

Tilman, R. 'Emergence of Black-Market Bureaucracy: Administration, Development and Corruption in the New States'. *Political Administration Review*. XXVIII, 5, 1968.

Tullis, L. *Beneficiaries of the Illicit Drug Trade: Political Consequences and International Policy at the Intersection of Supply and Demand*. Geneva: United Nations Research Institute for Social Development, 1991.

Tullis, L. *Unintended Consequences: Illicit Drugs and Drugs Policies in Nine Countries* Boulder, CO: Lynne Rienner, 1995.

Tullock, G. *Rent Seeking*. The Shaftesbury Papers, 2. Aldershot: Edward Elgar, 1993.

United Nations. *Bulletin on Narcotics V*, 2, New York: United Nations, 1953.

United Nations. *United Nations and Drug Control*. Vienna: Division of Narcotics Drugs, 1982a.

United Nations. *Piami* (Urdu) 6, Karachi: UNESCO/Hamdard Foundation, April 1982b.

United Nations. *Declaration on the Control of Drug Trafficking and Drug Abuse*. New York: United Nations, 1984a.

United Nations. *A Review of Narcotics Related Matters in NWFP*. Peshawar: Drug Control Programme, 1984b.

United Nations. *Dir District Development Project: Consultant Report/Draft Project Document* Peshawar: Drug Control Programme, 1991.

United Nations. *Dir District Development Project, Phase II: Planning Report*. Peshawar: Drug Control Programme, 1992.

United Nations. *Dir District Development Project: Project Document*. Peshawar: Drug Control Programme, 1994.

United Nations. *The Illicit Drug Problem in Southwest Asia: Briefing Note.* Islamabad: Drug Control Programme, June and November 1996a.

United Nations. *Trends in Poppy Harvest.* Islamabad: Drug Control Programme, 1996b.

United Nations. *Poppy Cultivation in Pakistan: Briefing Note.* Islamabad: Drug Control Programme, 1997.

Watt, G. *A Dictionary of the Economic Products of India.* London: W.H. Allen, 1893.

Wemkel, H. 'Narcotics Trafficking in Pakistan. *Workshop on Mass Media Orientation for Prevention of Drug Abuse.* Islamabad: PNCB, 22–27 October 1984.

Werter, F. *Cultural Values, Land Management and Land Degradation.* Saidu Swat: Malakand Social Forestry Project. 1994.

Westermeyer, J. 'The Pro-Heroin Effects of Anti-Opium Laws in Asia'. *Archives of General Psychiatry*, 33, 1976. pp1135–39.

World Bank. *Pakistan: Poverty Assessment Report.* Washington: Country Operation Division South Asia. Report No. 14397, 1995.

World Bank. *World Tables 1995.* Baltimore: Johns Hopkins University Press, 1995.

Wright, A.D. 'The History of Opium Transaction'. *Studies of the Royal College of Physicians of Philadelphia*, 29, 1, 1969. pp22–7.

Young, J. *The Drug Takers: The Social Meaning of Drug Use.* London: MacGibbon and Kee, 1971.

Zeuner, F.E. *Cultivation of Plants: A History.* Oxford: Oxford University Press, 1954.

Index